Cancers in Hepatology

Cancers in Hepatology

Editor: Eddie Goblin

AMERICAN
MEDICAL PUBLISHERS
www.americanmedicalpublishers.com

AMERICAN
MEDICAL PUBLISHERS
www.americanmedicalpublishers.com

Cataloging-in-Publication Data

Cancers in hepatology / edited by Eddie Goblin.
p. cm.
Includes bibliographical references and index.
ISBN 978-1-63927-956-2
1. Hepatology. 2. Gastrointestinal system--Cancer.
3. Gastroenterology. I. Goblin, Eddie.
RC846 .C36 2023
616.362--dc23

American Medical Publishers,
41 Flatbush Avenue,
1st Floor, New York,
NY 11217, USA

ISBN 978-1-63927-956-2 (Hardback)

Contents

Preface

Hepatology is a sub field of medicine that deals with the study, prevention, diagnosis, and treatment of diseases that affect the liver, gallbladder, biliary tree, and pancreas. Liver cancers are a group of cancers that develop in the liver. There are several forms of liver cancers including primary liver cancer, secondary liver cancer, and benign liver tumors. Hepatocellular carcinoma (HCC) is the major type of primary liver cancer that commonly develops in patients suffering from chronic liver diseases, such as cirrhosis. Intrahepatic cholangiocarcinoma is the second most common type of primary liver cancer that arises from cells lining the bile ducts. Secondary liver cancer is a cancerous tumor that has metastasized to the liver from a cancer in some other part of the body such as the stomach, breast, lung, or pancreas. This book includes some of the vital pieces of work being conducted across the world, on various topics related to cancers in hepatology. It will serve as a valuable source of reference for medical graduate and post graduate students.

After months of intensive research and writing, this book is the end result of all who devoted their time and efforts in the initiation and progress of this book. It will surely be a source of reference in enhancing the required knowledge of the new developments in the area. During the course of developing this book, certain measures such as accuracy, authenticity and research focused analytical studies were given preference in order to produce a comprehensive book in the area of study.

This book would not have been possible without the efforts of the authors and the publisher. I extend my sincere thanks to them. Secondly, I express my gratitude to my family and well-wishers. And most importantly, I thank my students for constantly expressing their willingness and curiosity in enhancing their knowledge in the field, which encourages me to take up further research projects for the advancement of the area.

Editor

1

Augmented Reality Navigation for Stereoscopic Laparoscopic Anatomical Hepatectomy of Primary Liver Cancer

Weiqi Zhang[1,2†], *Wen Zhu*[1,2†], *Jian Yang*[1,2], *Nan Xiang*[1,2], *Ning Zeng*[1,2], *Haoyu Hu*[1,2], *Fucang Jia*[3] *and Chihua Fang*[1,2*]

[1] *Department of Hepatobiliary Surgery, Zhujiang Hospital, Southern Medical University, Guangzhou, China,* [2] *Guangdong Provincial Clinical and Engineering Center of Digital Medicine, Guangzhou, China,* [3] *Research Laboratory for Medical Imaging and Digital Surgery, Shenzhen Institutes of Advanced Technology, Chinese Academy of Sciences, Shenzhen, China*

Correspondence:
Chihua Fang
fangch_dr@163.com

[†]*These authors have contributed equally to this work*

Background: Accurate determination of intrahepatic anatomy remains challenging for laparoscopic anatomical hepatectomy (LAH). Laparoscopic augmented reality navigation (LARN) is expected to facilitate LAH of primary liver cancer (PLC) by identifying the exact location of tumors and vessels. The study was to evaluate the safety and effectiveness of our independently developed LARN system in LAH of PLC.

Methods: From May 2018 to July 2020, the study included 85 PLC patients who underwent three-dimensional (3D) LAH. According to whether LARN was performed during the operation, the patients were divided into the intraoperative navigation (IN) group and the non-intraoperative navigation (NIN) group. We compared the preoperative data, perioperative results and postoperative complications between the two groups, and introduced our preliminary experience of this novel technology in LAH.

Results: There were 44 and 41 PLC patients in the IN group and the NIN group, respectively. No significant differences were found in preoperative characteristics and any of the resection-related complications between the two groups (All $P > 0.05$). Compared with the NIN group, the IN group had significantly less operative bleeding ($P = 0.002$), lower delta Hb% ($P = 0.039$), lower blood transfusion rate ($P < 0.001$), and reduced postoperative hospital stay ($P = 0.003$). For the IN group, the successful fusion of simulated surgical planning and operative scene helped to determine the extent of resection.

Conclusions: The LARN contributed to the identification of important anatomical structures during LAH of PLC. It reduced vascular injury and accelerated postoperative recovery, showing a potential application prospects in liver surgery.

Keywords: laparoscopic surgical navigation, augmented reality, three-dimensional laparoscopy, anatomical hepatectomy, primary liver cancer

INTRODUCTION

Primary liver cancer (PLC) is the fourth most common cause of cancer-related death worldwide (second in males), and its incidence is steadily increasing (1). Anatomical hepatectomy (AH) is one of the surgical methods for PLC, which refers to the resection of hepatic area innervated by portal vein (PV) and its branches (2). With the development of laparoscopic technique, an increasing number of AH can be performed under laparoscopy (3–5). The advent of three-dimensional (3D) laparoscopy provides surgeons with depth perception, however, laparoscopic anatomical hepatectomy (LAH) has its own technical difficulty in determining the anatomic landmark and surgical plane due to the lack of tactile feedback, limited operating space, and poor viewing angles. To alleviate these drawbacks, laparoscopic augmented reality navigation (LARN) systems, including video-based, projection-based, and see-through AR visualization methods, have been introduced to improve information on the position of intrahepatic tumors and vessels, thereby facilitating LAH (6, 7). Nevertheless, unlike rigid surgical navigation in orthopedics and neurosurgery, the impact of pneumoperitoneum, respiration, heartbeat and surgical manipulation will change the accuracy of liver surgical navigation, making it difficult to transform LARN into clinical practice (8–10).

Recently, our team developed a 3D LARN system (6). This system, combined with preoperative 3D surgical planning, provides simple, safe and real-time image navigation for LAH. In this study, the clinical outcomes of the IN group and the NIN group were compared to explore the application value of this new image navigation technology in 3D LAH of PLC.

METHODS

Patients

Between May 2018 and July 2020, a total of 85 consecutive PLC patients undergoing 3D LAH in the Department of Hepatobiliary Surgery, Zhujiang Hospital, Southern Medical University were enrolled in the study. Inclusion criteria: (1) age ≥ 18 years, regardless of gender; (2) PLC diagnosed by enhanced computed tomography (CT) or magnetic resonance imaging scan, and confirmed by pathological examination; (3) Child–Pugh class A or B liver function. Patients with main vascular invasion or extrahepatic metastasis were excluded from the study. In the intraoperative navigation (IN) group, PLC patients received 3D LAH using the LARN system. In the non-intraoperative navigation (NIN) group, PLC patients received 3D laparoscopic AH without assistance of the LARN system. All the operations were performed by the surgical group with more than 10 years of laparoscopic hepatic resection experience. The clinical data of the two groups were collected and analyzed, including sex, age, body mass index (BMI), history of hepatitis B, liver cirrhosis, Child-Pugh classification of liver function, preoperative α-fetoprotein (AFP), preoperative carbohydrate antigen 19-9 (CA19-9), preoperative total bilirubin (TBil), preoperative hemoglobin (Hb), preoperative albumin (ALB), preoperative blood platelet (PLT) count, tumor size, tumor number, operative details, perioperative results and recurrence patterns. The amount of intraoperative blood loss was calculated by adding the contents of suction containers to the weight of laparotomy sponges at the end of the surgery. Delta Hb% was defined as (Difference between preoperative Hb and postoperative lowest Hb/preoperative Hb)×100. Clavien-Dindo classification was used to evaluate postoperative complications (11). Liver failure was determined using the "50-50 criteria" (12).

Informed consent for clinical analysis was obtained from each patient, and the study was approved and supervised by the ethics committee of Zhujiang Hospital of Southern Medical University with the batch number of 2018-GDYK-003.

3D Model Reconstruction and Surgical Planning

All patients in the IN group were scanned with Philips Brilliance 64- or 256-multislice spiral CT scanner to collect four-phase CT data during plain scan phase, arterial phase, portal venous phase and delayed phase. The specific scanning parameters and methods were referenced to consensus recommendations of 3D visualization for diagnosis and management of liver diseases (13). The self-developed 3D visualization system (MI-3DVS, software copyright: No.2008SR18798) was used for 3D reconstruction, and several quality control criteria were followed: (1) Patients should be instructed to hold their breath during CT scan to avoid difficulties in image segmentation and registration between different phases; (2) quality of original CT images should meet the minimum standards of 3D visualization software; (3) 3D reconstruction should be performed by qualified personnel; (4) 3D models should be manually checked and modified by a senior surgeon and an imaging physician. According to the 3D models, the anatomy and spatial distribution of the targets, including liver, biliary tract, blood vessel, tumor were defined and delineated. Furthermore, residual liver volume calculation and stimulated hepatectomy were carried out to determine the surgical plane and extent of resection.

Laparoscopic Augmented Reality Navigation System

As described in our previous study, the LARN system consisted of preoperative model segmentation, real-time image surface reconstruction, intraoperative registration, and intraoperative posture tracking modules (Software copyright: No. 2018SR840555) (14). LARN was implemented in C^{++} and Python using the open source toolkit on the Windows 10 operating system, and the software interface is shown in **Figure 1**. The ORB-SLAM2 method was adopted to acquire the real-time camera pose and 3D information of the organ surface (15). Intraoperative real-time surgical images were collected by 3D laparoscopic (Karl Storz, Germany) camera, and the output video signal in Line-by-line format needed to be analyzed by video parser (E-hospital 3D embedded multimedia workstation GK310, China). Epiphan AV.io HD video capture card was input into the

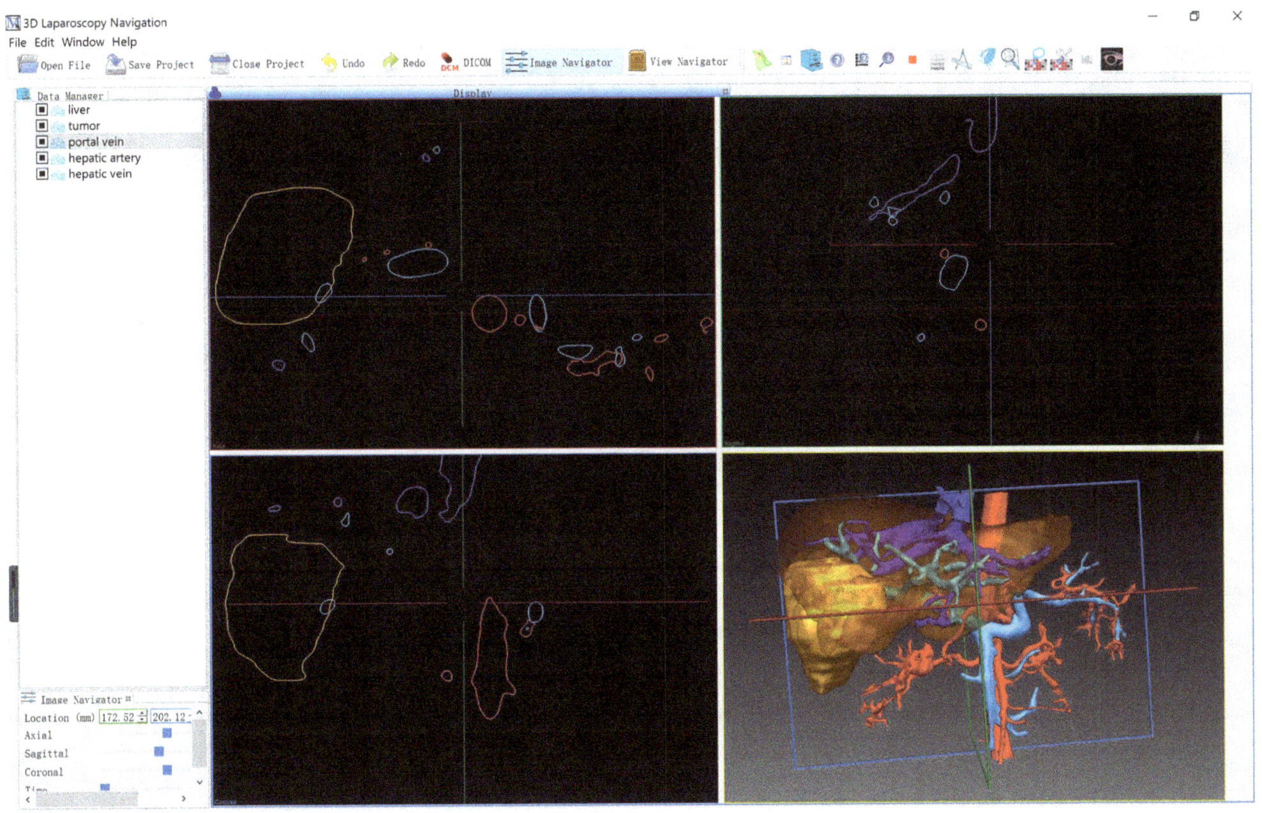

FIGURE 1 | 3D LARN software interface.

laptop to form the effect of AR image display and realize real-time fusion navigation.

The spatial transformation matrix between preoperative CT image space and intraoperative laparoscopic space was obtained by Go-ICP method to realize the registration of preoperative 3D visualization model and intraoperative video image (16). If the effect of automatic registration is not satisfactory, the system will provide manual registration function. The installation, debugging, 3D model introduction, positioning and image registration of the LARN system took an average of 10 minutes. 3D models including liver, gallbladder, tumor, hepatic artery, hepatic vein and PV were assigned brown, green, yellow, red, dark blue and sky blue, respectively. Two liver surface anatomical landmarks, the inferior vena cava fossa and the fundus of gallbladder, were selected for registration. While registering, the size alignment of the liver shape was taken into account, and the projection and fusion of the 3D model were further adjusted. LARN was not performed during liver mobilization. After dissociating ligaments, the liver would undergo morphological changes due to the effects of squeezing, flipping, lifting and pulling the liver tissue and pneumoperitoneal pressure. Therefore, when dissecting the first porta hepatis, we used the vessels of hepatic hilum (PV, hepatic artery or abdominal aorta) as the registration landmarks for real-time image navigation to understand the location relationship of vascular system.

Statistical Analysis

All statistical analyses were performed using SPSS 25.0 (IBM Corp., Armonk, NY, USA). Continuous variables were expressed as median (Range) and compared using Mann-Whitney U test. Category data were presented as number (Percentage) and compared with the $\chi 2$ test or the Fisher exact test. $P < 0.05$ was considered as indicative of statistical significance.

RESULTS

Patients Characteristics

The comparison of baseline data between the IN group and the NIN group is shown in **Table 1**. Between May 2018 and July 2020, a total of 85 PLC patients were enrolled into our study, including 34 cases of right hepatectomy, 21 cases of left hepatectomy, 13 cases of right posterior sectionectomy, 8 cases of left lateral sectionectomy, 7 cases of mesohepatectomy, and 2 cases of S5+6 segmentectomy. No significant differences were noted regarding age, sex, BMI, history of hepatitis B, Child-Pugh classification of liver function, preoperative AFP, preoperative CA19-9, preoperative TBIL, preoperative Hb, preoperative ALB, preoperative PLT, tumor size, tumor number, type of AH, extent of resection and pathological result between the two groups (All $P > 0.05$).

TABLE 1 | Patient Characteristics.

Characteristics	IN group (n = 44)	NIN group (n = 41)	*P* Value
Host factors			
Age, year, median (range)	53 (25-74)	61 (26-78)	0.381
Sex, n (%)			0.659
Male	36 (82)	35 (85)	
Female	8 (18)	6 (15)	
BMI, kg/m^2, median (range)	22.3 (17.4-27.2)	22.1 (15.4-29.0)	0.907
Hepatitis B, n (%)	34 (77)	25 (61)	0.103
Liver cirrhosis, n (%)	21 (48)	13 (32)	0.132
Child-Pugh classification, n (%)			0.738
Class A	40 (91)	39 (95)	
Class B	4 (9)	2 (5)	
Preoperative laboratory tests			
AFP, ng/mL, median (range)	10.1 (1.6-79776.0)	10.7 (1.4-166690.0)	0.076
CA19-9, U/mL, median (range)	16.6 (1.1-968.6)	27.5 (0.6-431800.0)	0.208
TBil, mg/dL, median (range)	0.8 (0.4-2.4)	0.9 (0.3-8.9)	0.208
Hb, g/L, median (range)	137 (97-170)	135 (99-185)	0.264
ALB, g/L, median (range)	37.8 (28.0-59.7)	39.5 (27.3-52.9)	0.335
PLT, 10^3/μL, median (range)	177 (14-469)	220 (30-539)	0.418
Tumor and surgical factors			
Tumor size	6.0 (0.6-16.0)	7.0 (1.3-18.0)	0.779
Tumor number, n (%)			
Solitary	41 (93)	38 (93)	1.000
2-3 nodules	3 (7)	2 (5)	1.000
>3 nodules	0	1 (2)	0.482
Anatomical resection, n (%)			
Left hepatectomy (S2, S3 and S4)	10 (23)	11 (27)	0.661
Right hepatectomy (S5, S6, S7 and S8)	19 (44)	15 (36)	0.535
Left lateral sectionectomy (S2+3)	2 (4)	6 (15)	0.222
Mesohepatectomy (S4, S5 and S8)	4 (9)	3 (7)	1.000
Right posterior sectionectomy (S6+7)	7 (16)	6 (15)	0.870
S5+6 segmentectomy	2 (4)	0 (0)	0.496
Extent of resection, n (%)			0.658
Minor[a]	11 (25)	12 (29)	
Major[b]	33 (75)	29 (71)	
Pathological findings, n (%)			0.843
Hepatocellular carcinoma	38 (86)	36 (88)	
Cholangiocarcinoma	6 (14)	5 (12)	

BMI, body mass index; AFP, α-fetoprotein; CA19-9, carbohydrate antigen 19-9; Hb, hemoglobin; TBil, total bilirubin; ALB, albumin; PLT, platelet.
[a]Removal of less than 3 hepatic segments.
[b]Removal of 3 or more adjacent hepatic segments.

Perioperative Outcomes and Recurrence Patterns

The operation time, blood loss, intraoperative blood transfusion, postoperative hospital stay, resection-related complications and recurrence patterns are described in **Table 2**. We found that the intraoperative blood loss, delta Hb% and blood transfusion rate were significantly higher in the NIN group than in the IN group ($P = 0.002$, $P = 0.039$ and $P < 0.001$, respectively). In addition, the length of postoperative hospital stay in the IN group was significantly shorter than that in the NIN group (P = 0.003). There was no significant difference in operative time and postoperative complications between the two groups (All P > 0.05). All patients recovered and discharged without liver failure or perioperative death.

The median follow-up for all patients was 16 months (Range, 1–32 months). By the end of follow-up, 27 patients (32%) had developed tumor recurrence, including 11 cases (25%) in the IN group and 16 cases (39%) in the NIN group. The results of overall, intrahepatic or extrahepatic recurrence were similar between the IN and NIN groups (All P > 0.05).

Right Hepatectomy

The case of right hepatectomy is shown in **Figure 2**. The upper abdomen enhanced CT indicated that the lesion was located in the right liver and was closely related to the right PV (**Figure 2A**). The 3D liver model clearly showed the location of the lesion and its anatomical relationship with the hepatic vessels (**Figure 2B**). Considering hepatocellular carcinoma (HCC), we planned to perform laparoscopic right hepatectomy. Based on simulated resection results, residual liver volume accounted for 47.1% of the total liver volume (Right liver volume = 558.15 ml) (**Figure 2C**). Intraoperatively, image fusion was performed to navigate the right hepatic artery (**Figure 2D**), the main PV and the right PV (**Figure 2E**). Under real-time image navigation, a hemi-hepatic ischemic line appeared on the surface of the liver after ligation of the right PV, and the hepatic parenchyma was incised and the right

TABLE 2 | Perioperative Outcomes and Recurrence Patterns.

	IN group (n = 44)	NIN group (n = 41)	*P* Value
Operation time, min, median (range)	300 (90-690)	300 (90-540)	0.061
Blood loss, mL, median (range)	200 (20-400)	300 (50-1000)	**0.002**
Delta Hb%[a], median (range)	12.1 (1.3-34.6)	14.1 (6.3-57.9)	**0.039**
Intraoperative blood transfusion, n (%)			**<0.001**
Yes	5 (10)	19 (42)	
No	39 (90)	22 (58)	
Resection-related complications, n (%)			
Total	18 (41)	19 (46)	0.614
Wound infection	0 (0)	1 (2)	0.482
Abdominal hemorrhage	0 (0)	1 (2)	0.482
Lung infection	2 (5)	3 (7)	0.935
Pleural effusion	12 (27)	12 (30)	0.838
Ascites	4 (9)	2 (5)	0.738
Liver failure	0 (0)	0 (0)	–
Clavien-Dindo classification of complications, n (%)			
Grade I or II	15 (32)	14 (33)	0.996
≥Grade III	3 (7)	5 (11)	0.634
Postoperative hospital stay, day, median (range)	8 (4-14)	10 (4-23)	**0.003**
Recurrence Patterns			
Overall recurrence, n (%)	11 (25)	16 (39)	0.165
Intrahepatic, n (%)	7 (16)	12 (29)	0.140
Extrahepatic, n (%)	1 (2)	2 (5)	0.950
Intrahepatic and extrahepatic, n (%)	3 (7)	2 (5)	1.000

[a](Difference between preoperative Hb and postoperative lowest Hb/preoperative Hb)×100.
Bold values indicate P < 0.05.

hepatic vein was carefully processed (**Figure 2F**). Postoperative pathological examination revealed HCC.

Right Posterior Sectionectomy

The case of right posterior sectionectomy is shown in **Figure 3**. 3D visualization model displayed that the lesion was located in the right posterior sector (**Figure 3A**). On the basis of simulated right posterior sectionectomy, the resected liver volume was 340.12 ml (41.33%) and the residual liver volume was 482.79 ml (58.67%) (**Figure 3B**). The hepatoduodenal ligament was dissected to isolate the main PV and the right hepatic artery (**Figures 3C, D**), and the right PV was suspended under the intraoperative image navigation (**Figure 3E**). By projecting the 3D vessel model, the right PV "fluoroscopically" traveled from the liver surface, and the right posterior PV branch was further dissected and severed (**Figures 3F, G**). According to the ischemic line, the dissection of hepatic parenchyma and the management of the hepatic veins in S6 and S7 were performed with the assistance of LARN (**Figure 3H**). Postoperative pathological examination revealed cholangiocarcinoma.

S5+6 Segmentectomy

The case of S5+6 segmentectomy is described in **Figure 4**. The abdominal contrast-enhanced CT showed a mixed density lesion in the right liver with heterogeneous enhancement (**Figure 4A**). 3D reconstruction and individualized liver segmentation demonstrated that the lesion was located in the S5 and S6 (**Figures 4B, C**), and the resected liver volume was 228.52 ml (26.57%) and the residual liver volume was 631.37 ml (73.43%) (**Figure 4C**). During the operation, the lesion was observed protruding from the liver surface. We projected the 3D models onto the liver surface to show the relationship between the lesion and PVs (**Figures 4D, E**). The right PV, the right anterior PV branch and right posterior PV branch were visualized through the fused 3D reconstructed models, and the PV branches of S5 (**Figure 4F**) and S6 (**Figure 4G**) were further separated and severed to complete the corresponding liver segment resection. Middle hepatic vein processing and the ligation of S5 hepatic vein were carried out under real-time image navigation (**Figure 4H**). Postoperative pathological examination revealed HCC.

DISCUSSION

Laparoscopic liver resection, which has progressed over the last 20 years, has become a feasible choice for various kinds of liver lesions owing to the development of high-tech surgical techniques and equipment (17). Due to the diversity of the lesion sites and the complicated relationship with great vessels, LAH of PLC is a high-risk procedure, and suggested to be performed by senior surgeons with adequate laparoscopic experiences (18). Overdependence on the skills of surgeons may lead to vascular injury, inaccurate tumor localization, and excessive resection of normal liver tissue. 3D visualization based on preoperative CT has been proven safe and effective for hepatic vessels classification, liver segmentation, simulated hepatectomy, and measurement of liver volume (13, 19). However, it mainly plays the role of pre-resection evaluation and cannot be fused into the surgical scene. Intraoperative visualization of preoperative image data has been a research issue of software engineers, computer scientists and clinicians to improve clinical outcomes for technically challenging LAH. AR allows a real-time updated 3D virtual model of anatomical structures beneath the tissue surface such as blood vessels, nerves, lesions, etc. to be

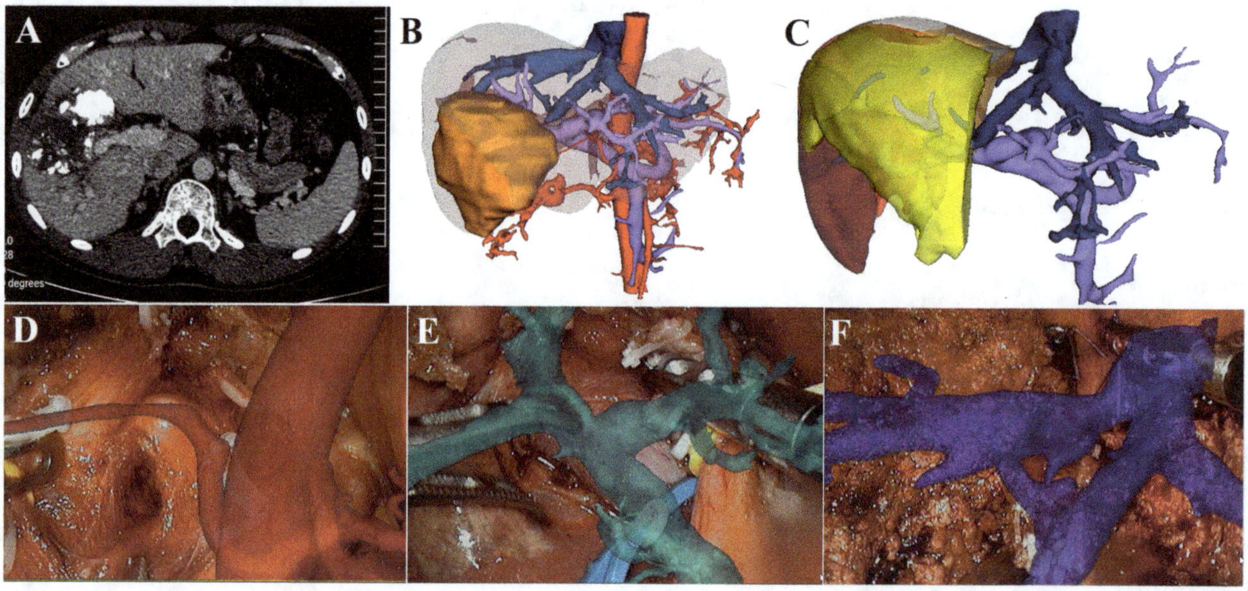

FIGURE 2 | LARN-assisted right hepatectomy. **(A)**, enhanced CT indicated that the lesion was in the right liver, and it was closely related to the right PV. Iodide oil deposition was found inside the lesion. **(B)**, The 3D reconstructed model showed the relationship between the lesion and hepatic vessels. **(C)**, simulated right hepatectomy was performed, and the residual liver volume ratio was 47.1%. **(D)**, intraoperative navigation of the right hepatic artery. **(E)**, intraoperative navigation of the main PV and the right PV. **(F)**, intraoperative navigation of right hepatic vein.

superimposed over the real-world scenario (20). Compared with AR display modes including see-through, 3D image overlay, and projector based methods (21–23), video see-through is more natural and convenient for surgeons to operate under the laparoscopic view and becomes the main form of LARN (6). Concerning the field of laparoscopic surgery, LARN based on video see-through has been gradually promoted to nephrectomy (24), pancreatoduodenectomy (25), esophagectomy (26). Because of the particularity of abdominal environment and the complexity of hepatic vascular structure, the application of LARN in liver surgery is still facing challenges. The LARN system reported in this study achieved real-time navigation of LAH by fusing the preoperative 3D models and contributed to the precise resection of PLC.

The literature on LARN in liver surgery is scarce, mainly in the form of case reports, video reports, and small series. In 2014, Kenngott et al. (27) reported a promising method of real-time image guidance in laparoscopic liver surgery by combining AR software guidance system with intraoperative C-arm cone-beam CT. In a publication by Hallet et al. (28), 3D virtual planning and AR were demonstrated to facilitate trans-thoracic approach for resection of lesions from the liver dome. Nevertheless, the above studies did not involve LAH and surgical details. In 2017, Phutane et al. (29) described a case of laparoscopic left hepatectomy with initial control of the left hepatic vein assisted by their new AR guidance system. According to their study, they completed 8 similar LARN-guided left hepatectomies with satisfactory results, showing potential application prospect of LARN in LAH. Recently, a case series including laparoscopic hemihepatectomy and segmentectomy suggested the feasibility and the potential interest of using the AR guidance software to achieve AR with a deformable model during laparoscopic hepatectomy to locate tumors (30). It was noteworthy that the AR system supplemented the tumor location information in 2 patients which was not displayed by laparoscopic ultrasonography. Due to the small sample size and the lack of control groups, comparative researches are needed to further assess the interest and efficacy of LARN during LAH.

Our proposed LARN system achieved similar functions as the above studies, and the accuracy of our LARN system has been assessed in previous pre-clinical studies on both ex vivo and vivo porcine livers (6). Preoperatively, 3D models were reconstructed using a homogeneous and standardized 3D visualization processing (13). Through a fast registration procedure, 3D images were integrated with the current patient and surgical instrument position into a unified coordinate space. The optical tracking system was used to track the position of surgical instruments (Polaris Spectra optical tracker, Northern Digital Inc., Waterloo, Ontario, Canada). The system presented an intuitive AR navigation visualization by superimposing liver, tumor and vascular models in different colors on laparoscopic images to provide detailed information for LAH. From our experience, a notable advantage of the LARN system is that the surgeons can constantly keep track of the surgical field without the distraction during critical portions of surgical procedure, which was helpful to solve the hand-eye incongruity problem of laparoscopic operation.

Massive bleeding is the major concern in LAH. So far, the main methods used to prevent and control intraoperative hemorrhage include blocking hepatic blood flow and reducing central venous pressure. However, prolonged blockade of the porta hepatis may cause hepatic ischemia-reperfusion injury and

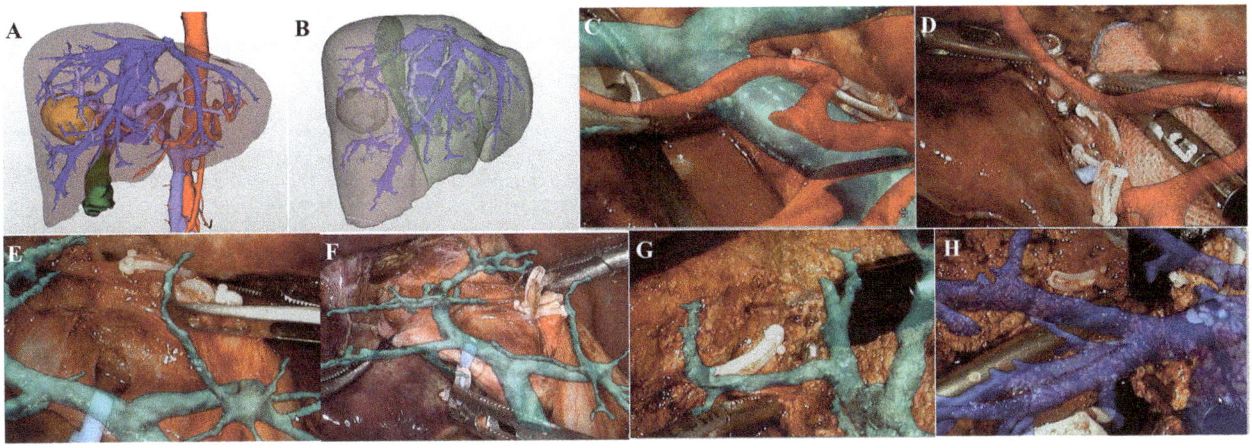

FIGURE 3 | LARN-assisted right posterior sectionectomy. **(A)**, the lesion was located in the right posterior sector from 3D visualization. **(B)**, the resected liver volume was calculated to be 340.12 ml (41.33%) based on simulated hepatectomy. **(C)**, intraoperative navigation of the main PV and hepatic artery. **(D)**, intraoperative navigation of the right hepatic artery. **(E)**, the right PV was suspended under the image navigation. **(F, G)**, the right posterior PV branch was dissected and severed with the assistance of LARN. **(H)**, intraoperative navigation of the hepatic veins in S6 and S7.

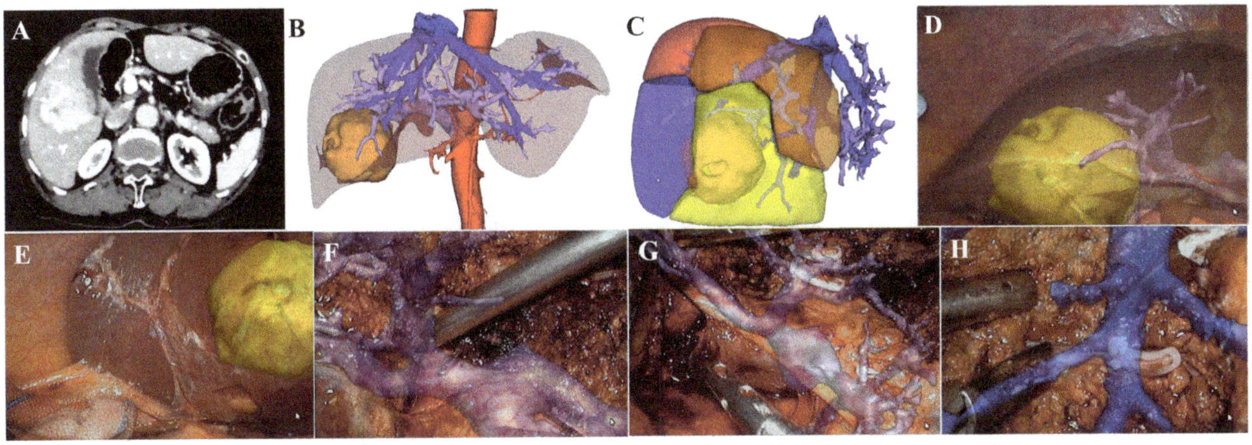

FIGURE 4 | LARN-assisted S5+6 segmentectomy. **(A)**, abdominal contrast-enhanced CT scan revealed a mixed density lesion in the right liver with heterogeneous enhancement. **(B)**, the lesion was located in the S5 and S6 from 3D visualization. **(C)**, the resected liver volume was 228.52 ml (26.57%) based on simulated hepatectomy. **(D, E)**, 3D models were projected onto the liver surface to show the relationship between the lesion and PVs. **(F)**, intraoperative navigation of the PV branch of S5. **(G)**, intraoperative navigation of the PV branch of S6. **(H)**, intraoperative navigation of middle hepatic vein.

increase the occurrence of postoperative liver failure (31). In our outcomes, intraoperative blood loss and blood transfusion rate were significantly reduced in the IN group than in the NIN group. For the patients in the IN group, LARN realized the real-time fusion of preoperative 3D reconstruction models with intraoperative surgical field, thus making the adjacent relationship between lesions and intrahepatic vascular structures more stereoscopic and visualized. At the same time, LARN predicted in advance the important vessels that were encountered in the resection plane, preventing accidental bleeding of hepatic venous system and hepatic ischemia caused by injuring PV branches. For instance, the bleeding-prone middle hepatic veins, short hepatic veins, and right hepatic vein roots were well protected during right hepatectomy under the navigation. Several studies have shown that increased intraoperative blood loss and blood transfusion decrease the overall survival and recurrence-free survival of patients with hepatocellular carcinoma treated with hepatectomy (32–34). Although there was no significant difference in postoperative recurrence between the two groups, the overall recurrence rate in the IN group was noted to be lower than that in the NIN group (25% versus 39%). The LARN system is expected to improve the long-term survival of patients with PLC undergoing LAH by reducing intraoperative bleeding and transfusion requirement.

Although there was no significant difference in resection-related complications between the two groups, the postoperative hospital stay in the IN group was significantly shorter than that in the NIN group. Previous studies have long demonstrated that excessive intraoperative blood loss and blood transfusion correlate with perioperative recovery (35, 36). We believed that the difference in postoperative hospital stay was due to the reduction of intraoperative blood loss and blood transfusion rate in LAH assisted by LARN system. In addition to the morphology of the liver, tumor, and vasculature, we also projected the preoperative scheme of LAH into the surgical scene. Through the analysis of the anatomy and variation of the hepatic vessels, the individualized liver segmentation were performed according to the topological relation of PV blood flow, and meanwhile, the volume calculation of PV branch drainage area were conducted. For all the patients in the IN group, the hepatic segment and simulated surgical plane were clearly fused with the actual operation. The successful intraoperative transformation of preoperative surgical planning improved preliminary identification of target hepatic segments.

Because the study is a retrospective case-control study with selective bias, a large sample prospective randomized controlled trial should be carried out to confirm the application value of LARN in 3D LAH. Besides, the present the LARN system is limited by a short time lag, and the preoperative 3D visualization results are not completely consistent with the liver displacement and deformation caused by pneumoperitoneum, respiration, heartbeat and surgical manipulation. It is therefore advised to combine the surgical navigation system with ultrasound in complex cases to identify the location of tumor and hepatic vessel. Soft tissue deformation and intraoperative image real-time analysis still need further research to improve the real-time and accuracy of navigation.

CONCLUSIONS

Despite the above limitations, the LARN system helped surgeons identify important anatomical structures during LAH. The unique advantages of LARN-assisted 3D LAH of PLC in our study included decreased intraoperative bleeding, transfusion requirements and length of hospital stay. The novel image navigation technology provides a reliable technical support for laparoscopic liver resection.

AUTHOR CONTRIBUTIONS

WQZ, WZ, FJ and CF contributed to conception and design of the study. WQZ organized the database. WQZ and HH performed the statistical analysis. WQZ wrote the first draft of the manuscript. JY, NX and NZ wrote sections of the manuscript. All authors contributed to the article and approved the submitted version.

ACKNOWLEDGMENTS

The authors wish to acknowledge the researchers of the Shenzhen Institute of Advanced Technology of the Chinese Academy of Science for their technical support of the laparoscopic augmented reality navigation system.

REFERENCES

1. Satriano L, Lewinska M, Rodrigues P, Banales JM, Andersen JB. Metabolic rearrangements in primary liver cancers: cause and consequences. *Nat Rev Gastroenterol Hepatol* (2019) 16(12):748–66. doi: 10.1038/s41575-019-0217-8
2. Makuuchi M, Hasegawa H, Yamazaki S. Ultrasonically guided subsegmentectomy. *Surg Gynecol Obstet* (1985) 161(4):346–50.
3. Xu Y, Chen M, Meng X, Lu P, Wang X, Zhang W, et al. Laparoscopic anatomical liver resection guided by real-time indocyanine green fluorescence imaging: experience and lessons learned from the initial series in a single center. *Surg Endosc* (2020) 34(10):4683–91. doi: 10.1007/s00464-020-07691-5
4. Homma Y, Honda G, Kurata M, Ome Y, Doi M, Yamamoto J. Pure laparoscopic right posterior sectionectomy using the caudate lobe-first approach. *Surg Endosc* (2019) 33(11):3851–7. doi: 10.1007/s00464-019-06877-w
5. Berardi G, Wakabayashi G, Igarashi K, Ozaki T, Toyota N, Tsuchiya A, et al. Full Laparoscopic Anatomical Segment 8 Resection for Hepatocellular Carcinoma Using the Glissonian Approach with Indocyanine Green Dye Fluorescence. *Ann Surg Oncol* (2019) 26(8):2577–8. doi: 10.1245/s10434-019-07422-8
6. Luo H, Yin D, Zhang S, Xiao D, He B, Meng F, et al. Augmented reality navigation for liver resection with a stereoscopic laparoscope. *Comput Methods Programs Biomed* (2020) 187:105099. doi: 10.1016/j.cmpb.2019.105099
7. Tang R, Ma LF, Rong ZX, Li MD, Zeng JP, Wang XD, et al. Augmented reality technology for preoperative planning and intraoperative navigation during hepatobiliary surgery: A review of current methods. *Hepatobiliary Pancreat Dis Int* (2018) 17(2):101–12. doi: 10.1016/j.hbpd.2018.02.002
8. Simpson A, Kingham T. Current Evidence in Image-Guided Liver Surgery. *J Gastrointest Surg* (2016) 20(6):1265–9. doi: 10.1007/s11605-016-3101-7
9. Zygomalas A, Kehagias I. Up-to-date intraoperative computer assisted solutions for liver surgery. *World J Gastrointest Surg* (2019) 11(1):1–10. doi: 10.4240/wjgs.v11.i1.1
10. Dilley JWR, Hughes-Hallett A, Pratt PJ, Pucher PH, Camara M, Darzi AW, et al. Perfect Registration Leads to Imperfect Performance: A Randomized Trial of Multimodal Intraoperative Image Guidance. *Ann Surg* (2019) 269 (2):236–42. doi: 10.1097/SLA.0000000000002793
11. Dindo D, Demartines N, Clavien PA. Classification of surgical complications: a new proposal with evaluation in a cohort of 6336 patients and results of a survey. *Ann Surg* (2004) 240(2):205–13. doi: 10.1097/01.sla.0000133083.54934.ae
12. Balzan S, Belghiti J, Farges O, Ogata S, Sauvanet A, Delefosse D, et al. The "50-50 criteria" on postoperative day 5: an accurate predictor of liver failure and death after hepatectomy. *Ann Surg* (2005) 242(6):824–8, discussion 828-9. doi: 10.1097/01.sla.0000189131.90876.9e
13. Fang C, An J, Bruno A, Cai X, Fan J, Fujimoto J, et al. Consensus recommendations of three-dimensional visualization for diagnosis and management of liver diseases. *Hepatol Int* (2020) 14(4):437–53. doi: 10.1007/s12072-020-10052-y
14. Zhang P, Luo H, Zhu W, Yang J, Zeng N, Fan Y, et al. Real-time navigation for laparoscopic hepatectomy using image fusion of preoperative 3D surgical plan and intraoperative indocyanine green fluorescence imaging. *Surg Endosc* (2020) 34(8):3449–59. doi: 10.1007/s00464-019-07121-1
15. Mahmoud N, Collins T, Hostettler A, Soler L, Doignon C, Montiel JMM. Live Tracking and Dense Reconstruction for Handheld Monocular Endoscopy. *IEEE Trans Med Imag* (2019) 38(1):79–89. doi: 10.1109/TMI.2018.2856109
16. Yang J, Li H, Campbell D, Jia Y. Go-ICP: A Globally Optimal Solution to 3D ICP Point-Set Registration. *IEEE Trans Pattern Anal Mach Intell* (2016) 38 (11):2241–54. doi: 10.1109/TPAMI.2015.2513405
17. Syn NL, Kabir T, Koh YX, Tan HL, Wang LZ, Chin BZ, et al. Survival Advantage of Laparoscopic Versus Open Resection For Colorectal Liver Metastases: A Meta-analysis of Individual Patient Data From Randomized

Trials and Propensity-score Matched Studies. *Ann Surg* (2020) 272(2):253–65. doi: 10.1097/SLA.0000000000003672

18. Xu W, Li H, Ji Z, Yan W, Zhang Y, Zhang X, et al. Retroperitoneal Laparoscopic Management of Paraganglioma: A Single Institute Experience. *PLoS One* (2016) 11(2):e0149433. doi: 10.1371/journal.pone.0149433
19. Fang C, Zhang P, Qi X. Digital and intelligent liver surgery in the new era: Prospects and dilemmas. *EBioMedicine* (2019) 41:693–701. doi: 10.1016/j.ebiom.2019.02.017
20. Lang H, Huber T. Virtual and Augmented Reality in Liver Surgery. *Ann Surg* (2020) 271(1):e8. doi: 10.1097/SLA.0000000000003601
21. Golab MR, Breedon PJ, Vloeberghs M. A wearable headset for monitoring electromyography responses within spinal surgery. *Eur Spine J* (2016) 25 (10):3214–9. doi: 10.1007/s00586-016-4626-x
22. Weiss CR, Marker DR, Fischer GS, Fichtinger G, Machado AJ, Carrino JA. Augmented reality visualization using Image-Overlay for MR-guided interventions: system description, feasibility, and initial evaluation in a spine phantom. *AJR Am J Roentgenol* (2011) 196(3):W305–7. doi: 10.2214/AJR.10.5038
23. Volonte F, Pugin F, Bucher P, Sugimoto M, Ratib O, Morel P. Augmented reality and image overlay navigation with OsiriX in laparoscopic and robotic surgery: not only a matter of fashion. *J Hepatobiliary Pancreat Sci* (2011) 18 (4):506–9. doi: 10.1007/s00534-011-0385-6
24. Teber D, Guven S, Simpfendorfer T, Baumhauer M, Güven EO, Yencilek F, et al. Augmented reality: a new tool to improve surgical accuracy during laparoscopic partial nephrectomy? Preliminary in vitro and in vivo results. *Eur Urol* (2009) 56(2):332–8. doi: 10.1016/j.eururo.2009.05.017
25. Onda S, Okamoto T, Kanehira M, Suzuki F, Ito R, Fujioka S, et al. Identification of inferior pancreaticoduodenal artery during pancreaticoduodenectomy using augmented reality-based navigation system. *J Hepatobiliary Pancreat Sci* (2014) 21(4):281–7. doi: 10.1002/jhbp.25
26. Kenngott HG, Neuhaus J, Muller-Stich BP, Wolf I, Vetter M, Meinzer HP, et al. Development of a navigation system for minimally invasive esophagectomy. *Surg Endosc* (2008) 22(8):1858–65. doi: 10.1007/s00464-007-9723-9
27. Kenngott HG, Wagner M, Gondan M, Nickel F, Nolden M, Fetzer A, et al. Real-time image guidance in laparoscopic liver surgery: first clinical experience with a guidance system based on intraoperative CT imaging. *Surg Endosc* (2014) 28(3):933–40. doi: 10.1007/s00464-013-3249-0
28. Hallet J, Soler L, Diana M, Mutter D, Baumert TF, Habersetzer F, et al. Trans-thoracic minimally invasive liver resection guided by augmented reality. *J Am Coll Surg* (2015) 220(5):e55–60. doi: 10.1016/j.jamcollsurg.2014.12.053
29. Phutane P, Buc E, Poirot K, Ozgur E, Pezet D, Bartoli A, et al. Preliminary trial of augmented reality performed on a laparoscopic left hepatectomy. *Surg Endosc* (2018) 32(1):514–5. doi: 10.1007/s00464-017-5733-4
30. Bertrand LR, Abdallah M, Espinel Y, Calvet L, Pereira B, Ozgur E, et al. A case series study of augmented reality in laparoscopic liver resection with a deformable preoperative model. *Surg Endosc* (2020) 34(12):5642–8. doi: 10.1007/s00464-020-07815-x
31. Chen H, Jia W. Progress in hepatectomy for hepatocellular carcinoma and peri-operation management. *Genes Dis* (2020) 7(3):320–7. doi: 10.1016/j.gendis.2020.02.001
32. Yamamoto J, Kosuge T, Takayama T, Shimada K, Yamasaki S, Ozaki H, et al. Perioperative blood transfusion promotes recurrence of hepatocellular carcinoma after hepatectomy. *Surgery* (1994) 115(3):303–9.
33. Katz S, Shia J, Liau K, Gonen M, Ruo L, Jarnagin WR, et al. Operative blood loss independently predicts recurrence and survival after resection of hepatocellular carcinoma. *Ann Surg* (2009) 249(4):617–23. doi: 10.1097/SLA.0b013e31819ed22f
34. Harada N, Shirabe K, Maeda T, Kayashima H, Ishida T, Maehara Y. Blood transfusion is associated with recurrence of hepatocellular carcinoma after hepatectomy in Child-Pugh class A patients. *World J Surg* (2015) 39(4):1044–51. doi: 10.1007/s00268-014-2891-6
35. Otsubo T. Control of the inflow and outflow system during liver resection. *J Hepatobiliary Pancreat Sci* (2012) 19(1):15–8. doi: 10.1007/s00534-011-0451-0
36. Nagao T, Inoue S, Goto S, Mizuta T, Omori Y, Kawano N, et al. Hepatic resection for hepatocellular carcinoma. Clinical features and long-term prognosis. *Ann Surg* (1987) 205(1):33–40. doi: 10.1097/00000658-198701000-00006

2

Development and Validation of a Nomogram for Differentiating Combined Hepatocellular Cholangiocarcinoma from Intrahepatic Cholangiocarcinoma

Tao Wang[1†], Wanxiang Wang[2†], Jinfu Zhang[1], Xianwei Yang[1], Shu Shen[1] and Wentao Wang[1]*

[1] *Department of Liver Surgery and Liver Transplantation Center, West China Hospital of Sichuan University, Chengdu, China,*
[2] *Department of Hepatobiliary, Pancreatic, and Splenic Surgery, The Affiliated Hospital of Inner Mongolia Medical University, Hohhot, China*

***Correspondence:**
Wentao Wang
wwtdoctor02@163.com

†These authors have contributed equally to this work

Objectives: To establish a nomogram based on preoperative laboratory study variables using least absolute shrinkage and selection operator (LASSO) regression for differentiating combined hepatocellular cholangiocarcinoma (cHCC) from intrahepatic cholangiocarcinoma (iCCA).

Methods: We performed a retrospective analysis of iCCA and cHCC patients who underwent liver resection. Blood signatures were established using LASSO regression, and then, the clinical risk factors based on the multivariate logistic regression and blood signatures were combined to establish a nomogram for a differential preoperative diagnosis between iCCA and cHCC. The differential accuracy ability of the nomogram was determined by Harrell's index (C-index) and decision curve analysis, and the results were validated using a validation set. Furthermore, patients were categorized into two groups according to the optimal cut-off values of the nomogram-based scores, and their survival differences were assessed using Kaplan-Meier curves.

Results: A total of 587 patients who underwent curative liver resection for iCCA or cHCC between January 2008 and December 2017 at West China Hospital were enrolled in this study. The cHCC score was based on the personalized levels of the seven laboratory study variables. On multivariate logistic analysis, the independent factors for distinguishing cHCC were age, sex, biliary duct stones, and portal hypertension, all of which were incorporated into the nomogram combined with the cHCC-score. The nomogram had a good discriminating capability, with a C-index of 0.796 (95% CI, 0.752–0.840). The calibration plot for distinguishing cHCC from iCCA showed optimal agreement between the nomogram prediction and actual observation in the training and validation sets. The decision curves indicated significant clinical usefulness.

Conclusion: The nomogram showed good accuracy for the differential diagnosis between iCCA and cHCC preoperatively, and therapeutic decisions would improve if it was applied in clinical practice.

Keywords: intrahepatic cholangiocarcinoma, combined hepatocellular cholangiocarcinoma, differential diagnosis, least absolute shrinkage and selection operator regression, nomogram

HIGHLIGHTS

cHCC is a rare, distinct entity different from iCCA. Using the clinical data obtained from West China Hospital, the authors discovered that the prognosis of the cHCC was significantly worse than that of iCCA. The novel validated nomogram presented herein is a tool that can effectively differentiate cHCC from iCCA preoperatively.

INTRODUCTION

Intrahepatic cholangiocarcinoma (iCCA) is the second most common primary liver cancer after hepatocellular carcinoma (1, 2). Combined hepatocellular cholangiocarcinoma (cHCC) is a rare malignant liver tumor containing components of both hepatocellular carcinoma (HCC) and intrahepatic cholangiocarcinoma (iCCA) (3, 4),accounting for 0.8%–14.3% of primary liver malignancies, with incidences widely varying among studies (5–7). Previous studies have classified cHCC and iCCA in the same category (8–10), but there is controversy about their clinical features and prognoses; for example, some studies have suggested that patients with cHCC have a poorer prognosis than those with iCCA (5, 11, 12), while other studies have reported the opposite conclusion (13).

An accurate differential diagnosis of cHCC and iCCA before surgery remains an important goal with prognostic significance because of differences in therapeutic strategies and prognoses between two; however, at present, the gold standard for cHCC diagnosis is still fine needle aspiration biopsy or a histopathological examination after surgery. With the development of radiological technology, there may be some features of imaging that imply cHCC; however, when cHCC has characteristics consistent with cholangiocarcinoma differentiation in variable proportion, cHCC is often easily misdiagnosed as iCCA (7, 14, 15). Thus, better preoperative noninvasive prediction models are needed to differentiate cHCC from iCCA. We retrospectively performed a comprehensive analysis of the clinicopathological characteristics and survival information of cHCC and iCCA patients in our single center. Furthermore, we established a feasible and straightforward simplified nomogram based on laboratory study variables selected by the least absolute shrinkage and selection operator (LASSO) regression analysis as well as other clinical risks obtained by multivariate logistic regression for the preoperative differential diagnosis between cHCC and iCCA. LASSO regression analysis was used to reduce high-dimensional data and choose the predictive factors in the differential diagnosis of cHCC and iCCA (16, 17).

METHODS

Patients and Study Design

This retrospective study was conducted on iCCA and cHCC patients who underwent curative liver resection between January 2008 and December 2017. Our selection criteria for patients in this study included the following (1) age ≥ 18 years (2); patients who underwent R0 resection, defined as the absence of microscopic or gross residual disease, pathology of the resection margin is was confirmed to be negative, and after the organ or tissue directly invaded by the tumor was combined with resection, the surgical margin was also negative (3); contrast-enhanced CT of the abdomen and laboratory study were performed less than 1 week prior to surgery; and (4) detailed clinical characteristics. Our exclusion criteria for this study were as follows:(1) postoperative pathology confirmed hepatocellular carcinoma (HCC) and R1 excision or tumor margin was not specified in detail (2); the patient had a history of other extrahepatic malignancies; and (3) poor clinical data integrity. In this study, the whole set was randomly divided into two sets: the training set(n=412, 70%) and the validation set (n=175, 30%). The flowchart of the present study selection is shown in **Figure 1** and the clinicopathologic characteristics of patients in the training and validation sets are listed in **Table 1**. This study was conducted in accordance with the Declaration of Helsinki and was approved by the ethics committee of Sichuan University West China Hospital. Informed consent was obtained from all the patients.

Data Collection and Follow-Up

The clinical medical data of cHCC and iCCA patients who underwent curative liver resection were retrospectively collected from our hospital and included demographics, comorbid illnesses, portal hypertension, preoperative routine blood tests, biochemistry tests, tumor marker tests, tumor imaging data and survival information. In general, all patients who received curative liver resection were prospectively followed up through outpatient clinic visits or telephone calls at intervals of 2–3 months during the first year after the operation and 3-6 months thereafter. Chest CT examination, bone scintigraphy and PET-CT were performed when extrahepatic tumor recurrence was suspected. Oncological survival outcomes, including overall survival (OS) and recurrence-free survival (RFS), were collected until December 31, 2019. OS was defined as the interval between resection and death, or the period up to the last follow-up. RFS was defined as the interval from after surgery to tumor recurrence, including intrahepatic tumor recurrence and extrahepatic metastasis, or the period up to the last observation endpoint.

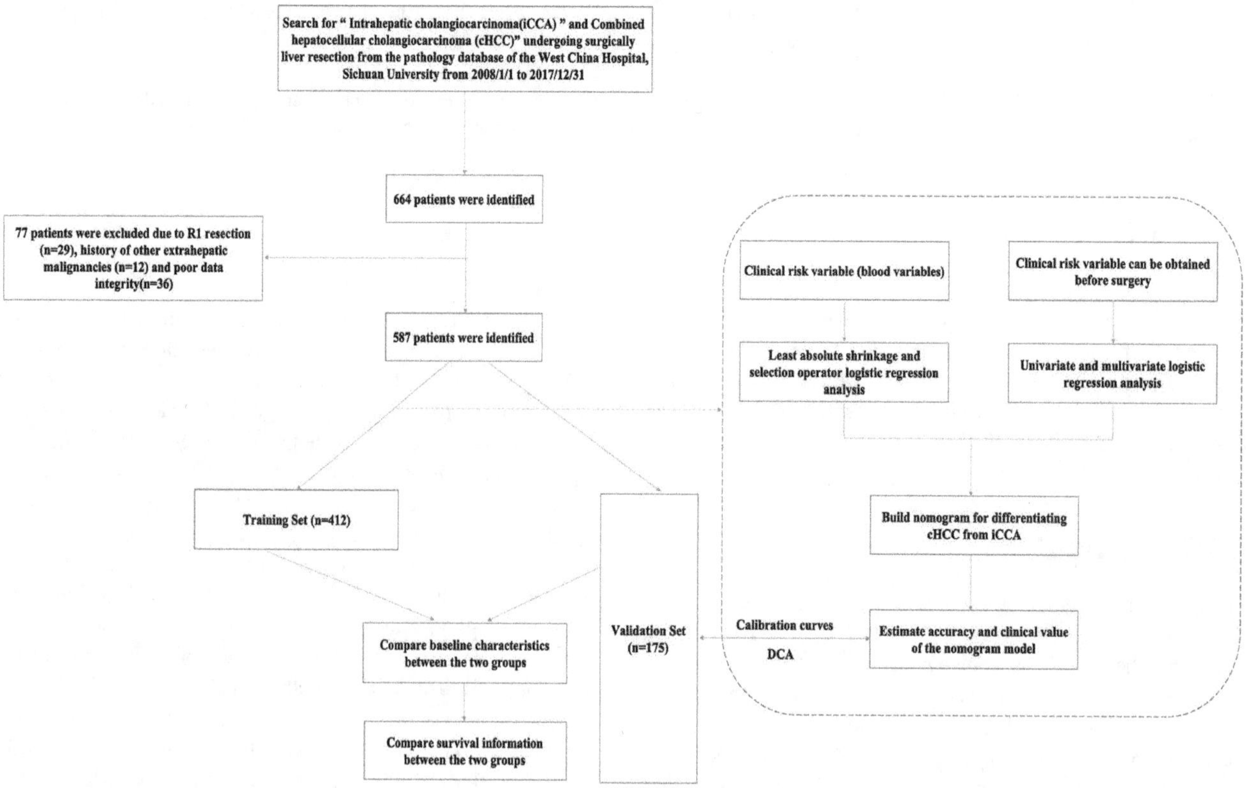

FIGURE 1 | The flowchart of patient selection.

Risk Factors for Presence of cHCC

Univariate logistic regression analysis was performed to estimate the impacts of demographics, comorbid illnesses and imaging features on distinguishing cHCC and iCCA in the training set. Stepwise multivariate logistic regression analysis was further performed to screen for independent risk factors at a significant level. The LASSO logistic regression model was used to build a prognostic classifier, which integrated all types of laboratory study variables that can be obtained before surgery, to differentiate iCCA from cHCC in the training set. Using the coefficients derived from the LASSO logistic regression models, we then constructed a formula to calculate a score for each patient. We used the receiver operating characteristic (ROC) curve with calculations of the area under the curve (AUC) to determine the optimal cut-off value of the blood signature score. Restricted cubic spline (RCS) was used to evaluate the relationship between the blood signature score obtained by LASSO logistic regression and the outcome of distinguishing cHCC from iCCA.

Construction, Assessment, and Internal Validation of Nomograms

Laboratory study variables chosen by LASSO regression and the results of multivariate logistic regression were included in the model. All possible diagnostic factors are performed to construct a simplified nomogram for the differential diagnosis of iCCA and cHCC. The differential accuracy of the models was measured using the C-index, quantifying the level of agreement between the predicted probabilities and the actual possibility of having the event of interest, and the bootstrap estimate of slope shrinkage (18). The bootstrap resampling method was chosen for the internal validation of the predictive models' selecting 1000 repetitions. Decision curve analysis (DCA) was used to determine the clinical application value of the nomogram by evaluating the net benefit (19). Clinical impact curves were further drawn to evaluate the clinical impact of the nomogram to help understand its importance more intuitively (20).

Statistical Analysis

The Mann-Whitney U test was used to compare continuous variables between two patient groups. The chi-squared test and two-tailed Fisher's exact test were used for the comparison of categorical variables between two groups. Continuous variables are expressed as the medians and interquartile ranges(*Q1-Q3*), and categorical variables are expressed as the numbers and percentages. R version 4.0.0 (http://www.r-project.org/) was used for ROC curve analysis, RCS, LASSO logistic regression, nomogram generation, C-index assessment, calibration plot generation, and DCA. The rest of the analyses were conducted using SPSS statistical software version 25.0 (IBM Corporation, Armonk, NY). In all analyses, $P < 0.05$ was considered to indicate statistical significance.

TABLE 1 | Baseline characteristics of patients in intrahepatic cholangiocarcinoma (iCCA) and combined hepatocellular cholangiocarcinoma (cHCC).

Variables	Patients					
	Training set			Validation set		
	iCCA group(n=280)	cHCC group(n=132)	*P-value*	iCCA group(n=118)	cHCC group(n=57)	*P-value*
Age (years), median (IQR)	57(48–64)	52(45–59)	0.005	58(50–64)	55(46.25–58)	0.004
Gender (male/female),	151/129	105/27	<0.001	55/63	50/7	<0.001
Portal hypertension, n (%)			0.003			<0.001
Yes	40(14.29%)	35(26.52%)		13(11.02%)	21(36.84%)	
No	240(85.71%)	97(73.48%)		105(88.98%)	36(63.16%)	
HBsAg positive, n (%)			<0.001			<0.001
Yes	88(31.43%)	105(79.55%)		38(32.20%)	40(70.18%)	
No	192(68.57%)	27(20.45%)		80(67.80%)	17(29.82%)	
Diabetes, n (%)			0.700			0.906
Yes	40(14.3%)	17(12.9%)		11(9.3%)	5(8.8%)	
No	240(85.7%)	115(87.1%)		107(90.7%)	52(91.2%)	
Biliary duct stones, n (%)			<0.001			0.024
Yes	45(16.1%)	5(3.8%)		21(17.8%)	3(5.3%)	
No	235(83.9%)	127(96.2%)		97(82.2%)	54(94.7%)	
Baseline laboratory investigations						
WBC count $\times 10^9$/L, median (IQR)	6.62(5.42–8.00)	5.78(4.74–7.16)	0.005	6.31(5.15–7.76)	5.76(4.56–7.80)	0.177
NEUT count $\times 10^9$/L, median (IQR)	4.24(3.33–5.65)	3.62(2.87–5.11)	0.018	3.94(3.06–5.37)	3.55(2.85–5.13)	0.068
PLT count ×109/L, median (IQR)	163.5(122–219)	142.5(99.25–192.5)	0.015	132(132–218.75)	139(83–15.5)	0.011
ALT (U/L), median (IQR)	30(18–47)	33(25–49)	0.033	24.5(16–36)	38(26.5–58)	<0.001
AST (U/L), median (IQR)	30(23–42)	35.5(27–53)	0.007	28.5(23–37)	35(27.5–50.5)	<0.001
GGT (U/L), median (IQR)	66(36–132.25)	71(41–135)	0.598	66(22.75–136.5)	61(38–120)	0.360
TBIL (umol/L), median (IQR)	13.45(9.93–17.18)	13.35(10.23–18.08)	0.970	11.7(9.38–14.73)	13.3(9.50–20.4)	0.148
ALB (g/L), median (IQR)	42.5(39.7–45.1)	41.7(38.03–44.5)	0.274	42.7(40.28–45.93)	42.8(39.35–46.6)	0.958
PT(s), median (IQR)	11.6(11.0–12.3)	12.0(11.4–12.9)	0.017	11.5(11–12.13)	11.9(11.3–13)	0.037
INR, median (IQR)	1.02(0.96–1.08)	1.05(1.01–1.13)	0.001	1.0(0.95–1.06)	1.04(0.98–1.15)	0.001
AFP, ng/ml median (IQR)	3.18(2.26–5.37)	75.84(6.35–621)	<0.001	3.24(2.16–5.68)	44.09(3.71–226.10)	<0.001
CA19-9 level(U/mL), median (IQR)	78.19(19.28–861.35)	31.17(14.32–95.89)	<0.001	57.13(13.77–493.98)	23.49(13.64–47.61)	<0.001
Tumor size (cm), median (range)	5.5(4.2–8)	5.5(3.7–7.8)	0.448	6(4.6–8.0)	5.3(3.1–7.05)	0.098
Tumor number (Multiple/solitary),			0.317			0.001
multiple	90(32.14%)	36(27.27%)		39(33.1%)	6(10.5%)	
solitary	190(67.86%)	96(72.73%)		79(66.9%)	51(89.5%)	
Tumor location			<0.001			0.004
Left lobe	116(41.43%)	28(21.21%)		46(39.0%)	21(36.8%)	
Right lobe	103(36.79%)	84(63.64%)		44(37.3%)	33(57.9%)	
Both lobes	61(21.78%)	20(15.15%)		28(23.7%)	3(5.3%)	
Extent of liver resection, n(%)			0.082			0.342
major	166(59.29%)	90(68.18%)		81(68.64%)	35(61.40%)	
minor	114(40.71%)	42(31.82%)		37(31.36%)	22(38.60%)	
MVI, n (%)			0.002			0.001
Yes	52(18.57%)	43(32.58%)		21(17.80%)	23(40.35%)	
No	228(81.43%)	89(67.42%)		97(82.20%)	34(59.65%)	
Macroscopic vascular invasion, n(%)			0.205			0.622
Yes	96(34.29%)	37(28.03%)		35(29.66%)	19(33.33%)	
No	184(65.71%)	95(71.97%)		83(70.34%)	38(66.67%)	
Satellite nodules, n(%)			0.411			0.432
Yes	42(15%)	24(18.18%)		21(17.80%)	13(22.81%)	
No	238(850%)	108(81.82%)		97(83.20%)	44(77.19%)	
Lymph node metastasis, n (%)			0.024			0.027
Present	70(25%)	20(15.15%)		32(27.12%)	7(12.28%)	
Absent	210(75%)	112(84.85%)		86(72.88%)	50(87.72%)	
Tumor encapsulation, n (%),			0.759			0.088
incomplete	153(54.64%)	70(53.03%)		74(62.71%)	28(49.12%)	
complete	127(45.36%)	62(46.97%)		44(37.29%)	29(50.88%)	

HBsAg, hepatitis B surface antigen; WBC, white blood cell; NEU, neutrophil; PLT, platelet; ALT, alanine aminotransferase; AST, aspartate transaminase; GGT, γ-glutamyl transferase; TBIL, total bilirubin; ALB, albumin; PT, Prothrombin time; INR, international normalized ratio; AFP, alpha fetoprotein; CA19-9, carbohydrate antigen 19-9; MVI, microvascular invasion.

RESULTS

Clinical Characteristics of the Study Patients

A total of 587 patients (361 men, 226 women) who underwent curative liver resection for iCCA and cHCC between January 2008 and December 2017 at West China Hospital were enrolled in this study. All iCCA and cHCC patients were followed up after initial treatment until December 2019. In the training set, a total of 412 patients, including 132 cHCC patients and 280 iCCA patients. For the validation set, 175 consecutive patients were studied, consisting of 57 cHCC patients and 118 iCCA patients. There were more males in the cHCC group than in the iCCA group. Portal hypertension and HBsAg positivity were more common in patients with cHCC. However, microvascular invasion (MVI) and lymph node metastasis were more common in the iCCA group. Patients with cHCC were younger and had higher serum alpha-fetoprotein (AFP) levels and lower serum CA19-9 levels than patients with iCCA. The baseline clinicopathologic characteristics of the patients are listed in **Supplementary Table 1**. Among the entire set, the median overall survival (OS) of 189 patients with cHCC was 16.2 months and that of the 398 patients with iCCA was 18.6 months. The patients in the cHCC group had poorer OS and RFS than those in the iCCA group. The 1-, 3-, and 5-year OS rates were 78.3%, 12.2%, and 3.2%, respectively, in patients with cHCC and 70.1%, 23.1%, and 7.8%, respectively, in patients with iCCA (**Figure 2**).

Constructing a Simplified Prediction Model and Internal Validation

To distinguish between cHCC and iCCA well before surgery and guide clinical decision making, univariate logistic regression analysis was performed to estimate the impacts of demographics, comorbid illnesses, and imaging features on the differential diagnosis of cHCC and iCCA in the training set. According to univariable logistic regression analysis, age, sex, biliary duct stones, and portal hypertension were associated with the possibility of cHCC diagnosis. Stepwise multivariate logistic regression analysis was further performed to identify significant independent risk factors. The multivariate analyses revealed that age (≥55 vs. <55 years, OR, 0.568, 95%CI, 0.366–0.882, P=0.012), sex (female vs. male, OR, 0.354, 95%CI, 0.215–0.582, P<0.001), biliary duct stones (yes vs. no, OR, 0.274, 95% CI, 0.103-0.729, P=0.010), and portal hypertension (present vs. absent, OR, 1.816, 95% CI, 1.066–3.095, P=0.028) were independent risk factors for distinguishing cHCC from iCCA (**Table 2**). Using the coefficients derived from the LASSO logistic regression models in the training set, we then constructed a formula to calculate for each patient. The LASSO coefficient profiles of the selected blood features are shown in **Figure 3**. The blood signature score was based on the personalized levels of the 7 blood features, as listed in **Supplementary Table 2**. Restrictive cubic spline functions of the blood-cHCC scores in the training and validation sets showed that the blood-cHCC score presented linear profiles (**Supplementary Figure 2**). Using the ROC curve, we classified patients into a type-cHCC$^{\text{low risk}}$ group and a type-cHCC$^{\text{high risk}}$ group with a blood signature score of -0.535 as the cut-off value (**Supplementary Figure 1A**). Based on the results of the blood signatures and multivariate logistic regression, a nomogram for distinguishing cHCC and iCCA was established (**Figure 4**). Point assignments and differential scores for each variable in the nomogram models are presented in **Supplementary Table 3**. According to the nomogram for distinguishing between cHCC and iCCA, the blood signature made the largest contribution. The calibration curve of the prediction nomogram for the differential diagnosis of cHCC and iCCA presented a good agreement in training and validation sets (**Figures 4B, C**). The Harrell's concordance index (C-index) for the nomogram for distinguishing cHCC and iCCA was 0.796 (95% CI, 0.752–0.840) for the training set and 0.824 (95% CI, 0.761–0.887) for the validation set, as detailed in **Supplementary Table 4**. After obtaining risk scores were obtained from the nomogram, risk classification of the differential diagnosis nomogram was conducted by ROC curve analysis. The patients were classified into low- and high-risk groups according to the optimal cut-off score of 119 on the cHCC nomogram (**Supplementary Figure 1B**). The high-risk group had a noticeably increased possibility of cHCC in the training set and validation set (**Figures 5E–H**). In addition, we performed survival analysis based on the cHCC nomogram risk score, and the high-risk groups had a worse prognosis in terms of RFS (**Supplementary Figure 3**). Hence, the nomogram could effectively distinguish between cHCC and iCCA before surgery but also predict prognosis after surgery to some extent.

DISCUSSION

Previous studies have classified cHCC and iCCA in the same category (7, 21), however, the prognosis of cHCC in comparison to iCCA remains controversial. Furthermore, treatment strategies for cHCC and iCCA differ. A previous study demonstrated that the molecular biology features of cHCC are more similar to those of hepatocellular carcinoma (HCC) than of iCCA, therefore, multitargeted inhibitors, including lenvatinib, regorafenib, and cabozantinib, may have potential for benefit in cHCC due to frequent alterations in RTK/Ras/PI3-kinase pathways (22). Moreover, liver transplantation might also bring potential survival benefits to patients with cHCC (23, 24). However, due to the current controversy over the value of liver transplantation for iCCA and the lack of indications for liver transplantation that meet the characteristics of the disease, liver transplantation has not been recommended as a routine treatment for iCCA. Since iCCA often metastasizes to distant sites in the early stage of the disease, which seriously affects long-term survival after transplantation, most centers in the West hold a conservative attitude towards the treatment of liver transplantation for iCCA (25). Curative liver resection is an important treatment for two types of resectable tumors. For resectable tumor, if we can distinguish the pathological type of the tumor before surgery, we can perform a comprehensive assessment to choose a wider surgical margin, anatomic liver resection. we could choose individualized treatment for each patient's condition especially for unresectable patients or

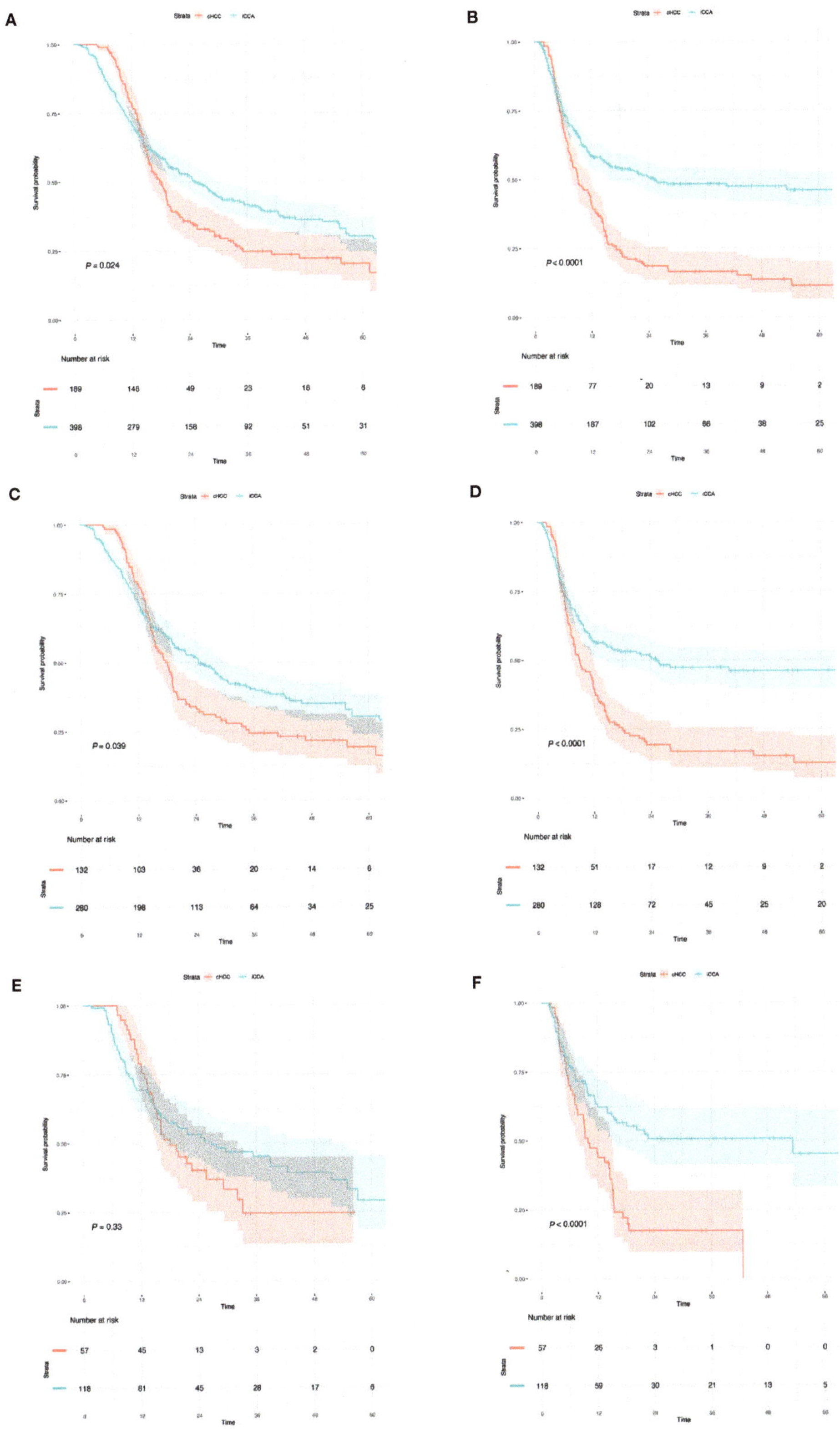

FIGURE 2 | (A, C, E) Kaplan–Meier analysis of overall survival for cHCC and iCCA in the whole sets, training sets and validation sets. **(B, D, F)** Kaplan–Meier analysis of recurrence-free survival and overall survival for cHCC and iCCA in the whole sets, training sets and validation sets. The number at risk refers to the number of patients who have not relapsed at the corresponding time point. cHCC, combined hepatocellular cholangiocarcinoma; iCCA, intrahepatic cholangiocarcinoma.

TABLE 2 | Logistic regression models of variables associated with distinguish combined hepatocellular cholangiocarcinoma (cHCC) from intrahepatic cholangiocarcinoma (iCCA) before surgery.

Variable	Univariate regression model			Multivariate regression model		
	Odds ratio	95% CI	*P* value	Odds ratio	95% CI	*P* value
Age (≥55 vs. <55 years)	**0.530**	**0.348–0.805**	**0.003**	**0.568**	**0.366–0.882**	**0.012**
Sex (female vs. male)	**0.301**	**0.186–0.488**	**<0.001**	**0.354**	**0.215–0.582**	**<0.001**
Diabetes (yes vs. no)	0.887	0.482–1.631	0.700			
Portal hypertension (present vs. absent)	**2.020**	**1.204–3.389**	**0.008**	**1.816**	**1.066–3.095**	**0.028**
Biliary duct stones (yes vs. no)	**0.206**	**0.080–0.531**	**0.001**	**0.274**	**0.103–0.729**	**0.010**
Maximum tumor size (>5 vs. ≤5cm)	0.900	0.593–1.365	0.620			
Tumor number (multiple vs. single)	0.792	0.501–1.251	0.317			
Macroscopic vascular invasion (yes vs. no)	0.746	0.475–1.174	0.206			

cHCC, combined hepatocellular carcinoma; iCCA, intrahepatic cholangiocarcinoma; CI, confidence interval.
Bold indicates statistically significant difference.

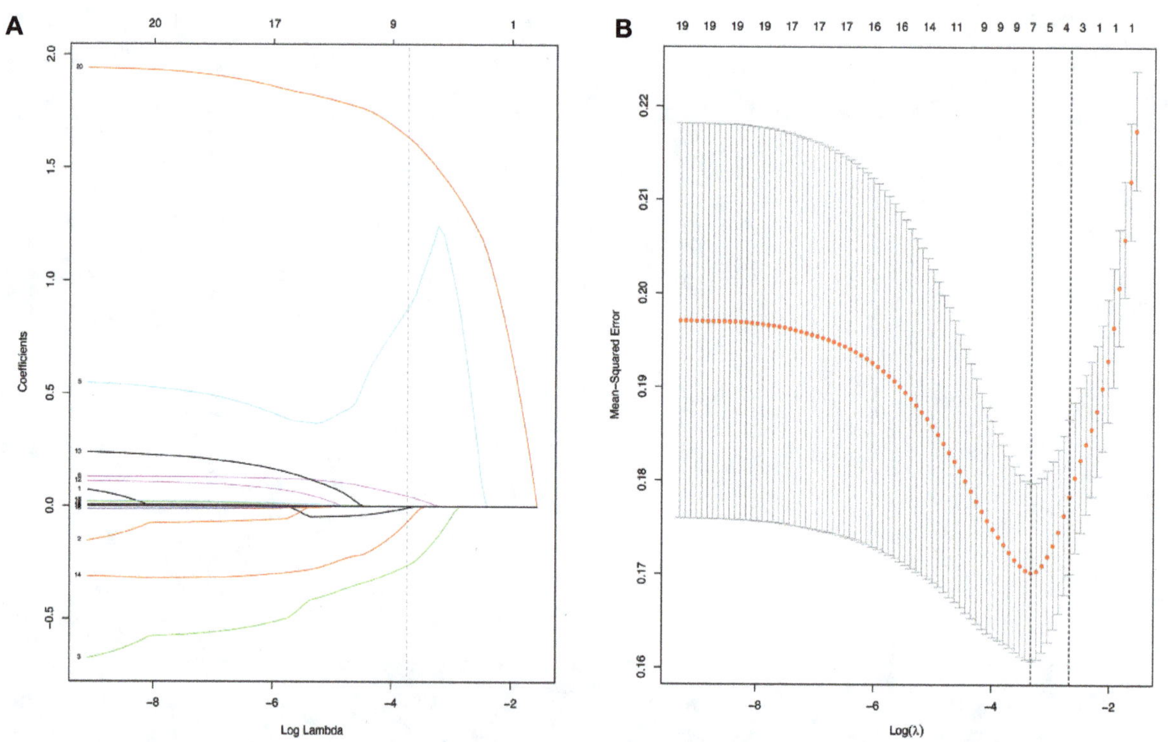

FIGURE 3 | Blood-cHCC score models selection using the least absolute shrinkage and selection operator (LASSO) binary logistic regression model in the training set **(A)**. LASSO coefficient profiles of the seven selected blood signatures for combined hepatocellular cholangiocarcinoma (cHCC). A dashed vertical line is drawn at the value (logγ=-3.3) chosen by 10-fold cross-validation. Vertical line was shown at the value selected using cross-validation, where the optimum lambda gave rise to seven features with nonzero coefficients **(B)**. Partial likelihood deviance for the LASSO coefficient profiles. The partial likelihood deviance (binomial deviance) curve was presented versus log (lambda). A light dashed vertical line stands for the minimum partial likelihood deviance. A dashed vertical line stands for the partial likelihood deviance at the value (logγ=-3.3).

patients who could not guarantee the R0 margin of surgery, which is in line with the current concept of precision liver cancer surgery (26). cHCC is associated with high risk of recurrence following surgical resection as compared with iCCA. Closely post-operative monitoring is highly recommended for cHCC patients. Simultaneously, it could aid clinicians in explaining the illness for patient counseling. For unresectable iCCA, chemotherapy with gemcitabine, platinum compounds, and fluoropyrimidines is the main treatment choice. A recent multicenter study reported that postoperative chemotherapy with gemcitabine prolonged the

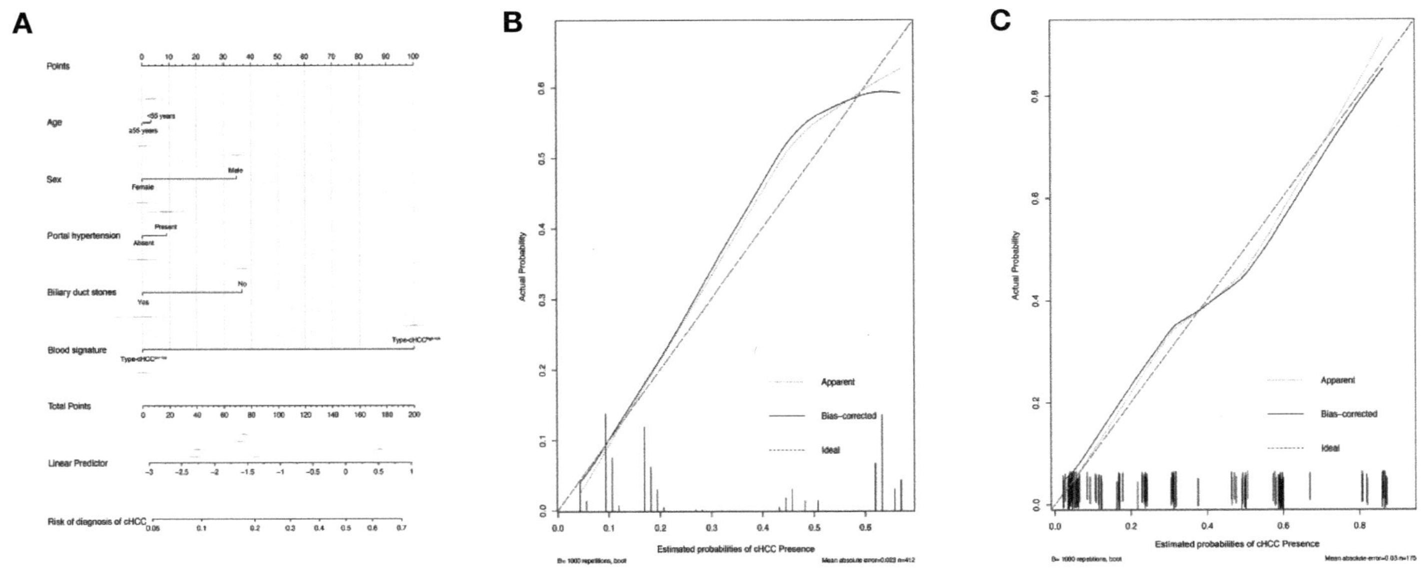

FIGURE 4 | Differential diagnosis nomograms for distinguishing combined hepatocellular cholangiocarcinoma (cHCC) and intrahepatic cholangiocarcinoma (iCCA) and the calibration plot **(A)**. The nomogram maps the distinguishing ability of cHCC and iCCA on a scale of 0 to 200. For each covariate, a vertical line is drawn upwards and the corresponding points are noted. This is repeated for each covariate, ending with a total point that corresponds to the differential diagnosis axes to seek the probability of cHCC at the bottom of the nomogram. The C-index value for the nomogram distinguishing cHCC from iCCA was 0.796 (95% CI, 0.752–0.840). The calibration curve for distinguishing cHCC and iCCA in the training set **(B)** and in the validation set **(C)**. Ideal line (blue), estimated probabilities correspond to the actual observed; apparent line (red), prediction capability of the model obtained after data analysis; bias-corrected line, prediction capability of the model obtained after bootstrap correction.

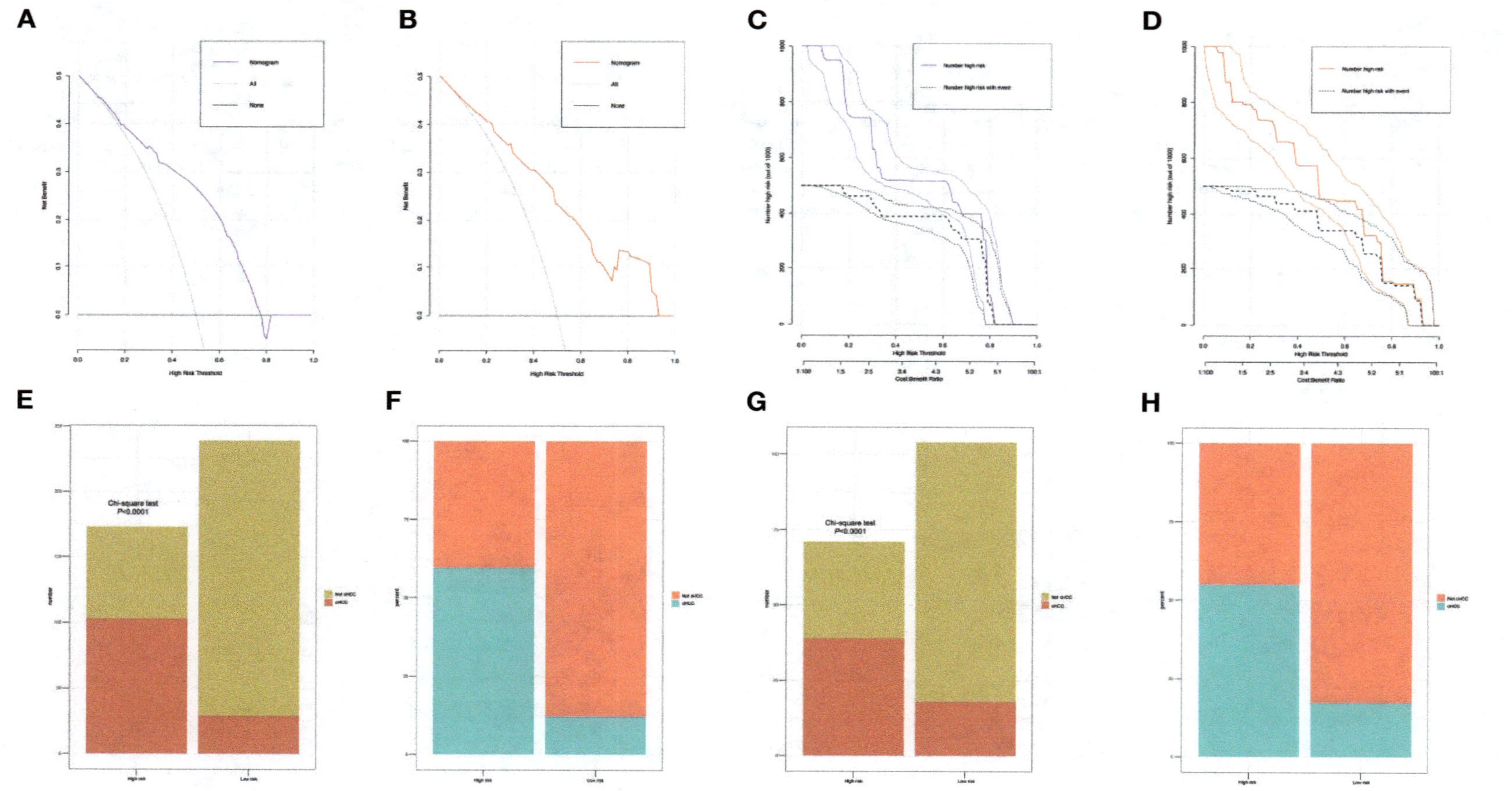

FIGURE 5 | The decision curves of the nomograms for distinguishing combined hepatocellular cholangiocarcinoma (cHCC) from intrahepatic cholangiocarcinoma (iCCA) in the training and validation sets. The Y-axis represents the net benefit. The X-axis shows the threshold probability. The horizontal solid black line represents the hypothesis that no patients experienced presence of cHCC, and the solid gray line represents the hypothesis that all patients met the endpoint **(A, B)**. Clinical impact curves of the nomogram for distinguishing cHCC from iCCA in the training and validation set **(C, D)**. At different threshold probabilities within a given population, the number of high-risk patients and the number of high- risk patients with the outcome are shown. Discriminatory power of the nomograms for cHCC status with bar charts. Risk classification of the differential diagnosis nomogram conducted by the Receiver operating characteristic (ROC) curve analysis, and the performance in distinguishing the cHCC from iCCA in the training and validation set **(E–H)**.

survival time of patients at high risk of recurrence and metastasis (27). However, systemic therapy or chemotherapy is not the standard option for advanced and unresectable cHCC (28), and a large sample size is still needed to distinguish cHCC from iCCA, and determine the value of other treatments for cHCC, which reflected the significance and importance of our research.

To data, the gold standard for the preoperative diagnosis of liver tumors is fine needle aspiration biopsy, but for tumors without a biopsy path or with a small-diameter tumors, biopsies are usually not available before surgery. In addition, the pathological data obtained at the morphological, phenotypical, and molecular levels from these tiny fragments by fine-needle aspiration biopsy may be incomplete or only partially representative, especially for cHCC patients with two components. The real risk of seeding and the oncologic prognosis by inserting a needle into a liver tumor lesion are still unclear (29–31). In recent years, with the development of imaging technology, the role of liver biopsy in the diagnosis of primary liver cancer (PLC) has been challenged over time by the ability of imaging techniques to conjecture the histologic status (32, 33). Imaging techniques could also help clinicians to understand more information, such as vascular invasion and lymph node metastasis, and even determine the most appropriate operative method (34). However, the diagnosis of cHCC and the differentiation of cHCC from other PLCs based on imaging findings can be challenging because of the histologic diversity and complexity of cHCC components and the overlapping imaging characteristics with those of iCCA (35–37). Moreover, their clinical value is limited due to the lack of costly high-resolution equipment and experienced radiologists especially in some developing areas. Therefore, a novel and noninvasive method is required to distinguish cHCC from iCCA before receiving various treatments.

To our knowledge, our research is the first large comprehensive comparison reported to date on the clinical characteristics and prognoses of cHCC and iCCA patients after surgery. Our study focused on distinguishing between cHCC and iCCA before liver resection using a simple predictive model that incorporated the clinical risk factors as well as laboratory blood indicators that could be used in daily clinical practice to accurately predict pathological information preoperatively, rather than being limited to the identification of clinicopathological risk factors in resected specimens.

In this study, we showed that the prognosis of cHCC was significantly worse than that of iCCA in both the training set and in the validation set. Differences in prognosis for iCCA and cHCC might be due to their distinct mechanisms of carcinogenesis and biological behaviors. It is increasingly believed that cHCC may originate from hepatic progenitor cells, which are intermediate stem cells capable of undergoing bidirectional differentiation into hepatocytes and bile duct epithelial cells (38, 39), causing cHCC to have significant heterogeneity and aggressive biological behavior. Coulouarn et al. determined that the occurrence of cHCC might be related to the microenvironment remodeling and the activation of TGFβ and Wnt/β-catenin were identified as the two major signaling pathways in cHCC (39). In addition, most patients with cHCC have a background of hepatitis B cirrhosis, which easily leads to tumor recurrence. However, for iCCA, the possible causative risk factors include biliary diseases such as biliary duct stones, hepatobiliary flukes, primary sclerosing cholangitis, and biliary tract cysts (40). Although our study found that the cHCC and iCCA groups had significant differences in MVI and lymph node metastasis, which might be the basis for distinguishing between cHCC and iCCA, the above information was obtained only through postoperative pathological specimens. In our study, we found that liver function and coagulation function indicators in cHCC patients were higher than those in iCCA patients which might be related to the facts that cHCC patients usually are infected with hepatitis virus. The above might become a potential blood predictor to distinguish cHCC from iCCA. Age (<55 years) and portal hypertension were positively related to cHCC, while biliary duct stones and female sex were positive factors in the iCCA differential nomogram. Our differential diagnosis nomogram demonstrated good agreement between predictions and observations in the training and validation sets. In addition, we found that the nomogram we established has better diagnostic performance than other clinical risk factors or blood signatures alone. With our nomogram, we can identify the cHCC patients who were previously misdiagnosed with iCCA. These patients could regain the chance to undergo liver transplantation or targeted therapy. Additionally, our nomogram might serve as a selection tool to assess neoadjuvant treatment for iCCA patients during randomized clinical trials in the future. Meaningfully, the Kaplan–Meier survival curves demonstrated that the nomograms could not only effectively distinguish between cHCC and iCCA regardless of individual values, but also successfully discriminate among different risk groups, thereby improving clinical decision making.

Although our research provided a new and simple method to distinguish between iCCA and cHCC, several limitations should be taken into consideration when interpreting our findings. Our study was conducted at a single-center study, and due to the characteristics of retrospective studies, there may be potential selection bias. The data for the training set and validation set were obtained from a single center, which might have hampered the identification of possibly important predictive factors. Moreover, although hepatitis virus infection is an important pathogenic factor in the carcinogenesis of PLC in China, however, in the West, hepatitis C virus infection and alcohol or metabolic factors are usually the causes of PLC. Whether this differential diagnosis nomogram is generalizable to patients in Western countries is still worth exploring, other western liver cancer centers are needed to recruit to build external validation.

CONCLUSION

In conclusion, the current study proves that patients with cHCC have a poorer prognosis than those with iCCA and that cHCC is a distinct tumor different from iCCA. Furthermore, we constructed and validated a nomogram that optimally differentiates cHCC from iCCA preoperatively by combining other clinical risk factors identified by logistic regression and blood signatures selected by the LASSO algorithm.

AUTHOR CONTRIBUTIONS

Study concept and design: TW, WXW, and WTW. Acquisition of data: TW, SS, and JZ. Statistical analysis of data: TW and XY. Drafting of the manuscript: TW and WXW. Critical revision of the manuscript: TW, WXW, SS, and WTW. All authors contributed to the article and approved the submitted version.

SUPPLEMENTARY MATERIAL

SUPPLEMENTARY FIGURE 1 | (A) Receiver operating characteristic (ROC) curve analysis of the blood signature for cHCC. The areas under the curve (AUCs) were 0.806. The optimal cut-off blood score was -0.535 **(B)** Receiver operating characteristic (ROC) curve analysis of the nomogram risk score for distinguishing cHCC. The areas under the curve (AUCs) were 0.799. The optimal cut-off the nomogram risk score was 119.

SUPPLEMENTARY FIGURE 2 | The restricted cubic spline of the blood-cHCC score in training and validation sets **(A, B)**. The restricted cubic spline of the nomogram risk score for distinguishing cHCC in training and validation sets **(C, D).**

SUPPLEMENTARY FIGURE 3 | Kaplan–Meier analysis of recurrence-free survival and overall survival according to risk score based on nomogram. The number at risk refers to the number of patients who have not relapsed at the corresponding time point.

REFERENCES

1. Bertuccio P, Malvezzi M, Carioli G, Hashim D, Boffetta P, El-Serag HB, et al. Global trends in mortality from intrahepatic and extrahepatic cholangiocarcinoma. *J Hepatol* (2019) 71(1):104–14. doi: 10.1016/j.jhep.2019.03.013
2. Wang T, Kong J, Yang X, Shen S, Zhang M, Wang W. Clinical features of sarcomatoid change in patients with intrahepatic cholangiocarcinoma and prognosis after surgical liver resection: A Propensity Score Matching analysis. *J Surg Oncol* (2020) 121(3):524–37. doi: 10.1002/jso.25815
3. Holzner ML, Tabrizian P, Parvin-Nejad FP, Fei K, Gunasekaran G, Rocha C, et al. Resection of Mixed Hepatocellular-Cholangiocarcinoma, Hepatocellular Carcinoma, and Intrahepatic Cholangiocarcinoma: A Western Center Experience. *Liver Transpl* (2020) 26(7):888–98. doi: 10.1002/lt.25786
4. Yamashita YI, Aishima S, Nakao Y, Yoshizumi T, Nagano H, Kuroki T, et al. Clinicopathological characteristics of combined hepatocellular cholangiocarcinoma from the viewpoint of patient prognosis after hepatic resection: High rate of early recurrence and its predictors. *Hepatol Res* (2020) 50(7):863–70. doi: 10.1111/hepr.13507
5. Lee JH, Chung GE, Yu SJ, Hwang SY, Kim JS, Kim HY, et al. Long-term prognosis of combined hepatocellular and cholangiocarcinoma after curative resection comparison with hepatocellular carcinoma and cholangiocarcinoma. *J Clin Gastroenterol* (2011) 45(1):69–75. doi: 10.1097/MCG.0b013e3181ce5dfa
6. Chantajitr S, Wilasrusmee C, Lertsitichai P, Phromsopha N. Combined hepatocellular and cholangiocarcinoma: clinical features and prognostic study in a Thai population. *J Hepato Biliary Pancreatic Surg* (2006) 13 (6):537–42. doi: 10.1007/s00534-006-1117-1
7. Kassahun WT, Hauss J. Management of combined hepatocellular and cholangiocarcinoma. *Int J Clin Pract* (2008) 62(8):1271–8. doi: 10.1111/j.1742-1241.2007.01694.x
8. Edge SB, Byrd DR, Carducci MA, Compton CC, Fritz A, Greene F. *AJCC cancer staging manual.* 7th ed. New York, NY: Springer (2010) p. 201–5.
9. Amin MB, Edge SB. *AJCC cancer staging manual.* 8th ed. New York, NY: Springer (2017) p. 288–92.
10. Brierley JD, Gospodarowicz MK, Wittekind C, eds. *TNM classification of malignant tumours.* 8th ed. New York, NY: Wiley Blackwell (2017) 83–84.
11. Yano Y, Yamamoto J, Kosuge T, Sakamoto Y, Yamasaki S, Shimada K, et al. Combined hepatocellular and cholangiocarcinoma: a clinicopathologic study of 26 resected cases. *Jpn J Clin Oncol* (2003) 33(6):283–7. doi: 10.1093/jjco/hyg056
12. Zuo HQ, Yan LN, Zeng Y, Yang JY, Luo HZ, Liu JW, et al. Clinicopathological characteristics of 15 patients with combined hepatocellular carcinoma and cholangiocarcinoma. *Hepatobiliary Pancreatic Dis Int HBPD Int* (2007) 6 (2):161–5.
13. Yin X, Zhang BH, Qiu SJ, Ren G, Zhou J, Chen XH, et al. Combined hepatocellular carcinoma and cholangiocarcinoma: clinical features, treatment modalities, and prognosis. *Ann Surg Oncol* (2012) 19(9):2869–76. doi: 10.1245/s10434-012-2328-0
14. Panjala C, Senecal DL, Bridges MD, Kim GP, Nakhleh RE, Nguyen JH, et al. The diagnostic conundrum and liver transplantation outcome for combined hepatocellular-cholangiocarcinoma. *Am J Transplant* 10(5):1263–7. doi: 10.1111/j.1600-6143.2010.03062.x
15. Gera S, Ettel M, Acosta-Gonzalez G, Xu R. Clinical features, histology, and histogenesis of combined hepatocellular-cholangiocarcinoma. *World J Hepatol* (2017) 9(6):300–9. doi: 10.4254/wjh.v9.i6.300
16. Sauerbrei W, Royston P, Binder H. Selection of important variables and determination of functional form for continuous predictors in multivariable model building. *Stat Med* (2007) 26(30):5512–28. doi: 10.1002/sim.3148
17. Friedman J, Hastie T, Tibshirani R. Regularization Paths for Generalized Linear Models via Coordinate Descent. *J Stat Softw* (2010) 33(1):1–22.
18. Iasonos A, Schrag D, Raj GV, Panageas KS. How to build and interpret a nomogram for cancer prognosis. *J Clin Oncol* (2008) 26(8):1364–70. doi: 10.1200/jco.2007.12.9791
19. Vickers AJ, Elkin EB. Decision curve analysis: a novel method for evaluating prediction models. *Med Decis Making* (2006) 26(6):565–74. doi: 10.1177/0272989x06295361
20. Kerr KF, Brown MD, Zhu K, Janes H. Assessing the Clinical Impact of Risk Prediction Models With Decision Curves: Guidance for Correct Interpretation and Appropriate Use. *J Clin Oncol* (2016) 34(21):2534–40. doi: 10.1200/jco.2015.65.5654
21. Sobin LH, Gospodarowicz MK, Wittekind C, eds. *TNM Classification of Malignant Tumours, 7th Edition.* New York, NY: Wiley Blackwell (2009) p. 108–10.
22. Joseph NM, Tsokos CG, Umetsu SE, Shain AH, Kelley RK, Onodera C, et al. Genomic profiling of combined hepatocellular-cholangiocarcinoma reveals similar genetics to hepatocellular carcinoma. *J Pathol* (2019) 248(2):164–78. doi: 10.1002/path.5243
23. Sapisochin G, de Lope CR, Gastaca M, de Urbina JO, López-Andujar R, Palacios F, et al. Intrahepatic cholangiocarcinoma or mixed hepatocellular-cholangiocarcinoma in patients undergoing liver transplantation: a Spanish matched cohort multicenter study. *Ann Surg* (2014) 259(5):944–52. doi: 10.1097/sla.0000000000000494
24. Lunsford KE, Court C, Seok Lee Y, Lu DS, Naini BV, Harlander-Locke MP, et al. Propensity-Matched Analysis of Patients with Mixed Hepatocellular-Cholangiocarcinoma and Hepatocellular Carcinoma Undergoing Liver Transplantation. *Liver Transpl* (2018) 24(10):1384–97. doi: 10.1002/lt.25058
25. Lee DD, Croome KP, Musto KR, Melendez J, Tranesh G, Nakhleh R, et al. Liver transplantation for intrahepatic cholangiocarcinoma. *Liver Transpl* (2018) 24(5):634–44. doi: 10.1002/lt.25052
26. Balachandran VP, Gonen M, Smith JJ, DeMatteo RP. Nomograms in oncology: more than meets the eye. *Lancet Oncol* (2015) 16(4):e173–80. doi: 10.1016/s1470-2045(14)71116-7
27. Reames BN, Bagante F, Ejaz A, Spolverato G, Ruzzenente A, Weiss M, et al. Impact of adjuvant chemotherapy on survival in patients with intrahepatic cholangiocarcinoma: a multi-institutional analysis. *HPB* (2017) 19(10):901–9. doi: 10.1016/j.hpb.2017.06.008

28. Feng M, Pan Y, Kong R, Shu S. Therapy of Primary Liver Cancer. *Innovation (N Y)* (2020) 1(2):100032. doi: 10.1016/j.xinn.2020.100032
29. Mulier S, Mulier P, Ni Y, Miao Y, Dupas B, Marchal G, et al. Complications of radiofrequency coagulation of liver tumours. *Br J Surg* (2002) 89(10):1206–22. doi: 10.1046/j.1365-2168.2002.02168.x
30. Yu J, Liang P, Yu XL, Cheng ZG, Han ZY, Dong BW. Needle track seeding after percutaneous microwave ablation of malignant liver tumors under ultrasound guidance: analysis of 14-year experience with 1462 patients at a single center. *Eur J Radiol* (2012) 81(10):2495–9. doi: 10.1016/j.ejrad.2011.10.019
31. Silva MA, Hegab B, Hyde C, Guo B, Buckels JA, Mirza DF. Needle track seeding following biopsy of liver lesions in the diagnosis of hepatocellular cancer: a systematic review and meta-analysis. *Gut* (2008) 57(11):1592–6. doi: 10.1136/gut.2008.149062
32. Di Tommaso L, Spadaccini M, Donadon M, Personeni N, Elamin A, Aghemo A, et al. Role of liver biopsy in hepatocellular carcinoma. *World J Gastroenterol* (2019) 25(40):6041–52. doi: 10.3748/wjg.v25.i40.6041
33. Zhang HC, Zhu T, Hu RF, Wu L. Contrast-enhanced ultrasound imaging features and clinical characteristics of combined hepatocellular cholangiocarcinoma: comparison with hepatocellular carcinoma and cholangiocarcinoma. *Ultrasonography* (2020) 30(4):356–66. doi: 10.14366/usg.19093
34. Lee WS, Lee KW, Heo JS, Kim SJ, Choi SH, Kim YI, et al. Comparison of combined hepatocellular and cholangiocarcinoma with hepatocellular carcinoma and intrahepatic cholangiocarcinoma. *Surg Today* (2006) 36(10):892–7. doi: 10.1007/s00595-006-3276-8
35. Wang Y, Yang Q, Li S, Luo R, Mao S, Shen J. Imaging features of combined hepatocellular and cholangiocarcinoma compared with those of hepatocellular carcinoma and intrahepatic cholangiocellular carcinoma in a Chinese population. *Clin Radiol* (2019) 74(5):407.e1–4e10. doi: 10.1016/j.crad.2019.01.016
36. Sammon J, Fischer S, Menezes R, Hosseini-Nik H, Lewis S, Taouli B, et al. MRI features of combined hepatocellular- cholangiocarcinoma versus mass forming intrahepatic cholangiocarcinoma. *Cancer Imaging* (2018) 18(1):8–8. doi: 10.1186/s40644-018-0142-z
37. Sagrini E, Iavarone M, Stefanini F, Tovoli F, Vavassori S, Maggioni M, et al. Imaging of combined hepatocellular-cholangiocarcinoma in cirrhosis and risk of false diagnosis of hepatocellular carcinoma. *U Eur Gastroenterol J* (2019) 7 (1):69–77. doi: 10.1177/2050640618815378
38. Yeh MM. Pathology of combined hepatocellular-cholangiocarcinoma. *J Gastroenterol Hepatol* (2010) 25(9):1485–92. doi: 10.1111/j.1440-1746.2010.06430.x
39. Coulouarn C, Cavard C, Rubbia-Brandt L, Audebourg A, Dumont F, Jacques S, et al. Combined hepatocellular-cholangiocarcinomas exhibit progenitor features and activation of Wnt and TGFbeta signaling pathways. *Carcinogenesis* (2012) 33(9):1791–6. doi: 10.1093/carcin/bgs208
40. Wang Q, Li J, Lei Z, Wu D, Si A, Wang K, et al. Prognosis of Intrahepatic Cholangiocarcinomas with HBV Infection is Better than Those with Hepatolithiasis After R0 Liver Resection: A Propensity Score Matching Analysis. *Ann Surg Oncol* (2017) 24(6):1579–87. doi: 10.1245/s10434-016-5751-9

3

Comparative Effectiveness of Adjuvant Treatment for Resected Hepatocellular Carcinoma

Ying Liu[1†], Yuzhu Wang[1†], Xinkun Guo[2], Yifeng He[3,4], Jian Zhou[3,4], Qianzhou Lv[1], Xiaowu Huang[3,4] and Xiaoyu Li[1*]*

[1] Department of Pharmacy, Zhongshan Hospital, Fudan University, Shanghai, China, [2] Deparment of Hepatic Oncology, Zhongshan Hospital, Fudan University, Xiamen, China, [3] Department of Liver Surgery and Transplantation, Liver Cancer Institute, Zhongshan Hospital, Fudan University, Shanghai, China, [4] Key Laboratory of Carcinogenesis and Cancer Invasion, Ministry of Education, Shanghai, China

***Correspondence:**
Xiaoyu Li
li.xiaoyu@zs-hospital.sh.cn
Xiaowu Huang
huang.xiaowu@zs-hospital.sh.cn

†These authors have contributed equally to this work

Background: It is controversial whether adjuvant treatment could be recommended for hepatocellular carcinoma (HCC) after curative hepatectomy. Thus, we performed a network meta-analysis (NMA) to assess adjuvant treatment's benefit and determine the optimal adjuvant regimen.

Methods: We systematically searched PubMed, Embase, and Cochrane Library for randomized controlled trials comparing adjuvant therapy *versus* no active treatment after curative hepatectomy among patients with HCC. Pooled data on recurrence and overall survival (OS) were analyzed within pairwise meta-analysis and NMA.

Results: Twenty-three eligible trials (3,940 patients) reporting eight treatments were included. The direct meta-analysis showed that adjuvant therapy prevented the recurrence (OR = 0.65; 95% CI: 0.55, 0.77; P = 0.177; I^2 = 21.7%) and contributed to OS (HR = 0.63; 95% CI: 0.54, 0.73; P = 0.087; I^2 = 31.1%) in comparison to the observation. In the NMA, internal radiotherapy (IRT; OR = 0.55; 95% CI: 0.39, 0.77; SUCRA = 87.7%) followed by hepatic artery infusion chemotherapy (HAIC; OR = 0.6; 95% CI: 0.36, 0.97; SUCRA = 77.8%), and HAIC (HR = 0.44; 95% CI: 0.21, 0.87; SUCRA = 82.6%) followed by IRT (HR 0.54; 95% CI:0.36, 0.81; SUCRA = 69.7%) were ranked superior to other treatments in terms of preventing recurrence and providing survival benefit, respectively.

Conclusions: The addition of adjuvant therapy lowers the risk of recurrence and provide survival benefit after surgical resection for HCC. HAIC and IRT are likely to be the two most effective adjuvant regimens.

Systematic Review Registration: https://inplasy.com/inplasy-2020-11-0039/.

Keywords: hepatocellular carcinoma, adjuvant treatment, network meta-analysis, hepatic artery infusion chemotherapy, internal radiotherapy

INTRODUCTION

Liver cancer ranks as the sixth most frequently diagnosed cancer and the fourth leading cause of cancer death worldwide in 2018, with an estimated 841,000 new cases and 782,000 deaths annually (1). Hepatocellular carcinoma (HCC) is the most common primary liver cancer, which comprises 90% of cases (2). Although multiple treatments are available for patients with HCC, tumor resection performed through partial resection or liver transplantation (LT), together with ablative therapies, is proven to be the potentially curative treatment (3). Given the shortage of available organ donors, huge costs, and the restrictive criteria to select the optimal recipient, LT is not the first choice for most patients (4). And the outcomes of ablative therapies are optimized in patients with tumors smaller than 2 cm. Therefore, partial surgical resection remains the initial treatment used for early-stage HCC (5).

Unfortunately, the 5-year recurrence rate for patients who ideally undergo surgical resection is relatively common, as high as 70% (6, 7). It has been widely accepted that recurrence occurs not because of inadequate resection, but due to the undetectable pre-existing microscopic tumor or disseminated malignant cells during operative manipulation. Recurrence of HCC generally occurs in two phases, namely, early intrahepatic metastases and late *de novo* formation of tumors (8, 9). Considering the high recurrence rate, a series of adjuvant therapies are essential to improve the prognosis of curative treatment for HCC (10, 11). Nevertheless, due to the lack of high-quality evidence, the European Association for the Study of the Liver (EASL) (12), the American Association for the Study of Liver Diseases (AASLD) (13), and the Asian Pacific Association for the Study of the Liver (APASL) (14) hold distinct recommendations on whether to take adjuvant therapies to prevent HCC recurrence. Asian guidelines generally take a positive view towards adjuvant therapies for patients with intermediate risk [single nodule >5 cm without microvascular invasion (MVI)] or high risk (single nodule >5 cm with MVI, or multiple nodules) of recurrence, while the EASL or AASLD guidelines currently do not recommend.

At present, there is no global consensus on whether the adjuvant therapies to be recommended for HCC after hepatectomy. And in the absence of direct head-to-head comparisons, the evidence proving the superiority of one adjuvant therapy over another is limited. Most published meta-analyses concerning adjuvant therapies after hepatectomy were carried out *via* traditional meta-analysis from randomized controlled trials (RCTs) and non-randomized controlled trials (NRCTs). Moreover, these studies have analyzed time-to-event outcomes using odds ratios (ORs) or relative risks (RRs) instead of hazard ratios (HRs) (15–17). A network meta-analysis (NMA) published in 2015 evaluated the efficacy of four adjuvant therapies and concluded that immunotherapy together with interferon was the most effective way to prevent recurrence, and interferon was the most efficacious therapy to prolong survival time (18). It failed to include adequate and updated trials published in the last few years, while emerging evidence of novel adjuvant therapies from RCTs is currently available. Therefore, we conducted an NMA of RCTs to compare the relative efficacy and the ranking probabilities of eight adjuvant therapies in previously curative resected patients with HCC.

MATERIALS AND METHODS

Search Strategy and Selection Criteria

This NMA was performed in accordance with the Preferred Reporting Items for Systematic Reviews and Meta-analysis (PRISMA) extension statement for Network Meta-analysis. The method and analysis were prespecified in advance and registered on the INPLASY website (2020110039). We systematically searched (up to July 1, 2020) PubMed, Embase, and Cochrane Library. We also manually searched the relevant systematic reviews for potentially eligible articles. The searches will be refined using the Boolean term "AND" between three parts: "liver cancer," "hepatocellular carcinoma," "HCC," "hepatic carcinoma," "hepatoma"; "adjuvant," "post-operative," "postoperative"; "randomized controlled trial." Studies were eligible for inclusion if they met the following criteria: (1) RCTs; (2) patients with HCC who had undergone a curative hepatectomy; and (3) reported at least one clinical outcome of interest including recurrence or overall survival (OS). The exclusion criteria were as follows: (1) duplications; (2) non-human studies; (3) NRCTs; (4) incomplete literature data; (5) review, meta-analysis, comment, and case; (6) trials not related to HCC; (7) patients with HCC who had undergone curative treatment with LT or ablative therapies; (8) adjuvant treatment with nucleos(t)ide analogues; or (9) studies focusing on irrelevant purpose.

Two authors (XG and YH) independently reviewed the titles and abstracts of selected studies, and any discrepancies were resolved through consensus with a third reviewer (YL). Full-text articles of potentially eligible studies were retrieved for further evaluation.

Data Extraction and Quality Assessment

Two reviewers (YL and YW) independently extracted the data from the eligible studies. The following data were collected: (1) characteristics of studies and patients (authors, publication year, details of treatment, sample size, sex, age, number of tumors, tumor size, Child-Pugh score, liver cirrhosis, virology, vascular invasion and Edmondson's grading); (2) statistics for meta-analysis [the number of recurrence in each treatment arm, the HR with 95% confidence interval (CI) for OS]. Seven items specifically developed from the Cochrane risk of bias tools were used by two reviewers (YL and YW) to assess the quality of the eligible studies. Any discrepancies in data extraction and quality assessment were resolved by discussion in the whole study groups.

Data Synthesis and Analysis

We synthesized all direct and indirect evidence to compare different treatments in terms of efficacy, reported as OR for recurrence and HR for OS, along with corresponding 95% CI.

A combined OR<1 or HR<1 implied preferable efficacy in the intervention group. And it was considered statistically significant if 95% CI for the combined OR or HR did not overlap 1.

First, a traditional pairwise meta-analysis that directly compared interventions with observation were performed using STATA (version 15.0). The statistical heterogeneity in each pairwise comparison was evaluated using I^2 statistic with p values. A random-effect model was used. Secondly, we used STATA (version 15.0) to generate the network meta diagram, in which edges and nodes revealed the head-to-head comparisons among interventions. The widths of edges were proportional to the number of studies comparing the two treatments. The sizes of the nodes were also proportional to the number of arms in the included studies that corresponded to the treatment. Thirdly, the NMA was conducted in the Bayesian framework with the statistical software R (version 3.6.2) and the R package "gemtc." Both random-effect model and fixed-effect model were performed, and the best was selected based on deviance information criteria (DIC). To assess recurrence and OS, 100,000 iterations per chain (four chains, 400,000 in total) were generated with 50,000 burn-ins and a thinning interval of 1. The convergence of iterations was assessed by the Brooks-Gelman-Rubin statistic and trace plots. Global and local inconsistencies in the network were not assessed due to lacking closed loops. Within the Bayesian approach, the probability of each intervention being the most effective treatment was calculated by surface under the cumulative ranking curve (SUCRA). For each outcome, the greater the SUCRA value, the better the rank of a certain therapy among the various treatment. In addition, publication bias was evaluated *via* observing the symmetry characteristics of funnel plots and the p-value of Egger test using the package "netmeta" in software R (version 3.6.2). The symmetrical and concentrated distribution of the dots indicates no obvious deviation.

RESULTS

Characteristics of Included Studies and Bias Assessment

After the initial search, 4,417 relevant records were identified, of which 102 potentially eligible articles were evaluated in full text (**Figure 1**). The baseline characteristics of included studies are reported in **Table 1**. Finally, 23 RCTs met the inclusion criteria with a total of 3,940 patients, among whom 2,171 patients were enrolled to receive eight different adjuvant treatments after curative surgery and 1,769 patients were treated with surgery alone. Among the included studies, patients treated with adoptive immunotherapy (AIT) in three trials, external radiotherapy (ERT) in one trial, hepatic artery infusion chemotherapy (HAIC) in two trials, Huaier in one trial, interferon (IFN) in five trials, internal radiotherapy (IRT) in four trials, oral chemotherapy (OCT) in three trials, and transarterial chemoembolization (TACE) in four trials. The risk-of-bias assessment was performed and outlined in **Figure 2** and **Supplementary Figure 1**. All the studies included were randomized, and the trial quality was generally high, with most studies evaluated as having a low risk of bias overall. However, blinding of participants and personnel were considered impractical because of the differences between the treatment methods or almost common adverse effect. And unclear assessments were common because several articles only stated randomization and allocation concealment without detailed methods. And it is not clear whether the participants who assessed the outcomes were blind.

Pairwise Meta-Analysis

The detailed forest plot of the results is presented in **Supplementary Figure 2** for recurrence and **Supplementary Figure 3** for OS. Original ORs with 95% CIs were reported in 22 studies (3,836 patients) for recurrence and HRs with 95% CIs in 21 studies (3,663 patients) were informed for OS. An overall OR of 0.65 (95% CI, 0.55, 0.77; P = 0.177; I^2 = 21.7%) and HR of 0.63 (95% CI, 0.54, 0.73; P = 0.087; I^2 = 31.1%) revealed the efficacy of adjuvant group over observation group. When compared to observation, HAIC [OR 0.50 (0.28, 0.89)], Huaier [OR 0.58 (0.44, 0.76)], and IRT [OR 0.41 (0.27, 0.64)] showed significantly lower risk of recurrence, and trended toward improvements were presented in AIT [OR 0.69 (0.45, 1.07)], ERT [OR 0.68 (0.33, 1.41)], IFN [OR 0.89 (0.66, 1.19)], OCT [OR 0.60 (0.27, 1.34)], and TACE [OR 0.71 (0.45, 1.14)]. Pooled HRs strongly favored the adjuvant treatment of AIT [HR 0.64 (0.43, 0.94)], HAIC [HR 0.45 (0.25, 0.79)], Huaier [HR 0.55 (0.33, 0.92)], IFN [HR 0.61 (0.39, 0.94)], IRT [HR 0.54 (0.38, 0.79)], and TACE [HR 0.63 (0.51, 0.78)] in significantly improving OS.

Network Meta-Analysis

Figure 3 presents the network of eligible comparisons for OS and the network diagram for recurrence is shown in **Supplementary Figure 4**. Most of the included studies have OS and recurrence as the endpoints, except Hui 2009 and Mazzaferro 2006 have the endpoint of recurrence, while Peng 2009 used OS as the endpoint. The consistency and inconsistency models were compared using the deviance information criterion, which indicated that the data was basically consistent.

As shown in **Figures 4** and **5**, indirect comparison by network meta-analysis suggested a lower risk of recurrence with the help of adjuvant therapy when compared to surgery alone group (observation group). Briefly, adjuvant treatment of IRT was ranked best in preventing recurrence [OR 0.55 (0.39, 0.77) and SUCRA = 87.7%], followed by HAIC [OR 0.6 (0.36, 0.97); SUCRA = 77.8%], Huaier [OR 0.66 (0.45, 0.97); SUCRA = 69%], ERT [OR 0.77 (0.41, 1.42); SUCRA = 48.9%], AIT [OR 0.79 (0.58, 1.07); SUCRA = 46.7%], OCT [OR 0.8 (0.54, 1.12); SUCRA = 44.7%], TACE [OR 0.82 (0.61, 1.07); SUCRA = 41.4%], and IFN [OR 0.9 (0.69, 1.14); SUCRA = 25.8%].

For improving OS, HAIC was superior to all other adjuvant treatment as compared to observation group with HR 0.44 (0.21, 0.87) and SUCRA = 82.6%, followed by IRT [HR 0.54 (0.36, 0.81); SUCRA = 69.7%], Huaier [HR 0.55 (0.26, 1.17); SUCRA = 64.6%], IFN [HR 0.62 (0.41, 0.9); SUCRA = 56%], TACE [HR 0.62 (0.44, 0.88); SUCRA = 54.5%], AIT (HR 0.64 (0.37, 1.1); SUCRA = 52.6%), ERT [HR 0.75 (0.29, 1.96); SUCRA = 40.2%], and OCT [HR 0.92 (0.53, 1.47); SUCRA = 20.1%].

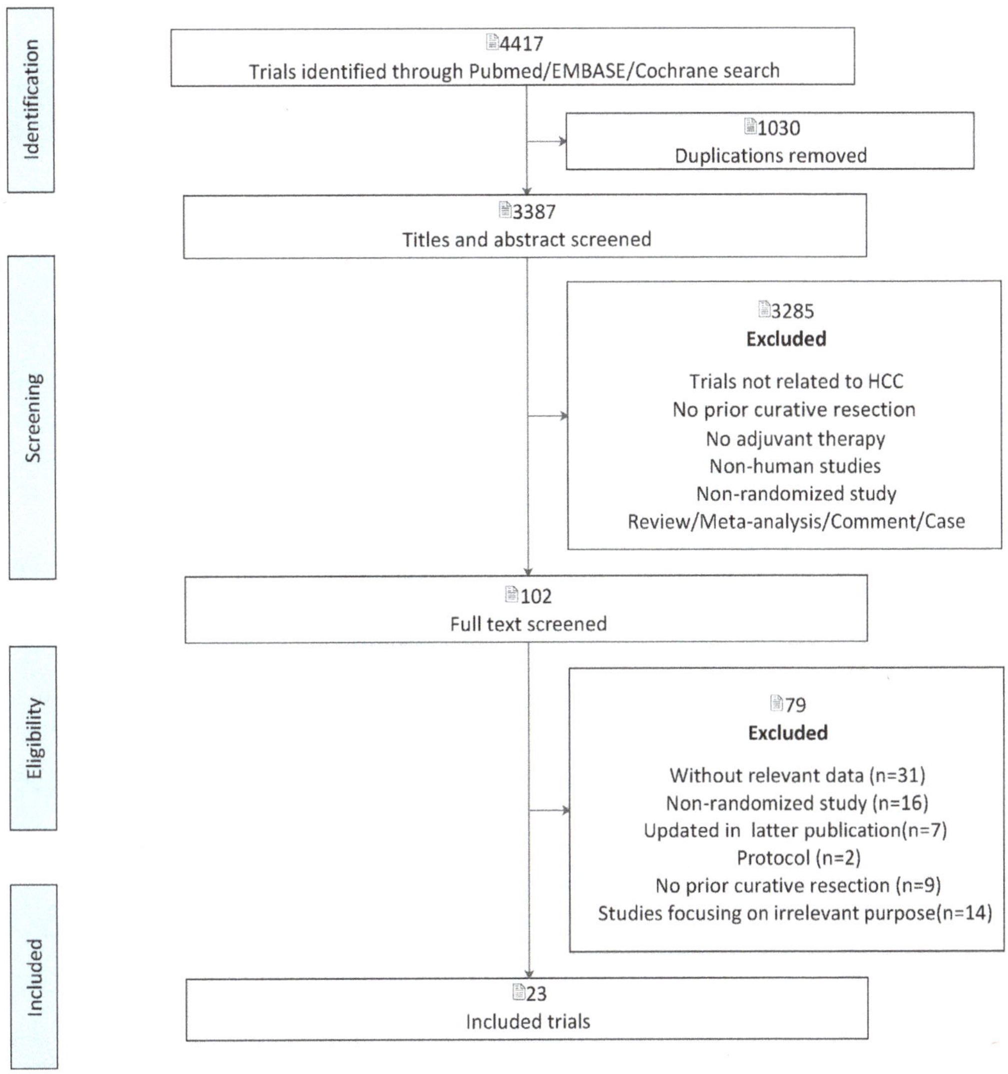

FIGURE 1 | PRISMA (Preferred Reporting Items for Systematic Reviews and Meta-Analyses) flow diagram.

Assessment of Publication Bias

As shown in **Supplementary Figure 5**, there was no significant asymmetry among the included studies in terms of recurrence and OS. The p-value of Egger's test for recurrence was 0.846 and for OS was 0.995. Hence, it can be concluded that there is less likelihood of publication bias.

DISCUSSION

Given that the benefits of adjuvant therapies compared to surgery alone after curative resection for HCC remains to be clearly defined, we combined direct and indirect evidence from 23 RCT comparing eight different adjuvant treatments with a total of 3,940 participants. The results suggested that adjuvant treatments provide survival benefits over surgery alone. HAIC and IRT probably provide the fewest recurrence and the best survival among all the post-operative therapeutic interventions evaluated, as evidenced by their SUCRA values.

Unlike systemic chemotherapy, HAIC can directly deliver chemotherapeutic drugs to the tumor supplying artery with increased local concentration, and thus achieve better inhibition of tumor recurrence and milder adverse effects, even for patients with marginal liver function (42). HAIC has attracted wide attention in Asia, especially in Japan, where HAIC is recommended as the standard therapy in the treatment of TACE-refractory patients and patients with portal branch tumor thrombus (PVTT) (43). Most published reports have observed that HAIC may reduce the risk of recurrence after hepatectomy for HCC patients with macroscopic PVTT. Patients with high-grade vascular invasion are good candidates for the adjuvant treatment of HAIC (44–46). A meta-analysis demonstrated that adjuvant

TABLE 1 | The baseline characteristics of included studies.

Study	Year	Treatment	Sample size (n)	Sex, M/F (n)	Age (year)	Number of tumors, 1/≥2 (n)	Tumor size (cm)	Liver cirrhosis (n)	Virology, HBV/HCV (n)	Child-Pugh, A/B (n)	Vascular invasion (n)	Edmondson's grading, I–II/III–IV (n)
Hui (19)	2009	AIT	84	63/21	NA	NA	NA	68	65/NA	68/16	36	NA
		Observation	43	34/9	NA	NA	NA	33	31/NA	34/9	23	NA
Takayama (20)	2000	AIT	76	NA	NA	51/25	NA	NA	15/50	54/22	NA	62/14
		Observation	74	NA	NA	53/21	NA	NA	14/49	50/24	NA	61/13
Xu (21)	2016	AIT	100	92/8	43 (38–56)	95/5	NA	55	84/NA	NA	2*	NA
		Observation	100	89/11	52 (43–60)	94/6	NA	58	87/NA	NA	1*	NA
Yu (22)	2014	ERT	58	51/7	53.1 ± 10.5	52/6	4.7 ± 2.6	51	53/1	NA	7	NA
		Observation	61	48/13	55.5 ± 10.7	53/8	5.6 ± 3.7	54	53/5	NA	8	NA
Huang (23)	2015	HAIC	42	31/11	59.1 ± 6.2	24/18	6.2 ± 1.5	NA	NA	24/18	NA	NA
		Observation	43	30/13	58.4 ± 5.7	23/20	5.7 ± 1.3	NA	NA	27/16	NA	NA
Li SH (24)	2020	HAIC	58	52/6	54 (25-69)	36/22	NA	32	54/2	NA	NA	23/35
		Observation	58	49/9	55.6 ± 1.6	42/16	NA	35	51/1	NA	NA	29/29
Chen (25)	2018	Huaier	686	565/ 121	NA	595/91	NA	473	544/8	643/43	NA	488/198
		Observation	316	255/61	NA	274/42	NA	198	234/5	291/25	NA	223/93
Chen (26)	2012	IFN	133	108/25	50 (48–54)	103/30	3.5 (3.04.0)	73	106/27	NA	41*	NA
		Observation	135	112/23	49 (46–51)	115/20	3.0 (2.5–3.5)	74	108/26	NA	33*	NA
Lo (27)	2007	IFN	40	31/9	49 (26–75)	33/7	5.5 (1.8–22)	19	38/1	NA	NA	NA
		Observation	40	34/6	54 (24–74)	29/11	5.7 (1.2–18)	19	39/2	NA	NA	NA
Mazzaferro (28)	2006	IFN	76	61/15	65 (41–74)	NA	NA	NA	NA	70/6	NA	NA
		Observation	74	51/23	67 (36–73)	NA	NA	NA	NA	70/4	NA	NA
Nishiguchi (29	2005	IFN	15	15/0	61.9 ± 5.8	NA	2.5 (1.9–3.5)	NA	NA	11/4	NA	10/5
		Observation	15	15/0	60.0 ± 4.8	NA	2.6 (2.4–3.5)	NA	NA	12/3	NA	8/7
Sun (30)	2006	IFN	118	106/12	52.2	102/16	4.3 ± 2.7	98	NA	NA	90*	86/32
		Observation	118	102/16	50.4	103/15	4.9 ± 3.0	104	NA	NA	89*	77/41
Chen (31)	2013	IRT	34	25/9	50.8 ± 6.8	30/4	6.24 ± 2.55	18	26/6	34/0	17*	22/12
		Observation	34	24/10	48.9 ± 7.3	31/3	5.65 ± 2.52	20	31/5	34/0	14*	23/11
Chung (32)	2013	IRT	51	41/10	65 (22–82)	NA	4.2 (0.4–30)	NA	29/NA	NA	NA	34/16
		Observation	52	45/7	63 (42–84)	NA	3.8 (1.4–18)	NA	32/NA	NA	NA	32/20
Lau (33)	1999	IRT	21	17/4	51 (23–71)	14/7	4.4 (1.4–11)	NA	19/NA	NA	1	17/2
		Observation	22	18/4	54 (24–75)	18/4	3.8 (1.5–10)	NA	19/NA	NA	1	18/2
Li J (34)	2020	IRT	78	58/20	53 (47–59)	73/5	4.9 (3.2–6.4)	42	66/0	NA	31	29/49
		Observation	78	61/17	53 (47–58)	74/4	5.3 (3.2–7.3)	45	60/3	NA	32	27/51
Hasegawa (35)	2006	OCT	79	60/19	65 (29–75)	53/26	3.3 (1.2–12)	42	14/58	68/11	18	NA
		Observation	80	65/15	64 (35–78)	58/22	3.4 (7–13)	38	15/56	70/10	17	NA
Xia (36)	2010	OCT	30	25/5	NA	25/5	7.27 ± 4.37	19	26/NA	NA	18	NA
		Observation	30	21/9	NA	26/4	6.34 ± 3.16	21	24/NA	NA	20	NA
Yamamoto (37)	1996	OCT	28	NA	NA	NA	NA	NA	NA	NA	NA	NA
		Observation	27	NA	NA	NA	NA	NA	NA	NA	NA	NA
Peng (38)	2009	TACE	51	46/5	46.2 ± 13.8	NA	9.04 ± 3.02	42	31/5	44/7	NA	NA
		Observation	53	50/3	50.2 ± 7.5	NA	8.39 ± 2.29	37	40/3	46/7	NA	NA
Wang (39)	2018	TACE	140	121/19	54.2 ± 9.7	102/38	NA	140	NA	NA	78*	81/59
		Observation	140	109/31	52.6 ± 10.3	109/31	NA	140	NA	NA	87*	80/60

(Continued)

TABLE 1 | Continued

Study	Year	Treatment	Sample size (n)	Sex, M/F (n)	Age (year)	Number of tumors, 1/≥2 (n)	Tumor size (cm)	Liver cirrhosis (n)	Virology, HBV/HCV (n)	Child-Pugh, A/B (n)	Vascular invasion (n)	Edmondson's grading, I–II/III–IV (n)
Wei (40)	2018	TACE	116	106/10	44 (18-75)	NA	NA	50	94	116/0	NA	NA
		Observation	118	106/12	48.5 (18-74)	NA	NA	42	101	116/2	NA	NA
Zhong (41)	2009	TACE	57	53/4	47.6 ± 10.4	13/44	9.5 ± 3.8	NA	53/NA	56/1	NA	35/22
		Observation	58	49/9	48.2 ± 11.2	16/42	9.7 ± 3.6	NA	52/NA	58/0	NA	34/24

*Microvascular invasion.
NA, Not Available.

HAIC improved PFS and OS after hepatectomy, especially in tumors larger than 7 cm (47). However, patients prefer TACE and oral anticancer drugs rather than HAIC due to the complexity of managing the implanted catheter system, so there is currently insufficient data of RCTs (48). And the optimal regimen for HAIC remains a controversial issue. Various regimens have been reported, including single or combined administration of cisplatin, 5-fluorouracil, oxaliplatin, doxorubicin, epirubicin, and mitomycin C (42).

During the last decade, HCC is generally considered to be a radiosensitive tumor (49). However, most international guidelines still do not recommend ERT to treat HCC with few exceptions due to the severe hepatotoxicity of the normal tissues after absorbing radiation more than 35 Gy. Since the early 1990s, radiotherapy (RT) has experienced tremendous technological advancements to develop IRT, which can precisely deliver very high tumoricidal dose to the tumor while preserving normal liver parenchyma (50). According to the pharmacokinetics of radionuclides, IRT can be properly indicated in HCC accompanied by PVTT with the OS reaching more than 20 months (51). A variety of radioisotopes, such as 131I-lipiodol for radioembolization (32, 33), 131I-metuximab for radioimmunotherapy (34), and iodine-125 for brachytherapy (31), have also been verified to be used as adjuvant therapies after curative hepatectomy. Side effects reported with IRT were generally moderate and manageable. Given the variability in radiosensitivity of the patient and the decisive role of absorption dose in the biological effects of IRT, the dosimetry of radionuclide therapy has gradually attracted much attention (52).

The strength of our research is that we used NMA to compare eight different adjuvant treatments for HCC simultaneously, while most of the previous analyses have been carried out *via* traditional meta-analysis from both RCTs and NRCTs. We excluded studies concerning nucleos(t)ide analogues, because the necessity of its administration for many years or for life in patients with HBV-related HCC has been discussed in many research (53, 54). In this NMA, the adjuvant treatments included are given for a finite duration. A previously published NMA of 14 trials by Zhu et al. in 2015 provided evidence for the superior survival benefit with the treatment of IFN. However, without adequate and updated trials, only AIT, IFN, IRT, and OCT have been taken into consideration for comparing the efficacy in the review (18). Consistent with earlier meta-analysis, results of our analysis suggested that adjuvant therapies contributed to OS, except for ERT and OCT. Contrast to some previous studies, administered with TACE and IFN showed no benefit of preventing recurrence. This result could be partly illustrated with the subgroup analysis by Huang et al. (55) and Xu et al. (56), which suggested that adjuvant IFN significantly reduces the recurrence of HCV-related HCC rather than HBV-related HCC. And some meta-analysis reported the clinical benefit of adjuvant TACE for HCC with risk factors (multiple nodules, tumors ≥5 cm or vascular invasion) (15, 57, 58).

Several limitations of this study deserve further discussion. First, though only RCTs were included, double-blind was considered impractical due to the difference between the adjuvant treatment methods or almost common adverse effect,

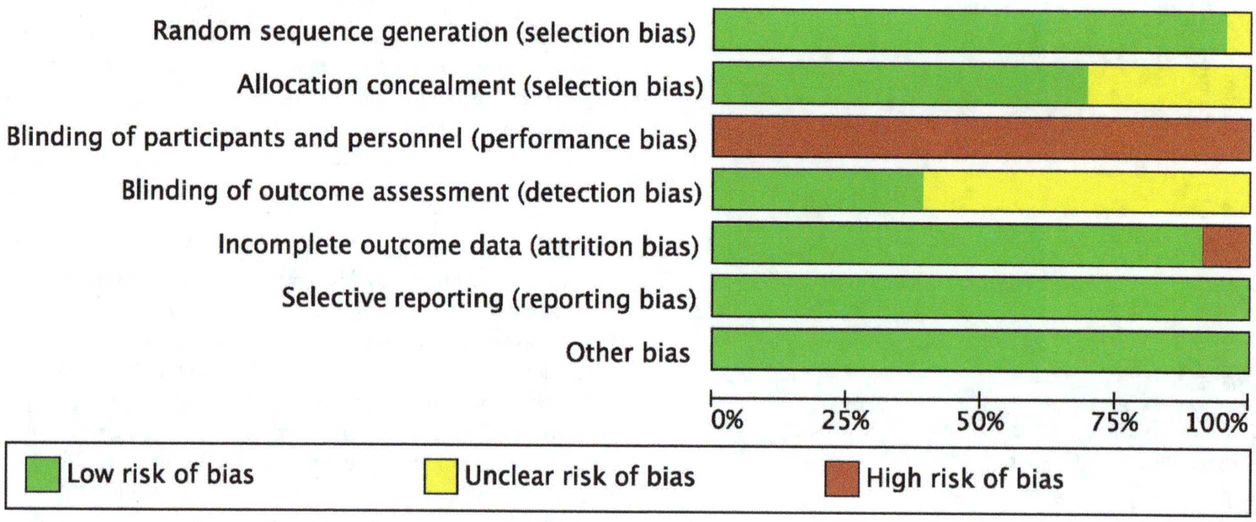

FIGURE 2 | Quality assessment of included studies using Cochrane Collaboration's Risk of Bias.

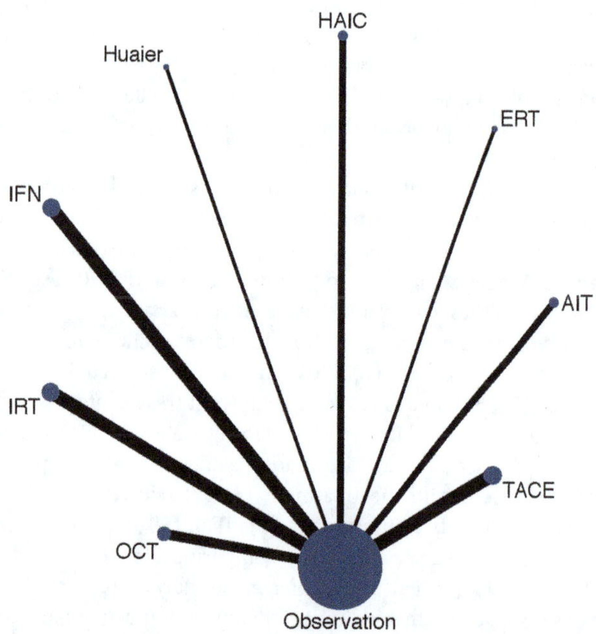

FIGURE 3 | Network diagram of eligible comparisons for OS. Each circular node represents a variety of interventions. The circle size is proportional to the number of randomly assigned participants. The width of lines between the nodes is proportional to the number of trials performing head-to-head comparisons. AIT, adoptive immunotherapy; ERT, external radiotherapy; HAIC, hepatic artery infusion chemotherapy; IFN, interferon; IRT, internal radiotherapy; OCT, oral chemotherapy; TACE, transarterial chemoembolization.

and some eligible studies showed unclear risk of bias, especially in terms of allocation concealment and blinding of outcome assessment. Second, it is impossible to precisely integrate or incorporate data from each study for all endpoints into the analysis in the absence of original data. As a well-recognized outcome in adjuvant trials, recurrence-free survival (RFS) takes account of whether and when the event occurred. However, some trials defined RFS as the time from randomization to the first recurrence or death due to any cause, while other trials defined RFS without the endpoint of death. Hence, recurrence instead of RFS was considered as the outcome. Since many studies did not provide HRs for OS, they were estimated from the reported log-rank p values and the events in each arm according to the procedure in the study by Tierney et al. (59). Third, unavoidable confounding factors remain in this NMA, manifesting in the difference of follow-up time, post-operative staging, HBV/HCV infection, and so on. However, it was not available to perform subgroup NMA for these confounding factors with limited reporting outcomes. A further stratified analysis will help us clarify the indications of adjuvant treatments. Fourth, in the absence of sufficient direct head-to-head comparisons, most treatments were compared indirectly, and the most direct evidence came from a single trial. In addition, some new methods for adjuvant therapy without comparing in any RCTs were not included, such as multitarget tyrosine kinase inhibitors (TKIs), immune checkpoint inhibitors (ICIs), or the combination of both.

Although TKIs and ICIs are generally used in patients with advanced-stage HCC, their use after curative resection is still controversial. The phase III STORM trial was designed to compare the efficacy and safety of sorafenib as adjuvant therapy in patients who have undergone curative surgery or local ablation. Sorafenib not only failed to show superiority over placebo in terms of RFS (HR=0.940; 95% CI: 0.780, 1.134; p=0.26), but it was also accompanied by an increased grade 3 or 4 adverse events (60). It is unclear that the dose of sorafenib lower than the intended 800 mg or eligible patients with a lower risk of recurrence was a contributing factor to the negative findings reported. Except for the STORM trial, there are

	Recurrence								
OS	**AIT**	0.98 (0.48, 1.93)	0.76 (0.42, 1.36)	0.85 (0.52, 1.38)	1.15 (0.76, 1.69)	0.71 (0.44, 1.1)	1.27 (0.93, 1.73)	1.02 (0.62, 1.6)	1.04 (0.68, 1.56)
	0.85 (0.28, 2.55)	**ERT**	0.78 (0.35, 1.73)	0.87 (0.42, 1.81)	1.18 (0.6, 2.29)	0.72 (0.36, 1.47)	1.3 (0.71, 2.46)	1.04 (0.5, 2.13)	1.06 (0.54, 2.1)
	1.46 (0.61, 3.62)	1.72 (0.53, 5.71)	**HAIC**	1.12 (0.6, 2.09)	1.52 (0.87, 2.65)	0.93 (0.51, 1.69)	1.68 (1.03, 2.79)	1.34 (0.72, 2.46)	1.37 (0.77, 2.43)
	1.15 (0.46, 2.91)	1.35 (0.41, 4.55)	0.79 (0.28, 2.14)	**Huaier**	1.36 (0.85, 2.1)	0.83 (0.49, 1.36)	1.51 (1.03, 2.2)	1.2 (0.69, 1.96)	1.23 (0.76, 1.95)
	1.03 (0.53, 2.06)	1.22 (0.44, 3.45)	0.71 (0.32, 1.57)	0.9 (0.39, 2.12)	**IFN**	0.61 (0.41, 0.93)	1.11 (0.87, 1.44)	0.88 (0.57, 1.34)	0.9 (0.63, 1.32)
	1.18 (0.6, 2.35)	1.39 (0.49, 3.93)	0.81 (0.36, 1.79)	1.02 (0.44, 2.4)	1.14 (0.64, 1.98)	**IRT**	1.81 (1.3, 2.56)	1.44 (0.87, 2.34)	1.47 (0.96, 2.3)
	0.64 (0.37, 1.1)	0.75 (0.29, 1.96)	0.44 (0.21, 0.87)	0.55 (0.26, 1.17)	0.62 (0.41, 0.9)	0.54 (0.36, 0.81)	**Observation**	0.8 (0.54, 1.12)	0.82 (0.61, 1.07)
	0.7 (0.34, 1.53)	0.82 (0.29, 2.5)	0.48 (0.21, 1.15)	0.6 (0.26, 1.55)	0.67 (0.37, 1.31)	0.59 (0.32, 1.18)	1.09 (0.68, 1.89)	**OCT**	1.02 (0.66, 1.64)
	1.02 (0.54, 1.96)	1.2 (0.43, 3.34)	0.7 (0.32, 1.51)	0.89 (0.39, 2.02)	0.99 (0.58, 1.64)	0.87 (0.51, 1.48)	1.6 (1.14, 2.27)	1.47 (0.76, 2.59)	**TACE**

FIGURE 4 | Pooled estimates of the network meta-analysis. Data in each cell are hazard or odds ratios (95% confidence intervals) for the comparison between the column defining intervention and the row defining intervention. For the lower triangle (overall survival), hazard ratios less than 1 favor the treatment in the corresponding column. For the upper triangle (recurrence), odds ratios less than 1 favor the treatment in the corresponding row. AIT, adoptive immunotherapy; ERT, external radiotherapy; HAIC, hepatic artery infusion chemotherapy; IFN, interferon; IRT, internal radiotherapy; OCT, oral chemotherapy; TACE, transarterial chemoembolization.

A

Treatment	SUCRA(%)
IRT	87.7
HAIC	77.8
Huaier	69.0
ERT	48.9
AIT	46.7
OCT	44.7
TACE	41.4
IFN	25.8
Observation	8.1

Recurrence

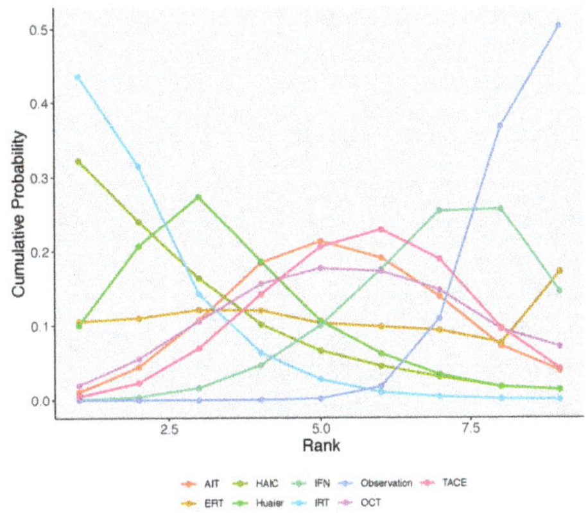

B

Treatment	SUCRA(%)
HAIC	82.6
IRT	69.7
Huaier	64.6
IFN	56.0
TACE	54.5
AIT	52.6
ERT	40.2
OCT	20.1
Observation	9.6

OS

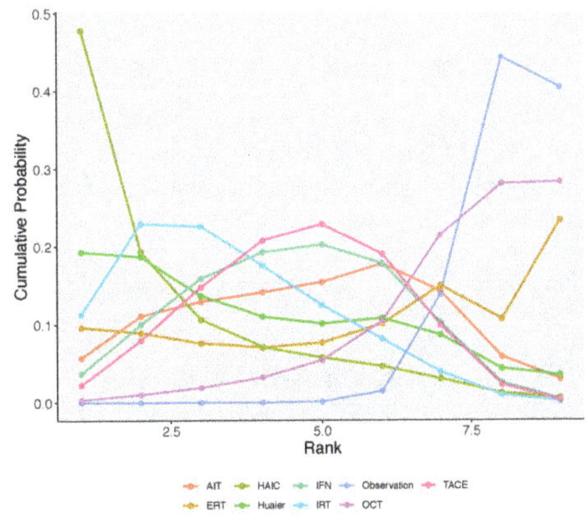

FIGURE 5 | Surface under the cumulative ranking curve (SUCRA) values for recurrence **(A)** and OS **(B)**. AIT, adoptive immunotherapy; ERT, external radiotherapy; HAIC, hepatic artery infusion chemotherapy; IFN, interferon; IRT, internal radiotherapy; OCT, oral chemotherapy; TACE, transarterial chemoembolization.

currently no published RCTs evaluating the efficacy of TKIs and ICIs as adjuvant therapy. NCT04227808 is an ongoing trial to evaluate the use of adjuvant lenvatinib in HCC. In CheckMate 9DX and KEYNOTE-937, nivolumab and pembrolizumab are being investigated in the adjuvant setting for patients with HCC, respectively. Numerous combination regimens for advanced HCC comprise PD-1/PD-L1 blockade plus antiangiogenic agents have demonstrated improved outcome data. In an NMA of 14 trials, the combination of atezolizumab and bevacizumab was found to be the most preferred therapy for patients with HCC compared with sorafenib (HR=0.58; 95% CI: 0.42–0.80), lenvatinib (HR=0.63; 95% CI: 0.44–0.89), and nivolumab (HR=0.68; 95% CI: 0.48–0.98) (61). Looking forward to the findings of the ongoing EMERALD-2 and IMbrave050 trials, which evaluated the combined efficacy of anti-PD-L1 antibody and VEGF antibody in adjuvant therapy.

CONCLUSION

Among people with previously resected HCC, HAIC and IRT are likely to be the most two effective adjuvant treatments to prevent recurrence and improve OS. However, these adjuvant regimens have not yet undergone a direct head-to-head comparison. The final decision on adjuvant therapy requires a multidisciplinary consultation, and the potential risks and benefits should be considered to prolonging the survival of HCC. Further clinical researches are warranted to confirm or condemn our findings and to predict patients with a higher likelihood of response to adjuvant therapy.

AUTHOR CONTRIBUTIONS

XL and XH designed the conception and wrote the protocol. XG and YH retrieved and reviewed the literature. YL and YW extracted the data and assessed its quality. JZ and QL guided the statistical analysis. YL and XG analyzed the data. YL wrote the manuscript. All authors contributed to the article and approved the submitted version.

REFERENCES

1. Bray F, Ferlay J, Soerjomataram I, Siegel RL, Torre LA, Jemal A. Global Cancer Statistics 2018: GLOBOCAN Estimates of Incidence and Mortality Worldwide for 36 Cancers in 185 Countries. *CA Cancer J Clin* (2018) 68:394–424. doi: 10.3322/caac.21492
2. Llovet JM, Kelley RK, Villanueva A, Singal AG, Pikarsky E, Roayaie S, et al. Hepatocellular Carcinoma. *Nat Rev Dis Primers* (2021) 7:6. doi: 10.1038/s41572-020-00240-3
3. Yang JD, Hainaut P, Gores GJ, Amadou A, Plymoth A, Roberts LR. A Global View of Hepatocellular Carcinoma: Trends, Risk, Prevention and Management. *Nat Rev Gastroenterol Hepatol* (2019) 16:589–604. doi: 10.1038/s41575-019-0186-y
4. Vibert E, Schwartz M, Olthoff KM. Advances in Resection and Transplantation for Hepatocellular Carcinoma. *J Hepatol* (2020) 72:262–76. doi: 10.1016/j.jhep.2019.11.017
5. Couri T, Pillai A. Goals and Targets for Personalized Therapy for HCC. *Hepatol Int* (2019) 13:125–37. doi: 10.1007/s12072-018-9919-1
6. Kim J, Kang W, Sinn DH, Gwak GY, Paik YH, Choi MS, et al. Substantial Risk of Recurrence Even After 5 Recurrence-Free Years in Early-Stage Hepatocellular Carcinoma Patients. *Clin Mol Hepatol* (2020) 26:516–28. doi: 10.3350/cmh.2020.0016
7. Tsilimigras DI, Bagante F, Moris D, Hyer JM, Sahara K, Paredes AZ, et al. Recurrence Patterns and Outcomes After Resection of Hepatocellular Carcinoma Within and Beyond the Barcelona Clinic Liver Cancer Criteria. *Ann Surg Oncol* (2020) 27:2321–31. doi: 10.1245/s10434-020-08452-3
8. Chawla A, Ferrone C. Hepatocellular Carcinoma Surgical Therapy: Perspectives on the Current Limits to Resection. *Chin Clin Oncol* (2018) 7:48. doi: 10.21037/cco.2018.08.12
9. Erstad DJ, Tanabe KK. Prognostic and Therapeutic Implications of Microvascular Invasion in Hepatocellular Carcinoma. *Ann Surg Oncol* (2019) 26:1474–93. doi: 10.1245/s10434-019-07227-9
10. Zhu XD, Li KS, Sun HC. Adjuvant Therapies After Curative Treatments for Hepatocellular Carcinoma: Current Status and Prospects. *Genes Dis* (2020) 7:359–69. doi: 10.1016/j.gendis.2020.02.002
11. Akateh C, Black SM, Conteh L, Miller ED, Noonan A, Elliott E, et al. Neoadjuvant and Adjuvant Treatment Strategies for Hepatocellular Carcinoma. *World J Gastroenterol* (2019) 25:3704–21. doi: 10.3748/wjg.v25.i28.3704
12. EASL Clinical Practice Guidelines. Management of Hepatocellular Carcinoma. *J Hepatol* (2018) 69:182–236. doi: 10.1016/j.jhep.2018.03.019
13. Marrero JA, Kulik LM, Sirlin CB, Zhu AX, Finn RS, Abecassis MM, et al. Diagnosis, Staging, and Management of Hepatocellular Carcinoma: 2018 Practice Guidance by the American Association for the Study of Liver Diseases. *Hepatology* (2018) 68:723–50. doi: 10.1002/hep.29913
14. Omata M, Cheng AL, Kokudo N, Kudo M, Lee JM, Jia J, et al. Asia-Pacific Clinical Practice Guidelines on the Management of Hepatocellular Carcinoma: A 2017 Update. *Hepatol Int* (2017) 11:317–70. doi: 10.1007/s12072-017-9799-9
15. Chen ZH, Zhang XP, Zhou TF, Wang K, Wang H, Chai ZT, et al. Adjuvant Transarterial Chemoembolization Improves Survival Outcomes in Hepatocellular Carcinoma With Microvascular Invasion: A Systematic Review and Meta-Analysis. *Eur J Surg Oncol* (2019) 45:2188–96. doi: 10.1016/j.ejso.2019.06.031
16. Zhang W, Song TQ, Zhang T, Wu Q, Kong DL, Li Q, et al. Adjuvant Interferon for Early or Late Recurrence of Hepatocellular Carcinoma and Mortality From Hepatocellular Carcinoma Following Curative Treatment: A Meta-Analysis With Comparison of Different Types of Hepatitis. *Mol Clin Oncol* (2014) 2:1125–34. doi: 10.3892/mco.2014.386
17. Jiang S, Liu Y, Wang L, Duan C, Liu M. A Meta-Analysis and Systematic Review: Adjuvant Interferon Therapy for Patients With Viral Hepatitis-Related Hepatocellular Carcinoma. *World J Surg Oncol* (2013) 11:240. doi: 10.1186/1477-7819-11-240
18. Zhu GQ, Shi KQ, Yu HJ, He SY, Braddock M, Zhou MT, et al. Optimal Adjuvant Therapy for Resected Hepatocellular Carcinoma: A Systematic Review With Network Meta-Analysis. *Oncotarget* (2015) 6:18151–61. doi: 10.18632/oncotarget.4098
19. Hui D, Qiang L, Jian W, Ti Z, Da-Lu K. A Randomized, Controlled Trial of Postoperative Adjuvant Cytokine-Induced Killer Cells Immunotherapy After Radical Resection of Hepatocellular Carcinoma. *Dig Liver Dis* (2009) 41:36–41. doi: 10.1016/j.dld.2008.04.007
20. Takayama T, Sekine T, Makuuchi M, Yamasaki S, Kosuge T, Yamamoto J, et al. Adoptive Immunotherapy to Lower Postsurgical Recurrence Rates of Hepatocellular Carcinoma: A Randomised Trial. *Lancet* (2000) 356:802–7. doi: 10.1016/s0140-6736(00)02654-4
21. Xu L, Wang J, Kim Y, Shuang ZY, Zhang YJ, Lao XM, et al. A Randomized Controlled Trial on Patients With or Without Adjuvant Autologous Cytokine-Induced Killer Cells After Curative Resection for Hepatocellular Carcinoma. *Oncoimmunology* (2016) 5:e1083671. doi: 10.1080/2162402x.2015.1083671
22. Yu W, Wang W, Rong W, Wang L, Xu Q, Wu F, et al. Adjuvant Radiotherapy in Centrally Located Hepatocellular Carcinomas After Hepatectomy With Narrow Margin (<1 Cm): A Prospective Randomized Study. *J Am Coll Surg* (2014) 218:381–92. doi: 10.1016/j.jamcollsurg.2013.11.030

23. Huang SX, Wu YL, Tang CW, Feng WM, Xu YQ, Bao Y, et al. Prophylactic Hepatic Artery Infusion Chemotherapy Improved Survival After Curative Resection in Patients With Hepatocellular Carcinoma. *Hepatogastroenterology* (2015) 62:122–5. doi: 10.5754/hge14885
24. Li S, Mei J, Wang Q, Guo Z, Lu L, Ling Y, et al. Postoperative Adjuvant Transarterial Infusion Chemotherapy With FOLFOX Could Improve Outcomes of Hepatocellular Carcinoma Patients With Microvascular Invasion: A Preliminary Report of a Phase III, Randomized Controlled Clinical Trial. *Ann Surg Oncol* (2020) 27:5183–90. doi: 10.1245/s10434-020-08601-8
25. Chen Q, Shu C, Laurence AD, Chen Y, Peng BG, Zhen ZJ, et al. Effect of Huaier Granule on Recurrence After Curative Resection of HCC: A Multicentre, Randomised Clinical Trial. *Gut* (2018) 67:2006–16. doi: 10.1136/gutjnl-2018-315983
26. Chen LT, Chen MF, Li LA, Lee PH, Jeng LB, Lin DY, et al. Long-Term Results of a Randomized, Observation-Controlled, Phase III Trial of Adjuvant Interferon Alfa-2b in Hepatocellular Carcinoma After Curative Resection. *Ann Surg* (2012) 255:8–17. doi: 10.1097/SLA.0b013e3182363ff9
27. Lo CM, Liu CL, Chan SC, Lam CM, Poon RT, Ng IO, et al. A Randomized, Controlled Trial of Postoperative Adjuvant Interferon Therapy After Resection of Hepatocellular Carcinoma. *Ann Surg* (2007) 245:831–42. doi: 10.1097/01.sla.0000245829.00977.45
28. Mazzaferro V, Romito R, Schiavo M, Mariani L, Camerini T, Bhoori S, et al. Prevention of Hepatocellular Carcinoma Recurrence With Alpha-Interferon After Liver Resection in HCV Cirrhosis. *Hepatology* (2006) 44:1543–54. doi: 10.1002/hep.21415
29. Nishiguchi S, Tamori A, Kubo S. Effect of Long-Term Postoperative Interferon Therapy on Intrahepatic Recurrence and Survival Rate After Resection of Hepatitis C Virus-Related Hepatocellular Carcinoma. *Intervirology* (2005) 48:71–5. doi: 10.1159/000082098
30. Sun HC, Tang ZY, Wang L, Qin LX, Ma ZC, Ye QH, et al. Postoperative Interferon Alpha Treatment Postponed Recurrence and Improved Overall Survival in Patients After Curative Resection of HBV-Related Hepatocellular Carcinoma: A Randomized Clinical Trial. *J Cancer Res Clin Oncol* (2006) 132:458–65. doi: 10.1007/s00432-006-0091-y
31. Chen K, Xia Y, Wang H, Xiao F, Xiang G, Shen F. Adjuvant Iodine-125 Brachytherapy for Hepatocellular Carcinoma After Complete Hepatectomy: A Randomized Controlled Trial. *PloS One* (2013) 8:e57397. doi: 10.1371/journal.pone.0057397
32. Chung AY, Ooi LL, Machin D, Tan SB, Goh BK, Wong JS, et al. Adjuvant Hepatic Intra-Arterial Iodine-131-Lipiodol Following Curative Resection of Hepatocellular Carcinoma: A Prospective Randomized Trial. *World J Surg* (2013) 37:1356–61. doi: 10.1007/s00268-013-1970-4
33. Lau WY, Leung TW, Ho SK, Chan M, Machin D, Lau J, et al. Adjuvant Intra-Arterial Iodine-131-Labelled Lipiodol for Resectable Hepatocellular Carcinoma: A Prospective Randomised Trial. *Lancet* (1999) 353:797–801. doi: 10.1016/s0140-6736(98)06475-7
34. Li J, Xing J, Yang Y, Liu J, Wang W, Xia Y, et al. Adjuvant (131)I-Metuximab for Hepatocellular Carcinoma After Liver Resection: A Randomised, Controlled, Multicentre, Open-Label, Phase 2 Trial. *Lancet Gastroenterol Hepatol* (2020) 5:548–60. doi: 10.1016/s2468-1253(19)30422-4
35. Hasegawa K, Takayama T, Ijichi M, Matsuyama Y, Imamura H, Sano K, et al. Uracil-Tegafur as an Adjuvant for Hepatocellular Carcinoma: A Randomized Trial. *Hepatology* (2006) 44:891–5. doi: 10.1002/hep.21341
36. Xia Y, Qiu Y, Li J, Shi L, Wang K, Xi T, et al. Adjuvant Therapy With Capecitabine Postpones Recurrence of Hepatocellular Carcinoma After Curative Resection: A Randomized Controlled Trial. *Ann Surg Oncol* (2010) 17:3137–44. doi: 10.1245/s10434-010-1148-3
37. Yamamoto M, Arii S, Sugahara K, Tobe T. Adjuvant Oral Chemotherapy to Prevent Recurrence After Curative Resection for Hepatocellular Carcinoma. *Br J Surg* (1996) 83:336–40. doi: 10.1002/bjs.1800830313
38. Peng BG, He Q, Li JP, Zhou F. Adjuvant Transcatheter Arterial Chemoembolization Improves Efficacy of Hepatectomy for Patients With Hepatocellular Carcinoma and Portal Vein Tumor Thrombus. *Am J Surg* (2009) 198:313–8. doi: 10.1016/j.amjsurg.2008.09.026
39. Wang Z, Ren Z, Chen Y, Hu J, Yang G, Yu L, et al. Adjuvant Transarterial Chemoembolization for HBV-Related Hepatocellular Carcinoma After Resection: A Randomized Controlled Study. *Clin Cancer Res* (2018) 24:2074–81. doi: 10.1158/1078-0432.ccr-17-2899
40. Wei W, Jian PE, Li SH, Guo ZX, Zhang YF, Ling YH, et al. Adjuvant Transcatheter Arterial Chemoembolization After Curative Resection for Hepatocellular Carcinoma Patients With Solitary Tumor and Microvascular Invasion: A Randomized Clinical Trial of Efficacy and Safety. *Cancer Commun (Lond)* (2018) 38:61. doi: 10.1186/s40880-018-0331-y
41. Zhong C, Guo RP, Li JQ, Shi M, Wei W, Chen MS, et al. A Randomized Controlled Trial of Hepatectomy With Adjuvant Transcatheter Arterial Chemoembolization Versus Hepatectomy Alone for Stage III a Hepatocellular Carcinoma. *J Cancer Res Clin Oncol* (2009) 135:1437–45. doi: 10.1007/s00432-009-0588-2
42. Song MJ. Hepatic Artery Infusion Chemotherapy for Advanced Hepatocellular Carcinoma. *World J Gastroenterol* (2015) 21:3843–9. doi: 10.3748/wjg.v21.i13.3843
43. Kokudo N, Takemura N, Hasegawa K, Takayama T, Kubo S, Shimada M, et al. Clinical Practice Guidelines for Hepatocellular Carcinoma: The Japan Society of Hepatology 2017 (4th JSH-HCC Guidelines) 2019 Update. *Hepatol Res* (2019) 49:1109–13. doi: 10.1111/hepr.13411
44. Niguma T, Mimura T, Tutui N. Adjuvant Arterial Infusion Chemotherapy After Resection of Hepatocellular Carcinoma With Portal Thrombosis: A Pilot Study. *J Hepatobiliary Pancreat Surg* (2005) 12:249–53. doi: 10.1007/s00534-004-0969-5
45. Kojima H, Hatano E, Taura K, Seo S, Yasuchika K, Uemoto S. Hepatic Resection for Hepatocellular Carcinoma With Tumor Thrombus in the Major Portal Vein. *Dig Surg* (2015) 32:413–20. doi: 10.1159/000437375
46. Hatano E, Uemoto S, Yamaue H, Yamamoto M. Significance of Hepatic Resection and Adjuvant Hepatic Arterial Infusion Chemotherapy for Hepatocellular Carcinoma With Portal Vein Tumor Thrombus in the First Branch of Portal Vein and the Main Portal Trunk: A Project Study for Hepatic Surgery of the Japanese Society of Hepato-Biliary-Pancreatic Surgery. *J Hepatobiliary Pancreat Sci* (2018) 25:395–402. doi: 10.1002/jhbp.574
47. Moran A, Ramos LF, Picado O, Pendola F, Sleeman D, Dudeja V, et al. Hepatocellular Carcinoma: Resection With Adjuvant Hepatic Artery Infusion Therapy *vs* Resection Alone. A Systematic Review and Meta-Analysis. *J Surg Oncol* (2019) 119:455–63. doi: 10.1002/jso.25338
48. Chiba T, Hiraoka A, Mikami S, Shinozaki M, Osaki Y, Obu M, et al. Japanese Patient Preferences Regarding Intermediate to Advanced Hepatocellular Carcinoma Treatments. *Patient Prefer Adherence* (2019) 13:637–47. doi: 10.2147/ppa.s198363
49. Bang A, Dawson LA. Radiotherapy for HCC: Ready for Prime Time? *JHEP Rep* (2019) 1:131–37. doi: 10.1016/j.jhepr.2019.05.004
50. Xu MJ, Feng M. Radiation Therapy in HCC: What Data Exist and What Data do We Need to Incorporate Into Guidelines? *Semin Liver Dis* (2019) 39:43–52. doi: 10.1055/s-0038-1676098
51. Garin E, Rolland Y, Edeline J, Icard N, Lenoir L, Laffont S, et al. Personalized Dosimetry With Intensification Using 90Y-Loaded Glass Microsphere Radioembolization Induces Prolonged Overall Survival in Hepatocellular Carcinoma Patients With Portal Vein Thrombosis. *J Nucl Med* (2015) 56:339–46. doi: 10.2967/jnumed.114.145177
52. Graves SA, Hobbs RF. Dosimetry for Optimized, Personalized Radiopharmaceutical Therapy. *Semin Radiat Oncol* (2021) 31:37–44. doi: 10.1016/j.semradonc.2020.07.008
53. Xiao C, Huang L, Xiao N, Lun J. Effect of Radical Resection Combined With Antiviral Therapy in Patients With Hepatitis B Virus-Associated Hepatocellular Carcinoma and Prognostic Analysis. *J buon.* (2020) 25:2576–83.
54. Hoshida Y. Risk of Recurrence in Hepatitis B-Related Hepatocellular Carcinoma: Impact of Viral Load in Late Recurrence. *J Hepatol* (2009) 51:842–4. doi: 10.1016/j.jhep.2009.08.003
55. Huang TS, Shyu YC, Chen HY, Yuan SS, Shih JN, Chen PJ. A Systematic Review and Meta-Analysis of Adjuvant Interferon Therapy After Curative Treatment for Patients With Viral Hepatitis-Related Hepatocellular Carcinoma. *J Viral Hepat* (2013) 20:729–43. doi: 10.1111/jvh.12096
56. Xu JB, Qi FZ, Xu G, Chen GF, Huang MD, Zhang JH. Adjuvant Interferon Therapy After Surgical Treatment for Hepatitis B/C Virus-Related Hepatocellular Carcinoma: A Meta-Analysis. *Hepatol Res* (2014) 44:209–17. doi: 10.1111/hepr.12109

57. Shen A, Liu M, Zheng D, Chen Q, Wu Z. Adjuvant Transarterial Chemoembolization After Curative Hepatectomy for Hepatocellular Carcinoma With Microvascular Invasion: A Systematic Review and Meta-Analysis. *Clin Res Hepatol Gastroenterol* (2020) 44:142–54. doi: 10.1016/j.clinre.2019.06.012

58. Chen W, Ma T, Zhang J, Zhang X, Chen W, Shen Y, et al. A Systematic Review and Meta-Analysis of Adjuvant Transarterial Chemoembolization After Curative Resection for Patients With Hepatocellular Carcinoma. *HPB (Oxford)* (2020) 22:795–808. doi: 10.1016/j.hpb.2019.12.013

59. Tierney JF, Stewart LA, Ghersi D, Burdett S, Sydes MR. Practical Methods for Incorporating Summary Time-to-Event Data Into Meta-Analysis. *Trials* (2007) 8:16. doi: 10.1186/1745-6215-8-16

60. Bruix J, Takayama T, Mazzaferro V, Chau GY, Yang J, Kudo M, et al. Adjuvant Sorafenib for Hepatocellular Carcinoma After Resection or Ablation (STORM): A Phase 3, Randomised, Double-Blind, Placebo-Controlled Trial. *Lancet Oncol* (2015) 16:1344–54. doi: 10.1016/s1470-2045(15)00198-9

61. Sonbol MB, Riaz IB, Naqvi SAA, Almquist DR, Mina S, Almasri J, et al. Systemic Therapy and Sequencing Options in Advanced Hepatocellular Carcinoma: A Systematic Review and Network Meta-Analysis. *JAMA Oncol* (2020) 6:e204930. doi: 10.1001/jamaoncol.2020.4930

4

Dose–Response Between Serum Prealbumin and All-Cause Mortality After Hepatectomy in Patients with Hepatocellular Carcinoma

Rong-Rui Huo†*, Hao-Tian Liu*†*, Zhu-Jian Deng*†*, Xiu-Mei Liang, Wen-Feng Gong, Lu-Nan Qi, Xue-Mei You, Bang-De Xiang, Le-Qun Li, Liang Ma* and Jian-Hong Zhong**

Hepatobiliary Surgery Department, Guangxi Liver Cancer Diagnosis and Treatment Engineering and Technology Research Center, Guangxi Medical University Cancer Hospital, Nanning, China

***Correspondence:**
Liang Ma
malianggxyd@163.com
Jian-Hong Zhong
zhongjianhong@gxmu.edu.cn;
zhongjianhong66@163.com

†These authors have contributed equally to this work

Background: The relationship between serum prealbumin and the risk of all-cause mortality after hepatectomy in patients with hepatocellular carcinoma (HCC) needs to be evaluated.

Methods: We conducted a retrospective study. A Cox proportional hazards regression model was used to adjust for potential confounders. Prealbumin level was transformed by Z-scores and categorized into quartiles (Q1: <147 mg/L, Q2: 147–194 mg/L, Q3: 194–239 mg/L, Q4: >239 mg/L). We assessed the dose-response relationship between serum prealbumin and the risk of all-cause mortality using a restricted cubic spline model.

Results: Data were included from 2,022 HCC patients who underwent hepatectomy at Guangxi Medical University Cancer Hospital in China between January 2006 and January 2016. The adjusted hazard ratios (HRs) for increasing quartiles of serum prealbumin were 0.78 [95% confidence interval (CI): 0.64–0.95] for Q2, 0.66 (0.53–0.81) for Q3, and 0.51 (0.41–0.64) for Q4 in the Cox model (all $P < 0.001$). Serum prealbumin showed an L-shaped, non-linear dose-response relationship with the risk of all-cause mortality ($P < 0.001$). Among patients whose serum prealbumin was below 250 mg/L, risk of all-cause mortality decreased by 27% (95% CI: 18–36%) per increase of one standard deviation (69.8 mg/L) in serum prealbumin.

Conclusions: Levels of serum prealbumin under 250 mg/L may be considered dangerous with respect to all-cause mortality after hepatectomy in HCC patients. Serum prealbumin may be useful as a prognostic marker in HCC patients undergoing hepatectomy.

Keywords: all-cause mortality, dose–response relationship, hepatocellular carcinoma, serum prealbumin, prognosis

HIGHLIGHTS

- Low serum prealbumin is associated with higher risk of all-cause mortality after hepatectomy in patients with hepatocellular carcinoma.
- Among these patients, levels of serum prealbumin under 250 mg/L may indicate elevated risk of all-cause mortality.

INTRODUCTION

Hepatocellular carcinoma (HCC) is a common malignant neoplasm (1). Hepatectomy is one of the main radical treatments for HCC. The 5-year recurrence rate of HCC is up to 70% (2), and the 5-year overall survival (OS) is only 37% for patients with portal hypertension, 30% for those with multiple tumors, and 18% for those suffering macrovascular invasion after hepatectomy (3). Therefore, it is important to explore reliable preoperative risk markers to predict the OS of such patients. Some preoperative variables, such as tumor number, tumor differentiation, tumor size, alpha-fetoprotein (AFP) level, liver function, and the presence of liver cirrhosis have been associated with OS of HCC patients after hepatectomy (4–7). Preoperative malnutritional status may also contribute to poor prognosis after hepatectomy (8–10).

Serum prealbumin synthesized by the liver is a common laboratory indicator of nutritional status. Serum prealbumin is less affected by liver diseases than other serum proteins (11, 12). In addition, the level of serum prealbumin is not significantly altered by blood transfusion or supplemental infusion of human albumin. Some studies reported a positive association between the level of serum prealbumin and prognosis in various cancers (13–15). However, few studies have investigated the association between the level of serum prealbumin and the risk of mortality after hepatectomy in patients with HCC. In our previous study, we found that serum prealbumin <200 mg/L was associated with mortality after hepatic resection in patients with HCC (16). Other studies found similar results (17, 18). However, these studies were limited to multivariate analysis of serum prealbumin treated as a categorical variable, so they could not determine whether the risk of death of patients with HCC changed to different degrees with slight changes in serum prealbumin level.

In the present study, we examined the dose-response relationship of serum prealbumin level with the risk of all-cause mortality after resection in patients with HCC. In order to capture the relationship in detail and to compensate for the statistical problems of treating serum prealbumin as a continuous or categorial variable (19, 20), we applied a restricted cubic spline (RCS) function. The RCS function has proven effective at characterizing dose-response correlations between a continuous exposure (such as serum prealbumin) and all-cause mortality, regardless of whether the relationship was linear or not (21). It has been used in several single studies and meta-analyses (22–24). Therefore, in this study, we evaluated the dose-response relationships of serum prealbumin level with the risk of all-cause mortality after resection in patients with HCC.

METHODS

Patients

We retrospectively reviewed records of patients who underwent hepatectomy for HCC between January 2006 and January 2016 at Guangxi Medical University Cancer Hospital, in Nanning, China. Eligible patients had to be admitted for initial HCC treatment at our hospital and had to have histologically confirmed HCC. Indications for hepatectomy was described as previous (2). No age restriction was applied during enrollment of patients in this study. HCC patients with distant metastasis or with other tumors were excluded, as were patients for whom preoperative serum prealbumin data were missing. Liver function indicators were assayed in blood collected at 6:00–7:00 a.m. on the second morning of hospitalization after overnight fasting. Hepatectomy was performed after 3 to 7 days of hospitalization. This study was conducted in accordance with the Declaration of Helsinki guidelines, and the protocol was approved by the Ethics Commitment of our hospital.

Assessment of Covariates

The following data were extracted from patient records: sex, age, liver function categorized according to Child-Pugh category criteria, Barcelona Clinic Liver Cancer (BCLC) stage, serum prealbumin, hepatitis B surface antigen (HBsAg), albumin (ALB), aspartate aminotransferase (AST), alanine aminotransferase (ALT), total bilirubin (TBIL), AFP, and pathology of HCC involving cirrhosis, tumor size and number, integrity of tumor capsule, and presence or absence of macrovascular invasion. All measurements were obtained before surgery. However, liver cirrhosis and macrovascular invasion were confirmed by postoperative histopathology.

In order to ensure the accuracy and reliability of data, measures for standard quality controls were planned before the start of study, such as a table for collection of patients' information and a code for replacement of categorical data. Two researchers independently collected and organized data; any discrepancies were corrected by a third reviewer.

Outcomes and Follow-Up

Follow-up was conducted starting from the first month after surgery, every 2 months during the first year, then every 6 months thereafter until May 31, 2019 or death or loss to follow-up. During follow-up appointments, data were collected about time to HCC recurrence, survival or death, and liver function. Follow-up was conducted by telephone and review of the hospital's data management system. The endpoint of the study was OS, defined as the interval from the date of hepatic resection until the date of last follow-up (May 31, 2019) or death.

Statistical Analysis

Before testing independent associations of serum prealbumin with the risk of all-cause mortality in patients with HCC, Z-scores were calculated, such that the resulting estimated effect size indicated the change in serum prealbumin in terms of the standard deviation (SD). The Z-score normalizes the mean parameter value to 0 and the parameter value at one SD to 1. In addition, we also categorized serum prealbumin into quartiles based on sample size. Other categorical covariates were classified based on clinical findings and were entered as dummy variables. Continuous covariates were transformed into categorical variables based on cut-off values routinely used in clinical practice.

We assessed potential associations between serum prealbumin (as a categorical variable) and other characteristics using a chi-squared test or Fisher's exact test. Survival curves were generated using the Kaplan-Meier method. The OS curves were compared between groups using the log-rank test. We tested associations of serum prealbumin with the risk of all-cause mortality using two Cox proportional hazards regression models: model 1 was adjusted for age and sex, while model 2 adjusted for age, sex, tumor size and number, tumor capsule, AFP, ALB, AST, ALT, TBIL, HBsAg, liver cirrhosis, liver function, and BCLC stage. From each fitted model, we searched for a linear trend by modeling the median value of each quartile to test ordered relations across the different serum prealbumin quartiles. Interactions between serum prealbumin and other factors were also examined using a likelihood ratio test, with a comparison of the log likelihood of the two models with or without the interaction terms. We calculated hazard ratios (HRs) for risk of all-cause mortality and the corresponding 95% confidence intervals (CIs).

We assessed the dose-response relationship between serum prealbumin (as a continuous variable) and the risk of all-cause mortality using RCS models. RCS assumes that the effect of the exposure on the outcome is a smooth, piecewise, cubic polynomial with linear tails (21). RCS models provide flexibility in fitting highly curved relationships, avoiding significant influences from outlying variables, and may provide better power than dichotomizing continuous variables (21). We used RCS models adjusted for the same potential confounders as in model 2, and plotted smooth curves with five knots at the 5th, 25th (reference level), 50th, 75th, and 95th percentiles of serum prealbumin. We further applied a two-piecewise linear regression model to examine the threshold effect of the serum prealbumin on all-cause mortality using a smoothing function (25, 26).

To ensure the stability of the results, we conducted two sensitivity analyses. In one, we repeated the analysis after excluding patients who died 3 months after follow-up began in order to avoid confounding due to premature death. In another, we separately examined patients with or without liver cirrhosis.

We performed all statistical analyses using R version 3.5.1 (https://www.r-project.org/). All P values were two-tailed, with a P value under 0.05 indicating statistical significance.

RESULTS

Baseline Characteristics

The patient records contained details of 2,060 patients with HCC who underwent curative hepatectomy at our institution during January 2006 to January 2016. Based on the inclusion criteria, 2,022 (98.1%) patients were enrolled. The mean age (SD) was 49.5 (11.2) years, and 1,739 patients (86.0%) were male. Among the 2,022 patients, 31% underwent major hepatectomy, while 69% underwent minor hepatectomy. During a median follow-up (range) of 59 months (3–115 months), 385 patients (19%) were lost to follow-up. Among the remaining patients, tumor recurrence and liver failure were the main causes of mortality. The mean level of serum prealbumin level (SD) was 195.5 (69.8) mg/L, and the median (interquartile range) was 193.5 (147.0–239.0) mg/L. **Table 1** presents the characteristics of the patients stratified by quartiles of serum prealbumin.

Cox Regression Analysis

To assess whether clinical variables contributed to the risk of all-cause mortality, we conducted a univariate Cox regression analysis of clinical characteristics (**Table 2**). We found that tumor size and number, BCLC stage, tumor capsule, ALB, AST, ALT, and AFP levels were related to the risk of all-cause mortality. In contrast, age, sex, liver cirrhosis, HBsAg, TBIL, and Child-Pugh were not related to the risk of all-cause mortality in our cohort. To control for any possible confounding factors affecting the association between serum prealbumin and the risk of all-cause mortality, subsequent multivariate Cox regression and RCS models were adjusted for age, sex, tumor size and number, tumor capsule, AFP, HBsAg, ALB, AST, ALT, TBIL, Child-Pugh, liver cirrhosis, and BCLC stage.

We analyzed the associations between serum prealbumin level and the risk of all-cause mortality (**Table 3**). In model 1, which was adjusted for age and sex, the HRs (95% CIs) of the risk of all-cause mortality across increasing quartiles of serum prealbumin were 1.00 for Q1, 0.68 (0.57–0.82) for Q2, 0.50 (0.41–0.60) for Q3, and 0.37 (0.30–0.45) for Q4 (P for trend < 0.001). The HR was 0.68 (0.63–0.73) per 1-SD increase in serum prealbumin. According to model 2, the HRs (95% CIs) were 1.00 for Q1, 0.78 (0.64–0.95) for Q2, 0.66 (0.53–0.81) for Q3, and 0.51 (0.41–0.64) for Q4 (P for trend < 0.001). In model 2, the HR was 0.77 (0.71–0.84) per 1-SD increase in serum prealbumin. Inclusion of a quadratic term for serum prealbumin in the Cox proportional hazard models suggested a linear correlation between serum prealbumin and all-cause mortality. However, RCS analysis showed this correlation to be non-linear.

Subgroup Analysis

When we analyzed serum prealbumin in correlation with all-cause mortality across subgroups of clinical characteristics (**Table 4**), we detected no significant subgroup interactions. In analyses stratified by age, sex, tumor capsule, tumor size, liver cirrhosis, HBsAg, AFP, ALT, AST, Child-Pugh, and BCLC stage, inclusion of a quadratic term for serum prealbumin in the Cox proportional hazard models revealed a linear correlation between serum prealbumin and all-cause mortality. However, this correlation was not linear in subsets of patients with tumor number >3, ALB ≤35 g/L, or TBIL >21 μmol/L (**Table 4**).

Dose–Response Analysis

We evaluated the potential dose-response relationship between serum prealbumin and the risk of all-cause mortality using an RCS model adjusted for potential confounders. Serum

TABLE 1 | Baseline characteristics by serum prealbumin quartiles.

Characteristic	Overall (n = 2,022)	Serum prealbumin quartiles (mg/L)				P value*
		Q1 (<147, n = 501)	Q2 (147~194, n = 510)	Q3 (194~239, n = 502)	Q4 (>239, n = 509)	
Age, y						0.004
≤60	1,683 (83.2)	391 (78.0)	433 (84.9)	422 (84.1)	437 (85.9)	
>60	339 (16.8)	110 (22.0)	77 (15.1)	80 (15.9)	72 (14.1)	
Gender						<0.001
Male	1,739 (86.0)	390 (77.8)	423 (82.9)	453 (90.2)	473 (92.9)	
Female	283 (14.0)	111 (22.2)	87 (17.1)	49 (9.8)	36 (7.1)	
Liver cirrhosis						0.044
No	863 (42.7)	204 (40.7)	202 (39.6)	214 (42.6)	243 (47.7)	
Yes	1,159 (57.3)	297 (59.3)	308 (60.4)	288 (57.4)	266 (52.3)	
Tumor number						0.067
≤3	1,887 (93.3)	455.0 (90.8)	480 (94.1)	470 (93.6)	482 (94.7)	
>3	135 (6.7)	46 (9.2)	30 (5.9)	32 (6.4)	27 (5.3)	
Tumor size, cm						<0.001
≤5	825 (40.8)	129 (25.7)	182 (35.7)	228 (45.4)	286 (56.2)	
>5	1,197 (59.2)	372 (74.3)	328 (64.3)	274 (54.6)	223 (43.8)	
BCLC stage						<0.001
0/A	1,282 (63.4)	272 (54.3)	312 (61.2)	339 (67.5)	359 (70.5)	
B	328 (16.2)	92 (18.4)	76 (14.9)	79 (15.7)	81 (15.9)	
C	412 (20.4)	137 (27.3)	122 (23.9)	84 (16.7)	69 (13.6)	
Tumor capsule						0.133
Complete	1,289 (63.7)	316 (63.1)	313 (61.4)	314 (62.5)	346 (68.0)	
Incomplete	733 (36.3)	185 (36.9)	197 (38.6)	188 (37.5)	163 (32.0)	
HBsAg						<0.001
Negative	226 (11.2)	29 (5.8)	47 (9.2)	69 (13.7)	81 (15.9)	
Positive	1,796 (88.8)	472 (94.2)	463 (90.8)	433 (86.3)	428 (84.1)	
ALB, g/L						<0.001
≤35	217 (10.7)	153 (30.5)	33 (6.5)	19 (3.8)	12 (2.4)	
>35	1,805 (89.3)	348 (69.5)	477 (93.5)	483 (96.2)	497 (97.6)	
AST, U/L						<0.001
≤40	1,082 (53.5)	181 (36.1)	253 (49.6)	300 (59.8)	348 (68.4)	
>40	940 (46.5)	320 (63.9)	257 (50.4)	202 (40.2)	161 (31.6)	
ALT, U/L						0.290
9≤40	1,198 (59.2)	283 (56.5)	305 (59.8)	293 (58.4)	317 (62.3)	
>40	824 (40.8)	218 (43.5)	205 (40.2)	209 (41.6)	192 (37.7)	
TBIL, μmol/L						<0.001
≤21	1,812 (89.6)	421 (84.0)	459 (90.0)	465 (92.6)	467 (91.7)	
>21	210 (10.4)	80 (16.0)	51 (10.0)	37 (7.4)	42 (8.3)	
Child-Pugh						<0.001
A	1,974 (97.6)	470 (93.8)	505 (99.0)	493 (98.2)	506 (99.4)	
B	48 (2.4)	31 (6.2)	5 (1.0)	9 (1.8)	3 (0.6)	
AFP, ng/ml						<0.001
≤400	1,174 (58.1)	252 (50.3)	289 (56.7)	304 (60.6)	329 (64.6)	
>400	848 (41.9)	249 (49.7)	221 (43.3)	198 (39.4)	180 (35.4)	

Data are n (%). Q, quartile; AFP, alpha-fetoprotein; ALB, serum albumin; ALT, alanine transaminase; AST, aspartate aminotransferase; BCLC, Barcelona Clinic Liver Cancer; HBsAg, hepatitis B surface antigen; TBIL, total bilirubin.

**Pearson's chi-squared test or Fisher's exact test, P value < 0.05 indicates a significant difference between quartiles.*

prealbumin showed an L-shape, non-linear dose-response relationship with the risk of all-cause mortality (P for non-linearity <0.001, **Figure 1A**). RCS analyses based on a two-piecewise linear regression model included a knot at 250 mg/L, and Kaplan-Meier survival plots showed significantly higher all-cause mortality in patients with serum prealbumin below 250 mg/L than in those with serum prealbumin above this threshold (P < 0.001, **Figure 2**). The risk of all-cause mortality decreased with serum prealbumin level over the threshold (HR per SD decrease: 0.73, 95% CI: 0.64–0.82, **Table 5**). Risk was no longer reduced when the serum prealbumin level was above the threshold (HR 1.15, 95% CI: 0.87–1.53).

Sensitivity Analysis

The exclusion of patients who died 3 months prior to follow-up did not substantially alter the results described above, suggesting that the findings are robust (**Table 3**, **Figure 1B**). Similarly, excluding patients with or without liver cirrhosis did not substantially affect the results (**Figures 1C, D**).

DISCUSSION

This is the first epidemiological study to investigate the dose-response association between serum prealbumin level and the

TABLE 2 | Risk of mortality associated with serum prealbumin*.

Variables	HR (95% CI)	P value
Age, y (>60 *vs* ≤60)	1.10 (0.92–1.32)	0.299
Sex (F *vs* M)	0.81 (0.66–1.01)	0.061
Liver cirrhosis (Yes *vs* No)	1.09 (0.95–1.26)	0.234
Tumor number (>3 *vs* ≤3)	2.20 (1.75–2.78)	<0.001
Tumor size,cm (>5 *vs* ≤5)	2.31 (1.98–2.70)	<0.001
BCLC stage		
B *vs* 0/A	1.93 (1.60–2.33)	<0.001
C *vs* 0/A	3.97 (3.39–4.66)	<0.001
Capsule (Incomplete *vs* Complete)	1.88 (1.63–2.16)	<0.001
HBsAg (Positive *vs* Negative)	1.04 (0.83–1.29)	0.755
ALB, g/L (>35 *vs* ≤35)	0.64 (0.52–0.79)	<0.001
AST, U/L (>40 *vs* ≤40)	1.99 (1.73–2.29)	<0.001
ALT, U/L (>40 *vs* ≤40)	1.32 (1.14–1.51)	<0.001
TBIL, μmol/L (>21 *vs* ≤21)	1.07 (0.85–1.34)	0.588
Child-Pugh B *vs* A	1.52 (1.01–2.28)	0.043
AFP, ng/ml (>400 *vs* ≤400)	1.48 (1.29–1.71)	<0.001

Data are HR (95% CI), unless otherwise specified.
**HRs for risk of all-cause mortality, and the corresponding 95% CIs were calculated by Cox proportional hazards regression model.*

TABLE 3 | Risk of mortality associated with serum prealbumin.

	Serum prealbumin quartiles (mg/L)				Per-SD	P for trend*
	Q1 (<147)	Q2 (147~194)	Q3 (194~239)	Q4 (>239)		
All patients						
Case	501	510	502	509	2,022	–
No. of death	259 (51.7%)	209 (41.0%)	176 (35.1%)	146 (28.7%)	790 (39.1%)	–
Model 1†	1.00 (ref)	0.68 (0.57–0.82)	0.50 (0.41–0.60)	0.37 (0.30–0.45)	0.68 (0.63–0.73)	<0.001
Model 2‡	1.00 (ref)	0.78 (0.64–0.95)	0.66 (0.53–0.81)	0.51 (0.41–0.64)	0.77 (0.71–0.84)	<0.001
Patients with OS >3 months						
Case	448	476	473	486	1,883	–
No. of death	229 (51.1%)	194 (40.8%)	165 (34.9%)	138 (28.4%)	726 (38.6%)	–
Model 1†	1.00 (ref)	0.70 (0.58–0.85)	0.52 (0.42–0.63)	0.38 (0.31–0.47)	0.70 (0.64–0.75)	<0.001
Model 2‡	1.00 (ref)	0.80 (0.65–0.98)	0.64 (0.52–0.80)	0.49 (0.39–0.63)	0.77 (0.71–0.84)	<0.001

Data are HR (95% CI), unless otherwise specified. ref, reference; Q, quartile.
**Tests for linear trend were done by modeling the median value of each quartile to test ordered relations across quartiles of serum prealbumin.*
†Adjusted for age and gender.
‡Adjusted for age, gender, tumor number, tumor size, tumor capsule, HBsAg, liver cirrhosis, AFP, ALB, AST, ALT, TBIL, Child-Pugh, and BCLC stage.

risk of all-cause mortality after hepatectomy in patients with HCC. In our large cohort study, we demonstrate that serum prealbumin level is independently associated with the risk of all-cause mortality. The association between serum prealbumin level and all-cause mortality was non-linear: among patients with serum prealbumin below 250 mg/L, risk fell by 27% per SD increase of 69.8 mg/L.

Although some studies have shown that serum prealbumin is associated with the prognosis of HCC patients after hepatectomy (16, 17), no study assessed its association with the risk of all-cause mortality. After controlling for potential confounders, quadratic terms for serum prealbumin in the Cox proportional hazard models suggested a linear association between serum prealbumin and all-cause mortality. However, RCS analysis showed the association to be non-linear. These findings were not substantially affected by potential confounding from premature death or presence of liver cirrhosis. The findings of this study suggest that lower levels of serum prealbumin might be associated with increased risk of all-cause mortality in HCC patients in a non-linear manner.

Since the reference values for what is considered a "normal" serum prealbumin level vary considerably, investigating the appropriate cut-off value of prealbumin for each particular type of cancer is important for predicting OS. Serum prealbumin level using a cut-off value of 170 mg/L could predict long-term OS after hepatectomy for patients with HCC (17). We have previously shown that serum prealbumin <182 mg/L is associated with poor prognosis based on maximally selected rank statistics, and therefore we consider serum prealbumin levels ≥182 mg/L as normal. However, the lower limit of the normal reference range is 200 mg/L in many hospitals (16, 18). Based on the non-linear effects of the serum prealbumin in our study, a serum prealbumin level over 250 mg/L may be considered safe. In

TABLE 4 | Stratified associations between serum prealbumin and all-cause mortality.

Characteristic	Serum prealbumin quartiles (mg/L)				P for trend*	P for interaction
	Q1 (<147, n = 501)	Q2 (147~194, n = 510)	Q3 (194~239, n = 502)	Q4 (>239, n = 509)		
Age, y						0.516
≤60	1.00 (ref)	0.74 (0.59–0.91)	0.59 (0.46–0.74)	0.48 (0.37–0.61)	<0.001	
>60	1.00 (ref)	0.90 (0.56–1.45)	0.80 (0.49–1.30)	0.48 (0.27–0.85)	0.015	
Gender						0.452
Male	1.00 (ref)	0.78 (0.63–0.97)	0.64 (0.51–0.80)	0.50 (0.39–0.63)	<0.001	
Female	1.00 (ref)	0.68 (0.40–1.14)	0.44 (0.21–0.91)	0.21 (0.08–0.57)	<0.001	
Liver cirrhosis						0.883
No	1.00 (ref)	0.75 (0.55–1.03)	0.55 (0.39–0.77)	0.47 (0.33–0.67)	<0.001	
Yes	1.00 (ref)	0.73 (0.57–0.94)	0.62 (0.48–0.82)	0.46 (0.34–0.62)	<0.001	
Tumor number						0.098
≤3	1.00 (ref)	0.76(0.62–0.93)	0.58 (0.46–0.72)	0.46 (0.36–0.59)	<0.001	
>3	1.00 (ref)	0.62 (0.30–1.29)	0.93 (0.47–0.86)	0.51 (0.24–1.07)	0.131	
Tumor size, cm						0.373
≤5	1.00 (ref)	0.60 (0.39–0.91)	0.53 (0.34–0.80)	0.43 (0.28–0.65)	<0.001	
>5	1.00 (ref)	0.83 (0.66–1.03)	0.67 (0.52–0.85)	0.49 (0.37–0.65)	<0.001	
BCLC stage						0.881
0/A	1.00 (ref)	0.76 (0.56–1.02)	0.60 (0.44–0.82)	0.50 (0.36–0.70)	<0.001	
B	1.00 (ref)	0.70 (0.43–1.13)	0.55 (0.35–0.87)	0.44 (0.26–0.75)	0.001	
C	1.00 (ref)	0.80 (0.58–1.11)	0.65 (0.45–0.95)	0.46 (0.30–0.70)	<0.001	
Tumor capsule						0.303
Complete	1.00 (ref)	0.89 (0.68–1.16)	0.59 (0.44–0.79)	0.58 (0.43–0.79)	<0.001	
Incomplete	1.00 (ref)	0.66 (0.49–0.88)	0.63 (0.47–0.85)	0.37 (0.26–0.53)	<0.001	
HBsAg						0.614
Negative	1.00 (ref)	0.86 (0.39–1.87)	0.57 (0.27–1.17)	0.39 (0.19–0.81)	0.003	
Positive	1.00 (ref)	0.75 (0.61–0.93)	0.60 (0.48–0.75)	0.49 (0.38–0.62)	<0.001	
ALB, g/L						0.595
≤35	1.00 (ref)	0.99 (0.54–1.81)	0.44 (0.20–1.00)	0.62 (0.21–1.80)	0.082	
>35	1.00 (ref)	0.75 (0.61–0.92)	0.63 (0.50–0.78)	0.47 (0.37–0.59)	<0.001	
AST, U/L						0.559
≤40	1.00 (ref)	0.81 (0.59–1.12)	0.56 (0.40–0.79)	0.44 (0.31–0.62)	<0.001	
>40	1.00 (ref)	0.72 (0.56–0.93)	0.67 (0.51–0.88)	0.50 (0.36–0.69)	<0.001	
ALT, U/L						0.626
≤40	1.00 (ref)	0.79 (0.61–1.03)	0.56 (0.42–0.76)	0.45 (0.33–0.62)	<0.001	
>40	1.00 (ref)	0.70 (0.52–0.94)	0.67 (0.50–0.90)	0.48 (0.34–0.68)	<0.001	
TBIL, μmol/L						0.174
≤21	1.00 (ref)	0.79 (0.64–0.97)	0.60 (0.48–0.75)	0.47 (0.37–0.59)	<0.001	
>21	1.00 (ref)	0.49 (0.25–0.94)	0.72 (0.34–1.50)	0.47 (0.21–1.04)	0.091	
AFP, ng/ml						0.962
≤400	1.00 (ref)	0.77 (0.58–1.02)	0.61 (0.45–0.82)	0.48 (0.35–0.65)	<0.001	
>400	1.00 (ref)	0.78 (0.59–1.03)	0.65 (0.48–0.87)	0.48 (0.34–0.68)	<0.001	

Data are HR (95% CI), unless otherwise specified. ref, reference; Q, quartile.
**Tests for linear trend were done by modeling the median value of each quartile to test ordered relations across quartiles of serum prealbumin.*
Adjusted for age, gender, tumor number, tumor size, tumor capsule, HBsAg, liver cirrhosis, AFP, ALB, AST, ALT, TBIL, Child-Pugh, and BCLC stage.

our cohort, all-cause mortality was significantly higher among patients with serum prealbumin below this threshold than among patients with levels above this threshold. Under this threshold, the risk of all-cause mortality decreased with increasing serum prealbumin level (HR per SD decrease: 0.73, 95% CI: 0.64–0.82).

Although how prealbumin may influence the prognosis of patients with HCC is not fully understood, a role for immunosuppression in the development of tumors has been widely accepted (27). Prealbumin promotes the production of lymphocytes, with lower serum level associated with reduced lymphocyte number, which leads to a suboptimal immune status (28). Prealbumin is an acute-phase liver protein with a half-life of only 2–3 days and can be used to reflect nutritional and inflammatory status as well as the liver's ability to synthesize protein (29). The nutritional status is closely related to postoperative recurrence and prognosis (30). Although albumin is more commonly used than prealbumin to detect protein malnutrition and assess liver function in the clinic (11, 31, 32), some studies suggest that prealbumin is more sensitive and specific (31, 33). Therefore, serum prealbumin may be a good indicator of nutritional status and prognosis, and may be preferable to albumin for predicting the risk of death after curative hepatectomy for HCC.

The strengths of our study include the relatively large cohort, relatively long follow-up, and our adjustment for HBsAg and liver cirrhosis. Moreover, we applied an RCS model to evaluate the dose-response relationship between

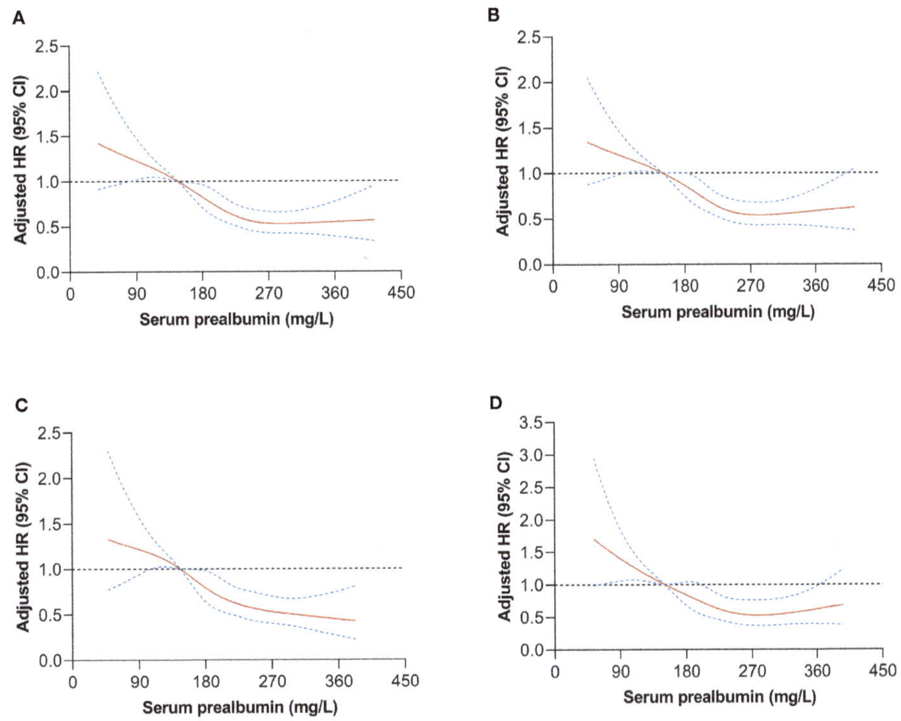

FIGURE 1 | | Dose–response relationship between serum prealbumin and the risk of mortality after hepatectomy in patients with hepatocellular carcinoma. Graphs show the hazard ratio (HR; *solid red lines*) and 95% confidence interval (CI, *dotted blue lines*) describing the association of serum prealbumin with the risk of mortality. Cox regression analysis with a restricted cubic spline approach was conducted to allow flexible, non-linear assessment of the HR for mortality in **(A)** all patients (n = 2,022), **(B)** patients with overall survival >3 months (n = 1,883), **(C)** patients with liver cirrhosis (n = 1,159), or **(D)** patients without liver cirrhosis (n = 863) (all $P < 0.001$). All models were adjusted for age, sex, HBsAg, liver cirrhosis, tumor size and number, tumor capsule, AFP, ALB, ALT, AST, TBIL, Child-Pugh, and BCLC stage.

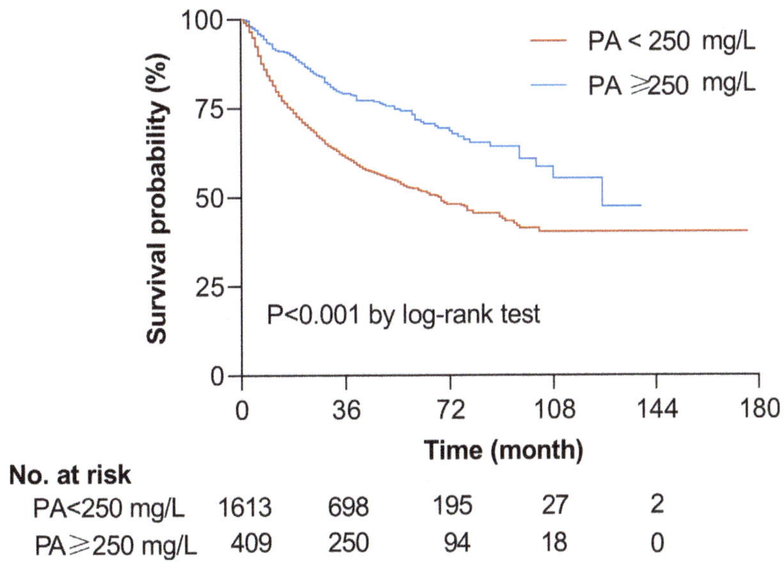

FIGURE 2 | | Unadjusted Kaplan-Meier curve of overall survival according to serum prealbumin (PA) level. The graph shows the survival probability according to serum prealbumin level in patients with a level above a threshold of 250 mg/L (*blue line*, n = 409) or below the threshold (*red line*, n = 1,613). The two groups differed significantly in survival, based on the log-rank test. The number of patients indicated in the table is the number of patients at risk at the indicated time.

TABLE 5 | Threshold effect analysis of serum prealbumin on all-cause mortality.

	Case	No. of death (%)	Per-SD	
			HR (95% CI)	P
PA<250 g/ml				
Model 1†	1,613	679 (42.1%)	0.64 (0.58–0.71)	<0.001
Model 2‡			0.73 (0.64–0.82)	<0.001
PA≥250 g/ml				
Model 1†	409	111 (27.1%)	1.09 (0.83–1.43)	0.533
Model 2‡			1.15 (0.87–1.53)	0.319

PA, Prealbumin.
†Adjusted for age and gender.
‡Adjusted for age, gender, tumor number, tumor size, tumor capsule, HBsAg, liver cirrhosis, AFP, ALB, AST, ALT, TBIL, Child-Pugh, and BCLC stage.

serum prealbumin and the risk of all-cause mortality in HCC patients. RCS models are powerful tools that can avoid the loss of information and statistical power caused by discretization of continuous variables (21). Nevertheless, our study has several limitations. First, it was retrospective, and thus, incomplete adherence to the post-resection follow-up protocol and potential confounders for OS are inevitable. In addition, although the multivariable analysis was adjusted for several covariates, we were unable to control for other unknown confounders for lack of data. For example, some inflammatory and nutritional factors such as neutrophil-lymphocyte ratio, platelet-lymphocyte ratio, and sarcopenia were not assessed (10, 34, 35). This may reduce the accuracy of our estimate of the association between serum prealbumin and all-cause mortality. On the other hand, our results are likely to be reliable given that they remained robust to several Cox regression models and sensitivity analyses. Third, we did not measure serum prealbumin in repeated samples in the same patients at different times and thus we could not correct for regression dilution, which could have led to underestimation of the association between serum prealbumin and the risk of all-cause mortality.

CONCLUSIONS

We provide evidence that serum prealbumin is non-linearly associated with all-cause mortality after hepatectomy in HCC patients. A serum prealbumin level under 250 mg/L is a risk factor of all-cause mortality in HCC patients after hepatectomy. Our results should be confirmed and extended in pooled analyses across large prospective cohorts of HCC patients, especially in China, where this cancer is highly prevalent.

AUTHOR CONTRIBUTIONS

J-HZ and LM conceived the study. R-RH, H-TL, Z-JD, X-ML, W-FG, L-NQ, XMY, and B-DX collected and analyzed the data. Z-JD and J-HZ analyzed the data. R-RH and H-TL drafted the manuscript. B-DX, L-QL, and LM revised the manuscript. All authors contributed to the article and approved the submitted version.

ACKNOWLEDGMENTS

The abstract of this study was submitted to the 3rd International Advanced Liver & Pancreas Surgery Symposium (ISLS 2019), October 10–12, 2019, Istanbul, Turkey, and published online (Zhong JH, et al. Dose-response between serum prealbumin and all-cause mortality in patients with hepatocellular carcinoma after hepatectomy. *Int J Surg*. 2020;75;Suppl:S9).

REFERENCES

1. Siegel RL, Miller KD, Jemal A. Cancer statistics, 2018. *CA Cancer J Clin* (2018) 68:7–30. doi: 10.3322/caac.21442
2. Zhong JH, Ke Y, Gong WF, Xiang BD, Ma L, Ye XP, et al. Hepatic resection associated with good survival for selected patients with intermediate and advanced-stage hepatocellular carcinoma. *Ann Surg* (2014) 260:329–40. doi: 10.1097/SLA.0000000000000236
3. Zhong JH, Ke Y, Wang YY, Li LQ. Liver resection for patients with hepatocellular carcinoma and macrovascular invasion, multiple tumours, or portal hypertension. *Gut* (2015) 64:520–1. doi: 10.1136/gutjnl-2014-308139
4. Lu SD, Wang YY, Peng NF, Peng YC, Zhong JH, Qin HG, et al. Preoperative Ratio of Neutrophils to Lymphocytes Predicts Postresection Survival in Selected Patients With Early or Intermediate Stage Hepatocellular Carcinoma. *Med (Baltimore)* (2016) 95:e2722. doi: 10.1097/MD.0000000000002722
5. Ganslmayer M, Hagel A, Dauth W, Zopf S, Strobel D, Muller V, et al. A large cohort of patients with hepatocellular carcinoma in a single European centre: aetiology and prognosis now and in a historical cohort. *Swiss Med Wkly* (2014) 144:w13900. doi: 10.4414/smw.2014.13900
6. Cucchetti A, Ercolani G, Vivarelli M, Cescon M, Ravaioli M, La Barba G, et al. Impact of model for end-stage liver disease (MELD) score on prognosis after hepatectomy for hepatocellular carcinoma on cirrhosis. *Liver Transpl* (2006) 12:966–71. doi: 10.1002/lt.20761
7. Franssen B, Alshebeeb K, Tabrizian P, Marti J, Pierobon ES, Lubezky N, et al. Differences in surgical outcomes between hepatitis B- and hepatitis C-related hepatocellular carcinoma: a retrospective analysis of a single North American center. *Ann Surg* (2014) 260:650–6; discussion 6-8. doi: 10.1097/SLA.0000000000000917
8. Cornet M, Lim C, Salloum C, Lazzati A, Compagnon P, Pascal G, et al. Prognostic value of sarcopenia in liver surgery. *J Visc Surg* (2015) 152:297–304. doi: 10.1016/j.jviscsurg.2015.08.001

9. Ji F, Liang Y, Fu S, Chen D, Cai X, Li S, et al. Prognostic value of combined preoperative prognostic nutritional index and body mass index in HCC after hepatectomy. *HPB (Oxford)* (2017) 19:695–705. doi: 10.1016/j.hpb.2017.04.008
10. Voron T, Tselikas L, Pietrasz D, Pigneur F, Laurent A, Compagnon P, et al. Sarcopenia Impacts on Short- and Long-term Results of Hepatectomy for Hepatocellular Carcinoma. *Ann Surg* (2015) 261:1173–83. doi: 10.1097/SLA.0000000000000743
11. Kuszajewski ML, Clontz AS. Prealbumin is best for nutritional monitoring. *Nursing* (2005) 35:70–1. doi: 10.1097/00152193-200505000-00056
12. Bernstein L, Pleban W. Prealbumin in nutrition evaluation. *Nutrition* (1996) 12:255–9. doi: 10.1016/s0899-9007(96)90852-7
13. Kawai H, Ota H. Low perioperative serum prealbumin predicts early recurrence after curative pulmonary resection for non-small-cell lung cancer. *World J Surg* (2012) 36:2853–7. doi: 10.1007/s00268-012-1766-y
14. Esfahani A, Makhdami N, Faramarzi E, Asghari Jafarabadi M, Ostadrahimi A, Ghayour Nahand M, et al. Prealbumin/CRP Based Prognostic Score, a New Tool for Predicting Metastasis in Patients with Inoperable Gastric Cancer. *Gastroenterol Res Pract* (2016) 2016:4686189. doi: 10.1155/2016/4686189
15. Mahlck CG, Grankvist K. Plasma prealbumin in women with epithelial ovarian carcinoma. *Gynecol Obstet Invest* (1994) 37:135–40. doi: 10.1159/000292542
16. Jia RR, Zhong JH, Huo RR, Su QB, Xiang X, Zhao FL, et al. Correlation between serum prealbumin and prognosis of patients with hepatocellular carcinoma after hepatectomy. *J Surg Oncol* (2019) 119:794–800. doi: 10.1002/jso.25378
17. Li JD, Xu XF, Han J, Wu H, Xing H, Li C, et al. Preoperative prealbumin level as an independent predictor of long-term prognosis after liver resection for hepatocellular carcinoma: a multi-institutional study. *HPB (Oxford)* (2019) 21:157–66. doi: 10.1016/j.hpb.2018.06.1803
18. Liao YY, Teng CL, Peng NF, Jia RR, Cui J, Chen K, et al. Serum Prealbumin is Negatively Associated with Survival in Hepatocellular Carcinoma Patients after Hepatic Resection. *J Cancer* (2019) 10:3006–11. doi: 10.7150/jca.30903
19. Zhao LP, Kolonel LN. Efficiency loss from categorizing quantitative exposures into qualitative exposures in case-control studies. *Am J Epidemiol* (1992) 136:464–74. doi: 10.1093/oxfordjournals.aje.a116520
20. Altman DG, Royston P. The cost of dichotomising continuous variables. *BMJ* (2006) 332:1080. doi: 10.1136/bmj.332.7549.1080
21. Desquilbet L, Mariotti F. Dose-response analyses using restricted cubic spline functions in public health research. *Stat Med* (2010) 29:1037–57. doi: 10.1002/sim.3841
22. Lee W, Han HS, Ahn S, Yoon YS, Cho JY, Choi Y. Correlation between Resection Margin and Disease Recurrence with a Restricted Cubic Spline Model in Patients with Resected Hepatocellular Carcinoma. *Dig Surg* (2018) 35:520–31. doi: 10.1159/000485805
23. Beal EW, Tumin D, Kabir A, Moris D, Zhang XF, Chakedis J, et al. Trends in the Mortality of Hepatocellular Carcinoma in the United States. *J Gastrointest Surg* (2017) 21:2033–8. doi: 10.1007/s11605-017-3526-7
24. Grosso G, Micek A, Godos J, Pajak A, Sciacca S, Galvano F, et al. Dietary Flavonoid and Lignan Intake and Mortality in Prospective Cohort Studies: Systematic Review and Dose-Response Meta-Analysis. *Am J Epidemiol* (2017) 185:1304–16. doi: 10.1093/aje/kww207
25. Vieth E. Fitting piecewise linear regression functions to biological responses. *J Appl Physiol (1985)* (1989) 67:390–6. doi: 10.1152/jappl.1989.67.1.390
26. Nakamura T. BMDP program for piecewise linear regression. *Comput Methods Programs Biomed* (1986) 23:53–5. doi: 10.1016/0169-2607(86)90080-5
27. Qi Q, Geng Y, Sun M, Wang P, Chen Z. Clinical implications of systemic inflammatory response markers as independent prognostic factors for advanced pancreatic cancer. *Pancreatology* (2015) 15:145–50. doi: 10.1016/j.pan.2014.12.004
28. Delhem N, Carpentier A, Morales O, Miroux C, Groux H, Auriault C, et al. Regulatory T-cells and hepatocellular carcinoma: implication of the regulatory T lymphocytes in the control of the immune response. *Bull Cancer* (2008) 95:1219–25. doi: 10.1684/bdc.2008.0761
29. Li B, Liu HY, Guo SH, Sun P, Gong FM, Jia BQ. Impact of early enteral and parenteral nutrition on prealbumin and high-sensitivity C-reactive protein after gastric surgery. *Genet Mol Res* (2015) 14:7130–5. doi: 10.4238/2015.June.29.6
30. Meng J, Zhong J, Zhang H, Zhong W, Huang Z, Jin Y, et al. Pre-, peri-, and postoperative oral administration of branched-chain amino acids for primary liver cancer patients for hepatic resection: a systematic review. *Nutr Cancer* (2014) 66:517–22. doi: 10.1080/01635581.2013.780628
31. Devoto G, Gallo F, Marchello C, Racchi O, Garbarini R, Bonassi S, et al. Prealbumin serum concentrations as a useful tool in the assessment of malnutrition in hospitalized patients. *Clin Chem* (2006) 52:2281–5. doi: 10.1373/clinchem.2006.080366
32. Beck FK, Rosenthal TC. Prealbumin: a marker for nutritional evaluation. *Am Fam Phys* (2002) 65:1575–8.
33. Collins N. The difference between albumin and prealbumin. *Adv Skin Wound Care* (2001) 14:235–6. doi: 10.1097/00129334-200109000-00009
34. Zhao Z, Liu J, Wang J, Xie T, Zhang Q, Feng S, et al. Platelet-to-lymphocyte ratio (PLR) and neutrophil-to-lymphocyte ratio (NLR) are associated with chronic hepatitis B virus (HBV) infection. Int. *Immunopharmacol* (2017) 51:1–8. doi: 10.1016/j.intimp.2017.07.007
35. Wang Y, Peng C, Cheng Z, Wang X, Wu L, Li J, et al. The prognostic significance of preoperative neutrophil-lymphocyte ratio in patients with hepatocellular carcinoma receiving hepatectomy: A systematic review and meta-analysis. *Int J Surg* (2018) 55:73–80. doi: 10.1016/j.ijsu.2018.05.022

5

Resection vs. Sorafenib for Hepatocellular Carcinoma with Macroscopic Vascular Invasion: A Real World, Propensity Score Matched Analytic Study

Jie Mei[1,2,3†], *Shao-Hua Li*[1,2,3†], *Qiao-Xuan Wang*[2,3,4†], *Liang-He Lu*[1,2,3], *Yi-Hong Ling*[2,3,5], *Jing-Wen Zou*[1,2,3], *Wen-Ping Lin*[1,2,3], *Yu-Hua Wen*[1,2,3], *Wei Wei*[1,2,3*†] and *Rong-Ping Guo*[1,2,3*†]

[1] *Department of Hepatobiliary Oncology, Sun Yat-sen University Cancer Center, Guangzhou, China,* [2] *State Key Laboratory of Oncology in South China, Guangzhou, China,* [3] *Collaborative Innovation Center for Cancer Medicine, Guangzhou, China,* [4] *Department of Radiation Oncology, Sun Yat-sen University Cancer Center, Guangzhou, China,* [5] *Department of Pathology, Sun Yat-sen University Cancer Center, Guangzhou, China*

***Correspondence:**
Wei Wei
weiwei@sysucc.org.cn
Rong-Ping Guo
guorp@sysucc.org.cn

† *These authors have contributed equally to this work*

Background: Macroscopic vascular invasion (MVI) commonly occurs in patients with advanced hepatocellular carcinoma (HCC) for which resection and sorafenib are the common therapies prescribed. Here, we aimed to compare the survival outcomes of these two therapies in HCC patients with MVI.

Methods: In total, 496 patients diagnosed with HCC and MVI without extrahepatic metastasis, treated with resection (resection-based group, $n = 388$) and sorafenib (sorafenib-based group, $n = 108$) were included in this study. A one-to-one propensity score-matching analysis (PSM) was performed to minimize the effect of potential confounders.

Results: The median OS in the resection- and sorafenib-based group was 20.7 months (95% CI: 16.9–24.5) and 11.6 months (95% CI: 8.4–14.9) ($p < 0.001$), respectively. The median PFS was 4.7 months (95% CI: 3.8–5.5) in the resection-based group and 4.4 months (95% CI: 3.6–5.2) in the sorafenib-based group ($p < 0.001$). After PSM, 72 patients from each group were matched. The median OS was 27.2 months (95% CI: 16.4–38.0) in the resection-based group and 13.0 months (95% CI: 9.6–16.3) in the sorafenib-based group ($p < 0.001$). The median PFS was 5.3 months (95% CI: 3.2–7.4) in the resection-based group and 4.8 months (95% CI: 3.6–6.0) in the sorafenib-based group ($p = 0.061$).

Conclusion: Findings from this study showed that, compared with sorafenib-based treatment, surgical resection might be associated with better survival benefits to HCC patients with MVI.

Keywords: hepatocellular carcinoma, macroscopic vascular invasion, resection, sorafenib, propensity score matched

INTRODUCTION

Hepatocellular carcinoma (HCC) is one of the most common malignancies, and the fourth leading cause of cancer-related deaths worldwide (1). Because of its concealed onset, HCC often progresses to macroscopic vascular invasion (MVI) at the time of diagnosis (2). Before new targeted drugs such as lenvatinib and immune checkpoint inhibitors were available, the first-line of treatment for HCC patients with MVI recommended by the Barcelona guideline was systemic therapy with sorafenib (3) and had a median overall survival (mOS) ranging from 5.6 to 8.1 months (4, 5). However, in the Asia-Pacific region, some patients with MVI, especially those without extrahepatic metastases, could still benefit from survival through resection, with mOS ranging from 8.9 to 33 months (6–11). Therefore, the optimal choice between the two therapies for HCC patients with MVI was controversal.

To date, only a few studies have investigated the prognosis of surgical resection in comparison to sorafenib in HCC patients with MVI and inconsistent results have been reported, possibly, due to imbalanced patients characteristics between the investigated cohorts and a limited number of enrolled patients (8, 12). Nowadays, the vast majority of patients with MVI were not in the initial treatment state when receiving surgery or sorafenib. Late-stage HCC patients are referred to combined therapies, instead of surgery or sorafenib alone. Therefore, relevant clinical researches were valuable.

The purpose of this study was to compare the prognoses of HCC patients with MVI undergoing surgical resection and sorafenib, aiming to provide a reference for the treatment of advanced HCC patients.

MATERIALS AND METHODS

This study was conducted according to the ethical guidelines of the 1975 Declaration of Helsinki. The analysis of the patient data was reviewed and approved by the Institutional Review Board and Human Ethics Committee at the Sun Yat-sen University Cancer Center (SYSUCC; Guangzhou, China).

Patients

The medical records of patients diagnosed with HCC and MVI without extrahepatic metastasis who underwent surgical resection or were prescribed sorafenib as part of standard therapy at the Department of Liver Surgery (SYSUCC), between 2005 and 2017, were reviewed for eligibility. Some patients were excluded based on the following criteria: (a) diagnosed with malignant diseases other than HCC; (b) aged >80 or <18; (c) had a performance status score >1; (d) had incomplete follow-up or medical information; (e) had sorafenib treatment for <2 months. Those who first received surgical resection treatment were classified into a resection-based group, while those who first received sorafenib-based treatment were classified into a sorafenib-based group. The patient enrolment and categorization flow chart is shown in **Figure 1**. All laboratory serum test data was collected within 3 days before treatment (resection or sorafenib). Preoperative imaging examinations included contrast-enhanced computed tomography (CT) or magnetic resonance imaging (MRI) within a week before treatment.

Treatment Procedure

Hepatic resection was performed as previously described (13). Intraoperative ultrasound was routinely performed to evaluate the tumor burden, remnant liver, and possibility of a negative resection margin. Anatomic hepatectomy with mass tumor thrombectomy was the preferred method of liver resection. Depending on its location and extent, the tumor thrombus was removed by en-bloc resected with the tumor tissue or extracted from the lumen of the blood vessel. Tumor thrombus was confirmed by rinsing with normal saline, and the absence of tumor thrombus formation was confirmed by intraoperative ultrasound.

Sorafenib (Bayer, Leverkusen, Germany) was initially orally administered 200 or 400 mg twice daily and continued for at least 2 months. Withdrawal and reduction of the drug depended on unacceptable toxicities or untreatable disease progression.

The final follow-up ended on July 31, 2019. Enhanced CT or MRI was performed every 2 or 3 months after surgery or sorafenib according to subsequent therapies. Follow-ups were performed as previously described (14), unless judged otherwise by the treating physicians.

Diagnosis and Definitions

The diagnosis of MVI was based on standard radiological imaging prior to treatment (resection or sorafenib prescription) (15, 16). Portal vein tumor thrombus (PVTT) was graded according to the classification suggested by the Liver Cancer Study Group of Japan (17). Based on liver vessel structure and prognosis for different location of vascular tumor thrombus (18), we combined hepatic vein tumor thrombus (HVTT) into PVTT classification, based on which, Vp1 represented the invasion of a third-order branch or distal to the second branch of the portal vein; Vp2, invasion of a second-order branch of the portal vein, or branch of the hepatic vein; Vp3, invasion of in the first branch of the portal vein, or hepatic vein trunk or the short hepatic vein; Vp4, invasion of the main trunk/controlateral branch of the portal vein, or inferior vena cava. Overall survival (OS) was defined as the time interval from treatment initiation to cancer-related death. Progression-free survival (PFS) was defined as the time interval from treatment initiation to tumor progression. For the resection-based group, tumor progression was defined as intrahepatic recurrence or new intrahepatic or extrahepatic lesions developed. For the sorafenib-based group, progression was defined as progressive disease (PD) according to the modified response evaluation criteria in solid tumors (mRECIST) (19), progressive intrahepatic tumor thrombus or extrahepatic metastasis.

Statistical Analysis

Categorical variables in baseline characteristics were compared using the Pearson's χ^2 test or Fisher's exact test. To minimize the influence of selection bias produced by preoperative factors between the two groups, propensity score matching (PSM)

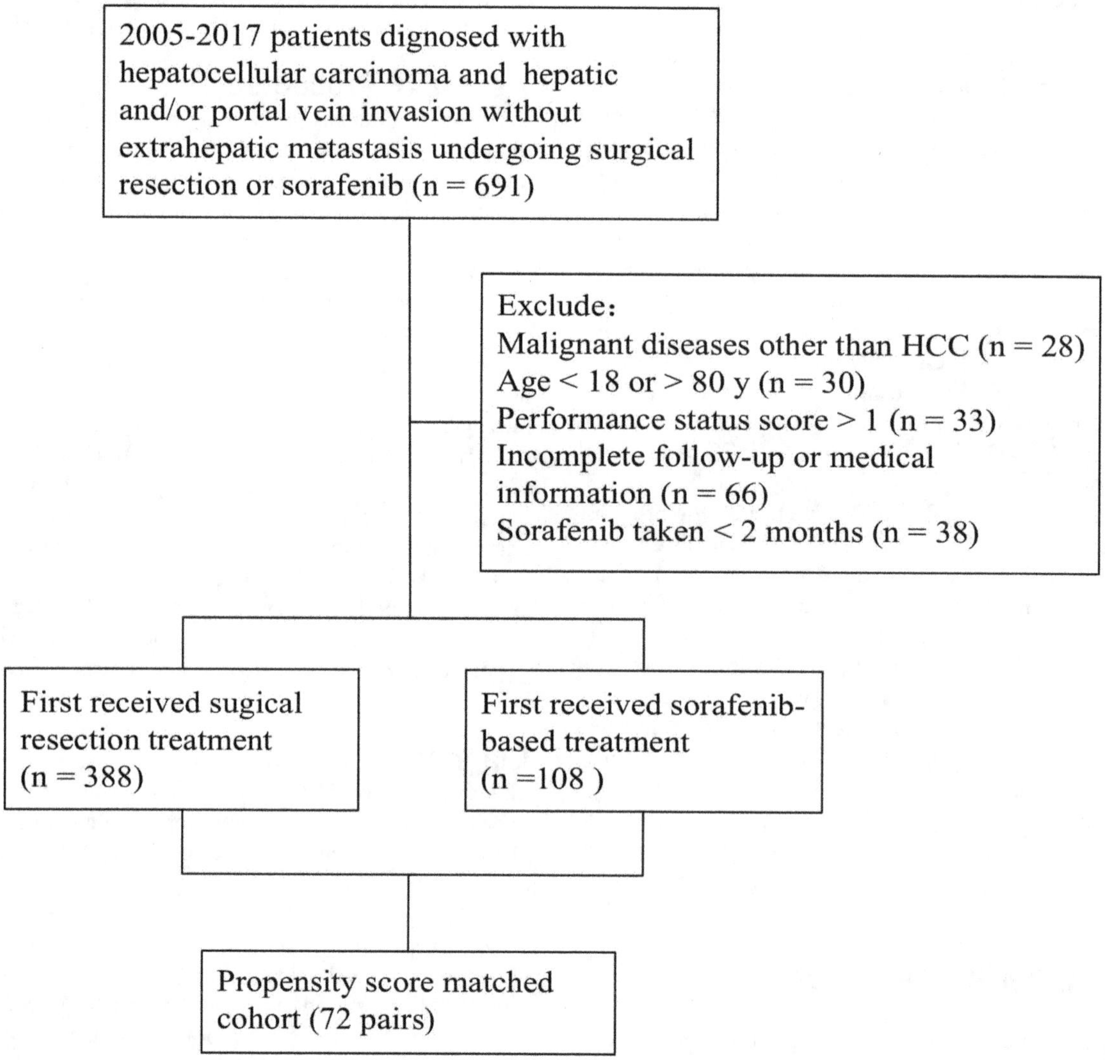

FIGURE 1 | Patient enrolment and categorization flow chart.

was conducted using a logistic regression model (20, 21). Pre-treatment variables were entered into the PSM, comprising of age (≤/>50 years old), gender (male/female), hepatitis B surface antigen DNA (HBs DNA) (≤103/>103), liver cirrhosis (None or mild/Moderate or severe), aspartate aminotransferase (AST) (≤50/>50 U/L), albumin (ALB) (≤40/>40 g/L), total bilirubin (TBIL) (≤20.5/>20.5 μmol/L), prothrombin time (PT) (≤13.5/>13.5 s), Child-Pugh score (5/>5), tumor number (1/>1), largest nodule (<5/5-10/>10 cm), distribution (Uni-lobar/Bi-lobar), tumor thrombus (Vp1/2/3/4). PSM was performed by a 1:1 matching method with a caliper width of 0.1. Survival analyses were calculated using the Kaplan-Meier method and differences in survival curves were analyzed using the log-rank test. All variables with a $P < 0.1$ in univariate analyses were used in multivariate analyses using the Cox's proportional hazards models. The hazard ratio (HR) and confidence intervals (CI) were also calculated. A value of two-tailed $P < 0.05$ was considered statistically significant. All data analyses were performed using SPSS 25.0 software (SPSS Inc., Chicago, IL) and GraphPad Prism (version 8.0; GraphPad, Inc.).

RESULTS

Identification of Study Patients

From 2005 to 2017, 488 patients with HCC who underwent surgical resection ($n = 388$) or sorafenib ($n = 108$) treatment after a diagnosis of MVI without extrahepatic metastasis were identified. Of note, all patients in the sorafenib-based group were treated since January 2009 because sorafenib was available only from that year. In the resection-based group, 88 (22.7%) patients underwent surgical resection before January 2009 and the rest after January 2009.

TABLE 1 | Baseline clinical characteristics of patients before PSM.

Characteristic*	Resection-based (n = 388)	Sorafenib-based (n = 108)	*P*-value
Age (y)			0.064
≤50	215 (55.4)	49 (45.4)	
>50	173 (44.6)	59 (54.6)	
Gender			0.831
Female	23 (6.0)	7 (6.5)	
Male	365 (94.0)	101 (93.5)	
HBsAg			0.675
Negative	64 (16.5)	16 (14.8)	
Positive	324 (83.5)	92 (85.2)	
HBVDNA			0.032
≤ 10^3	181 (46.6)	63 (58.3)	
> 10^3	207 (53.4)	45 (41.7)	
Cirrhosis			< 0.001
None or mild	190 (49.0)	23 (21.3)	
Moderate or severe	198 (51.0)	85 (78.7)	
Ascites			0.542
Absent or mild	359 (92.5)	98 (90.7)	
Moderate or severe	29 (7.5)	10 (9.3)	
PLT (10E9/L)			0.192
≤100	37 (9.5)	15 (13.9)	
>100	351 (90.5)	93 (86.1)	
ALT (U/L)			0.720
≤50	248 (63.9)	67 (62.0)	
>50	140 (36.1)	41 (38.0)	
AST (U/L)			0.008
≤40	151 (38.9)	27 (25.0)	
>40	237 (61.1)	81 (75.0)	
ALB (g/L)			< 0.001
≤40	117 (30.2)	52 (48.1)	
>40	271 (69.8)	56 (51.9)	
TBIL (μmol/L)			< 0.001
≤20.5	335 (86.3)	77 (71.3)	
>20.5	53 (13.7)	31 (28.7)	
PT (s)			0.094
≤13.5	323 (83.2)	97 (89.8)	
>13.5	65 (16.8)	11 (10.2)	
AFP (ng/ml)			0.336
≤400	135 (34.8)	43 (39.8)	
>400	253 (65.2)	65 (60.2)	
Child-pugh score			< 0.001
5	344 (88.7)	82 (75.9)	
6	39 (10.0)	24 (22.2)	
>6	5 (1.3)	2 (1.9)	
Number of tumor (s)			< 0.001
Single	263 (67.8)	35 (32.4)	
Multiple	125 (32.2)	73 (67.6)	
Tumor distribution			< 0.001
Uni-lobar	351 (90.5)	53 (49.1)	
Bi-lobar	37 (9.5)	55 (50.9)	

(Continued)

TABLE 1 | Continued

Characteristic*	Resection-based (n = 388)	Sorafenib-based (n = 108)	*P*-value
Size of largest nodule (cm)			0.172
<5	56 (14.4)	23 (21.3)	
5–10	214 (55.2)	51 (47.2)	
>10	118 (30.4)	34 (31.5)	
Tumor thrombus			
Vp1	22 (5.7)	1 (0.9)	< 0.001
Vp2	111 (28.6)	9 (8.3)	
VP3	237 (61.1)	57 (52.8)	
Vp4	18 (4.6)	41 (38.0)	
Pre-treatment			
None	306 (78.9)	40 (37.0)	
Surgery	7 (1.8)	12 (11.1)	
TACE	54 (13.9)	94 (87.0)	
RFA/PMCT	6 (1.5)	14 (13.0)	
HAIC	15 (3.9)	16 (14.8)	
Follow-up treatment			
Surgery	7 (1.8)	3 (2.8)	
TACE	169 (43.6)	41 (38.0)	
RFA/PMCT	51 (13.1)	12 (11.1)	
TAI	12 (3.1)	15 (13.9)	
Radiotherapy	7 (1.8)	6 (5.6)	
Sorafenib	25 (6.4)	–	

**No. (%).*
PSM, propensity score matching; HBsAg, hepatitis B surface antigen; PLT, blood platelet; ALT, alanine aminotransferase; AST, aspartate aminotransferase; ALB, albumin; TBIL, total bilirubin; PT, prothrombin time; AFP, alpha fetoprotein; TACE, transcatheter arterial chemoembolization; RFA, radiofrequency ablation; PMCT, percutaneous microwave coagulation therapy; HAIC, hepatic artery infusion chemotherapy.

Characteristics of the Study Patients

Between 2005 and 2017, 691 patients were reviewed for eligibility and 496 patients were ultimately included in this study (388 in resection-based group, 108 in sorafenib-based group).

The clinical pre-treatment characteristics of the patients in the resection-based and sorafenib-based groups are summarized in **Table 1**. In general, patients who underwent surgical resection had smaller tumor burden and better liver function. In the resection-based group, a smaller proportion of patients had severer liver cirrhosis (51.0 vs. 78.7%, $p < 0.001$), higher child-pugh score (11.3 vs. 24.1%, $p < 0.001$), higher AST (61.1 vs. 75.0%, $p = 0.008$), and higher TBIL (13.7 vs. 28.7, $p < 0.001$), as compared to the sorafenib-based group. Meanwhile, larger proportion of patients in the sorafenib-based group were with multiple (67.6 vs. 32.2%, $p < 0.001$) or bilateral tumors (50.9 vs. 9.5%, $p < 0.001$), and had higher tumor thrombus grade (Vp3 and Vp4, 90.8 vs. 65.7%, $p < 0.001$). 313(80.7%) patients received surgical resection as their first treatment in the resection-based group, while only 40 (37.0%) patients were first treated with sorafenib in sorafenib-based treatment. In this study, 25 (6.6%) patients received subsequent sorafenib treatment in

TABLE 2 | Baseline clinical characteristics of patients after PSM.

Characteristic*	Therapy		*P*-value
	Resection-based ($n = 72$)	Sorafenib-based ($n = 72$)	
Age (y)			0.238
≤50	27 (37.5)	34 (47.2)	
>50	45 (62.5)	38 (52.8)	
Gender			1.000
Female	5 (6.9)	5 (6.9)	
Male	67 (93.1)	67 (93.1)	
HBsAg			0.061
Negative	19 (26.4)	10 (13.9)	
Positive	53 (73.6)	62 (86.1)	
HBVDNA			0.133
$\leq 10^3$	33 (45.8)	42 (58.3)	
$>10^3$	39 (54.2)	30 (41.7)	
Cirrhosis			0.218
None or mild	28 (38.9)	21 (29.2)	
Moderate or severe	44 (61.1)	51 (70.8)	
Ascites			0.275
Absent or mild	70 (97.2)	66 (91.7)	
Moderate or severe	2 (2.8)	6 (8.3)	
PLT (10E9/L)			0.614
≤100	8 (11.1)	10 (13.9)	
>100	64 (88.9)	62 (86.1)	
ALT (U/L)			0.590
≤50	51 (70.8)	48 (66.7)	
>50	21 (29.2)	24 (33.3)	
AST (U/L)			0.230
≤40	31 (43.1)	24 (33.3)	
>40	41 (56.9)	48 (66.7)	
ALB (g/L)			0.053
≤40	19 (26.4)	30 (41.7)	
>40	53 (73.6)	42 (58.3)	
TBIL (μmol/L)			0.533
≤20.5	59 (81.9)	56 (77.8)	
>20.5	13 (18.1)	16 (22.2)	
PT (s)			0.532
≤13.5	68 (94.4)	65 (90.3)	
>13.5	4 (5.6)	7 (9.7)	
AFP (ng/ml)			0.230
≤400	24 (33.3)	31 (43.1)	
>400	48 (66.7)	41 (56.9)	
Child-pugh score			0.386
5	61 (84.7)	57 (79.2)	
>5	11 (15.3)	15 (20.8)	
Number of tumor (s)			0.736
Single	30 (41.7)	32 (44.4)	
Multiple	42 (58.3)	40 (55.6)	
Tumor distribution			0.278
Uni-lobar	53 (73.6)	47 (65.3)	
Bi-lobar	19 (26.4)	25 (34.7)	
Size of largest nodule (cm)			0.974
<5	17 (23.6)	16 (22.2)	
5-10	34 (47.2)	34 (47.2)	
>10	21 (29.2)	22 (30.6)	
Tumor thrombus			0.143
Vp1	2 (2.8)	1 (1.4)	
Vp2	10 (13.9)	9 (12.5)	
VP3	51 (70.8)	42 (58.3)	
VP4	9 (12.5)	20 (27.8)	
Pre-treatment			
None	50 (69.4)	20 (27.8)	
Surgery	0 (0)	12 (16.7)	
TACE	13 (18.1)	42 (58.3)	
RFA/PMCT	2 (2.8)	12 (16.7)	
HAIC	9 (12.5)	11 (15.3)	
Follow-up treatment			
Surgery	2 (2.8)	3 (4.2)	
TACE	27 (37.5)	26 (36.1)	
RFA/PMCT	6 (8.3)	9 (12.5)	
TAI	7 (9.7)	13 (18.1)	
Sorafenib	4 (5.6)	–	

*No. (%).
PSM, propensity score matching; HBsAg, hepatitis B surface antigen; PLT, blood platelet; ALT, alanine aminotransferase; AST, aspartate aminotransferase; ALB, albumin; TBIL, total bilirubin; PT, prothrombin time; AFP, alpha fetoprotein; TACE, transcatheter arterial chemoembolization; RFA, radiofrequency ablation; PMCT, percutaneous microwave coagulation therapy; HAIC, hepatic artery infusion chemotherapy.

the resection-based group, while 3 (2.8%) patients chose surgical resection afterward in the sorafenib-based group.

After a 1:1 PSM, 72 pairs of patients were selected. The basic clinical characteristics between the two groups were almost consistent (**Table 2**). Initially treated patients still differed, for 50 (69.4%) in the resection-based group and 20 (27.8%) in the sorafenib-based group. As for additional treatments, 4 patients received sorafenib after surgery and 3 patients received surgical resection after sorafenib treatment.

Overall Survival Analysis

Before PSM, the median OS was 20.7 months (95% CI: 16.9–24.5) in the resection-based group and 11.6 months (95% CI: 8.4–14.9) in the sorafenib-based group ($p < 0.001$). The median PFS was 4.7 months (95% CI: 3.8–5.5) in the resection-based group and 4.4 months (95% CI: 3.6–5.2) in the sorafenib-based group ($p < 0.001$). The 6-, 12-, and 24-month OS rates in the resection-based group were 74.0, 55.0, and 33.9%, respectively, and in the sorafenib-based group they were 71.3, 45.4, and 13.0%, respectively. The 6-, 12-, and 24-month PFS rates in the resection-based group were 41.8, 28.4, and 20.5%, respectively, and in the sorafenib-based group they were 33.3, 13.0, and 3.7%, respectively. Survival graphs of the different groups of patients are shown in **Figure 2**.

Survival Analysis in the Matching Cohort

After PSM, the median OS was 27.2 months (95% CI: 16.4–38.0) in the resection-based group and 13.0 months (95% CI: 9.6–16.3) in the sorafenib-based group ($p < 0.001$). The median PFS was 5.3 months (95% CI: 3.2–7.4) in the resection-based group and 4.8 months (95% CI: 3.6–6.0) in the sorafenib-based group ($p = 0.061$). The 6-, 12-, and 24-month OS rates in the resection-based group were 80.6, 56.9, and 25.0%, respectively, and in the sorafenib-based group, they were 72.2, 47.2, and 15.3%, respectively. The 6-, 12-, and 24-month PFS rates in the resection-based group were 48.6, 26.4, and 11.1%, respectively, and in the sorafenib-based group, they were 38.9, 13.9, and 5.6%, respectively. Survival graphs are shown in **Figure 3**. Forest plot analyses of factors associated with OS showed that resection provided a superior clinical benefit in most pre-planned subgroups except in female patients and those with tumor size <5 cm and Vp4 thrombus (**Figure 4**), as compared to sorafenib. ForPFS, resection only benefited patients with a single tumor (**Figure S1**).

Prognostic Factors Analysis of Matched Patients

The risk factors for OS and PFS were analyzed in the matched cohorts (**Tables S1, S2**). Multivariate analyses identified male (HR = 4.199, 95% CI: 1.023–17.234, $p = 0.046$), patients with ALB > 40 g/L (HR = 0.563, 95% CI: 0.357–0.889, $p = 0.014$), and sorafenib-based treatment (HR = 2.310, 95% CI: 1.481–3.587, $p < 0.001$) as three significant factors associated with OS. Sorafenib-based treatment (HR = 1.391, 95% CI: 0.982–1.968, p

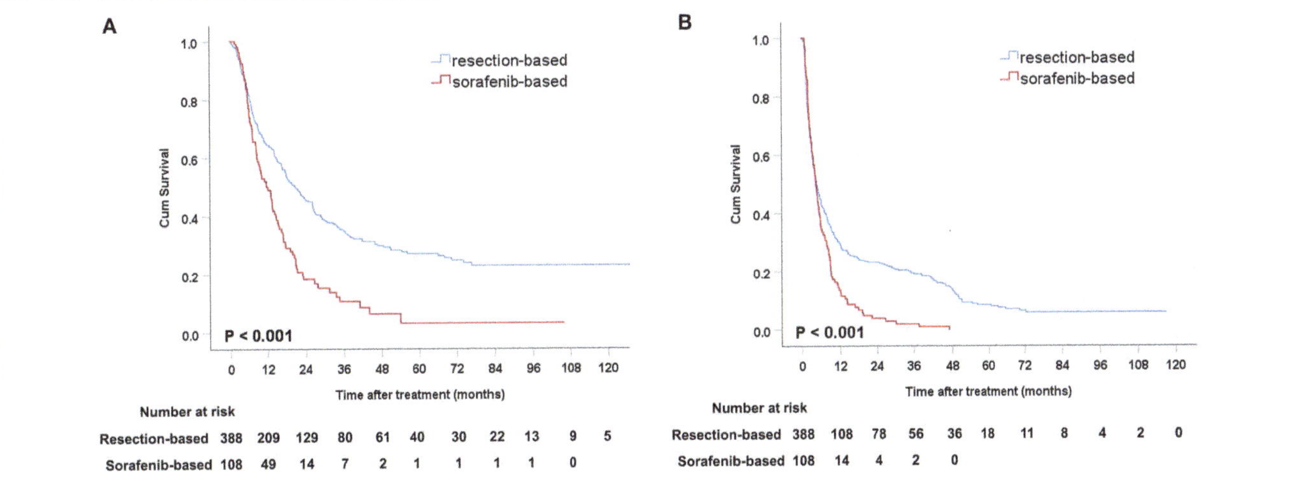

FIGURE 2 | Kaplan-Meier curves of survival outcomes after resection and sorafenib treatment in all patients. **(A)** Overall survival and **(B)** progression-free survival.

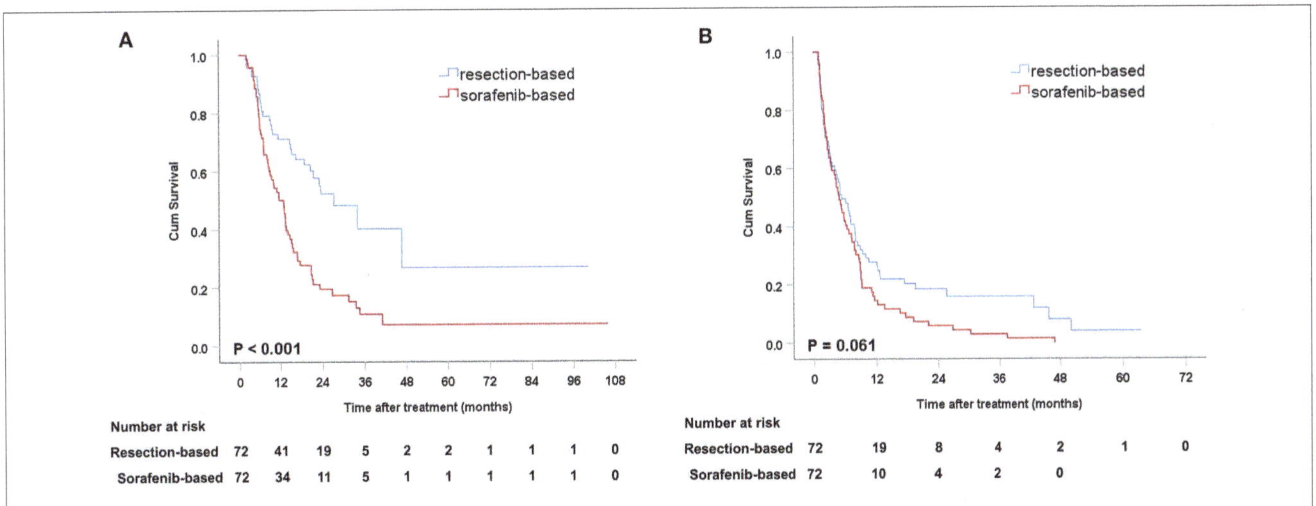

FIGURE 3 | Kaplan-Meier curves of survival outcomes after resection and sorafenib treatment in matched patients. **(A)** Overall survival and **(B)** progression-free survival.

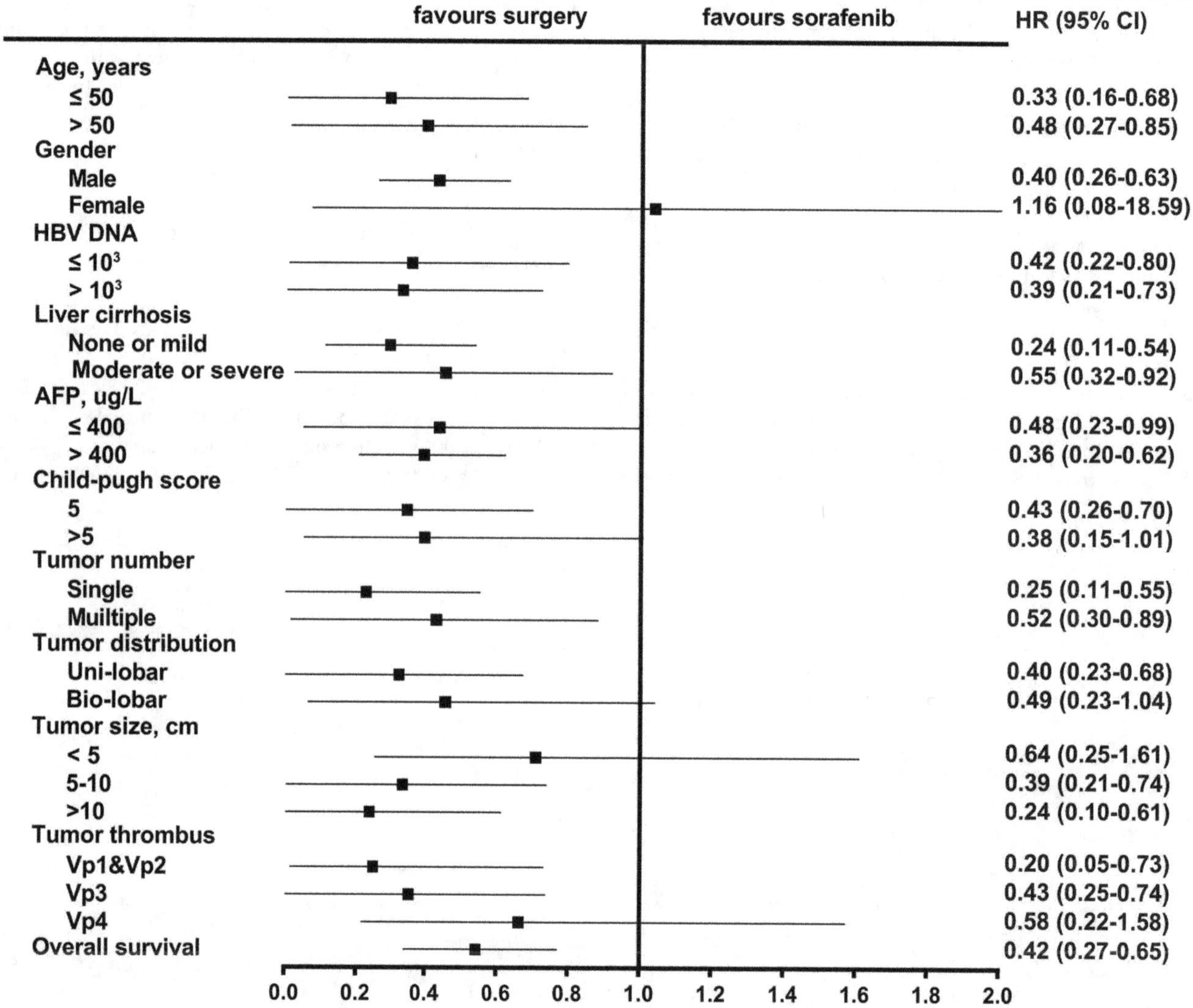

FIGURE 4 | Forest plot for overall survival of the matched cohorts of patients.

= 0.063) was a unique factor for RFS in both the univariate and multivariate analysis.

Progression Analysis of Matched Patients

The position of assessable tumor progression was analyzed in the matched cohorts (**Table S3**). Patients treated with sorafenib tended to have more intrahepatic progression (91.2 vs. 68.5%, $p = 0.003$). However, there was no statistically significant difference for extrahepatic progression between patients who underwent resection and sorafenib treatment (40.7 vs. 26.3%, $p = 0.107$).

Survival Analysis of Confounding Factors

Due to the actual treatment, the proportion of initial treated patients in the two groups was inconsistent. Thus, we further explore the prognosis of primary and non-primary patients in the two groups. Patients who underwent non-primary resection had better OS (mOS, 34.0 vs. 18.2 months, $p = 0.005$) but similar PFS (mPFS, 4.1 vs. 4.8 months, $p = 0.885$) as compared to those who received primary resection (**Figure S2**). No significant survival difference was found between patients received primary and non-primary sorafenib treatment (mOS, 13.6 vs. 10.1 months, $p = 0.565$; mPFS, 5.0 vs. 3.9 months, $p = 0.407$; **Figure S3**). In the resection-based group, 25 patients were treated with sorafenib after surgical resection and our findings showed that they had no superior OS or PFS (mOS, 24.1 vs. 20.7 months, $p = 0.900$; mPFS, 3.7 vs. 4.7 months, $p = 0.077$) than those who did not take sorafenib during the follow-up treatment (**Figure S4**).

DISCUSSION

At present, the optimal therapy for advanced HCC remained uncertain. Although most European guidelines recommend targeted therapy as the first-line therapy, there were still a large number of studies confirming that surgery could bring survival benefit (6–8, 17, 22). Our study proved that in the real world, for some selected patients with good liver function and low tumor burden, surgical resection could have significant benefits of survival and disease control. After PSM, in the two groups of patients with similar baseline levels, surgery was still associated with significant increase in OS.

To our knowledge, there are currently a few studies comparing the efficacy of surgery with sorafenib. Costentin CE reported that OS of patients with HCC and MVI undergoing surgical resection was similar to that treated with sorafenib in a multicenter retrospective study, but the tumor states of patients after matching were not consistent and the result was based on a small sample of patients (46 patients vs. 39 patients) (12). Lee et al. and Wang et al. suggested that surgery offered more survival benefits to advanced HCC patients than other treatments including sorafenib and TACE (8, 23). Kokudo et al. reported their results of surgery in a large cohort of more than 2,000 HCC patients with PVTT (17). The mOS in the resection group was 0.88 years longer than that in the non-resection group (2.45 vs. 1.57 years) in a propensity score-matched cohort. However, sorafenib was not included in the non-surgical treatments.

This study included initially treated and non-initially treated HCC patients with MVI. In our study, there were more initially treated patients who received resection than those who received sorafenib, which was in line with the actual treatment process for HCC patients in the Asia-Pacific region. In the sorafenib-based group, initially or non-initially treatment had no effect on OS and PFS. Several researchers indicated that proper therapies prior to sorafenib led to better survival outcomes for HCC patients (24, 25). It implied that in the treatment strategy of advanced HCC, multiple combinations of locoreginal and systemic modalities treatment could be applied, which may have a beneficial therapeutic impact. For the resection-based group, patients who received non-first-line resection had better prognosis. This might suggest that those patients who could undergo surgery could benefit from preoperative neoadjuvant therapies.

Multivariate analysis showed that indicators of liver function seemed to have a greater impact on prognosis than tumor burden, distribution, and tumor thrombus levels. It was confirmed by other researches that attention should be not only paid to tumor-related conditions, but also to the liver function of patients (26, 27).

The results of subgroup analyses showed that almost all subgroups of patients could have greater overall survival benefits from surgery, except for female patients. This was possibly due to the limited number of identifiable and enrollable cases. Patients with all tumor thrombus levels except Vp4 could benefit from surgery and therefore, systemic therapy would be recommendable for advanced patients with PVTT reaching the main portal vein or HVTT reaching the inferior vena cava. It was confusing that patients with tumor size within 5 centimeters had not a significant OS benefit from surgical resection. Given the relatively small number of patients with small tumors in the analyzed two groups (resection vs. sorafenib, 17 vs. 16), it might accidentally cause statistical bias. The wide range of CI (0.25–1.61) indicated the poor sample representation, which probably could not reveal a true clinical phenomenon. Thus, more cases needed to be accumulated to confirm this part of the issue.

In this study, 25 patients received sorafenib after surgery but their prognosis (mOS, 24.1 months, mPFS, 3.7 months) was not significantly different from those who did not take post-operative sorafenib. Bruix Jordi's phase 3, double-blind, placebo-controlled study showed sorafenib is not an effective intervention in the adjuvant setting for HCC following resection or ablation (28). So, the application of post-operative sorafenib was controversial.

To note, the characteristics showed that patients with a higher tumor burden and more severe liver pathology were given sorafenib-based treatment. This was also reflected by the result that sorafenib-treatment as a negative prognostic factor for this group of patients. So resection shall be given careful evaluation for advanced HCC patients.

This study had some limitations. First, this was a retrospective study and although PSM was applied, there may still be some inevitable selection biases. Second, due to multidisciplinary comprehensive treatment strategy for HCC with MVI, patients included in this study had strong heterogeneity. The final result could not get rid of the influence of confounding factors including previous, concomitant and subsequent treatment after surgery and sorafenib. In addition, after the PSM, the number of cases was relatively small. Findings from this study should be further expanded to multicenter to obtain higher-level medical evidence. Besides, it was worth noting that the analyzed patients were coming from an Asia-Pacific region which was known to have a high incidence of hepatitis B virus (HBV) associated HCCs. Given the high prevalence of HBV associated HCC in Caucasians, Hong Kong Liver Cancer (HKLC) score could be operation-prone due to a better stratification for these patients, where BCLC score might be conservative and unbefitting (29, 30). To better manage the treatment for patients with advanced HCC, especially in Caucasian, HKLC score was expected to applied.

In conclusion, our study indicated that, compared with sorafenib, surgical resection might be associated with better survival benefits in resectable HCC patients with MVI and adequate liver function, and should be considered as an important reliable therapy.

AUTHOR CONTRIBUTIONS

JM, WW, and R-PG conceived and designed the experiments. JM, S-HL, Q-XW, J-WZ, L-HL, and Y-HL collected the data. JM, W-PL, and Y-HW analyzed the data. JM wrote the paper. All authors have read and approved the final version of the manuscript.

REFERENCES

1. Bray F, Ferlay J, Soerjomataram I, Siegel RL, Torre LA, Jemal A. Global cancer statistics 2018: GLOBOCAN estimates of incidence and mortality worldwide for 36 cancers in 185 countries. *CA Cancer J Clin.* (2018) 68:394–424. doi: 10.3322/caac.21492
2. Wei W, Jian PE, Li SH, Guo ZX, Zhang YF, Ling YH, et al. Adjuvant transcatheter arterial chemoembolization after curative resection for hepatocellular carcinoma patients with solitary tumor and microvascular

invasion: a randomized clinical trial of efficacy and safety. *Cancer Commun.* (2018) 38:61. doi: 10.1186/s40880-018-0331-y
3. European Association for the Study of the Liver. Electronic address:easloffice@easloffice.eu; European Association for the Study of the Liver. EASL clinical practice guidelines: management of hepatocellular carcinoma. *J Hepatol.* (2018) 69:182–236. doi: 10.1016/j.jhep.2018.03.019
4. Bruix J, Raoul JL, Sherman M, Mazzaferro V, Bolondi L, Craxi A, et al. Efficacy and safety of sorafenib in patients with advanced hepatocellular carcinoma: subanalyses of a phase III trial. *J Hepatol.* (2012) 57:821–9. doi: 10.1016/j.jhep.2012.06.014
5. Cheng AL, Guan Z, Chen Z, Tsao CJ, Qin S, Kim JS, et al. Efficacy and safety of sorafenib in patients with advanced hepatocellular carcinoma according to baseline status: subset analyses of the phase III sorafenib Asia-pacific trial. *Eur J Cancer.* (2012) 48:1452–65. doi: 10.1016/j.ejca.2011.12.006
6. Liang L, Chen TH, Li C, Xing H, Han J, Wang MD, et al. A systematic review comparing outcomes of surgical resection and non-surgical treatments for patients with hepatocellular carcinoma and portal vein tumor thrombus. *HPB.* (2018) 20:1119–29. doi: 10.1016/j.hpb.2018.06.1804
7. Peng ZW, Guo RP, Zhang YJ, Lin XJ, Chen MS, Lau WY. Hepatic resection versus transcatheter arterial chemoembolization for the treatment of hepatocellular carcinoma with portal vein tumor thrombus. *Cancer.* (2012) 118:4725–36. doi: 10.1002/cncr.26561
8. Lee JM, Jang BK, Lee YJ, Choi WY, Choi SM, Chung WJ, et al. Survival outcomes of hepatic resection compared with transarterial chemoembolization or sorafenib for hepatocellular carcinoma with portal vein tumor thrombosis. *Clin Mol Hepatol.* (2016) 22:160–7. doi: 10.3350/cmh.2016.22.1.160
9. Aldrighetti L, Pulitano C, Catena M, Arru M, Guzzetti E, Halliday J, et al. Liver resection with portal vein thrombectomy for hepatocellular carcinoma with vascular invasion. *Ann Surg Oncol.* (2009) 16:1254. doi: 10.1245/s10434-009-0383-y
10. Zhang X-P, Wang K, Li N, Zhong CQ, Wei XB, Cheng YQ, et al. Survival benefit of hepatic resection versus transarterial chemoembolization for hepatocellular carcinoma with portal vein tumor thrombus: a systematic review and meta-analysis. *BMC Cancer.* (2017) 17:902. doi: 10.1186/s12885-017-3895-z
11. Omata M, Lesmana LA, Tateishi R, Chen PJ, Lin SM, Yoshida H, et al. Asian pacific association for the study of the liver consensus recommendations on hepatocellular carcinoma. *Hepatol Int.* (2010) 4:439–74. doi: 10.1007/s12072-010-9165-7
12. Decaens T, Laurent A, Nault JC, Paule B, Letoublon C, Luciani A, et al. Sorafenib vs surgical resection for hepatocellular carcinoma with macrovascular invasion: a propensity score analysis. *Liver Int.* (2017) 37:1869–76. doi: 10.1111/liv.13491
13. Shi M, Guo RP, Lin XJ, Zhang YQ, Chen MS, Zhang CQ, et al. Partial hepatectomy with wide versus narrow resection margin for solitary hepatocellular carcinoma: a prospective randomized trial. *Ann Surg.* (2007) 245:36–43. doi: 10.1097/01.sla.0000231758.07868.71
14. He W, Zheng Y, Zou R, Shen J, Yang J, Qiu J, et al. Long- versus short-interval follow-up after resection of hepatocellular carcinoma: a retrospective cohort study. *Cancer Commun.* (2018) 38:26. doi: 10.1186/s40880-018-0296-x
15. Kim JH, Lee JM, Yoon JH, Lee DH, Lee KB, Han JK, et al. Portal vein thrombosis in patients with hepatocellular carcinoma: diagnostic accuracy of gadoxetic acid-enhanced mr imaging. *Radiology.* (2016) 279:773–83. doi: 10.1148/radiol.2015150124
16. Choi JY, Lee JM, Sirlin CB. CT and MR imaging diagnosis and staging of hepatocellular carcinoma: part I. Development, growth, and spread: key pathologic and imaging aspects. *Radiology.* (2014) 272:635–54. doi: 10.1148/radiol.14132361
17. Kokudo T, Hasegawa K, Matsuyama Y, Takayama T, Izumi N, Kadoya M, et al. Survival benefit of liver resection for hepatocellular carcinoma associated with portal vein invasion. *J Hepatol.* (2016) 65:938–43. doi: 10.1016/j.jhep.2016.05.044
18. Ikai I, Yamamoto Y, Yamamoto N, Terajima H, Hatano E, Shimahara Y, et al. Results of hepatic resection for hepatocellular carcinoma invading major portal and/or hepatic veins. *Surg Oncol Clin N Am.* (2003) 12:65–75, ix. doi: 10.1016/S1055-3207(02)00082-0
19. Lencioni R, Llovet JM. Modified RECIST (mRECIST) assessment for hepatocellular carcinoma. *Semin Liver Dis.* (2010) 30:52–60. doi: 10.1055/s-0030-1247132
20. Austin PC. Optimal caliper widths for propensity-score matching when estimating differences in means and differences in proportions in observational studies. *Pharm Stat.* (2011) 10:150–61. doi: 10.1002/pst.433
21. Austin PC. A tutorial and case study in propensity score analysis: an application to estimating the effect of in-hospital smoking cessation counseling on mortality. *Multivariate Behav Res.* (2011) 46:119–51. doi: 10.1080/00273171.2011.540480
22. Kokudo T, Hasegawa K, Yamamoto S, Shindoh J, Takemura N, Aoki T, et al. Surgical treatment of hepatocellular carcinoma associated with hepatic vein tumor thrombosis. *J Hepatol.* (2014) 61:583–8. doi: 10.1016/j.jhep.2014.04.032
23. Wang JH, Kuo YH, Wang CC, Chen CL, Cheng YF, Hsu HC, et al. Surgical resection improves the survival of selected hepatocellular carcinoma patients in Barcelona clinic liver cancer stage C. *Dig Liver Dis.* (2013) 45:510–5. doi: 10.1016/j.dld.2012.10.019
24. Geschwind JF, Kudo M, Marrero JA, Venook AP, Chen XP, Bronowicki JP, et al. TACE treatment in patients with sorafenib-treated unresectable hepatocellular carcinoma in clinical practice: final analysis of GIDEON. *Radiology.* (2016) 279:630–40. doi: 10.1148/radiol.2015150667
25. Abdel-Rahman O. Impact of baseline characteristics on outcomes of advanced HCC patients treated with sorafenib: a secondary analysis of a phase III study. *J Cancer Res Clin Oncol.* (2018) 144:901–8. doi: 10.1007/s00432-018-2610-z
26. Mei J, Li SH, Wang QX, Zhong XP, Lu LH, Kan A, et al. A novel treatment strategy using indocyanine green for transarterial chemoembolization in BCLC stage C hepatocellular carcinoma. *Cancer Med.* (2019) 62–76. doi: 10.1002/cam4.2671
27. Doyle A, Marsh P, Gill R, Rodov M, Mohsen W, Varma P, et al. Sorafenib in the treatment of hepatocellular carcinoma: a multi-centre real-world study. *Scand J Gastroenterol.* (2016) 51:979–85. doi: 10.3109/00365521.2016.1166518
28. Bruix J, Takayama T, Mazzaferro V, Chau G-Y, Yang J, Kudo M, et al. Adjuvant sorafenib for hepatocellular carcinoma after resection or ablation (STORM): a phase 3, randomised, double-blind, placebo-controlled trial. *Lancet Oncol.* (2015) 16:1344–54. doi: 10.1016/S1470-2045(15)00198-9
29. Yau T, Tang VY, Yao TJ, Fan ST, Lo CM, Poon RT. Development of hong kong liver cancer staging system with treatment stratification for patients with hepatocellular carcinoma. *Gastroenterology.* (2014) 146:1691–700.e3. doi: 10.1053/j.gastro.2014.02.032
30. Wallace MC, Huang Y, Preen DB, Garas G, Adams LA, MacQuillan G, et al. HKLC triages more hepatocellular carcinoma patients to curative therapies compared to BCLC and is associated with better survival. *Dig Dis Sci.* (2017) 62:2182–92. doi: 10.1007/s10620-017-4622-y

6

Transarterial Chemoembolization in Treatment-Naïve and Recurrent Hepatocellular Carcinoma

Yiming Liu[1,2†], Yanqiao Ren[1,2†], Sangluobu Ge[1,2], Bin Xiong[1,2], Guofeng Zhou[1,2], Gansheng Feng[1,2], Songlin Song[1,2] and Chuansheng Zheng[1,2*]*

[1] *Department of Radiology, Union Hospital, Tongji Medical College, Huazhong University of Science and Technology, Wuhan, China,*
[2] *Hubei Provinve Key Laboratory of Molecular Imaging, Wuhan, China*

***Correspondence:**
Songlin Song
song9413lin@sina.cn
Chuansheng Zheng
hqzcsxh@sina.com*

†These authors have contributed equally to this work

Objectives: The purpose of this study was to evaluate the efficacy and safety of transarterial chemoembolization (TACE) in the treatment of patients with treatment-naïve hepatocellular carcinoma (TN-HCC) and recurrent HCC (R-HCC). In addition, risk signature analysis was performed to accurately assess patients' recurrence and survival.

Methods: This retrospective study assessed the consecutive medical records of TN-HCC and R-HCC patients from January 2014 to December 2018. In order to reduce the patient selection bias, propensity score matching (PSM) analysis was applied. Conditional inference tree was used to establish a risk signature.

Results: A total of 401 eligible patients were included in our study, including 346 patients in the TN-HCC group and 55 patients in the R-HCC group. Forty-seven pairs of patients were chosen after the PSM analysis. Before the PSM analysis, the objective tumor regression (ORR) and disease control rate (DCR) of R-HCC patients were better than that of TN-HCC patients; however, after the PSM analysis, there was no significant difference in the ORR and DCR between the two groups (P>0.05). Before the PSM analysis, the median overall survival (OS) and progression-free survival (PFS) in the R-HCC group were significantly greater than those of the TN-HCC group (OS: 24 months *vs.* 18 months, *P* =0.004; PFS: 9 months *vs.* 6 months, *P* =0.012). However, after the PSM analysis, the median OS and PFS in the R-HCC group were inferior to those in the TN-HCC group (OS: 24 months *vs.* 33 months, *P*= 0.0035; PFS: 10 months vs. 12 months, *P* = 0.01). The conditional inference tree divided patients into different subgroups according to tumor size, BCLC stage, and TACE sessions and shared different hazards ratio to recurrence or survival.

Conclusion: Patients with R-HCC treated with TACE achieved satisfactory results, although survival after the PSM analysis was not as good as in the TN-HCC group. In addition, risk signature based on conditional inference tree analysis can more accurately predict the recurrence and survival in both groups of patients.

Keywords: hepatocellular carcinoma, transarterial chemoembolization, liver resection, recurrence, propensity score matching

INTRODUCTION

Hepatocellular carcinoma (HCC) is the fifth most common cancer and one of the most frequent causes of cancer-related death (1). Globally, and especially in China, the prognosis of HCC patients remains a depressing issue. Currently, therapies such as liver resection (LR) and liver transplantation have the potential to cure patients with preserved liver function, but these curative therapies only benefit a quarter of HCC patients (2, 3). In addition, intrahepatic recurrence and *de novo* tumor emergence in the liver remnant after LR are common, with a 5-year recurrence rate of up to 70%-80% (4). Although this is a common clinical manifestation, there is still no consensus on the treatment of recurrent HCC (R-HCC) after LR, which remains a thorny issue that currently confounds clinicians and patients.

When intrahepatic tumors recur, re-resection or salvage liver transplantation remains the best way to cure the patient. However, not all recurrent patients are eligible for surgical treatment due to the limited reserve of liver function in the residual liver, postoperative adhesion, or lack of a liver donor (5, 6). As a result, only a small number of patients benefit from curative treatments, which may create an incentive to try other therapies and approaches.

Transarterial chemoembolization (TACE) combines targeted chemotherapy with arterial embolization, which is the main palliative method for the treatment of HCC (7). Two randomized controlled trials (2, 8) established the status of TACE in BCLC stage B HCC patients, for whom TACE is recommended as the standard of care. Meanwhile, TACE has also been reported in patients with BCLC stage C HCC, and the results indicated that TACE can benefit these patients (9, 10). Currently, most studies have assessed the efficacy of TACE in patients with treatment-naïve HCC (TN-HCC), but it is also worth exploring whether TACE can benefit patients with R-HCC after LR compared with patients with TN-HCC.

Since TACE is not limited by tumor size, location and number of lesions, it is suitable for most types of HCC and is widely used in patients with R-HCC after LR (11). Therefore, the purpose of this study was to evaluate the efficacy and safety of TACE in patients with TN-HCC and R-HCC after LR by propensity score matching (PSM) analysis. Furthermore, prognostic factors influencing the efficacy of TACE in both groups were also analyzed. Meanwhile, the conditional inference tree analysis was constructed to assess recurrence and survival in both groups after TACE.

METHODS

Study Design and Patient Selection

We reviewed the electronic medical records of 2158 consecutive patients who received TACE in our medical center from January 2014 to December 2018 for HCC, including patients with TN-HCC and with R-HCC after LR. Prior to these patients received initial TACE, the treatment plan was nominated by the multidisciplinary tumor board. This retrospective study was approved by the institutional review board of the Union Hospital, Tongji Medical College, Huazhong University of Science and Technology. Written informed consent for the patients' data to be used for research purposes was obtained from all patients prior to treatment.

The diagnosis of HCC depended on the guidelines of the European Association for the Study of Liver and the American Association for the Study of Liver Disease (12). A total of 401 patients in this study met the inclusion criteria: (1) age > 18 years; (2) Child-Pugh class A or B; (3) Eastern Cooperative Oncology Group (ECOG) performance status of 0–1. The exclusion criteria were: (1) Incomplete clinical information; (2) main portal vein obstruction; (3) BCLC stage D; (4) ECOG>1; (5) Severe medical comorbidities, including hepatic dysfunction (total bilirubin serum levels > 3 mg/dL, serum albumin level < 2.0 mg/dL, INR > 1.5), renal impairment (serum creatinine level >2 mg/dL) and severe coagulation disorders (prothrombin activity<40% or platelet count<30X10^9/L); (6) Uncontrolled infection (**Figure 1**).

TACE Procedure

TACE was performed based on our institutional standard protocol and has been described previously (13, 14). Briefly, angiography was performed to determine tumor staining and tumor-supplying vessels, and a 5-F catheter (Cook, Bloomington, Indiana, USA) or 3-F microcatheter (Progreat, Terumo, Tokyo, Japan) was inserted as far as possible into the tumor supplying vessels. Then, an emulsion of 2–20 mL iodized oil (Lipiodol Ultra-Fluid; Laboratoire Andre Guerbet, Aulnay-sous-Bois, France) and 20–60 mg doxorubicin hydrochloride was injected into the target vessels. Finally, gelatin sponge particles (300–700μm, Alicon, Hangzhou, China) were injected for additional embolization until the stasis of arteries flow was achieved. After embolization, reexamination angiography of the feeding artery was performed to confirm the devascularization.

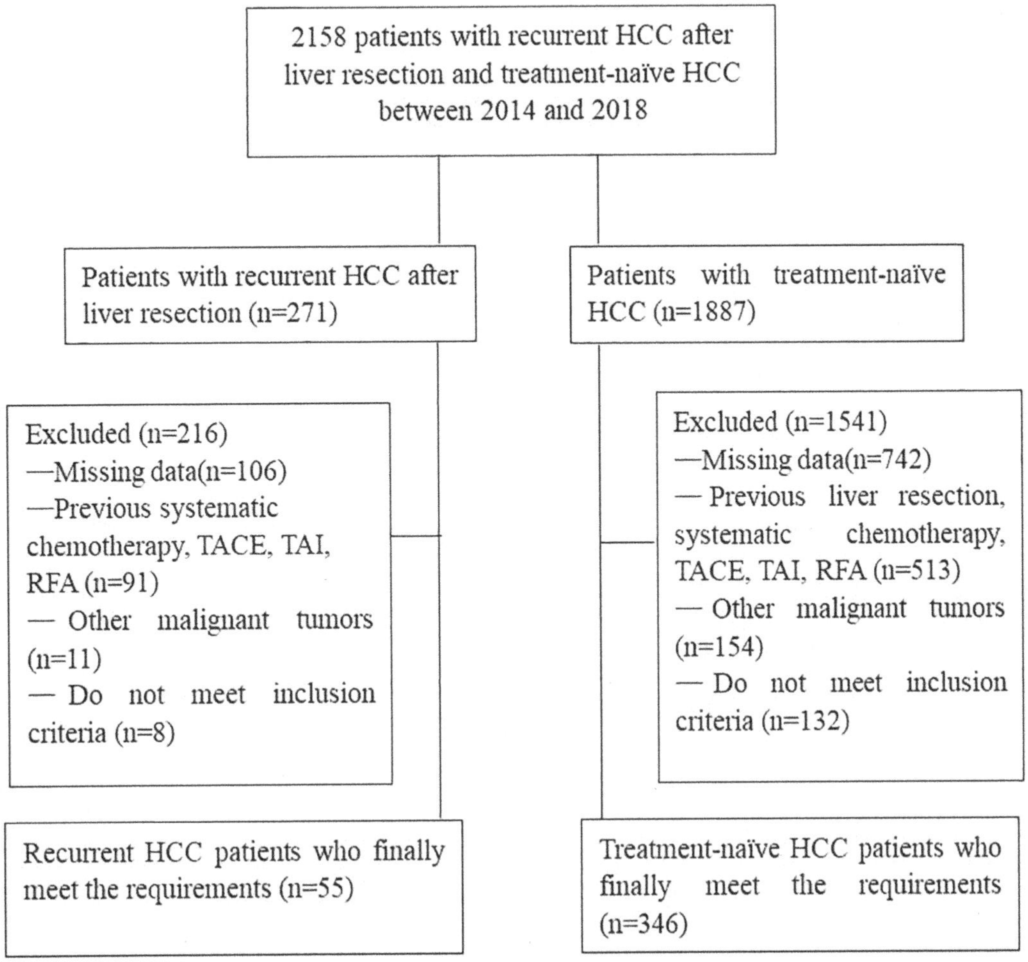

FIGURE 1 | Flow chart shows the screening procedure for patients with recurrent HCC after liver resection and treatment-naïve HCC.

Definition and Evaluation of Data

Overall survival (OS) and progression-free survival (PFS) were compared between TN-HCC and R-HCC groups. OS referred to the time from the initial TACE procedure to death or last follow-up. PFS was defined as the interval between the date of the first TACE procedure and the date of progression for patients who displayed radiologic evidence of disease progression or the date of death or last follow-up. Modified Response Evaluation Criteria in Solid Tumors was used to assess tumor response 1 month after initial TACE. Objective tumor regression (ORR) referred to complete response (CR) or partial response (PR). Disease control rate (DCR) represented CR, PR or stable disease (SD). The safety of TACE was evaluated by the Society of Interventional Radiology classification system (15). Those complications that lead to death and disability were defined as major complications that significantly increase the level of care or extend the length of hospital stay. Also, complications such as fever, vomiting and so on were considered minor.

Early recurrence was defined as a time interval of less than 2 years from curative LR to tumor recurrence, and a time interval of more than 2 years was considered as late recurrence. Curative LR meant that all tumor nodules were completely removed, the resection margin was clean, histological examination showed that there was no tumor on the cut surface, and no residual cancer in liver remnants was examined by abdominal contrast-enhanced computed tomography (CT) or magnetic resonance (MR) 1 month after the surgery (16).

Follow-Up and Repeated TACE

All patients were followed up 6-8 weeks after initial TACE. Follow-up evaluations included laboratory tests (including hematology and biochemical analyses) and abdominal contrast-enhanced CT or MR. Repeated TACE was performed in patients with residual viable or recurrent tumor in the liver on contrast-enhanced CT or MR imaging and with preserved liver function. If tumors were completely necrotic, abdominal contrast-enhanced CT or MR imaging and laboratory examination were performed every 2-3 months. Patients were followed until death or the end point of the study (December 31, 2020).

PSM Analysis

To reduce the patient selection bias and balance the variables between TN-HCC and R-HCC patients, a balanced cohort was assembled using a PSM analysis with a 1:1 ratio, and the value of the caliper was 0.05. The baseline variables including age, gender, Child–Pugh class, BCLC stage, tumor size, tumor number, TACE sessions, HBV infection, platelet, alanine aminotransferase, aspartate aminotransferase, prothrombin activity, total bilirubin, alpha-fetoprotein (AFP) level, and albumin were matched in our model.

Statistical Analysis

Discrete variables were represented by numbers with percentages and were calculated by Chi-square test, and continuous variables were presented as mean ± standard deviation and were calculated by Student's t-test. Kaplan-Meier method was used to evaluate the differences of PFS and OS between the two groups. The 95% confidence interval (CI) was calculated for median OS, median PFS, and hazard ratio (HR). A Cox proportional hazard regression model was used to analyze the potential prognostic factors affecting OS and PFS. Potential risk factors identified in univariate Cox model ($P<0.1$) were then entered into the multivariate Cox model. Conditional inference trees were constructed to further evaluate the association between RFS/OS and the associated risk factors. All analyses were performed using R (Version 3.6.1; R Foundation for Statistical Computing, Vienna, Austria; https://www.r-project.org/) and RStudio (Version 1.2.1335; RStudio, Inc., Boston, MA; https://www.rstudio.com/). All statistical tests were two-tailed, with $P < 0.05$ indicating a significant difference.

RESULTS

Study Population and Patient Characteristics

From January 2014 to December 2018, a total of 401 patients were included in our study, including 346 TN-HCC patients and 55 patients with R-HCC. Before the initial TACE, the mean tumor size of R-HCC patients was significantly smaller than that of the TN-HCC patients ($P<0.001$), and there were significant differences in BCLC stage, Child-Pugh class, alanine transaminase, and aspartate aminotransferase between the two groups ($P<0.05$). In addition, there was no significant difference in the other baseline characteristics between the two groups. Baseline demographics and characteristics of the 401 patients are shown in **Table 1**. The median follow-up duration was 18.0 months (range, 2–69 months) in the TN-HCC group and 22.0 months (range, 4–71 months) in the R-HCC group. At the end of follow-up, 226 (65.3%) patients in the TN-HCC group and 31 (56.4%) patients in the R-HCC group died.

Complications or Adverse Events

In TN-HCC group, 7 patients (2%) had serious complications. Three patients presented with biloma and four with liver abscess, and their symptoms improved gradually through percutaneous bile duct or abscess drainage. In R-HCC group, 1 patient (1.8%) developed biloma, and the symptom was improved by percutaneous bile duct drainage. There was no significant difference in the incidence of major complications between the two groups. Common minor complications such as fever, nausea and vomiting, abdominal pain, abnormal liver function, and scanty ascites occurred in 96 patients (27.7%) in TN-HCC group and 12 patients (21.8%) in R-HCC group.

Efficacy Comparison Between the Patients of TN-HCC and R-HCC

The morphological response of the target lesion was verified by abdominal contrast-enhanced CT or MR imaging. The ORR of TN-HCC patients was 61.6%, and that of R-HCC patients was 76.4% (P=0.034). In addition, the DCR of TN-HCC patients was 81.5%, and that of R-HCC patients was 90.9% (P=0.086). Hence, compared with TN-HCC patients, R-HCC patients had better ORR.

Median OS was 18 months (95% CI 16 months, 20 months) in the TN-HCC group and 24 months (95% CI 19 months, 54 months) in the R-HCC group (P=0.004) (**Figure 2A**). Median PFS was 6 months (95% CI 5 months, 7 months) in the TN-HCC group and 9 months (95% CI 6 months, 16 months) in the R-HCC group (P =0.012) (**Figure 2B**).

PSM Analysis

As baseline characteristics of TN-HCC patients were different from those of R-HCC patients, a PSM analysis was performed. After the PSM analysis, 47 pairs were selected (**Table 1**). The ORR of TN-HCC patients was 78.7%, and that of R-HCC patients was 72.3%, with no statistical difference between the two groups (P=0.472). Similarly, there was no statistically significant difference in DCR between the two groups (91.5% *vs* 87.2%, P=0.503).

The median OS in the TN-HCC group and the R-HCC group were 33 months (95% CI, 23-) and 24 months (95% CI, 19–54), respectively, and the difference between the two groups was significantly different (P= 0.0035) (**Figure 3A**). Multivariable analysis indicated that BCLC C and hepatitis B were independent risk factors for OS, while TACE sessions were associated with better OS (**Table 2**).

Median PFS was 12.0 months (95% CI: 6 months, 60 months) in the TN-HCC group and 10.0 months (95% CI: 4 months, 25 months) in the R-HCC group (P = 0.01) (**Figure 3B**). Univariate analyses showed that AFP level and platelet were significantly associated with PFS (**Table 3**), but there was no independent risk factor in multivariate analyses for PFS.

Decision Tree Model and Subgroup Analysis

To establish a risk signature that can classify patients into homogeneous subpopulations according to PFS and OS, we further constructed the conditional inference tree analysis using PFS and OS as predictive endpoints, respectively. After pruning the decision trees using the postpruning method, 5 terminal nodes (subpopulations) representing a recurrence signature were identified (**Figures 4A, B**). Furthermore, 6 subgroups representing

TABLE 1 | Baseline characteristics of patients between the two groups before and after PSM analysis.

Characteristics	Before PSM (No, %; Mean±SD)		*P* value	After PSM (No, %; Mean±SD)		*P* value
	TACE for R-HCC (n=55)	TACE for TN-HCC (n=346)		TACE for R-HCC (n =47)	TACE for TN-HCC (n =47)	
Age (years)	52.7±10.48	55.14±11. 63	0. 136	54.43±12.21	54. 64±9. 09	
Gender			0. 808			0. 924
Male	46 (83 6%)	281 (81.2%)		40 (81.6%)	40 (81.6%)	
Female	9 (16.4%)	65 (18.8%)		7 (14.9%)	7 (14.9%)	
ECOG performance			0.778			1
0	44 (80%)	271 (78.3%)		40 (81.6%)	40 (81.6%)	
1	11 (20%)	75 (21.7%)		7 (14.9%)	7 (14.9%)	
Child-Pugh class			0. 016			1
A	53 (96.4%)	291 (84.1%)		45 (95.7%)	45 (95.7%)	
B	2(3.6%)	55 (15.9%)		2 (4.3%)	2 (4.3%)	
BCLC stage			<0. 001			0. 869
A	4 (7.3%)	48 (13.9)		4 (8.5%)	4 (8.5%)	
B	43 (78.2%)	168 (48.6)		33 (70.2%)	35 (74.5%)	
C	8 (14.5%)	130 (37.6)		10 (21.3%)	8 (17.0%)	
HBV infection			0.448			0.55
Yes	47 (85.5%)	277 (80.1%)		42 (89.4%)	39 (83.0%)	
No	8 (14.5%)	69 (19.9%)		5 (10.6%)	8 (17%)	
AFP (ng/m,)			0. 645			0. 822
>400	18 (32.7%)	128 (37%)		15 (31.9%)	13 (27.7%)	
≤400	37 (67.3%)	218 (63%)		32 (68.1%)	34 (72.3%)	
ALT(IU/L)	33.20±20.69	60.40±86.13	0. 02	35.47±19.44	33.21±21.83	0.598
AST (IU /L)	3816±42.60	69.21±80.05	0. 005	49.00±45.58	39.57±45. 93	0. 321
Total bilirubin (μmol/L)	96.11±76.81	99.87±63.45	0.692	93.23±61.72	93.89±77.84	0.964
Platelet count(109/L)	139.85 (70.40)	152.64 (88.87)	0.31	131.83±69.38	141.85±74.38	0.501
Albumin (g/dL)	38.88± 3.89	36.39±5.64	0.515	39.31±5.11	38.96± 4.01	0. 712
Prothrombin time, INR	14.05±1.39	14.24±1.49	0. 354	14.11±0.92	14. 06±1.49	0. 848
Number of tumors			0. 144			>0. 999
1	13 (23.6%)	120 (34.7%)		13 (27.7%)	12 (25.5%)	
>1	42 (76.4%)	226 (65.3%)		34 (72.3)	35(74.5)	
Maximal tumor diameter (cm)	2. 96±1.71	7.42±4. 64	<0. 001	3.16±2. 17	3.09±1.73	0. 879
TACE sessions	9. 13+3.07	8.50+3.56	0.22	8.89±3.57	9.17+3.30	0. 697

PSM, propensity score matching; SD, standard deviation; R-HCC, recurrent hepatocellular carcinoma; TN-HCC, treatment-naive hepatocellular carcinoma; ECOG, Eastern Cooperative Oncology Grou, BCLC, Barcelona Clinic Liver Cancer; HBV, hepatitis B; AFP, alpha-fetoprotein; ALT, alanine transaminase; AST, aspartate aminotransferase; TACE, transarterial chemoembolization.

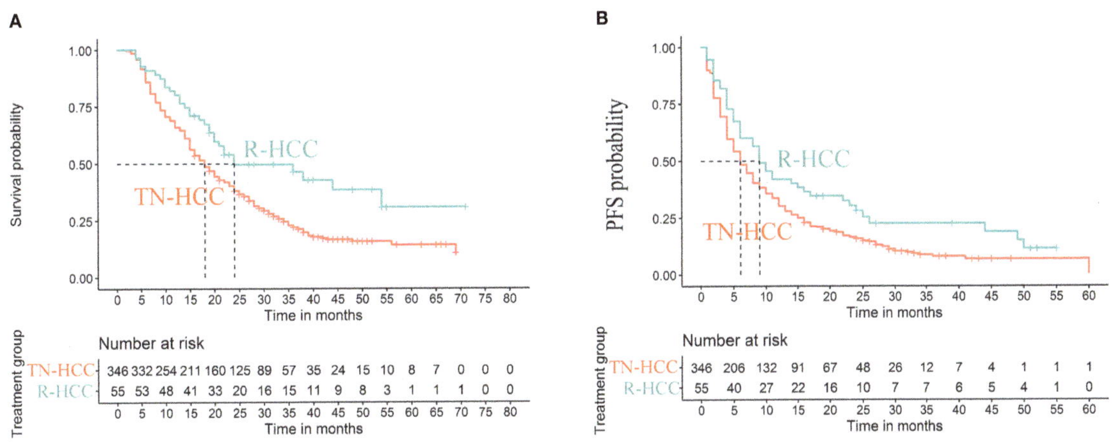

FIGURE 2 | Kaplan-Meier curves of cumulative survival **(A)** and progression-free survival (PFS) **(B)** in patients with recurrent HCC after liver resection and treatment-naïve HCC before propensity score matching.

a survival signature were identified (**Figure 5A, B**). Patients entered into different subgroups according to tumor size, BCLC stage, and TACE sessions and shared different hazards ratio to recurrence or survival (**Table 4**).

DISCUSSION

In this study, compared with R-HCC patients, TN-HCC patients showed poor baseline characteristics at the time of the first

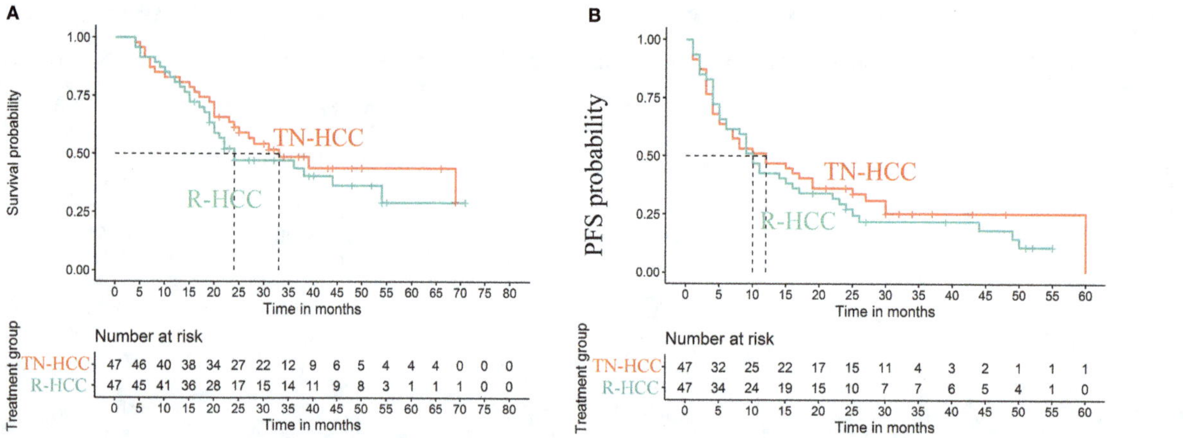

FIGURE 3 | Kaplan-Meier curves of cumulative survival **(A)** and progression-free survival (PFS) **(B)** in patients with recurrent HCC after liver resection and treatment-naïve HCC after propensity score matching.

TABLE 2 | Univariate and multivariate analysis of prognostic factors for overall survival (OS) after PSM analysis.

Variable	Univariate analysis		Multivariate analysis	
	HR(95%CI)	***P* value**	**HR(95%CI)**	***P* value**
Age	0.996 (0.972~1.020)	0.7208		
Sex		0.6777		
Male	Reference			
Female	1.165 (0.567~2.393)			
Number of tumors		0.0254		0.16
1	Reference		Reference	
>1	0.525 (0.299~0.924)		0.631 (0.332~1.199)	
HBV infection		0.3032		
No	Reference			
Yes	1.570 (0.665~3.705)			
Child-Pugh class		0.5148		
A	Reference			
B	1.603 (0.387~6.637)			
BCLC stage				
A	Reference		Reference	
B	0.438 (0.191~1.005)	0.0514	0.948 (0.347~2.593)	0.9178
C	1.711 (0.686~4.267)	0.2496	2.814 (1.051~7.535)	0.0396
AFP (ng/ml)				
≤400	Reference		Reference	
>400	1.693 (0.962~2.980)	0.0678	1.953 (1.092~3.493)	0.024
TACE sessions	0.887 (0.824~0.955)	0.0015	0.890 (0.818~0.968)	0.0068
Maximal tumor diameter (cm)	1.056 (0.917~1.215)	0.449		
Platelet count (10^9/L)	1.003 (0.999~1.007)	0.1947		
ALT(IU/L)	1.003 (0.990~1.017)	0.6313		
AST (IU/L)	1.000 (0.994~1.006)	0.9553		
Albumin (g/dL)	0.960 (0.904~1.021)	0.1919		
Total bilirubin (μmol/L)	1.002 (0.998~1.005)	0.415		
Prothrombin time, INR	0.961 (0.744~1.242)	0.7616		
Group				
TN-HCC	Reference			
R-HCC	1.243 (0.723~2.138)	0.4311		

PSM, propensity score matching; HR, hazard ratio; CI, confidence interval; BCLC, Barcelona Clinic Liver Cancer; HBV, hepatitis B; AFP, alpha-fetoprotein; ALT, alanine transaminase; AST, aspartate aminotransferase; TACE, transarterial chemoembolization; TN-HCC, treatment-naïve hepatocellular carcinoma; R-HCC, recurrent hepatocellular carcinoma.

TACE. Accordingly, the results of our study indicated that patients in the R-HCC group had better tumor response, OS and PFS than patients in the TN-HCC group before the PSM analysis. However, after PSM, patients in the TN-HCC group had better OS and PFS than patients in the R-HCC group, which further indicates that the recurrence of tumor after LR leads to unsatisfactory long-term survival and thus death of HCC patients (16, 17).

TABLE 3 | Univariate and multivariate analysis of prognostic factors for progression-free survival (PFS) after PSM analysis.

Variable	Univariate analysis		Multivariate analysis	
	HR (95%CI)	*P* value	HR (95%CI)	*P* value
Age	1.000 (0.979~1.022)	0.9847		
Sex		0.5752		
Male	Reference			
Female	1.187 (0.651~2.165)			
Number of tumors		0.3973		
1	Reference			
>1	0.803 (0.483~1.334)			
HBV infection		0.4748		
No	Reference			
Yes	1.276 (0.654~2.489)			
Child-Pugh class		0.7022		
A	Reference			
B	1.254 (0.393~4.002)			
C				
BCLC stage				
A	Reference			
B	0.704 (0.318~1.559)	0.387		
C	1.290 (0.521~3.190)	0.5818		
AFP (ng/ml)		0.0313	1.591 (0.955~2.651)	0.0744
≤400	Reference			
>400	1.735 (1.051~2.866)			
TACE sessions	0.975 (0.909~1.046)	0.4842		
Maximal tumor diameter (cm)	1.027 (0.907~1.164)	0.6711		
Platelet count (10^9/L)	1.003 (1.000~1.007)	0.0488	1.003(0.999~1.006)	0.1187
ALT(IU/L)	0.999 (0.987~1.011)	0.88		
AST (IU/L)	1.000 (0.995~1.005)	0.9608		
Albumin (g/dL)	0.993 (0.944~1.044)	0.7742		
Total bilirubin (µmol/L)	0.999 (0.996~1.002)	0.5925		
Prothrombin time, INR	0.951 (0.770~1.175)	0.6426		
Group				
TN-HCC	1.142 (0.718~1.816)	0.5756		
R-HCC				

PSM, propensity score matching; HR, hazard ratio; CI, confidence interval; BCLC, Barcelona Clinic Liver Cancer; HBV, hepatitis B; AFP alpha-fetoprotein; ALT, alanine transaminase; AST, aspartate aminotransferase; TACE, transarterial chemoembolization; TN-HCC, treatment-naïve hepatocellular carcinoma; R-HCC, recurrent hepatocellular carcinoma.

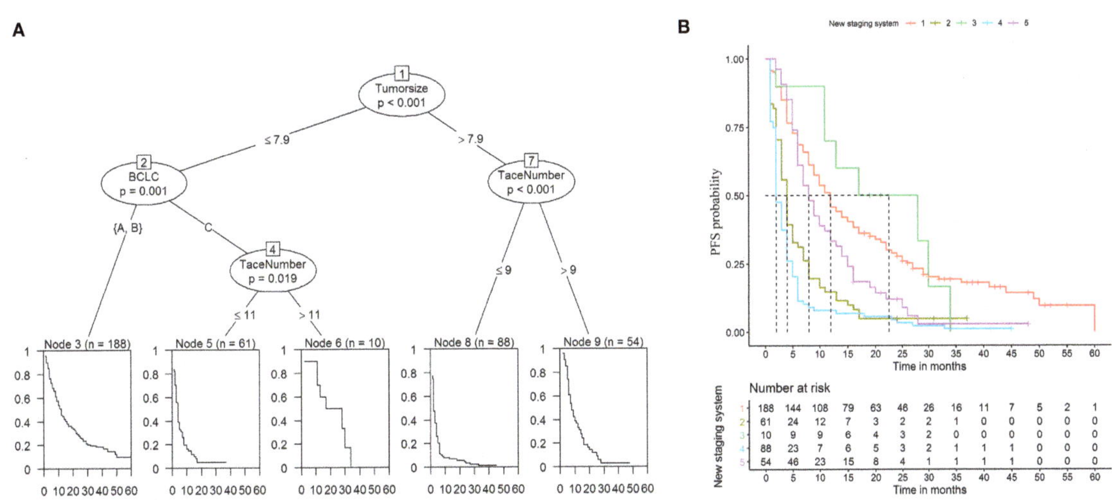

FIGURE 4 | Prediction of progression-free survival (PFS) **(A)** and Kaplan-Meier curves of PFS **(B)** based on decision tree results.

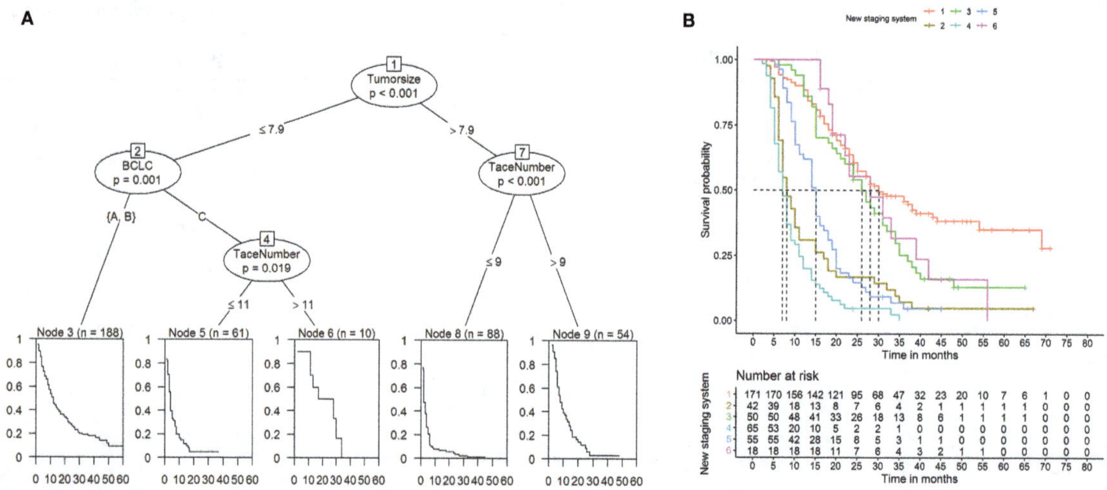

FIGURE 5 | Prediction of overall survival (OS) **(A)** and Kaplan-Meier curves of OS **(B)** based on decision tree results.

TABLE 4 | The Cox regression analysis of progression-free survival (PFS) or overall survival (OS) according to new stage.

Categorical variable	HR (95%CI)	*P* value
PFS		
1 Tumor size <=7.9 & BCLC ="A/B"	Reference	
2 Tumor size <=7.9 & BCLC="C"& Number of TACE <=11	2.68 (1.97, 3.65)	<0.001
3 Tumor size<=7.9 & BCLC="C")& Number of TACE >11	0.80 (0.39, 1.64)	0.546
4 Tumor size >7.9 & Number of TACE <=9	3.96 (3.02, 5.21)	<0.001
5 Tumor size >7.9 & Number of TACE >9	1.48 (1.07, 2.04)	0.018
OS		
1 BCLC ="A/B"& Tumor size <=6.9	Reference	
2 BCLC ="A/B"& Tumor size > 6.9 & Number of TACE <=8	4.35 (2.99, 6.31)	<0.001
3 BCLC ="A/B"& Tumor size > 6.9 & Number of TACE >8	1.57 (1.09, 2.27)	0.016
4 BCLC ="C"& Number of TACE <= 8	8.37 (5.98, 11.72)	<0.001
5 BCLC ="C"& 11>=Number of TACE > 8	3.50 (2.48, 4.95)	<0.001
6 BCLC ="C"& Number of TACE >11	1.36 (0.76, 2.42)	0.305

HR, hazard ratio; CI, confidence interval; BCLC, Barcelona Clinic Liver Cancer; TACE, transarterial chemoembolization.

So far, intrahepatic recurrence remains a thorny problem, and the choice of treatment after recurrence is extremely important. For patients with recurrence, resection or ablation is the optimal therapeutic option, provided that the liver function of these patients is Child-Pugh class A or B, adequate liver reserve, and appropriate tumor location, etc. (18). If these conditions are not met, TACE may be the treatment of choice. In our study, patients were eligible to receive TACE because most had multiple recurrent tumors or inadequate liver reserve or the tumor location was unsuitable for ablation. Nevertheless, the 1, 3-year OS rates in recurrent patients treated with TACE in this study were not inferior to the 1, 3-year OS rates reported in patients undergoing repeat resection or ablation. It has been reported that the 1- and 3-year OS rates of patients with recurrent HCC after LR were 71–94% and 41–75% (19–21), respectively, while the 1- and 3-year OS rates of patients undergoing radiofrequency ablation were 82% and 47-54% (22, 23), respectively. Similar to these reports, the 1 - and 3-year OS rates in our study after PSM were 80.9% and 43.9%, respectively.

At the same time, this study compared the efficacy between the two groups of TN-HCC patients treated with TACE and those patients with R-HCC. Currently, TACE has been recognized as the standard method for unresectable HCC patients and a significant number of studies have confirmed the therapeutic effect of TACE on TN-HCC patients (3, 24). However, to date, few studies (25) have reported the outcomes of TACE for R-HCC patients. Therefore, this study compared the therapeutic effects of TACE on the two groups of patients, and the results demonstrated that OS and PFS of R-HCC patients were slightly inferior to TN-HCC patients after PSM analysis. Hence, based on the results of PSM analysis, we believe that early dynamic detection of R-HCC can significantly improve the prognosis of patients.

Recurrence and survival after TACE in both groups are critical to the prognosis of patients. Zhuang et al. (26) incorporated seven prognostic factors to construct a prognostic nomogram, and concluded that TACE combining with RFA was beneficial in patients with recurrent HCC in the low-risk group after LR, while TACE alone was sufficient for patients in the medium/high-risk group. Meanwhile, Lu et al. (27) retrospectively analyzed clinical data from 597 HCC patients treated with TACE, suggesting that elevated platelet was associated with poor survival in HCC patients. In our study, in order to establish a risk signature that divides patients into homogeneous subgroups according to PFS and OS, the conditional inference tree analysis were constructed. Then, the prognosis of the two groups of patients was accurately determined according to the tumor diameter, BCLC stage and TACE sessions of patients.

Our study indicated that TACE procedure was well tolerated in patients with TN-HCC or R-HCC, and the 2% serious complication rate increases the number of literatures (28, 29) supporting chemoembolization as a safe method. In this study, the symptoms of patients with biloma and liver abscess were gradually improved after percutaneous drainage. Similar to other studies (30–33), postembolism syndrome such as fever, vomiting, and abdominal pain were the most common complications in the current study, and most of them are self-limiting.

This study had certain limitations. Retrospective and non-randomized design is one of the limitations. Although the PSM analysis was applied, there is still the risk of selection bias. In addition, the data in this study came from a single-center with a small sample size. Therefore, an adequately powered multi-center prospective randomized controlled trial is necessary to verify our results.

In conclusion, patients with R-HCC treated with TACE achieved satisfactory results, although survival after PSM was not as good as in the TN-HCC group. In addition, the conditional inference tree was used to construct a risk signature that divides patients into homogeneous subgroups according to PFS and OS, which can more accurately predict the prognosis of patients in the two groups.

AUTHOR CONTRIBUTIONS

YL, YR, and LB collected the patients' data. YL and YR drafted the manuscript. BX, GZ, GF, SS, and CZ revised the manuscript. YL, YR, LB, and SS analyzed and interpreted the data. BX and GZ made substantial contributions to the conception of the work. SS and CZ made substantial contributions to the design of the work and have revised the manuscript substantively. All authors contributed to the article and approved the submitted version.

ACKNOWLEDGMENTS

We are very grateful to Ms. Qin for her help in the statistical analysis of this study.

REFERENCES

1. European Association for the Study of the Liver. EASL Clinical Practice Guidelines: Management of Hepatocellular Carcinoma. *J Hepatol* (2018) 69:182–236. doi: 10.1016/j.jhep.2018.03.019
2. Llovet JM, Real MI, Montana X, Planas R, Coll S, Aponte J, et al. Arterial Embolisation or Chemoembolisation Versus Symptomatic Treatment in Patients With Unresectable Hepatocellular Carcinoma: A Randomised Controlled Trial. *Lancet* (2002) 359:1734–39. doi: 10.1016/S0140-6736(02)08649-X
3. Llovet JM, Bruix J. Systematic Review of Randomized Trials for Unresectable Hepatocellular Carcinoma: Chemoembolization Improves Survival. *Hepatology* (2003) 37:429–42. doi: 10.1053/jhep.2003.50047
4. Maluccio M, Covey A. Recent Progress in Understanding, Diagnosing, and Treating Hepatocellular Carcinoma. *CA Cancer J Clin* (2012) 62:394–9. doi: 10.3322/caac.21161
5. Jeon MY, Kim HS, Lim TS, Han DH, Kim BK, Park JY, et al. Refractoriness to Transarterial Chemoembolization in Patients With Recurrent Hepatocellular Carcinoma After Curative Resection. *PloS One* (2019) 14:e0214613. doi: 10.1371/journal.pone.0214613
6. Koh PS, Chan AC, Cheung TT, Chok KS, Dai WC, Poon RT, et al. Efficacy of Radiofrequency Ablation Compared With Transarterial Chemoembolization for the Treatment of Recurrent Hepatocellular Carcinoma: A Comparative Survival Analysis. *HPB (Oxford)* (2016) 18:72–8. doi: 10.1016/j.hpb.2015.07.005
7. Na SK, Choi GH, Lee HC, Shin YM, An J, Lee D, et al. The Effectiveness of Transarterial Chemoembolization in Recurrent Hepatocellular-Cholangiocarcinoma After Resection. *PloS One* (2018) 13:e0198138. doi: 10.1371/journal.pone.0198138
8. Lo CM, Ngan H, Tso WK, Liu CL, Lam CM, Poon RT, et al. Randomized Controlled Trial of Transarterial Lipiodol Chemoembolization for Unresectable Hepatocellular Carcinoma. *Hepatology* (2002) 35:1164–71. doi: 10.1053/jhep.2002.33156
9. Kan X, Liang B, Zhou G, Xiong B, Pan F, Ren Y, et al. Transarterial Chemoembolization Combined With Apatinib for Advanced Hepatocellular Carcinoma: A Propensity Score Matching Analysis. *Front Oncol* (2020) 10:970. doi: 10.3389/fonc.2020.00970
10. Lee SW, Lee TY, Peng YC, Yang SS, Yeh HZ, Chang CS. The Therapeutic Benefits of Combined Sorafenib and Transarterial Chemoembolization for Advanced Hepatocellular Carcinoma. *J Dig Dis* (2020) 21:287–92. doi: 10.1111/1751-2980.12866
11. Shim JH, Kim KM, Lee YJ, Ko GY, Yoon HK, Sung KB, et al. Complete Necrosis After Transarterial Chemoembolization Could Predict Prolonged Survival in Patients With Recurrent Intrahepatic Hepatocellular Carcinoma After Curative Resection. *Ann Surg Oncol* (2010) 17:869–77. doi: 10.1245/s10434-009-0788-7
12. Bruix J, Sherman M. Management of Hepatocellular Carcinoma. *Hepatology* (2005) 42:1208–36. doi: 10.1002/hep.20933
13. Ren Y, Cao Y, Ma H, Kan X, Zhou C, Liu J, et al. Improved Clinical Outcome Using Transarterial Chemoembolization Combined With Radiofrequency Ablation for Patients in Barcelona Clinic Liver Cancer Stage A or B Hepatocellular Carcinoma Regardless of Tumor Size: Results of a Single-Center Retrospective Case Control Study. *BMC Cancer* (2019) 19(1):983. doi: 10.1186/s12885-019-6237-5
14. Ren Y, Chen L, Huang S, Zhou C, Liu J, Shi Q, et al. Transarterial Chemoembolization of Unresectable Systemic Chemotherapy Refractory Liver Metastases: A Retrospective Single-Center Analysis. *Abdom Radiol (NY)* (2020) 459:2862–70. doi: 10.1007/s00261-020-02584-6
15. Ahmed M, Solbiati L, Brace CL, Breen DJ, Callstrom MR, Charboneau JW, et al. Image-Guided Tumor Ablation: Standardization of Terminology and Reporting Criteria–a 10-Year Update. *Radiology* (2014) 273:241–60. doi: 10.1148/radiol.14132958
16. Wang Z, Ren Z, Chen Y, Hu J, Yang G, Yu L, et al. Adjuvant Transarterial Chemoembolization for HBV-Related Hepatocellular Carcinoma After Resection: A Randomized Controlled Study. *Clin Cancer Res* (2018) 24:2074–81. doi: 10.1158/1078-0432.CCR-17-2899
17. Zhang X, Li C, Wen T, Yan L, Li B, Yang J, et al. Appropriate Treatment Strategies for Intrahepatic Recurrence After Curative Resection of Hepatocellular Carcinoma Initially Within the Milan Criteria: According to the Recurrence Pattern. *Eur J Gastroenterol Hepatol* (2015) 27:933–40. doi: 10.1097/MEG.0000000000000383
18. Zu QQ, Liu S, Zhou CG, Yang ZQ, Xia JG, Zhao LB, et al. Chemoembolization of Recurrent Hepatoma After Curative Resection: Prognostic Factors. *AJR Am J Roentgenol* (2015) 204:1322–8. doi: 10.2214/AJR.14.13343
19. Minagawa M, Makuuchi M, Takayama T, Kokudo N. Selection Criteria for Repeat Hepatectomy in Patients With Recurrent Hepatocellular Carcinoma. *Ann Surg* (2003) 238:703–10. doi: 10.1097/01.sla.0000094549.11754.e6
20. Itamoto T, Nakahara H, Amano H, Kohashi T, Ohdan H, Tashiro H, et al. Repeat Hepatectomy for Recurrent Hepatocellular Carcinoma. *Surgery* (2007) 141:589–97. doi: 10.1016/j.surg.2006.12.014
21. Huang ZY, Liang BY, Xiong M, Zhan DQ, Wei S, Wang GP, et al. Long-Term Outcomes of Repeat Hepatic Resection in Patients With Recurrent Hepatocellular Carcinoma and Analysis of Recurrent Types and Their

Prognosis: A Single-Center Experience in China. *Ann Surg Oncol* (2012) 19:2515–25. doi: 10.1245/s10434-012-2269-7

22. Peng ZW, Zhang YJ, Liang HH, Lin XJ, Guo RP, Chen MS. Recurrent Hepatocellular Carcinoma Treated With Sequential Transcatheter Arterial Chemoembolization and RF Ablation Versus RF Ablation Alone: A Prospective Randomized Trial. *Radiology* (2012) 262:689–700. doi: 10.1148/radiol.11110637
23. Choi D, Lim HK, Kim MJ, Lee SH, Kim SH, Lee WJ, et al. Recurrent Hepatocellular Carcinoma: Percutaneous Radiofrequency Ablation After Hepatectomy. *Radiology* (2004) 230:135–41. doi: 10.1148/radiol.2301021182
24. Camma C, Schepis F, Orlando A, Albanese M, Shahied L, Trevisani F, et al. Transarterial Chemoembolization for Unresectable Hepatocellular Carcinoma: Meta-Analysis of Randomized Controlled Trials. *Radiology* (2002) 224:47–54. doi: 10.1148/radiol.2241011262
25. Kim DS, Lim TS, Jeon MY, Kim BK, Park JY, Kim DY, et al. Transarterial Chemoembolization in Treatment-Naïve and Recurrent Hepatocellular Carcinoma: A Propensity-Matched Outcome Analysis. *Dig Dis Sci* (2019) 64:3660–8. doi: 10.1007/s10620-019-05701-8
26. Zhuang H, Zhou Z, Ma Z, Huang S, Gong Y, Zhang Z, et al. Prognostic Stratification Based on a Novel Nomogram for Solitary Large Hepatocellular Carcinoma After Curative Resection. *Front Oncol* (2020) 10:556489. doi: 10.3389/fonc.2020.556489
27. Lu L, Zhang Y, Zheng P, Wu Z, Wang X, Chen Y, et al. Elevated Platelet Count Is Associated With Poor Survival After Transarterial Chemoembolization Treatment in Patients With Hepatocellular Carcinoma: A Cohort Study. *J Hepatocell Carcinoma* (2020) 7:191–9. doi: 10.2147/JHC.S274349
28. Ngo A, von Stempel C, Corbo B, Bandula S, Shiu KK, Raja J, et al. Transarterial Chemoembolisation of Colorectal Liver Metastases With IrinotecanLoaded Beads: A Bi-Institutional Analysis of 125 Treatments in 53 Patients. *Cardiovasc Intervent Radiol* (2019) 42:979–90. doi: 10.1007/s00270-019-02219-4
29. Malagari K, Moschouris H, Kiakidis T, Harward S, Kelekis A, Vrakas S, et al. Five-Years Outcome Analysis of 142 Consecutive Hepatocellular Carcinoma Patients Treated With Doxorubicin Eluting Microspheres 30-60μm: Results From a Single-Centre Prospective Phase II Trial. *Cardiovasc Intervent Radiol* (2019) 42:1551–62. doi: 10.1007/s00270-019-02260-3
30. Vogl TJ, Naguib NN, Nour-Eldin NE, Eichler K, Zangos S, Gruber-Rouh T. Transarterial Chemoembolization (TACE) With Mitomycin C and Gemcitabine for Liver Metastases in Breast Cancer. *Eur Radiol* (2010) 20:173–80. doi: 10.1007/s00330-009-1525-0
31. Bhagat N, Reyes DK, Lin M, Kamel I, Pawlik TM, Frangakis C, et al. Phase II Study of Chemoembolization With Drug-Eluting Beads in Patients With Hepatic Neuroendocrine Metastases: High Incidence of Biliary Injury. *Cardiovasc Intervent Radiol* (2013) 36:449–59. doi: 10.1007/s00270-012-0424-y
32. Aal AKA, Moawad S, Lune PV, El Khudari H, Hanaoka MM, Abouldahab N, et al. Survival Outcomes of Very Small Drug-Eluting Beads Used in Chemoembolization of Unresectable Hepatocellular Carcinoma. *J Vasc Interv Radiol* (2019) 30:1325–1334.e2. doi: 10.1016/j.jvir.2019.05.006
33. Mokkarala M, Noda C, Malone C, Ramaswamy R, Akinwande O. Comparison of Response and Outcomes of Drug-eluting Bead Chemoembolization (DEB-TACE) Radioembolization (TARE) for Patients With Colorectal Cancer Liver Metastases. *Anticancer Res* (2019) 39:3071–7. doi: 10.21873/anticanres.13442

7

Enhanced Recovery After Surgery in Patients with Hepatocellular Carcinoma Undergoing Laparoscopic Hepatectomy

Jiamin Zhou[1,2†], *Xigan He*[1,2†], *Miao Wang*[1,2], *Yiming Zhao*[1,2], *Ning Zhang*[1,2], *Longrong Wang*[1,2], *Anrong Mao*[1,2*] *and Lu Wang*[1,2*]

[1] *Department of Hepatic Surgery, Shanghai Cancer Center, Fudan University, Shanghai, China,* [2] *Department of Oncology, Shanghai Medical College, Fudan University, Shanghai, China*

Correspondence:
Anrong Mao
13020143060@163.com
Lu Wang
wang.lu99@hotmail.com

† *These authors have contributed equally to this work*

Objective: To compare the effectiveness and safety of enhanced recovery after surgery (ERAS) in patients with hepatocellular carcinoma (HCC) undergoing laparoscopic hepatectomy.

Methods: From September 2016 to June 2019, 282 patients were enrolled, and ERAS was implemented since March 2018. All indicators related to surgery, liver function, and postoperative outcomes were included in the analysis. Propensity score matching (PSM) identified 174 patients for further comparison.

Results: After PSM, the clinicopathological baselines were well-matched. The group showed significantly less intraoperative blood loss (100.00 [100.00–200.00] vs. 200.00 [100.00–300.00] ml, $P = 0.001$), fewer days before abdominal drainage tube removal (4.00 [3.00–4.00] days vs. 4.00 [3.00–5.00] days, $P = 0.023$), shorter hospital stay after surgery (6.00 [5.00–6.00] days vs. 6.00 [6.00–7.00] days, $P < 0.001$), and reduced postoperative morbidity (18.39 vs. 34.48%, $P = 0.026$). The proportion of patients with a pain score ≥ 4 was significantly lower in the ERAS group within the first 2 days after surgery (1.15 vs. 13.79% and 8.05 vs. 26.44%, $P = 0.002$ and $P = 0.001$, respectively). Pringle maneuver was performed more frequently in the ERAS group (70.11 vs. 18.39%, $P < 0.001$), and a significantly higher postoperative alanine aminotransferase level was also observed (183.40 [122.85–253.70] vs. 136.20 [82.93–263.40] U/l, $P = 0.026$). The 2-year recurrence-free survival was similar between the two groups (72 vs. 71%, $P = 0.946$).

Conclusions: ERAS programs are feasible and safe and do not influence mid-term recurrence in HCC patients undergoing laparoscopic hepatectomy.

Keywords: enhanced recovery after surgery, hepatocellular carcinoma, hepatectomy, laparoscopy, liver function

INTRODUCTION

Since enhanced recovery after surgery (ERAS) programs were introduced by Kehlet in the 1990's, they have been widely applied in gastrointestinal, urologic, gynecological, orthopedic surgery, and many other surgical fields to minimize perioperative pain and stress, reduce morbidity, and accelerate postoperative recovery worldwide (1–11). Furthermore, the concept of ERAS is constantly being updated with continuous clinical practice (4).

Although the implementation of ERAS programs in hepatic surgery was slightly later than in other surgical fields (12), many randomized controlled trials (RCTs), meta-analyses, and guidelines and consensus have been performed or established specifically focusing on hepatectomy (13–20). However, most of the studies have only focused on the hepatectomy itself, while the type of liver tumors and the type of surgical approach used in these studies were always mixed.

Hepatocellular carcinoma (HCC) is still one of the leading causes of cancer-related mortality, especially in China. Most cases of hepatitis B virus (HBV)-related HCC occur in patients with cirrhosis (21, 22). In several previous studies, ERAS programs were considered to be beneficial to HCC patients, especially in patients with cirrhosis that may partly be attributed to the omission of overnight fasting and carbohydrate loading, which may lessen the nutritional stress (23, 24). However, only a few studies have focused on this field.

Since the second international consensus conference for laparoscopic liver resection in 2014, laparoscopic minor hepatectomy was the standard surgical practice (25). In addition, laparoscopic major hepatectomy was gradually accepted for its safety, feasibility, and good short- and long-term outcomes, including in HCC patients with cirrhosis in recent years (26, 27). Although many previous studies have explored the recovery of patients undergoing both ERAS programs and laparoscopic hepatectomy (LH), their results did not seem to be consistent (16, 23, 28, 29). The results might also be due to the mismatch of the type of liver tumors and the ratio of LH among these studies. Thus, it is meaningful to focus on the role of ERAS programs in patients with HCC undergoing LH.

Therefore, this study aimed to compare the effectiveness and safety of ERAS in patients with HCC undergoing LH.

MATERIALS AND METHODS

The inclusion criteria were as follows: (1) patients were pathologically confirmed to have HCC after surgery; (2) all surgical procedures were successfully performed by laparoscopy; (3) radical resection was achieved; and (4) preoperative liver function was Child-Pugh A or B. The exclusion criteria were as follows: (1) patients underwent laparoscopic radiofrequency ablation alone, and (2) laparoscopic surgery was converted to open surgery for any reason. From September 2016 to June 2019, 282 eligible patients in the Department of Hepatic Surgery, Shanghai Cancer Center, Fudan University, were enrolled in the study retrospectively. ERAS programs were implemented in our center on March 1, 2018. All the patients who were suitable for undergoing LH routinely followed the ERAS protocol. Therefore, 108 patients from September 2016 to February 2018 were enrolled in the control group, and the subsequent 174 patients were enrolled in the ERAS group. All surgical operations were performed by the team of Prof. Lu Wang. This study was approved by the Research Ethics Committee of Shanghai Cancer Center, Fudan University.

Enhanced recovery after surgery (ERAS) management measures at our center were introduced in our previous study (30) and are briefly described in **Table 1**. The underlying diseases of the patients were defined as cardiovascular disease, cerebrovascular disease, hypertension, diabetes, and other chronic diseases, namely, chronic bronchitis, chronic kidney disease, and rheumatoid arthritis. HBV infection referred to patients with HBsAg positivity, regardless of whether the HBV DNA was replicating or not. The tumor stage was defined according to the Barcelona Clinic Liver Cancer (BCLC) staging. Postoperative complications were defined and classified according to the Clavien–Dindo classification criteria. The pain score was classified according to the visual analog scale, and a score $\geq$ 4 was defined as severe pain requiring analgesic treatment. Four liver function-related indicators, namely, alanine aminotransferase (ALT), total bilirubin (TB), prothrombin time (PT), and prealbumin (PAB), were used to express the postoperative recovery of liver function, all of which were recorded before the surgery and on the 3rd day after surgery. Abdominal contrast-enhanced computed tomography scanning or magnetic resonance imaging, serum alpha-fetoprotein levels, and chest radiographs were monitored at an interval of 3 months after liver resection within the first 2 years. Recurrence-free survival (RFS) was defined as the interval between surgery and recurrence. If recurrence was not diagnosed, patients were censored on the date of death or the last follow-up. Two years was generally set as the cutoff value to define early recurrence (31).

Propensity score matching (PSM) analysis was performed in this study to reduce bias in patient selection using SPSS 22.0 for Windows (SPSS Inc., Chicago, IL, USA). The variables in the clinicopathological baseline that were not balanced and might affect the results, namely, age, sex, underlying diseases, HBV infection, American Society of Anesthesiologists (ASA) score, body mass index (BMI), preoperative level of ALT, TB, PT, PAB, and type of hepatectomy were included in the calculation. The propensity score was generated using logistic regression with these variables, and the caliper value was set to 0.02. The patients were selected using nearest-neighbor matching without replacement at a ratio of 1:1. A two-sample Student's t-test or Mann–Whitney U-test was performed to compare quantitative variables. For data analyzed with a two-sample Student's t-test, the data were presented as mean $\pm$ standard error, and for data analyzed with Mann–Whitney U test, the data were presented as median (interquartile range). Pearson's χ^2 test or Fisher's exact test was used to comparing qualitative variables. Statistical analyses were performed using the SPSS 22.0. Plot analysis was performed using GraphPad Prism 5 for Windows (GraphPad Software, Inc. San Diego, CA, USA). Statistical significance was set at $P < 0.05$.

TABLE 1 | Enhanced recovery after surgery (ERAS) programs in our center.

	ERAS programs
Preoperative management	ERAS programs are introduced during preoperative education
	NRS-2002 evaluation scale is used to determine preoperative nutritional assessment and support
	No preoperative bowel preparation
	Patients were fasted for 6 h and drink was forbidden for 2 h before surgery
	Child-Pugh liver function grading evaluation
	Accurate liver resection planning under three-dimensional reconstruction and ERAS management risk evaluation and control
	Routine evaluation and prevention training, focusing on the risk evaluation of deep venous thrombosis and respiratory function exercise
Intraoperative management	Routine usage of prophylactic antibiotics
	Multi-mode individualized anesthesia program
	Low central venous pressure (CVP) technique [CVP < 5 mmHg, systolic blood pressure (SBP) > 90 mmHg] + perioperative goal directed fluid therapy
	Individualized liver blood flow control technique
	Perioperative body temperature higher than 36.0°C (insulation blanket + warm distilled water rinse)
	Open/laparoscopy + delicate liver parenchyma dissection technique
Postoperative management	Selective indwelling drainage tube, no routine nasogastric tube, early removal of catheters
	Comprehensive, quantitative and dynamic evaluation + preventive multi-mode analgesic management (routine analgesic pump 1 d, supplemented by opioids, non-steroidal anti-inflammatory drugs and epidural anesthesia)
	PONV risk evaluation and multi-mode PONV prevention (such as 5-HT3 receptor antagonist and glucocorticoid)
	Patients were encouraged to drink water 4–6 h after surgery and to take a liquid or semi-liquid diet 1 d after surgery, gradually to a normal diet
	Mobilization was started at 1 d after surgery. Establish daily activity goals and increase activity levels gradually.
	In addition to routine care and symptomatic treatment, focusing on coagulation dysfunction (routine low-molecular heparin)/liver failure/bile leakage/ascites/hydrothorax and other complications
	Discharge as soon as possible in accordance with the criteria: basic self-care; pain relief or oral pain relievers can control pain well; normally diet without intravenous fluids support; normal flatus and defecation; the Child-Pugh liver function grade A or bilirubin returned to normal or nearly normal; good wound healing and no infection; no need to wait for removing stitches; the patient agreed and wished to be discharged.

PONV, Postoperative nausea and vomiting.

RESULTS

A total of 282 patients were recruited for this study. Among these, 108 patients (38.30%) received traditional perioperative care in the control group, and 174 patients (61.70%) received ERAS programs in the ERAS group. The clinicopathological characteristics of these cohorts are summarized in **Table 2**. The sex, HBV infection, BMI, preoperative TB, PT, PAB, type of hepatectomy, and BCLC stage of patients in these two groups were balanced. However, a significantly higher proportion of elderly patients ($P = 0.025$), patients with underlying diseases ($P = 0.010$), higher ASA scores ($P = 0.017$), and lower preoperative ALT levels ($P = 0.032$) were observed in the ERAS group.

The operative results and postoperative outcomes in the entire patient population are shown in **Table 3**. As for the operation-related indicators, significantly less intraoperative blood loss was observed in the ERAS group (200.00 [100.00–400.00] vs. 175.00 [100.00–275.00] ml, $P = 0.009$). Although the proportion of intraoperative blood transfusion was similar (5.56 vs. 3.45%, $P = 0.545$) in the two groups, the type of hepatectomy was different (control group: segmentectomy 3 and local resection 3 vs. ERAS group: extensive hemihepatectomy 1, segmentectomy 4, and local resection 1). The use of the Pringle maneuver was also significantly more frequent in the ERAS group (66.10 vs. 17.59%, $P < 0.001$). As an indicator of postoperative liver function recovery, the TB level was significantly lower in the ERAS group (24.00 [18.00–35.00] vs. 27.25 [22.68–41.63] μmol/l, $P = 0.002$), while the ALT, PT, and PAB levels showed no significant difference between these two groups. The postoperative outcomes, namely, the days that semiliquid diet was allowed after surgery and hospital stay after surgery, were significantly less in the ERAS group (2.00 [2.00–2.00] days vs. 3.00 [3.00–4.00] days and 6.00 [5.00–6.00] days vs. 6.00 [6.00–7.00] days, both $P < 0.001$). In terms of pain score, the proportion of patients with a score ≥ 4 was significantly lower in the ERAS group within the first 2 days after surgery (2.87 vs. 12.96% and 9.77 vs. 24.07%, both $P < 0.001$). There was no significant difference in the abdominal drainage tube indwelling duration and the hospital costs between these two groups were also similar (47,069.39 [40,980.86–54,488.74] CNY vs. 49,498.55 [42,812.30–57,936.92] CNY, $P = 0.158$). The incidence of complications was not significantly different between the two groups (25.29 vs. 36.11%, $P = 0.182$). Furthermore, the 2-year RFS was similar between the two groups (71 vs. 72%, $P = 0.887$).

After PSM, the clinicopathological baselines of the two groups were well-matched (**Table 2**). In the operation-related indicators, the ERAS group showed significantly

TABLE 2 | The clinicopathological characteristics of patients.

Variables	Before propensity score matching			After propensity score matching		
	Control group (n = 108)	ERAS group (n = 174)	P	Control group (n = 87)	ERAS group (n = 87)	P
Age, years	54.00 (47.00–62.50)	59.00 (49.00–65.00)	**0.025**	55.22 ± 1.09	54.89 ± 1.28	0.843
Sex, %			0.732			0.463
Male	87 (80.56%)	143 (82.18%)		70 (80.46%)	66 (75.86%)	
Female	21 (19.44%)	31 (17.82%)		17 (19.54%)	21 (24.14%)	
Underlying diseases, %			**0.010**			0.339
Yes	29 (26.85%)	73 (41.95%)		27 (31.03%)	33 (37.93%)	
No	79 (73.15%)	101 (58.05%)		60 (68.97%)	54 (62.07%)	
HBV infection, %			0.521			0.517
Yes	90 (83.33%)	146 (83.91%)		76 (87.36%)	73 (83.91%)	
No	18 (16.67%)	28 (16.09%)		11 (12.64%)	14 (16.09%)	
ASA score*, %			**0.017**			0.091
I	31 (29.81%)	33 (19.76%)		24 (27.59%)	20 (22.99%)	
II	65 (62.50%)	129 (77.25%)		55 (63.22%)	65 (74.71%)	
III	8 (7.69%)	4 (2.40%)		8 (9.20%)	2 (2.30%)	
IV	0 (0.00%)	1 (0.60%)		-	-	
BMI	23.78 ± 0.32	24.03 ± 0.25	0.553	23.74 ± 0.34	23.93 ± 0.35	0.703
Preoperative indicators						
ALT, U/l	29.60 (19.90–43.45)	25.10 (17.55–34.95)	**0.032**	27.90 (19.30–39.80)	26.70 (17.60–35.40)	0.519
TB, μmol/l	13.00 (9.90–16.45)	11.60 (8.90–15.15)	0.050	12.90 (9.20–16.20)	12.20 (9.60–16.60)	0.892
PT, s	13.40 (13.05–14.15)	13.30 (12.85–14.00)	0.059	13.40 (13.10–14.00)	13.30 (12.80–14.10)	0.442
PAB, mg/l	238.00 (206.00–277.00)	241.00 (206.50–287.50)	0.240	241.00 (206.00–277.00)	238.00 (197.00–277.00)	0.813
Type of hepatectomy, %			0.599			0.341
Extensive hemihepatectomy	0 (0.00%)	2 (1.15%)		-	-	
Hemihepatectomy	6 (5.56%) left 5, right 1	9 (5.17%) left 5, right 4		5 (5.75%) left 5	1 (1.15%) left 1	
Segmentectomy	46 (42.59%) VII 4, right posterior 6	84 (48.28%) I 1, VII 4, right posterior 7		41 (47.13%) VII 3, right posterior 6	43 (49.43%) I 1, VII 2, right posterior 2	
Local recection	56 (51.85%) VII 7	79 (45.40%) VII 21		41 (47.13%) VII 6	43 (49.43%) VII 12	
BCLC stage, %						
0	12 (11.11%)	17 (9.77%)		11 (12.64%)	9 (10.34%)	
A	84 (77.78%)	135 (77.59%)		65 (74.71%)	71 (81.61%)	
B	9 (8.33%)	18 (10.34%)		8 (9.20%)	7 (8.05%)	
C	3 (2.78%)	4 (2.30%)		3 (3.45%)	0 (0.00%)	

HBV, Hepatitis B virus; ASA, American society of anestheiologists; BMI, Body mass index; ALT, Alanine aminotransferase; TB, Total bilirubin; PT, Prothrombin time; PAB, Prealbumin; BCLC, Barcelona Clinic Liver Cancer.

**partial value of ASA score was missing. The bold P values were used to highlight the variables with P < 0.05.*

less intraoperative blood loss than the control group (100.00 [100.00–200.00] vs. 200.00 [100.00–300.00] ml, $P = 0.001$). The proportion of patients with intraoperative blood transfusion was slightly more in the control group (4.60 vs. 2.30%, $P = 0.682$) and the type of hepatectomy between the two groups was similar (control group: segmentectomy 2 and local resection 2 vs. ERAS group: segmentectomy 1 and local resection 1). The operative duration and intraoperative blood transfusion did not demonstrate any obvious differences. The Pringle maneuver was performed more frequently in the ERAS group (70.11 vs. 18.39%, $P < 0.001$). Impressively, in the liver function recovery indicators, the ALT level in the ERAS group was significantly higher than that in the control group (183.40 [122.85–253.70] vs. 136.20 [82.93–263.40] U/l, $P = 0.026$), which was completely consistent with the results of our previous study (30). On the contrary, the TB level in the ERAS group was lower than that in the control group, although the difference was not significant (24.90 [18.10-35.38] vs. 27.25 [22.85–38.78] U/l, $P = 0.073$). PT and PAB levels were also similar between the two groups.

In the postoperative outcomes, the ERAS group showed significantly fewer days that a semiliquid diet was allowed (2.00 [2.00–2.00] days vs. 3.00 [3.00–4.00] days, $P < 0.001$), abdominal

TABLE 3 | The operative results and postoperative outcomes.

Variables	Before propensity score matching			After propensity score matching		
	Control group (*n* = 108)	ERAS group (*n* = 174)	*P*	Control group (*n* = 87)	ERAS group (*n* = 87)	*P*
Operative duration, mins	128.00 (100.00–174.25)	126.50 (101.25–170.00)	0.259	125.50 (96.25–176.50)	121.50 (98.50–163.00)	0.127
Blood loss, ml	200.00 (100.00–400.00)	175.00 (100.00–275.00)	**0.009**	200.00 (100.00–300.00)	100.00 (100.00–200.00)	**0.001**
Intraoperative blood transfusion, %			0.545			0.682
Yes	6 (5.56%) Segmentectomy 3, local resection 3	6 (3.45%) Extensive hemihepatectomy 1, Segmentectomy 4, local resection 1		4 (4.60%) Segmentectomy 2, local resection 2	2 (2.30%) Segmentectomy 1, local resection 1	
No	102 (94.44%)	168 (96.55%)		83 (95.40%)	85 (97.70%)	
Pringle maneuver			**<0.001**			**<0.001**
Yes	19 (17.59%)	115 (66.10%)		16 (18.39%)	61 (70.11%)	
No	89 (82.41%)	59 (33.91%)		71 (81.61%)	26 (29.89%)	
Postoperative indicators						
ALT, U/l	146.15 (85.18–254.48)	174.10 (109.80–261.53)	0.195	136.20 (82.93–263.40)	183.40 (122.85–253.70)	**0.026**
TB, μmol/l	27.25 (22.68–41.63)	24.00 (18.00–35.00)	**0.002**	27.25 (22.85–38.78)	24.90 (18.10–35.38)	0.073
PT, s	14.90 (14.40–15.70)	14.75 (14.00–15.68)	0.935	14.90 (14.40–15.68)	14.90 (14.20–15.68)	0.649
PAB, mg/l	126.57 ± 3.15	128.41 ± 2.88	0.677	125.74 ± 3.38	126.41 ± 3.79	0.896
Pain score ≥ 4, yes/no, %						
POD 1	14/94 (12.96%)	5/169 (2.87%)	**0.001**	12/75 (13.79%)	1/86 (1.15%)	**0.002**
POD 2	26/82 (24.07%)	17/157 (9.77%)	**0.001**	23/64 (26.44%)	7/80 (8.05%)	**0.001**
POD 3	12/96 (11.11%)	9/165 (5.17%)	0.065	10/77 (11.49%)	4/83 (4.60%)	0.094
POD 4	7/101 (6.48%)	6/168 (3.45%)	0.255	5/82 (5.75%)	4/83 (4.60%)	1.000
POD 5	2/106 (1.85%)	0/174 (0.00%)	0.146	2/85 (2.30%)	0/87 (0.00%)	0.497
Semiliquid diet after surgery, days	3.00 (3.00–4.00)	2.00 (2.00–2.00)	**< 0.001**	3.00 (3.00–4.00)	2.00 (2.00–2.00)	**< 0.001**
Abdominal drainage tube removal, days	4.00 (3.00–5.00)	4.00 (3.00–5.00)	0.053	4.00 (3.00–5.00)	4.00 (3.00–4.00)	**0.023**
Hospital stay after surgery, days	6.00 (6.00–7.00)	6.00 (5.00–6.00)	**< 0.001**	6.00 (6.00–7.00)	6.00 (5.00–6.00)	**< 0.001**
Hospital costs, CNY	49498.55 (42812.30–57936.92)	47069.39 (40980.86–4488.74)	0.158	49397.18 (42749.59–56975.35)	46219.98 (41353.38–51841.06)	0.123
Complications, %			0.182			**0.026**
No	69 (63.89%)	130 (74.71%)		57 (65.52%)	71 (81.61%)	
Grade I	18 (16.67%)	24 (13.79%)		13 (14.94%)	11 (12.64%)	
Grade II	18 (16.67%)	15 (8.62%)		15 (17.24%)	5 (5.75%)	
Grade III	3 (2.78%)	4 (2.30%)		2 (2.30%)	0 (0.00%)	
Grade IV	0 (0.00%)	1 (0.57%)		-	-	

POD, Postoperative day. The bold P values were used to highlight the variables with P < 0.05.

drainage tube removal (4.00 [3.00–4.00] days vs. 4.00 [3.00–5.00] days, $P = 0.023$), and hospital stay after surgery (6.00 [5.00–6.00] days vs. 6.00 [6.00–7.00] days, $P < 0.001$) than in the control group. Similar to that before PSM, the proportion of patients with a pain score ≥ 4 was significantly lower in the ERAS group within the first 2 days after surgery (1.15 vs. 13.79% and 8.05 vs. 26.44%, $P = 0.002$ and $P = 0.001$, respectively). In the patient population after PSM, there was also no significant difference in the hospital costs between these two groups (46,219.98 [41,353.38–51,841.06] CNY vs. 49,397.18 [42,749.59–56,975.35] CNY, $P = 0.123$). Interestingly, the ERAS group demonstrated significantly less postoperative morbidity (18.39 vs. 34.48%, $P = 0.026$) after PSM. Furthermore, after PSM, 2-year RFS was similar in these two groups (72 vs. 71%, $P = 0.946$).

DISCUSSION

Laparoscopic hepatectomy (LH) has been considered as a landmark development in the progression of a surgical treatment since it was gradually introduced to cure liver lesions in the 1990s (32, 33). LH was first applied to a patient with HCC in 1998 (34). The majority of HCC patients were infected with HBV (appropriate 85% of patients in this study), which caused cirrhosis or at least an inflammatory background in the liver. Thus, the surgical risk of LH correspondingly increased. Compared with open hepatectomy, LH showed better surgical safety, faster postoperative recovery, and comparable long-term survival (35). LH itself could be regarded as an ERAS approach to reduce the impact of surgery on HCC patients (20, 36, 37). The combination of LH and ERAS programs seemed to demonstrate lower postoperative morbidity and more satisfactory functional recovery than open surgery in both minor and major liver resections (37, 38), although several meta-analyses have yielded inconsistent conclusions (15, 16, 28, 29, 39).

In this study, PSM was performed to minimize the confounding bias of the baselines due to the retrospective design. Early abdominal drainage tube removal, better pain control, shorter hospital stay, and lower postoperative morbidity after ERAS were confirmed. These results proved the effectiveness of ERAS programs in patients with HCC who had undergone LH. Furthermore, alterations in postoperative liver function and mid-term recurrence were also investigated in these patients. Several representative indicators, namely, ALT, TB, and PT were selected, and these indicators generally peaked on the 3rd day after surgery. The postoperative ALT level was significantly higher in the ERAS group. Conversely, the TB level was lower in the ERAS group, although the difference was not statistically significant. The PT levels were also not affected. Similar results were also observed in LH, but not open surgery, in our previous study (30). These indicators reflected that liver function was stable and trended to recover faster. The increasing level of ALT revealed that laparoscopic surgery combined with controlled low central venous pressure (CVP) according to the ERAS programs might enhance the ischemia-reperfusion injury (IRI) of the liver. Laparoscopic pneumoperitoneum can also cause hepatic IRI as a result of the temporary decrease in blood inflow into the portal vein (40, 41). Above all, the Pringle maneuver was performed more frequently in the ERAS group. Laparoscopic Pringle maneuver combined with low CVP obviously decreased intraoperative blood loss and tended to reduce the proportion of blood transfusion, which made LH safer. Meanwhile, low inflow and easy outflow reduce the amount of residual blood in the liver, which inevitably increases the severity of IRI (42, 43). The enrollment design of this study had a chronological sequence and the appropriate laparoscopic Pringle maneuver was gradually determined and more frequently used in the development of LH in our center, which made the Pringle maneuver used more in the ERAS group. Regardless of enhanced IRI, the laparoscopic Pringle maneuver might be considered as a step in ERAS programs.

Few studies have explored the role of ERAS programs in long-term or mid-term survival. Recently, stage III gastric cancer patients undergoing laparoscopic radical gastrectomy were verified to have a survival benefit from ERAS implementation (44). In colon cancer, laparoscopic surgery combined with ERAS has a longer overall survival than open surgery combined with ERAS (45). The potential explanations are as follows: (1) reducing stress might improve antitumor immunity and (2) quick recovery reduces delayed adjuvant therapy. Two years after surgery is a significant recurrence timing of HCC, and 2-year recurrence has an obvious influence on long-term prognosis (31). Our results showed no difference in 2-year RFS between the two groups. The potential explanation is that there is no standard adjuvant therapy for HCC, and thus, the implementation of adjuvant therapy would not be affected by ERAS. At the same time, both groups in this study were laparoscopic surgery groups, in which the role of the ERAS program alone on prognosis might be limited. In fact, ERAS implementation did not improve patient survival in all tumors (46).

Generally, in HCC patients undergoing LH, ERAS programs were verified to improve postoperative recovery significantly but did not show their role in 2-year recurrence. Although hepatic IRI might be enhanced, laparoscopic Pringle maneuver combined with low CVP might make LH safer by improving intraoperative blood loss, which should be considered as a step of ERAS programs. Although PSM was used to reduce confounding bias and make the conclusion more convincing, a following prospective RCT is still necessary to further confirm the conclusion.

AUTHOR CONTRIBUTIONS

Study concept: AM and LW. Data collection: JZ and XH. First draft: JZ. Data analysis and review and editing: All authors.

REFERENCES

1. Kehlet H. Multimodal approach to control postoperative pathophysiology and rehabilitation. *Br J Anaesth.* (1997) 78:606–17. doi: 10.1093/bja/78.5.606
2. Kehlet H, Dahl JB. Anaesthesia, surgery, and challenges in postoperative recovery. *Lancet.* (2003) 362:1921–8. doi: 10.1016/S0140-6736(03)14966-5
3. Kehlet H, Wilmore DW. Evidence-based surgical care and the evolution of fast-track surgery. *Ann Surg.* (2008) 248:189–98. doi: 10.1097/SLA.0b013e31817f2c1a
4. Schultz NA, Larsen PN, Klarskov B, Plum LM, Frederiksen HJ, Kehlet H, et al. Second generation of a fast-track liver resection programme. *World J Surg.* (2018) 42:1860–6. doi: 10.1007/s00268-017-4399-3
5. Muehling B, Schelzig H, Steffen P, Meierhenrich R, Sunder-Plassmann L, Orend KH. A prospective randomized trial comparing traditional and fast-track patient care in elective open infrarenal aneurysm repair. *World J Surg.* (2009) 33:577–85. doi: 10.1007/s00268-008-9892-2
6. Kim JW, Kim WS, Cheong JH, Hyung WJ, Choi SH, Noh SH. Safety and efficacy of fast-track surgery in laparoscopic distal gastrectomy for gastric cancer: a randomized clinical trial. *World J Surg.* (2012) 36:2879–87. doi: 10.1007/s00268-012-1741-7
7. Gustafsson UO, Scott MJ, Hubner M, Nygren J, Demartines N, Francis N, et al. Guidelines for perioperative care in elective colorectal surgery: enhanced recovery after surgery (ERAS((R))) society recommendations: 2018. *World J Surg.* (2019) 43:659–95. doi: 10.1007/s00268-018-4844-y
8. Hu ZC, He LJ, Chen D, Li XB, Feng ZH, Fu CW, et al. An enhanced recovery after surgery program in orthopedic surgery: a systematic review and meta-analysis. *J Orthop Surg Res.* (2019) 14:77. doi: 10.1186/s13018-019-1116-y
9. Macones GA, Caughey AB, Wood SL, Wrench IJ, Huang J, Norman M, et al. Guidelines for postoperative care in cesarean delivery: Enhanced Recovery After Surgery (ERAS) Society recommendations (part 3). *Am J Obstet Gynecol.* (2019) 221:247.e1–247.e9. doi: 10.1016/j.ajog.2019.04.012
10. Moschini M, Stabile A, Mattei A, Montorsi F, Cathelineau X, Sanchez-Salas R. Enhanced recovery after surgery (ERAS) in radical cystectomy patients: from consensus to evidences. *Int Braz J Urol.* (2019) 45:655–7. doi: 10.1590/s1677-5538.ibju.2019.04.02
11. Pache B, Joliat GR, Hubner M, Grass F, Demartines N, Mathevet P, et al. Cost-analysis of enhanced recovery after surgery (ERAS) program in gynecologic surgery. *Gynecol Oncol.* (2019) 154:388–93. doi: 10.1016/j.ygyno.2019.06.004

12. van Dam Hendry PO, Coolsen MME, Bemelmans MHA, Lassen K, Revhaug A, Fearon KCH, et al. Initial experience with a multimodal enhanced recovery programme in patients undergoing liver resection. *Brit J Surg.* (2008) 95:969–75. doi: 10.1002/bjs.6227
13. Qi S, Chen G, Cao P, Hu J, He G, Luo J, et al. Safety and efficacy of enhanced recovery after surgery (ERAS) programs in patients undergoing hepatectomy: A prospective randomized controlled trial. *J Clin Lab Anal.* (2018) 32:e22434. doi: 10.1002/jcla.22434
14. Ni CY, Wang ZH, Huang ZP, Zhou H, Fu LJ, Cai H, et al. Early enforced mobilization after liver resection: A prospective randomized controlled trial. *Int J Surg.* (2018) 54:254–8. doi: 10.1016/j.ijsu.2018.04.060
15. Liang X, Ying H, Wang H, Xu H, Liu M, Zhou H, et al. Enhanced recovery care versus traditional care after laparoscopic liver resections: a randomized controlled trial. *Surg Endosc.* (2018) 32:2746–57. doi: 10.1007/s00464-017-5973-3
16. Rouxel P, Beloeil H. Enhanced recovery after hepatectomy: A systematic review. *Anaesth Crit Care Pain Med.* (2019) 38:29–34. doi: 10.1016/j.accpm.2018.05.003
17. Damania R, Cocieru A. Impact of enhanced recovery after surgery protocols on postoperative morbidity and mortality in patients undergoing routine hepatectomy: review of the current evidence. *Ann Transl Med.* (2017) 5:341. doi: 10.21037/atm.2017.07.04
18. Wang C, Zheng G, Zhang W, Zhang F, Lv S, Wang A, et al. Enhanced recovery after surgery programs for liver resection: a meta-analysis. *J Gastrointest Surg.* (2017) 21:472–86. doi: 10.1007/s11605-017-3360-y
19. Melloul E, Hubner M, Scott M, Snowden C, Prentis J, Dejong CH, et al. Guidelines for perioperative care for liver surgery: enhanced recovery after surgery (ERAS) society recommendations. *World J Surg.* (2016) 40:2425–40. doi: 10.1007/s00268-016-3700-1
20. Jia W, Liu W, Qiao X. Chinese expert consensus on enhanced recovery after hepatectomy (Version 2017). *Asian J Surg.* (2019) 42:11–8. doi: 10.1016/j.asjsur.2018.01.007
21. Kulik L, El-Serag HB. Epidemiology and management of hepatocellular carcinoma. *Gastroenterology.* (2019) 156:477–91.e1. doi: 10.1053/j.gastro.2018.08.065
22. Sayiner M, Golabi P, Younossi ZM. Disease burden of hepatocellular carcinoma: a global perspective. *Dig Dis Sci.* (2019) 64:910–7. doi: 10.1007/s10620-019-05537-2
23. Chong CCN, Chung WY, Cheung YS, Fung AKY, Fong AKW, Lok HT, et al. Enhanced recovery after surgery for liver resection. *Hong Kong Med J.* (2019) 25:94–101. doi: 10.12809/hkmj187656
24. Kaibori M, Matsui K, Ishizaki M, Iida H, Yoshii K, Asano H, et al. Effects of implementing an "enhanced recovery after surgery" program on patients undergoing resection of hepatocellular carcinoma. *Surg Today.* (2017) 47:42–51. doi: 10.1007/s00595-016-1344-2
25. Wakabayashi G, Cherqui D, Geller DA, Buell JF, Kaneko H, Han HS, et al. Recommendations for laparoscopic liver resection: a report from the second international consensus conference held in Morioka. *Ann Surg.* (2015) 261:619–29. doi: 10.1097/SLA.0000000000001184
26. Xu HW, Liu F, Li HY, Wei YG, Li B. Outcomes following laparoscopic versus open major hepatectomy for hepatocellular carcinoma in patients with cirrhosis: a propensity score-matched analysis. *Surg Endosc.* (2018) 32:712–9. doi: 10.1007/s00464-017-5727-2
27. Shehta A, Han HS, Yoon YS, Cho JY, Choi Y. Laparoscopic liver resection for hepatocellular carcinoma in cirrhotic patients: 10-year single-center experience. *Surg Endosc.* (2016) 30:638–48. doi: 10.1007/s00464-015-4253-3
28. Liang X, Ying H, Wang H, Xu H, Yu H, Cai L, et al. Enhanced recovery program versus traditional care in laparoscopic hepatectomy. *Medicine (Baltimore).* (2016) 95:e2835. doi: 10.1097/MD.0000000000002835
29. Li L, Chen J, Liu Z, Li Q, Shi Y. Enhanced recovery program versus traditional care after hepatectomy: A meta-analysis. *Medicine (Baltimore).* (2017) 96:e8052. doi: 10.1097/MD.0000000000008052
30. Zhou JM, He XG, Wang M, Zhao YM, Shu L, Wang LR, et al. Enhanced recovery after surgery program in the patients undergoing hepatectomy for benign liver lesions. *Hepatobiliary Pancreat Dis Int.* (2020) 19:122–8. doi: 10.1016/j.hbpd.2019.12.012
31. Wang MD, Li C, Liang L, Xing H, Sun LY, Quan B, et al. Early and late recurrence of Hepatitis B virus-associated hepatocellular carcinoma. *Oncologist.* (2020) 25:e1541–51. doi: 10.1634/theoncologist.2019-0944
32. Klotz HP, Schlumpf R, Weder W, Largiader F. Minimal invasive surgery for treatment of enlarged symptomatic liver cysts. *Surg Laparosc Endosc.* (1993) 3:351–3.
33. Kaneko H, Takagi S, Shiba T. Laparoscopic partial hepatectomy and left lateral segmentectomy: technique and results of a clinical series. *Surgery.* (1996) 120:468–75. doi: 10.1016/S0039-6060(96)80065-1
34. Mizoe A, Tomioka T, Inoue K, Azuma T, Fujioka H, Furui J, et al. Systematic laparoscopic left lateral segmentectomy of the liver for hepatocellular carcinoma. *J Hepatobiliary Pancreat Surg.* (1998) 5:173–8. doi: 10.1007/s005340050029
35. Chen K, Pan Y, Zhang B, Liu XL, Maher H, Zheng XY. Laparoscopic versus open surgery for hepatocellular carcinoma: a meta-analysis of high-quality case-matched studies. *Can J Gastroenterol Hepatol.* (2018) 2018:1746895. doi: 10.1155/2018/1746895
36. Ratti F, Cipriani F, Reineke R, Catena M, Comotti L, Beretta L, et al. Impact of ERAS approach and minimally-invasive techniques on outcome of patients undergoing liver surgery for hepatocellular carcinoma. *Dig Liver Dis.* (2016) 48:1243–8. doi: 10.1016/j.dld.2016.06.032
37. Pagano D, Ricotta C, Barbàra M, Cintorino D, di Francesco F, Tropea A, et al. ERAS protocol for perioperative care of patients treated with laparoscopic nonanatomic liver resection for hepatocellular carcinoma: the ISMETT experience. *J Laparoendosc Adv Surg Tech A.* (2020) 30:1066–71. doi: 10.1089/lap.2020.0445
38. Ratti F, Cipriani F, Reineke R, Comotti L, Paganelli M, Catena M, et al. The clinical and biological impacts of the implementation of fast-track perioperative programs in complex liver resections: A propensity score-based analysis between the open and laparoscopic approaches. *Surgery.* (2018) 164:395–403. doi: 10.1016/j.surg.2018.04.020
39. He F, Lin X, Xie F, Huang Y, Yuan R. The effect of enhanced recovery program for patients undergoing partial laparoscopic hepatectomy of liver cancer. *Clin Transl Oncol.* (2015) 17:694–701. doi: 10.1007/s12094-015-1296-9
40. Hasegawa Y, Nitta H, Takahara T, Katagiri H, Kanno S, Umemura A, et al. Glucocorticoid use and ischemia-reperfusion injury in laparoscopic liver resection: Randomized controlled trial. *Ann Gastroenterol Surg.* (2020) 4:76–83. doi: 10.1002/ags3.12298
41. Lai H, Mo X, Yang Y, Xiao J, He K, Chen J, et al. Association between duration of carbon dioxide pneumoperitoneum during laparoscopic abdominal surgery and hepatic injury: a meta-analysis. *PLoS ONE.* (2014) 9:e104067. doi: 10.1371/journal.pone.0104067
42. Xia F, Wang S, Chen M, Wang X, Feng X, Dong J. Protective effect of Verapamil on hepatic ischemia-reperfusion injury during hepatectomy in the cirrhotic patients with hepatocellular carcinoma. *Langenbecks Arch Surg.* (2009) 394:1041–6. doi: 10.1007/s00423-009-0491-y
43. Hughes MJ, Ventham NT, Harrison EM, Wigmore SJ. Central venous pressure and liver resection: a systematic review and meta-analysis. *HPB.* (2015) 17:863–71. doi: 10.1111/hpb.12462
44. Tian YL, Cao SG, Liu XD, Li ZQ, Liu G, Zhang XQ, et al. Short- and long-term outcomes associated with enhanced recovery after surgery protocol vs conventional management in patients undergoing laparoscopic gastrectomy. *World J Gastroenterol.* (2020) 26:5646–60. doi: 10.3748/wjg.v26.i37.5646
45. Curtis NJ, Taylor M, Fraser L, Salib E, Noble E, Hipkiss R, et al. Can the combination of laparoscopy and enhanced recovery improve long-term survival after elective colorectal cancer surgery? *Int J Colorectal Dis.* (2018) 33:231–4. doi: 10.1007/s00384-017-2935-0
46. Ziegelmueller BK, Jokisch JF, Buchner A, Grimm T, Kretschmer A, Schulz GB, et al. Long-term follow-up and oncological outcome of patients undergoing radical cystectomy for bladder cancer following an enhanced recovery after surgery (ERAS) protocol: results of a large randomized, prospective, single-center study. *Urol Int.* (2020) 104:55–61. doi: 10.1159/000504236

8

Prognostic Impact of Surgical Margin in Hepatectomy on Patients with Hepatocellular Carcinoma

Yeting Lin [1†], Jiaxuan Xu [2†], Jiaze Hong [2], Yuexiu Si [3], Yujing He [2] and Jinhang Zhang [4]*

[1] Anesthesiology Department, Ningbo Yinzhou No. 2 Hospital, Ningbo, China, [2] The Second Clinical Medical College, Zhejiang Chinese Medical University, Hangzhou, China, [3] School of Basic Medical Sciences, Zhejiang Chinese Medical University, Hangzhou, China, [4] Surgery Department, Fenghua Hospital of Traditional Chinese Medicine, Ningbo, China

***Correspondence:**
Jinhang Zhang
george202110@163.com

† These authors have contributed equally to this work and share first authorship

Objective: This study aims to comprehensively evaluate the prognostic impact of the surgical margin in hepatectomy on patients diagnosed with hepatocellular carcinoma (HCC).

Methods: A comprehensive and systematic search for eligible articles published in English before July 2021 was conducted across PubMed, Cochrane Library, Web of Science, and Embase electronic databases. The overall survival (OS) and disease-free survival (DFS) were the primary endpoints.

Results: In total, 37 observational studies with 12,295 cases were included in this meta-analysis. The results revealed that a wide surgical margin (≥1 cm) was associated with better OS (hazard ration (HR), 0.70; 95% confidence interval (CI), 0.63–0.77) and DFS (HR, 0.66; 95% CI, 0.61–0.71) compared to a narrow surgical margin (<1 cm). Subgroup analyses were conducted based on median follow-up time, gender, country, hepatitis B surface antigen (HBsAg) status, tumor number, and liver cirrhosis. The prognostic benefit of a wide surgical margin was consistent in most subgroups, however, analysis of studies from Western countries showed that margin width was not associated with prognosis.

Conclusion: In summary, a surgical margin wider than 1 cm prolongs the long-term prognosis of HCC patients compared to a surgical margin narrower than 1 cm.

Keywords: hepatocellular carcinoma, hepatectomy, surgical margin, prognosis, meta-analysis

INTRODUCTION

Although hepatocellular carcinoma (HCC) has the 5th highest incidence across the globe, it is currently the 3rd leading cause of cancer-related deaths (1, 2). So far, liver transplantation, hepatic resection and radiofrequency ablation are the few treatment strategies for HCC. Although hepatectomy is the first-line therapeutic intervention, the prognosis of patients is unsatisfactory due to the high risk of recurrence (70% in the 5th year after surgery) and metastasis (3).

The long-term prognosis of patients with HCC is influenced by several factors, among them, liver cirrhosis is a main factor, and the surgical margin is considered a potential prognostic factor (4, 5). Curative hepatectomy is complete resection of all visible tumors without residual tumor cells at the resection margin (6). As such, an adequate resection margin is vital in preventing tumor recurrence (7). Nonetheless, minimizing the removal of the non-malignant parenchyma tissue and protecting the residual liver of liver resection is necessary for many HCC patients with liver cirrhosis or other liver diseases. This is because the capacity for liver regeneration is impaired among these patients and excessive liver tissue removal leads to severe consequences including liver failure (8, 9). Thus, controversies on the width of the surgical margin have been reported under the premise of R0 resection. Many studies reveal that the width of the resection margin narrower than 1 cm is a risk factor for the long-term prognosis of HCC patients after surgery (4, 10). Nevertheless, a number of articles found that a wide surgical margin did not improve the prognosis of HCC patients after hepatectomy (11, 12).

Therefore, this meta-analysis seeks to assess the correlation between surgical margins (a surgical margin wider than 1 cm; a surgical margin narrower than 1 cm) and long-term prognosis of HCC patients after hepatectomy.

METHODS

Literature Search Strategy

This meta-analysis adhered to the guidelines from the Preferred Reporting Items for Systematic Review and Meta-Analysis (13). A comprehensive and systematic literature search for articles published in English before July 2021 was conducted in four online electronic databases including PubMed, Cochrane Library, Web of Science, and Embase. The search terminologies included: "Hepatocellular Carcinoma" OR "Liver Cell Carcinomas" OR "Hepatoma" OR "HCC" AND "Resection Margin" OR "Surgical Margin" OR "Margin Width." Besides, reference lists of all retrieved papers were inspected to identify potentially eligible but uncaptured literature in the primary search.

Inclusion Criteria

Studies were included if they met the following criteria: (1) The cancer type was primary HCC and hepatectomy was performed on patients; (2) Patients received different surgical margins in the study (a wide surgical margin, ≥1 cm) and control (a narrow surgical margin, <1 cm) groups; (3) The study was original, including retrospective and prospective observational studies (OBS); (4) Extractable outcomes were in the studies.

Abbreviations: HCC, hepatocellular carcinoma; OS, overall survival; DFS, disease-free survival; HR, hazard ratio; CI, confidence interval; HBsAg, hepatitis B surface antigen; OBS, observational study; AFP, alpha-fetoprotein; NOS, Newcastle-Ottawa Scale; HBV, hepatitis B virus; PSM, propensity score matching; MVI, microvascular invasion.

Exclusion Criteria

The exclusion criteria for this meta-analysis included: (1) HCC was recurrent; (2) The patients received palliative hepatectomy or had extrahepatic metastases; (3) The study did not divide the study group and the control group into larger than 1 cm and smaller than 1 cm; (4) Duplicate article or repeat analyses using similar data.

Data Extraction and Quality Evaluation

Data extracted from eligible studies included study characteristics (author, country, publication year, study design, median follow-up time, and mentioned outcome measures), demographic data of patients (age, gender, and the number of patients), and clinicopathological features (liver cirrhosis, virus status, tumor number and size, and serum alpha-fetoprotein (AFP), and survival outcomes.

The quality of incorporated OBSs was evaluated using the Newcastle-Ottawa Scale (NOS) based on three aspects i.e., patient selection, comparability of groups, and outcome evaluation. The scores of papers >6 were considered high-quality.

Statistical Analysis

To evaluate the relationship between surgical margins and HCC prognosis, the overall survival (OS) and disease-free survival (DFS) in the wide surgical margin group vs. the narrow surgical margin group was compared using a pooled hazard ratio (HR) with its corresponding 95% confidence interval (CI). The degree of heterogeneity across included literature was assessed using the I^2 statistic. Considering the potential heterogeneity, random-effect model was applied to all analyses. To assess the robustness of conclusions, a sensitivity analysis was conducted. $P < 0.05$ was considered statistically significant.

RESULTS

Data Collection and Characteristics

A total of 6,864 records were initially identified by the literature search. Out of these, 4,743 records were excluded because of duplication, and 2,050 records were eliminated after evaluating their titles or abstracts. The remaining 71 records were carefully inspected by full-text reading. Finally, 37 articles (4, 5, 7, 10–12, 14–44) were included. The comprehensive search and selection process is shown in (**Figure 1**).

The comprehensive characteristics of the included studies are summarized in (**Table 1-1**). The included articles were published between 1993 and 2021. A total of 12,295 patients from Western and Asian countries were enrolled in 37 OBSs; two studies of these were prospective, while the rest were retrospective. The majority of articles were from Asia, with China representing the most (24 articles). The demographic and clinicopathological characteristics of patients are presented in (**Table 1-2**). Based on a qualitative assessment by NOS criteria, the results revealed that all included OBSs were of higher quality (**Supplementary Table 1**).

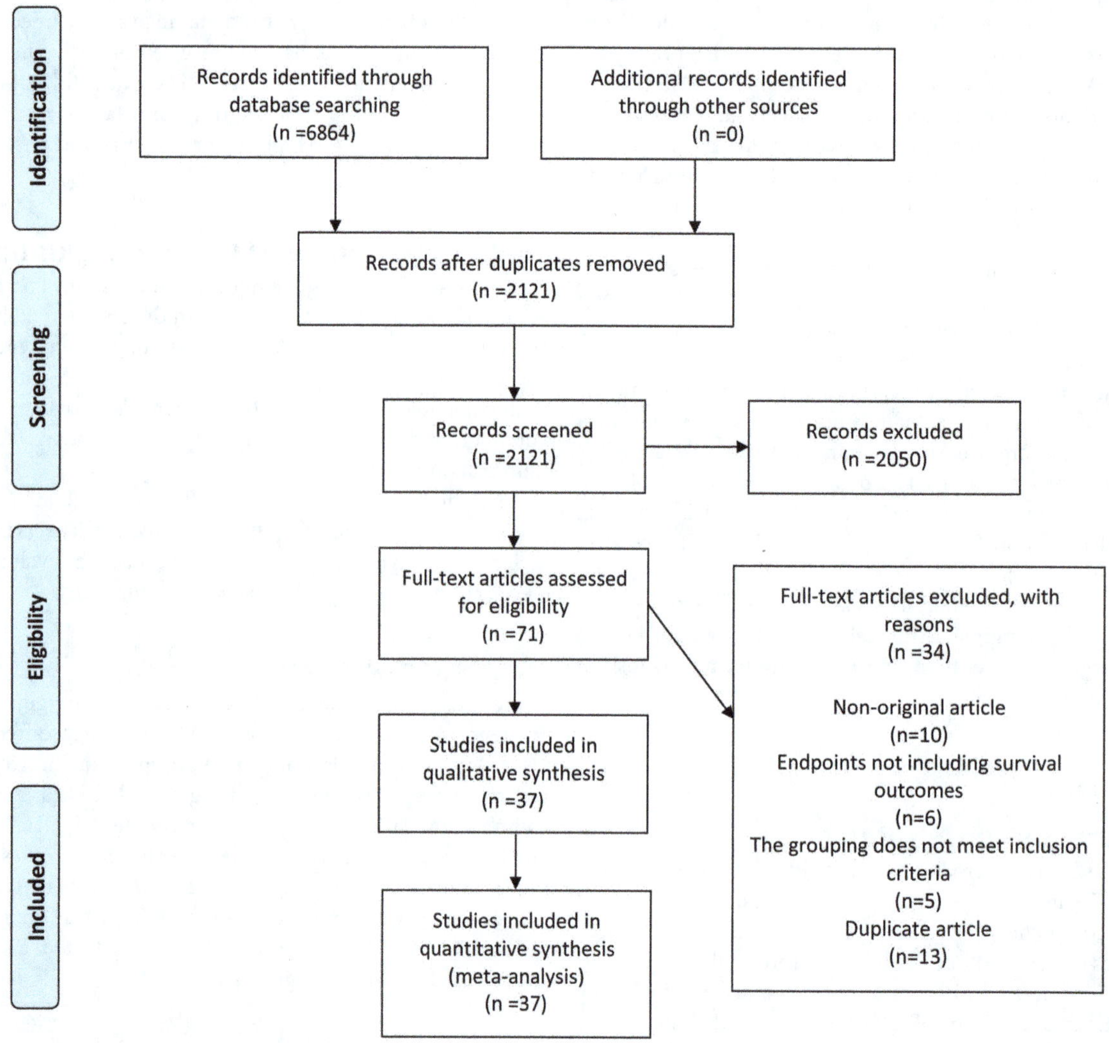

FIGURE 1 | A schematic flow for selecting the articles included in the meta-analysis.

Correlation Between Surgical Margin and OS

A total of 28 studies reported on OS outcomes and pooling analysis of these data revealed that a wide surgical margin is associated with better OS (HR, 0.70; 95% CI, 0.63–0.77) compared to a narrow surgical margin (**Figure 2**). Subgroups analyses were conducted to explore the potential factors that might affect the impact of the surgical margin on the prognosis (**Table 2**). This was based on the reported median follow-up time. The studies were divided into 3-year OS and 5-year OS subgroups. The result showed that patients who received a wide resection margin had better mid-and long-term prognosis than those who received a narrow resection margin. Moreover, the gender factor in the subgroups was analyzed and the findings revealed that a narrow surgical margin was a risk factor for OS of patients regardless of men and women. For patients from China or Non-Chinese Asian countries, a wide resection margin was associated with better OS than a narrow resection margin. However, a pooled analysis of three studies from western countries showed that margin width was not associated with prognosis. Additionally, the wide surgical margin group obtained greater OS than that of the narrow surgical margin group in subgroups of hepatitis B surface antigen status (HBsAg) positive/negative and single/multiple tumors.

Correlation Between Surgical Margin and DFS

A pooled analysis of DFS data from 27 studies including 9,443 patients revealed that a wide surgical margin was related to better DFS (HR, 0.66; 95% CI, 0.61–0.71) (**Figure 3**). Further, subgroup analyses were performed based on reported median follow-up time (3-year DFS/5-year DFS), gender (male/female), country (China/Non-Chinese Asian countries/Western countries), HBsAg status (positive/negative), tumor number

TABLE 1-1 | Characteristics of all the studies included in the meta-analysis.

Author	Year	Country	Number of patients		Median follow-up (months)	Study design	Survival outcomes
			Wide resection margin (>1 cm)	Narrow resection margin (<1 cm)			
Belli	2011	Italy	56	9	29.0	Retrospective	DFS
Chang	2012	China	478		29.5	Retrospective	DFS
Chen	2003	China	174	68	11.8	Retrospective	OS
Chen	2015	China	114	82	NA	Retrospective	OS
Chen	2021	China	176	238	>60.0	Retrospective	OS
Dong	2016	China	351	235	46.8	Retrospective	DFS
Han	2019	China	302	147	56.3	Retrospective	OS, DFS
Hirokawa	2014	Japan	10	10	46.0	Retrospective	DFS
Hsiao	2017	China	154	67	NA	Retrospective	OS
Huang	2013	China	528	512	42.0	Retrospective	OS, DFS
Huang	2015	China	71	159	72.0	Retrospective	OS, DFS
Laurent	2005	France	61	41	23.0	Retrospective	OS, DFS
Lee	1996	China	38	10	>60.0	Retrospective	OS
Lee	2007	Korea	44	56	31.0	Retrospective	OS, DFS
Lee	2012	China	142	156	73.0	Retrospective	OS, DFS
Lee	2018	Korea	186	233	37.5	Retrospective	OS, DFS
Lee	2019	China	143	391	66.3	Retrospective	OS, DFS
Lise	1998	Italy	72	15	29.0	Retrospective	OS, DFS
Liu	2016	China	186	37	26.1	Retrospective	DFS
Liu	2020	China	134	106	55.2	Retrospective	OS, DFS
Park	2018	Korea	61	31	28.0	Retrospective	OS, DFS
Poon	2000	China	138	150	27.0	Prospective	OS, DFS
Sasaki	2006	Japan	176	241	>120.0	Retrospective	DFS
Shi	2019	China	177	99	44.0	Retrospective	OS, DFS
Shimada	2008	Japan	32	85	62.0	Retrospective	OS
Shin	2018	Korea	55	61	66.7	Retrospective	DFS
Su	2021	China	45	114	61.2	Retrospective	OS, DFS
Takano	2000	Japan	244	56	NA	Retrospective	OS
Torii	1993	Japan	25	34	25.0	Retrospective	OS
Tsilimigras	2020	Multicenter	78	326	28.5	Retrospective	OS, DFS
Wang	2010	China	404	34	21.0	Retrospective	OS
Yang	2014	China	126	959	NA	Retrospective	OS, DFS
Zeng	2020	China	155	544	NA	Retrospective	OS, DFS
Zhang	2014	China	216	86	26.0	Prospective	DFS
Zhang	2021	China	305	120	26.0	Retrospective	DFS
Zhou	2020	China	92	217	NA	Retrospective	OS, DFS
Zhou	2021	China	325	492	NA	Retrospective	OS

OS, overall survival; DFS, disease-free survival; NA, not available.

(single/multiple), liver cirrhosis (patients with/without). As a consequence, a wide surgical margin provided patients with better DFS compared to a narrow surgical margin (**Table 2**).

Sensitivity Analysis

After careful selection of studies in sequence, sensitivity analysis outcomes confirmed the excellent robustness of the conclusion that a wide surgical margin could benefit the OS and DFS of patients (**Supplementary Figures 1, 2**).

DISCUSSION

The findings of this meta-analysis revealed that surgical margins correlate with the prognosis of HCC patients; besides, a wide surgical margin ($\geq$1 cm) could improve long-term prognosis compared to a narrow surgical margin (<1 cm). This is in line with the results reported in previous articles (39, 40). Through subgroups analyses, we found that the above outcome showed a similar phenomenon in different subgroups except for studies from Western countries. In this analysis, a wide surgical margin

TABLE 1-2 | Characteristics of all the studies included in the meta-analysis.

Author	Year	Age (years)	Gender (male/female)	Liver cirrhosis (numbers)	HBV/HCV status (numbers)	Number of tumor (solitary/multiple)	AFP (ng/ml)	Tumor size (cm)
Belli	2011	63.2	38/27	65	NA	53/12	56 cases≤400, 9 cases>400	3.8
Chang	2012	59.3	403/75	NA	313/77	171/307	110	7.5
Chen	2003	196 cases≤65, 46 cases>65	186/56	0	172/NA	161/81	58 cases≤20, 184 cases>20	19 cases≤2, 223 cases>2
Chen	2015	155 cases≤60, 41 cases>60	156/40	124	178/NA	111/85	94 cases≤200, 102 cases>200	50 cases≤5, 146 cases>5
Chen	2021	332 cases≤60, 82 cases>60	340/74	288	355/NA	362/52	295 cases≤400, 119 cases>400	271 cases≤5, 143 cases>5
Dong	2016	55.2	486/100	536	504/16	586/0	305 cases≤20, 281 cases>20	408 cases≤5, 178 cases>5
Han	2019	NA	394/55	300	415/11	NA	110 cases≤400, 339 cases>400	321 cases≤5, 128 cases>5
Hirokawa	2014	66	17/3	6	17/10	20/0	121	4.6
Hsiao	2017	NA	177/44	86	108/63	117/104	NA	101 cases≤5, 120 cases>5
Huang	2013	946 cases≤65, 94 cases>65	914/126	NA	1040/NA	NA	453 cases≤100, 587 cases>100	629 cases≤5, 411 cases>5
Huang	2015	102 cases≤56, 128 cases>56	173/57	99	152/59	NA	19.8	190 cases≤5, 40 cases>5
Laurent	2005	64	89/19	0	9/12	NA	65 cases≤10, 37 cases>10	NA
Lee	1996	55	42/6	40	NA	NA	9 cases≤20, 39 cases>20	3.3
Lee	2007	47	77/23	NA	83/NA	80/20	59 cases≤1000, 41 cases>1000	13.3
Lee	2012	205 cases≤65, 93 cases>65	222/76	200	146/90	209/86	240 cases≤400, 53 cases>400	NA
Lee	2018	58.4	326/93	249	302/28	376/43	NA	NA
Lee	2019	56.4	428/106	235	280/128	NA	354 cases≤200, 140 cases>200	4.8
Lise	1998	60.2	86/14	78	NA	NA	37 cases≤10, 58 cases>10	5
Liu	2016	54	189/34	199	174/2	168/55	NA	86 cases≤5, 137 cases>5
Liu	2020	NA	208/32	174	183/NA	205/35	137 cases≤20, 107 cases>20	101 cases≤5, 139 cases>5
Park	2018	59	75/17	NA	51/6	69/23	0.103	2.5
Poon	2000	NA	238/50	133	232/NA	NA	NA	124 cases≤5, 164 cases>5
Sasaki	2006	298 cases≤65, 119 cases>65	317/100	272	66/351	318/99	245 cases≤100, 172 cases>100	256 cases≤3, 161 cases>3
Shi	2019	145 cases≤60, 131 cases>60	238/38	140	249/NA	NA	175 cases≤400, 101 cases>400	46 cases≤3, 230 cases>3
Shimada	2008	63	87/30	54	23/78	86/31	23	2.5
Shin	2018	56.4	92/24	82	81/12	116/0	11.9	2.3
Su	2021	59.1	112/47	85	87/47	159/0	11.8	1.58
Takano	2000	60.8	235/65	NA	55/235	265/35	1.616	83 cases≤5, 217 cases>5
Torii	1993	57.7	48/11	56	NA	59/0	NA	30 cases≤2, 29 cases>2
Tsilimigras	2020	66	299/185	148	93/117	NA	8	4.3

(Continued)

TABLE 1-2 | Continued

Author	Year	Age (years)	Gender (male/female)	Liver cirrhosis (numbers)	HBV/HCV status (numbers)	Number of tumor (solitary/multiple)	AFP (ng/ml)	Tumor size (cm)
Wang	2010	50	380/58	NA	NA	374/54	NA	108 cases≤5, 272 cases>5
Yang	2014	NA	877/208	NA	210/NA	NA	NA	NA
Zeng	2020	36	615/84	355	699/NA	565/134	141 cases≤10, 558 cases>10	5.8
Zhang	2014	48.9	253/49	253	302/NA	238/64	90 cases≤20, 212 cases>20	120 cases≤5, 182 cases>5
Zhang	2021	53.8	357/68	260	376/2	354/71	54.4	3.5
Zhou	2020	NA	278/31	170	274/NA	228/81	203 cases≤400, 106 cases>400	NA
Zhou	2021	683 cases≤60, 134 cases>60	695/122	360	713/NA	NA	452 cases≤400, 365 cases>400	272 cases≤5, 545 cases>5

NA, not available; HBV, hepatitis B virus; HCV, hepatitis C virus.

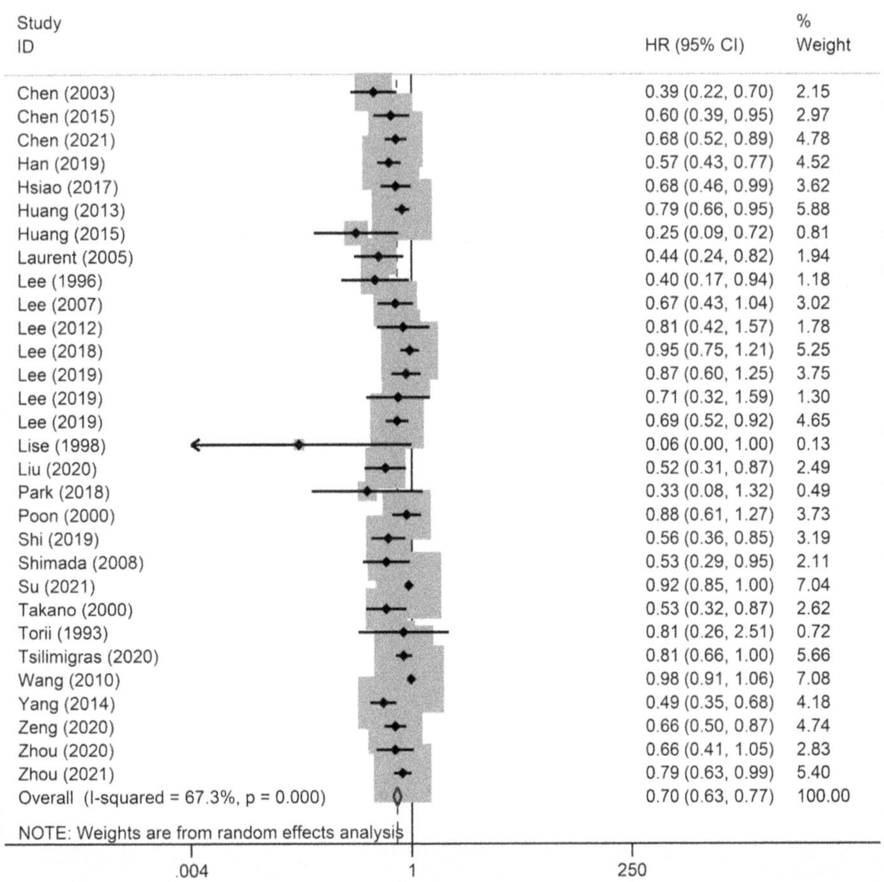

FIGURE 2 | Forest plot of OS of HCC patients receiving wide surgical margin.

TABLE 2 | Subgroup analysis of the resection margin on the prognosis of patients with HCC.

	Overall survival (OS)			Disease-free survival (DFS)		
	No. of studies	HR	95%CI	No. of studies	HR	95%CI
3-year survival	5	0.67	0.54–0.82	8	0.57	0.48–0.67
5-year survival	23	0.70	0.63–0.79	19	0.70	0.65–0.76
Male	18	0.68	0.59–0.78	18	0.66	0.60–0.72
Female	9	0.75	0.64–0.89	9	0.66	0.55–0.78
China	19	0.70	0.62–0.78	17	0.67	0.62–0.72
Non-Chinese Asian countries	6	0.68	0.51–0.91	4	0.64	0.46–0.88
Western countries	3	0.54	0.26–1.12	4	0.45	0.30–0.66
HBsAg positive	10	0.71	0.65–0.78	11	0.64	0.57–0.72
HBsAg negative	14	0.66	0.57–0.78	14	0.70	0.64–0.77
Single tumor	9	0.80	0.71–0.92	10	0.67	0.59–0.77
Multiple tumors	7	0.60	0.49–0.73	7	0.66	0.57–0.78
Liver cirrhosis	-	-	-	4	0.71	0.60–0.84
Non-liver cirrhosis	-	-	-	18	0.64	0.58–0.71

HBsAg, hepatitis B surface antigen; HCC, hepatocellular carcinoma; HR, hazard ratio; CI, confidence interval.

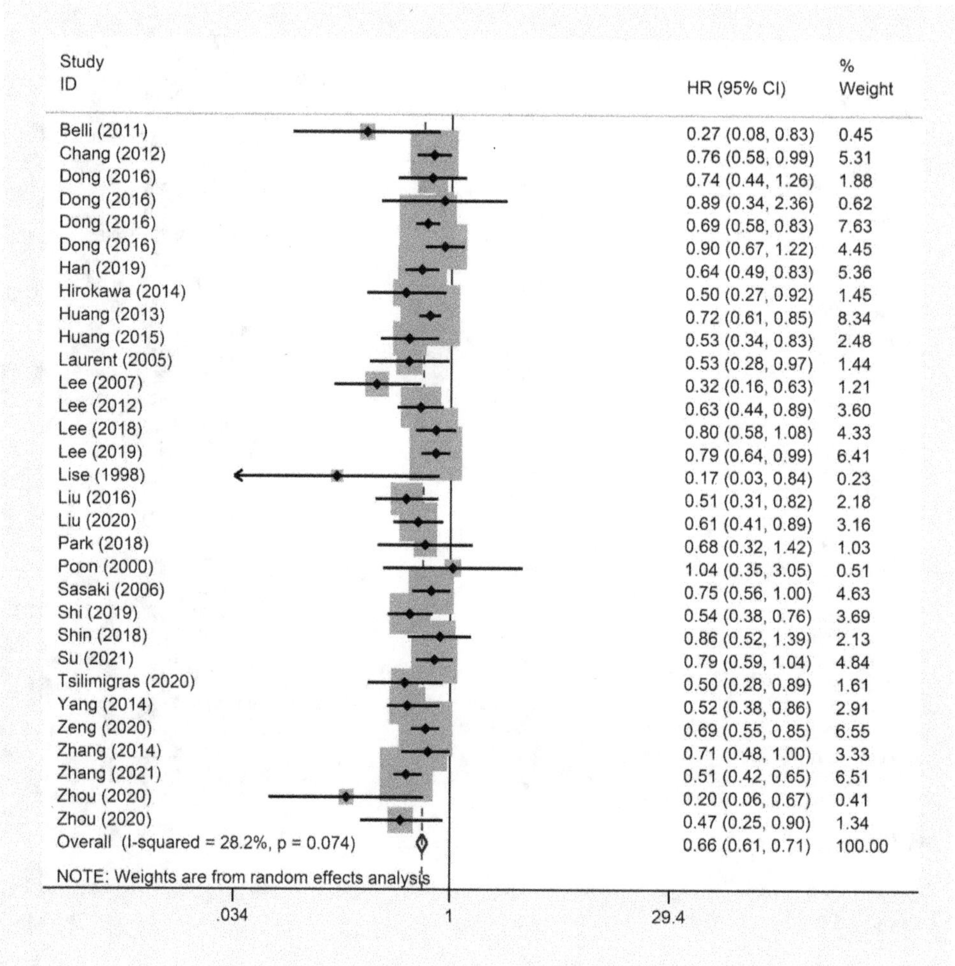

FIGURE 3 | Forest plot of DFS of HCC patients receiving wide surgical margin.

did not prolong the OS of patients compared to a narrow surgical margin. This is potentially attributed to the inclusion of a small number of studies (five articles).

No consensus has been reached in academia on whether gender is an independent risk factor for the prognosis of HCC patients after hepatectomy (45). Although there is no direct evidence that gender is a risk factor for HCC prognosis, men have higher smoking rates, alcohol consumption rates, and tumor burden than women (46). A different study found that women have a better long-term prognosis than men, but without statistical difference among patients with HCC lesions maximum size<3 cm or with solitary HCC (47).

Notably, regional factors were also considered in subgroup analysis. The etiology of HCC in different regions is remarkably different. Asian countries, specifically East Asia are dominated by viral hepatitis, whereas HCC etiology in Western countries is mostly related to alcohol (48). Subgroup analyses revealed that despite HCC patients with/without hepatitis B virus (HBV) and liver cirrhosis, a wide surgical margin prolonged the prognosis of patients than a narrow surgical margin. HBV-liver cirrhosis-HCC progression is a vital approach for HCC occurrence. High HBsAg level, lack of antiviral treatment, severe liver cirrhosis are risk factors affecting this process (49–51). However, in single or multiple HCC populations, the wide surgical margin group still yields a better prognosis than the narrow surgical margin group. Nevertheless, a study on a patients with solitary HCC lesions revealed that a wide surgical margin was not a prognostic factor. However, after propensity score matching (PSM), a wide surgical margin still prolongs the prognosis of patients (44). This is possibly because PSM could reduce the confounding bias of OBS and improve the research efficacy by omitting the unmatched study subjects.

Microvascular invasion (MVI) is the presence of tumor emboli in vascular spaces rowed by endothelial cells from the tumor capsule into the liver parenchyma (either hepatic vein or portal vein branches) (52). Based on the distribution and number of MVI, MVI is classified into the following grades, M0: no MVI; M1 (low risk): MVI <5 and the distance from adjacent liver tissues ≤1 cm; and M2 (high risk): MVI >5 or the distance from adjacent liver tissues >1 cm (53). Researchers attempted to develop a preoperative model integrating laboratory examinations and imaging examinations to predict MVI. However, its accuracy requires additional validation by large-scale prospective multi-center studies (54). At present, MVI can only be diagnosed by postoperative histopathological examination; this significantly limits the application of MVI in guiding diagnosis and treatment. From MVI to macrovascular invasion, the malignant degree of HCC cells gradually increases and destroys the surrounding tissues; the chance of radical surgery is lost if a macrovascular invasion is formed (55). Therefore, effective surgical plans and postoperative adjuvant treatment can be adopted if timely interventions are implemented at the MVI stage of HCC. This thus minimizes metastasis and HCC recurrence as well as significantly improves the prognosis of patients.

To survive and metastasize, cancer cells must evade the immune system. After cancer cells invade the bloodstream, the classic hematological mechanism believes that platelets, leukocytes, and endothelial cells mediate the related process of metastasis and recurrence (56). New research indicates that MVI provides another path for HCC recurrence and metastasis; besides, HCC cell clusters obtain endothelial coating by protruding into the vessels. This enables evasion of the immune surveillance mechanism and thereby preventing the activation of the coagulation cascade (57–60). Thus, if a liver resection with a narrower surgical margin is performed on patients, theoretically, the residual micrometastasis increases the risk of recurrence (37). Besides, 90% of MVI occurs in the range narrower than 1 cm from the edge of the tumor. If a wider margin is achieved, the incidence of MVI can be reduced, hence significantly preventing tumor recurrence and metastasis (61). However, due to data unavailability, we were unable to analyze the influence of MVI on the results in subgroup analysis. On the other hand, the liver status may be another mechanism of the prognostic influence of the resection margin. Patients who received a wide resection margin tend to have better liver reserves than patients who received a narrow resection margin. Therefore, compared with the narrow surgical margin group, the wide surgical margin group could achieve better OS and DFS.

The surgical margin should however not be blindly enlarged for preventing the recurrence and metastasis of HCC after surgery. Because of the excessively wide surgical margin, more normal liver parenchyma will be removed, causing serious postoperative complications including liver failure, and eventually death (8, 9, 11, 12). Poon et al. (12) revealed that the relatively healthy liver parenchyma should not be sacrificed for obtaining the wider margin, particularly in cirrhotic patients with limited hepatic functional reserves. Another study (25) showed that a wide surgical margin did not improve the OS of patients compared to a narrow surgical margin. This was because of different baselines of the study group and the control group. This was largely reflected in liver cirrhosis, large and multiple tumors.

Previous research evaluated the relationship between surgical margins and prognosis by systematic review and meta-analysis (62, 63). The findings (62) are inconsistent with this meta-analysis and suggests that prognostic benefits are not achieved in patients receiving a resection margin≥1 cm. A small number of articles (5 articles) included a potential reason. The study by Zhong et al. (63) lacked sensitivity analysis, therefore, the reliability and stability of its findings are uncertain. Yet, its results were consistent with this paper's findings. However, it had its limitations. Primarily, although the number of included studies is more than that of previous studies, it is still a relatively small amount when compared to the number of studies in our article (37 articles vs. 7 articles). Besides, subgroup analysis was not performed by Zhong et al. (63). It, therefore, remains unknown whether the conclusion (the prognostic benefit of a wide surgical margin) is affected by other factors.

Our study has worth-mentioning limitations. Firstly, because of the limited number of related studies, comprehensive analysis of different resection margin width could not be performed. Secondly, the study population is from Asia, therefore the results cannot be directly applied to the population in Western countries. Thirdly, most of the included literature is retrospective, thereby hinting a possibility of the potential risk of information bias. Fourthly, because of the non-availability of relevant data, we were unable to perform additional subgroup analyses including MVI and kind of resection (anatomical vs. non-anatomical).

CONCLUSION

In conclusion, our meta-analysis revealed that a wide surgical margin (≥1 cm) potentially prolongs the long-term prognosis of HCC patients than a narrow surgical margin (<1 cm). This meta-analysis conducted various subgroup analyses, and the results remained consistent across most factors of median follow-up time, gender, country, hepatitis B surface antigen status, tumor number, and liver cirrhosis.

AUTHOR CONTRIBUTIONS

JZ designed the research process. JX and YL searched the database for corresponding articles and drafted the meta-analysis. JH extracted useful information from the articles above. YS used statistical software for analysis. YH polished this article. All authors had read and approved the manuscript and ensured that this was the case.

SUPPLEMENTARY MATERIAL

Supplementary Figure 1 | Sensitivity analysis of OS for HCC patients receiving wide surgical margin.

Supplementary Figure 2 | Sensitivity analysis of DFS for HCC patients receiving wide surgical margin.

Supplementary Table 1 | Quality assessment of studies included.

REFERENCES

1. Torre LA, Bray F, Siegel RL, Ferlay J, Lortet-Tieulent J, Jemal A. Global cancer statistics, 2012. *CA Cancer J Clin.* (2015) 65:87–108. doi: 10.3322/caac.21262
2. Siegel RL, Miller KD, Jemal A. Cancer statistics, 2015. *CA Cancer J Clin.* (2015) 65:5–29. doi: 10.3322/caac.21254
3. Tabrizian P, Jibara G, Shrager B, Schwartz M, Roayaie S. Recurrence of hepatocellular cancer after resection: patterns, treatments, and prognosis. *Ann Surg.* (2015) 261:947–55. doi: 10.1097/SLA.0000000000000710
4. Chen B, Shen S, Wu J, Hua Y, Kuang M, Li S, et al. CISD2 associated with proliferation indicates negative prognosis in patients with hepatocellular carcinoma. *Int J Clin Exp Pathol.* (2015) 8:13725–38.
5. Huang WJ, Jeng YM, Lai HS, Sheu FY, Lai PL, Yuan RH. Tumor size is a major determinant of prognosis of resected stage I hepatocellular carcinoma. *Langenbecks Arch Surg.* (2015) 400:725–34. doi: 10.1007/s00423-015-1329-4
6. Hermanek P, Wittekind C. The pathologist and the residual tumor (R) classification. *Pathol Res Pract.* (1994) 190:115–23. doi: 10.1016/S0344-0338(11)80700-4
7. Lee JC, Cheng CH, Wang YC, Wu TH, Lee CF, Wu TJ, et al. Clinical relevance of alpha-fetoprotein in determining resection margin for hepatocellular carcinoma. *Medicine.* (2019) 98:e14827. doi: 10.1097/MD.0000000000014827
8. Madkhali AA, Fadel ZT, Aljiffry MM, Hassanain MM. Surgical treatment for hepatocellular carcinoma. *Saudi J Gastroenterol.* (2015) 21:11–7. doi: 10.4103/1319-3767.151216
9. Du ZG, Li B, Wei YG, Yin J, Feng X, Chen X. A new scoring system for assessment of liver function after successful hepatectomy in patients with hepatocellular carcinoma. *Hepatobiliary Pancreat Dis Int.* (2011) 10:265–9. doi: 10.1016/S1499-3872(11)60044-1
10. Chen MF, Tsai HP, Jeng LB, Lee WC, Yeh CN, Yu MC, Hung CM. Prognostic factors after resection for hepatocellular carcinoma in noncirrhotic livers: univariate and multivariate analysis. *World J Surg.* (2003) 27:443–7. doi: 10.1007/s00268-002-6708-7
11. Lee KT, Wang SN, Su RW, Chen HY, Shi HY, Ker CG, et al. Is wider surgical margin justified for better clinical outcomes in patients with resectable hepatocellular carcinoma? *J Formos Med Assoc.* (2012) 111:160–70. doi: 10.1016/j.jfma.2011.02.002
12. Poon RT, Fan ST, Ng IO, Wong J. Significance of resection margin in hepatectomy for hepatocellular carcinoma: a critical reappraisal. *Ann Surg.* (2000) 231:544–51. doi: 10.1097/00000658-200004000-00014
13. Moher D, Liberati A, Tetzlaff J, Altman DG. Preferred reporting items for systematic reviews and meta-analyses: the PRISMA statement. *BMJ.* (2009) 339:b2535. doi: 10.1136/bmj.b2535
14. Belli G, Fantini C, Belli A, Limongelli P. Laparoscopic liver resection for hepatocellular carcinoma in cirrhosis: long-term outcomes. *Dig Surg.* (2011) 28:134–40. doi: 10.1159/000323824
15. Chang WT, Kao WY, Chau GY, Su CW, Lei HJ, Wu JC, et al. Hepatic resection can provide long-term survival of patients with non-early-stage hepatocellular carcinoma: extending the indication for resection? *Surgery.* (2012) 152:809–20. doi: 10.1016/j.surg.2012.03.024
16. Chen ZH, Zhang XP, Feng JK, Li LQ, Zhang F, Hu YR, Zhong CQ, et al. Actual long-term survival in hepatocellular carcinoma patients with microvascular invasion: a multicenter study from China. *Hepatol Int.* (2021) 15:642–50. doi: 10.1007/s12072-021-10174-x
17. Dong S, Wang Z, Wu L, Qu Z. Effect of surgical margin in R0 hepatectomy on recurrence-free survival of patients with solitary hepatocellular carcinomas without macroscopic vascular invasion. *Medicine.* (2016) 95:e5251. doi: 10.1097/MD.0000000000005251
18. Han J, Li ZL, Xing H, Wu H, Zhu P, Lau WY, et al. The impact of resection margin and microvascular invasion on long-term prognosis after curative resection of hepatocellular carcinoma: a multi-institutional study. *HPB.* (2019) 21:962–71. doi: 10.1016/j.hpb.2018.11.005
19. Hirokawa F, Hayashi M, Miyamoto Y, Asakuma M, Shimizu T, Komeda K, et al. Outcomes and predictors of microvascular invasion of solitary hepatocellular carcinoma. *Hepatol Res.* (2014) 44:846–53. doi: 10.1111/hepr.12196
20. Hsiao JH, Tsai CC, Liang TJ, Chiang CL, Liang HL, Chen IS, et al. Adjuvant hepatic arterial infusion chemotherapy is beneficial for selective patients with hepatocellular carcinoma undergoing surgical treatment. *Int J Surg.* (2017) 45:35–41. doi: 10.1016/j.ijsu.2017.07.071
21. Huang G, Yang Y, Shen F, Pan ZY, Fu SY, Lau WY, et al. Early viral suppression predicts good postoperative survivals in patients with hepatocellular carcinoma with a high baseline HBV-DNA load. *Ann Surg Oncol.* (2013) 20:1482–90. doi: 10.1245/s10434-012-2803-7
22. Laurent C, Blanc JF, Nobili S, Sa Cunha A, le Bail B, Bioulac-Sage P, et al. Prognostic factors and longterm survival after hepatic resection for hepatocellular carcinoma originating from noncirrhotic liver. *J Am Coll Surg.* (2005) 201:656–62. doi: 10.1016/j.jamcollsurg.2005.05.027
23. Lee CS, Sheu JC, Wang M, Hsu HC. Long-term outcome after surgery for asymptomatic small hepatocellular carcinoma. *Br J Surg.* (1996) 83:330–3. doi: 10.1002/bjs.1800830310
24. Lee SG, Hwang S, Jung JP, Lee YJ, Kim KH, Ahn CS. Outcome of patients with huge hepatocellular carcinoma after primary resection and treatment of recurrent lesions. *Br J Surg.* (2007) 94:320–6. doi: 10.1002/bjs.5622
25. Lee W, Han HS, Ahn S, Yoon YS, Cho JY, Choi Y. Correlation between resection margin and disease recurrence with a restricted cubic spline model in patients with resected hepatocellular carcinoma. *Dig Surg.* (2018) 35:520–31. doi: 10.1159/000485805
26. Lise M, Bacchetti S, Da Pian P, Nitti D, Pilati PL, Pigato P. Prognostic factors affecting long term outcome after liver resection for hepatocellular carcinoma: results in a series of 100 Italian patients. *Cancer.* (1998) 82:1028–36.

27. Liu L, Shui Y, Yu Q, Guo Y, Zhang L, Zhou X, et al. Narrow-margin hepatectomy resulted in higher recurrence and lower overall survival for R0 resection hepatocellular carcinoma. *Front Oncol.* (2020) 10:610636. doi: 10.3389/fonc.2020.610636
28. Liu Y, Wang ZX, Cao Y, Zhang G, Chen WB, Jiang CP. Preoperative inflammation-based markers predict early and late recurrence of hepatocellular carcinoma after curative hepatectomy. *Hepatobiliary Pancreat Dis Int.* (2016) 15:266–74. doi: 10.1016/S1499-3872(16)60094-2
29. Park JH, Kim DH, Kim SH, Kim MY, Baik SK, Hong IS. The clinical implications of liver resection margin size in patients with hepatocellular carcinoma in terms of positron emission tomography positivity. *World J Surg.* (2018) 42:1514–22. doi: 10.1007/s00268-017-4275-1
30. Sasaki Y, Yamada T, Tanaka H, Ohigashi H, Eguchi H, Yano M, et al. Risk of recurrence in a long-term follow-up after surgery in 417 patients with hepatitis B- or hepatitis C-related hepatocellular carcinoma. *Ann Surg.* (2006) 244:771–80. doi: 10.1097/01.sla.0000225126.56483.b3
31. Shi F, Zhou Z, Huang X, Liu Q, Lin A. Is anatomical resection necessary for early hepatocellular carcinoma? A single institution retrospective experience. *Future Oncol.* (2019) 15:2041–51. doi: 10.2217/fon-2019-0117
32. Shimada K, Sakamoto Y, Esaki M, Kosuge T. Role of the width of the surgical margin in a hepatectomy for small hepatocellular carcinomas eligible for percutaneous local ablative therapy. *Am J Surg.* (2008) 195:775–81. doi: 10.1016/j.amjsurg.2007.06.033
33. Shin S, Kim TS, Lee JW, Ahn KS, Kim YH, Kang KJ. Is the anatomical resection necessary for single hepatocellular carcinoma smaller than 3 cm?: single-center experience of liver resection for a small HCC. *Ann Hepatobiliary Pancreat Surg.* (2018) 22:326–34. doi: 10.14701/ahbps.2018.22.4.326
34. Su CM, Chou CC, Yang TH, Lin YJ. Comparison of anatomic and non-anatomic resections for very early-stage hepatocellular carcinoma: The importance of surgical resection margin width in non-anatomic resection. *Surg Oncol.* (2021) 36:15–22. doi: 10.1016/j.suronc.2020.11.009
35. Takano S, Oishi H, Kono S, Kawakami S, Nakamura M, Kubota N, et al. Retrospective analysis of type of hepatic resection for hepatocellular carcinoma. *Br J Surg.* (2000) 87:65–70. doi: 10.1046/j.1365-2168.2000.01308.x
36. Torii A, Nonami T, Harada A, Yasui M, Nakao A, Takagi H. Extent of hepatic resection as a prognostic factor for small, solitary hepatocellular carcinomas. *J Surg Oncol.* (1993) 54:13–7. doi: 10.1002/jso.2930540106
37. Tsilimigras DI, Sahara K, Moris D, Hyer JM, Paredes AZ, Bagante F, et al. Effect of surgical margin width on patterns of recurrence among patients undergoing R0 hepatectomy for T1 hepatocellular carcinoma: an international multi-institutional analysis. *J Gastrointest Surg.* (2020) 24:1552–60. doi: 10.1007/s11605-019-04275-0
38. Wang J, Xu LB, Liu C, Pang HW, Chen YJ, Ou QJ. Prognostic factors and outcome of 438 Chinese patients with hepatocellular carcinoma underwent partial hepatectomy in a single center. *World J Surg.* (2010) 34:2434–41. doi: 10.1007/s00268-010-0664-4
39. Yang J, Li C, Wen TF, Yan LN, Li B, Wang WT, et al. Is hepatectomy for huge hepatocellular carcinoma ($\geq$ 10 cm in diameter) safe and effective? A single-center experience. *Asian Pac J Cancer Prev.* (2014) 15:7069–77. doi: 10.7314/APJCP.2014.15.17.7069
40. Zeng J, Lin K, Liu H, Huang Y, Guo P, Zeng Y, et al. prognosis factors of young patients undergoing curative resection for hepatitis B virus-related hepatocellular carcinoma: a multicenter study. *Cancer Manag Res.* (2020) 12:6597–606. doi: 10.2147/CMAR.S261368
41. Zhang H, Liu F, Wen N, Li B, Wei Y. Patterns, timing, and predictors of recurrence after laparoscopic liver resection for hepatocellular carcinoma: results from a high-volume HPB center. *Surg Endosc.* (2022) 36:1215–23. doi: 10.1007/s00464-021-08390-5
42. Zhang XF, Wei T, Liu XM, Liu C, Lv Y. Impact of cigarette smoking on outcome of hepatocellular carcinoma after surgery in patients with hepatitis B. *PLoS ONE.* (2014) 9:e85077. doi: 10.1371/journal.pone.0085077
43. Zhou KQ, Sun YF, Cheng JW, Du M, Ji Y, Wang PX, et al. Effect of surgical margin on recurrence based on preoperative circulating tumor cell status in hepatocellular carcinoma. *EBioMedicine.* (2020) 62:103107. doi: 10.1016/j.ebiom.2020.103107
44. Zhou Z, Qi L, Mo Q, Liu Y, Zhou X, Zhou Z, et al. Effect of surgical margin on postoperative prognosis in patients with solitary hepatocellular carcinoma: a propensity score matching analysis. *J Cancer.* (2021) 12:4455–62. doi: 10.7150/jca.57896
45. El-Serag HB. Epidemiology of viral hepatitis and hepatocellular carcinoma. *Gastroenterology.* (2012) 142:1264–73.e1261. doi: 10.1053/j.gastro.2011.12.061
46. Ladenheim MR, Kim NG, Nguyen P, Le A, Stefanick ML, Garcia G, et al. Sex differences in disease presentation, treatment and clinical outcomes of patients with hepatocellular carcinoma: a single-centre cohort study. *BMJ Open Gastroenterol.* (2016) 3:e000107. doi: 10.1136/bmjgast-2016-000107
47. Dohmen K, Shigematsu H, Irie K, Ishibashi H. Longer survival in female than male with hepatocellular carcinoma. *J Gastroenterol Hepatol.* (2003) 18:267–72. doi: 10.1046/j.1440-1746.2003.02936.x
48. Akinyemiju T, Abera S, Ahmed M, Alam N, Alemayohu MA, Allen C, et al. the burden of primary liver cancer and underlying etiologies from 1990 to 2015 at the global, regional, and national level: results from the global burden of disease study 2015. *JAMA Oncol.* (2017) 3:1683–91. doi: 10.1001/jamaoncol.2017.3055
49. Chien J, Liu J, Lee MH, Jen CL, Batrla-Utermann R, Lu SN, et al. Risk and predictors of hepatocellular carcinoma for chronic hepatitis B patients with newly developed cirrhosis. *J Gastroenterol Hepatol.* (2016) 31:1971–7. doi: 10.1111/jgh.13422
50. Bonino F, Oliveri F, Colombatto P, Brunetto MR. Impact of interferon-alpha therapy on the development of hepatocellular carcinoma in patients with liver cirrhosis: results of an international survey. *J Viral Hepat.* (1997) 4(Suppl. 2):79–82. doi: 10.1111/j.1365-2893.1997.tb00183.x
51. Shim JJ, Oh CH, Kim JW, Lee CK, Kim BH. Liver cirrhosis stages and the incidence of hepatocellular carcinoma in chronic hepatitis B patients receiving antiviral therapy. *Scand J Gastroenterol.* (2017) 52:1029–36. doi: 10.1080/00365521.2017.1335773
52. Poté N, Cauchy F, Albuquerque M, Voitot H, Belghiti J, Castera L, et al. Performance of PIVKA-II for early hepatocellular carcinoma diagnosis and prediction of microvascular invasion. *J Hepatol.* (2015) 62:848–54. doi: 10.1016/j.jhep.2014.11.005
53. Cong WM, Bu H, Chen J, Dong H, Zhu YY, Feng LH, et al. Practice guidelines for the pathological diagnosis of primary liver cancer: 2015 update. *World J Gastroenterol.* (2016) 22:9279–87. doi: 10.3748/wjg.v22.i42.9279
54. Lei Z, Li J, Wu D, Xia Y, Wang Q, Si A, et al. Nomogram for preoperative estimation of microvascular invasion risk in hepatitis B virus-related hepatocellular carcinoma within the milan criteria. *JAMA Surg.* (2016) 151:356–63. doi: 10.1001/jamasurg.2015.4257
55. EASL-EORTC clinical practice guidelines: management of hepatocellular carcinoma. *J Hepatol.* (2012) 56:908–43. doi: 10.1016/j.jhep.2011.12.001
56. Kappelmayer J, Nagy B Jr. The interaction of selectins and PSGL-1 as a key component in thrombus formation and cancer progression. *Biomed Res Int.* (2017) 2017:6138145. doi: 10.1155/2017/6138145
57. Ding T, Xu J, Zhang Y, Guo RP, Wu WC, Zhang SD, et al. Endothelium-coated tumor clusters are associated with poor prognosis and micrometastasis of hepatocellular carcinoma after resection. *Cancer.* (2011) 117:4878–89. doi: 10.1002/cncr.26137
58. Mitsunobu M, Toyosaka A, Oriyama T, Okamoto E, Nakao N. Intrahepatic metastases in hepatocellular carcinoma: the role of the portal vein as an efferent vessel. *Clin Exp Metastasis.* (1996) 14:520–9. doi: 10.1007/BF00115112
59. Rodríguez-Perálvarez M, Luong TV, Andreana L, Meyer T, Dhillon AP, Burroughs AK. A systematic review of microvascular invasion in hepatocellular carcinoma: diagnostic and prognostic variability. *Ann Surg Oncol.* (2013) 20:325–39. doi: 10.1245/s10434-012-2513-1
60. Sugino T, Yamaguchi T, Hoshi N, Kusakabe T, Ogura G, Goodison S, et al. Sinusoidal tumor angiogenesis is a key component in hepatocellular carcinoma metastasis. *Clin Exp Metastasis.* (2008) 25:835–41. doi: 10.1007/s10585-008-9199-6
61. Feng LH, Dong H, Lau WY, Yu H, Zhu YY, Zhao Y, et al. Novel microvascular invasion-based prognostic nomograms to predict survival outcomes in patients after R0 resection for hepatocellular carcinoma. *J Cancer Res Clin Oncol.* (2017) 143:293–303. doi: 10.1007/s00432-016-2286-1

62. Tang YH, Wen TF, Chen X. Resection margin in hepatectomy for hepatocellular carcinoma: a systematic review. *Hepatogastroenterology.* (2012) 59:1393–7. doi: 10.5754/hge10600
63. Zhong FP, Zhang YJ, Liu Y, Zou SB. Prognostic impact of surgical margin in patients with hepatocellular carcinoma: a meta-analysis. *Medicine.* (2017) 96:e8043. doi: 10.1097/MD.0000000000008043

9

Do Elderly Patients with Stage I–II Hepatocellular Carcinoma Benefit from More Radical Surgeries?

Qiu-Qiang Zhang [1,2†], Pan-Yi-Sha Wu [1,2†], Mugahed ALBahde [1,2†], Lu-Fei Zhang [1,2], Zhu-Ha Zhou [3], Hua Liu [4], Yu-Feng Li [1,2] and Wei-Lin Wang [1,2,5,6,7]*

[1] Department of Hepatobiliary and Pancreatic Surgery, The Second Affiliated Hospital, Zhejiang University School of Medicine, Hangzhou, China, [2] Clinical Medicine Innovation Center of Precision Diagnosis and Treatment for Hepatobiliary and Pancreatic Disease of Zhejiang University, Hangzhou, China, [3] Department of General Surgery, School of Medicine, Sir Run Run Shaw Hospital, Zhejiang University, Hangzhou, China, [4] Department of Hepatobiliary and Pancreatic Surgery, The First Affiliated Hospital, Zhejiang University School of Medicine, Hangzhou, China, [5] Key Laboratory of Precision Diagnosis and Treatment for Hepatobiliary and Pancreatic Tumor of Zhejiang Province, Hangzhou, China, [6] Research Center of Diagnosis and Treatment Technology for Hepatocellular Carcinoma of Zhejiang Province, Hangzhou, China, [7] Clinical Research Center of Hepatobiliary and Pancreatic Diseases of Zhejiang Province, Hangzhou, China

***Correspondence:**
Wei-Lin Wang
wam@zju.edu.cn

† These authors have contributed equally to this work

Background and Aims: The best treatment modalities for elderly patients with stage I–II HCC (hepatocellular carcinoma) remain controversial in an era of a shortage of liver donors.

Methods: From the SEER database (Surveillance, Epidemiology, and End Results program), 2,371 elderly patients were sampled as Cohort 1. OS (Overall Survival) and CSS (Cancer-Specific Survival) were compared between the Non-surgery and Surgery groups. A stratification analysis in a CSS Cox model was also conducted among sub-groups, and propensity score matching was performed to generate Cohort 2 (746 pairs), reducing the influences of confounders.

Results: For Cohort 1, the median follow-up times of the Non-surgery and Surgery groups were 11 months (95% CI, confidence interval: 9.74–12.26) vs. 49 months (44.80–53.21) in OS, and 14 months (12.33–15.67) vs. 74 months (64.74–83.26) in CSS, respectively. In the stratification analysis, for the elderly patients (age >= 70 years), Larger Resection was associated with a higher HR (hazard ratio) than Segmental Resection: 0.30 (95% CI, confidence interval: 0.22–0.41) vs. 0.29 (0.21–0.38) in 70–74 year-olds; 0.26 (0.18–0.38) vs. 0.23 (0.16–0.32) in 75–79 year-olds; 0.32 (0.21–0.49) vs. 0.21 (0.13–0.32) in those 80+ years old. For Cohort 2, a similar result could be seen in the CSS Cox forest plot. The HRs of Larger Resection and Segmental Resection were 0.27 (0.21–0.33) and 0.25 (0.20–0.31), respectively.

Conclusions: It is cautiously recommended that, when liver transplantation is not available, segmental or wedge liver resection is the better treatment choice for elderly patients with stage I–II HCC (AJCC edition 6), especially those over 70 years old, compared with other surgeries, based on the SEER data.

Keywords: SEER, early stage, surgery, geriatric, survival

INTRODUCTION

Hepatocellular carcinoma (HCC) is considered worldwidely to be one of the most malignant tumors (1). Today, with the increasingly aging global population, the proportion of elderly patients (age >= 65 years) with HCC is also becoming higher and higher each year (2). Elderly patients with HCC usually have worse prognostic survivals than younger patients do due to their poor health status or comorbidities, such as COPD (chronic obstructive pulmonary disease), cerebral stroke, and organ dysfunctions (3). It is therefore very challenging to find the best treatments of geriatric patients with HCC. And there are really some very special and distinctive characteristics in nursing and surgeries, especially for those diagnosed with stage I–II HCC (AJCC edition 6). On the one hand, there are many therapy options for them (4), including surgeries (e.g., segmental liver resection, hemihepatectomy, liver transplantation), radiation, and chemotherapy; on the other hand, controversy remains over which kinds of treatments are better for them, offering longer survival and less invasiveness, in an era of liver donor shortage (5). It is also undetermined whether these elderly patients benefit substantially more from the more radical surgical therapies, e.g., hemihepatectomy or liver transplantation, compared with the less invasive surgeries, such as radio-frequency ablation or segmental liver resection. For the present, there are few studies that investigate this issue with convincing and dependable huge-scale data such as ours (6, 7).

As of now, the large Surveillance, Epidemiology, and End Results (SEER) database in the USA, which covers almost 28% of the US population (8), is an ideal and perfect data pool for oncologic studies worldwide (9, 10). In this study, we sampled the elderly patients (age >= 65 years, stage I–II HCC) from the SEER database to try to determine whether more radical surgeries should be suggested for them and to explore the highest-impact and key factors for survival, particularly when liver transplantation is not available.

PATIENTS AND METHODS

Data Source

The SEER database (version 2019) is a public, free clinical records platform (11, 12) that comprises demographic and oncologic information of cancer patients from 18 registries across the USA, renewed online every year. In this research, we used SEER-stat software (version 8.3.5) to obtain the clinical data of those patients who were age >= 65 years, diagnosed as stage I–II HCC (AJCC edition 6), and hospitalized between January 1, 2004, and December 31, 2011. The overall regime of our research design is shown in the flowchart in **Supplementary Figure 1**.

Study Cohort

A total of 2,371 patients were finally sampled as Cohort 1. Since some variables, such as the specific surgery, tumor size, grade of morphology, and age, are highly involved in the prognostic outcome of HCC treatments, we excluded patients without complete data on these variables. Besides, follow-up months, overall vital status, and the cause-specific death variable were vital for the OS (overall survival) and CSS (cancer-specific survival) analysis, so we also ruled out patients without complete ascertainment and definite information on these parameters. Patients who did not have HCC diagnosis as their only or first of more than one tumors were also excluded. In order to reduce the influence of the confounding factors further, we used the PSM (propensity score matching) method to mimic randomized controlled trials (RCT) by producing a more balanced new dataset, Cohort 2, with 1,492 patients (746 pairs) in all. The PSM was based on logistic regression analysis of the variables in Cohort 1, which covered nearly all items except the grouping variable, Specific Surgery.

Demographic and Clinical Data Pretreatment

The patients were divided broadly into Non-surgery and Surgery groups. Some layers of the variables from the original data were merged. For example, the Larger Resection group was the integration of the lobectomy and the extended lobectomy in SEER. Furtherly, we regrouped the patients by Specific Surgery, which was composed of None, Local Destruction (local tumor destruction, e.g., Radio-Frequency Ablation), Segmental Resection (covering wedge resection), Larger Resection (including lobectomy and extended lobectomy), and Liver Transplantation. Although there is very limited information about the Radiation and Chemotherapy of the patients in SEER, we attempted to cover these variables by transforming them into binaries with two levels (No and Yes). AFP and Fibrosis score data were also collected in our study.

Statistical Analysis

The baseline demographic data for Non-surgery and Surgery groups were compared through the Student's *t*-test or $\chi 2$ test. Patients still alive at December 31, 2011, were censored in the OS analysis, while, in the CSS analysis, those who died from other disease causes except HCC were also censored. The accumulated OS and CSS probabilities were plotted, respectively, and the differences between the two groups were compared by the Kaplan-Meier method with a log-rank test. Cox proportional hazards regression analyses were performed with both a univariate model and a multivariate model in Cohort 1. Besides, the stratification analyses of Age, Grade of morphology, Tumor size, and HCC Stage were wholly conducted in a cross-table by Specific Surgery (including five sub-groups). In addition, a forest plot of hazard ratios was made from the multivariate CSS Cox analysis in Cohort 2.

All statistical tests were evaluated by the significance criterion $P < 0.05$ (two-sided), and the hazard ratios with 95% confidence interval (CI) are also shown in the study. All statistical analyses were conducted using SPSS 23.0 for Windows (SPSS, Chicago, IL, USA) and R software (version × 64 3.5.3). The Institutional Ethics Committee of The Second Affiliated Hospital of Zhejiang University School of Medicine considered the study exempt.

RESULTS

In our study, 2,371 patients with an affirmative diagnosis of stage I–II HCC and older than 64 years old were selected from the SEER database as Cohort 1. Among these cases, there were 1,283 patients who received surgical treatments, including Local Destruction (LD), Segmental Resection (SR), Larger Resection (LR), Liver Transplantation (LT), while 1,088 cases did not. The baseline demographic characteristics are shown in **Table 1**. Those who received surgical treatments were a little younger than the Non-surgery patients, 72.1(±5.73) years old vs. 75.1(±6.84) years old, $P < 0.001$. There were no statistical differences ($P > 0.05$) between the Non-surgery and Surgery groups in some variables, namely Gender, Year at diagnosis, and Stage (AJCC edition 6), while the statistical differences can be seen in the other variables. The median follow-up times of the Non-surgery and Surgery groups were 11 months (95% CI: 9.74–12.26) vs. 49 months (44.80–53.21) in OS, and 14 months (12.33–15.67) vs. 74 months (64.74–83.26) in CSS, respectively. As shown in both OS ($P < 0.0001$) and CSS ($P < 0.0001$) plots (**Supplementary Figure 2**), the Surgery group had a higher survival curve than the Non-surgery group. In the CSS survival Cox proportional hazard ratio models of both univariate analysis (UVA) and multivariate analysis (MVA), it was demonstrated that the survival probabilities were robustly associated with certain factors, e.g., Surgery overall (MVA: HR, hazard ratio, 0.76; 95% CI: 0.76–0.76; $P < 0.001$), Tumor size (>= 1 cm and <3 cm) (MVA: HR, 1.66; 95% CI: 1.44–1.92; $P < 0.001$), and Poor differentiation (MVA: HR, 1.57; 95% CI: 1.34–1.83; $P < 0.001$) (**Table 2**). Intriguingly, the variable Age was statistically correlated with worse CSS survival only in the univariate Cox model (UVA: HR, 1.04; 95% CI: 1.03–1.05; $P < 0.001$), while the Stage (AJCC edition 6) factor became associated with worse CSS survival only in the multivariate Cox model (MVA: HR, 1.25; 95% CI: 1.11–1.40; $P < 0.001$). Further, in the stratification analyses (Age, Tumor size, Grade of Morphology, and Stage) of the univariate CSS Cox model (**Table 3**), it was shown that Liver Transplantation had the best survival in nearly all ages bands: HR 0.13 (CI: 0.09–0.20) in 65–69, HR 0.06 (CI: 0.03–0.15) in 70–75, HR 0.11 (CI: 0.02–0.78) in 80+. Meanwhile, Larger Resection had better survival than Segmental Resection only in the 65–69 age band, HR 0.33 (CI: 0.24–0.44) vs. HR 0.38 (CI: 0.29–0.50). However, unexpectedly, at Age >= 70, Larger Resection did not show better survival than Segmental Resection. Similar results could be noticed in some other variables, e.g., Tumor size >= 1 cm and Stage II (**Table 3**).

After PSM, in Cohort 2 with 1,492 cases (746 pairs), the distributions became more balanced in nearly all of the variables (**Supplementary Table 1**), and more detailed survival plots were completed on OS and CSS. As depicted, the Non-surgery group had a lower survival curve than the Surgery group did, and Liver Transplantation had the highest survival curve ($P < 0.0001$) (**Figure 1**). It is also shown that Larger Resection had a better survival curve than Local Destruction but a worse one than Segmental Resection and Liver Transplantation, both in the OS ($P < 0.0001$) and CSS ($P < 0.0001$). The results of the multivariate CSS Cox analysis of Cohort 2

TABLE 1 | Baseline characteristics.

Terms	No. of Patients (%)		*P*-value
	Non-surgery (*N* = 1088)	Surgery (*N* = 1283)	
Age (years)			<0.001
mean (SD)	75.1 (6.84)	72.1 (5.73)	
Age group			<0.001
65-69 years	276 (25.4)	520 (40.5)	
70-74 years	273 (25.1)	366 (28.5)	
75-79 years	232 (21.3)	239 (18.6)	
>= 80 years	307 (28.1)	158 (12.3)	
Gender			0.827
Female	348 (32.0)	405 (31.6)	
Male	740 (68.0)	878 (68.4)	
Year at diagnosis			0.351
2004–2006	315 (29.0)	401 (31.3)	
2007–2009	439 (40.3)	484 (37.7)	
2010–2011	334 (30.7)	398 (31.0)	
Race			<0.001
White	759 (69.8)	822 (64.1)	
Black	107 (9.8)	93 (7.2)	
A.I./A.N.*	14 (1.3)	10 (0.8)	
Asian / P.I.$^{\Delta}$	207 (19.0)	356 (27.7)	
Unknown	1 (0.1)	2 (0.2)	
Marital status			<0.001
Unmarried	447 (41.1)	403 (31.4)	
Married	607 (55.8)	849 (66.2)	
Unknown	34 (3.1)	31 (2.4)	
Stage (AJCC 6th)			0.427
I	761 (69.9)	878 (68.4)	
II	327 (30.1)	405 (31.6)	
Grade of morphology			<0.001
Well	501 (46.0)	416 (32.4)	
Moderately	415 (38.1)	644 (50.2)	
Poorly	160 (14.7)	197 (15.4)	
Undifferentiated	12 (1.1)	26 (2.0)	
Tumor size			<0.001
<1 cm	864 (79.4)	1166 (90.9)	
>=1 and <3 cm	212 (19.5)	114 (8.9)	
>=3 cm	12 (1.1)	3 (0.2)	
Radiation			<0.001
None	1017 (93.5)	1257 (98.0)	
Yes	71 (6.5)	26 (2.0)	
Chemotherapy			<0.001
None	636 (58.5)	1031 (80.4)	
Yes	452 (41.5)	252 (19.6)	
AFP			0.002
Negative	273 (25.1)	410 (32.0)	
Borderline	2 (0.2)	2 (0.2)	
Positive	534 (49.1)	554 (43.2)	
Unknown	279 (25.6)	317 (24.7)	
Fibrosis score			<0.001
0-4	52 (4.8)	175 (13.6)	
5-6	147 (13.5)	229 (17.8)	
Unknown	889 (81.7)	879 (68.5)	

*American Indian/Alaska Native; $^{\Delta}$, Asian/Pacific Islander.

TABLE 2 | Univariate and multivariate analysis of CSS Cox model.

Terms	Univariate Cox analysis			Multivariate Cox analysis		
	HR	(95% CI)	*P*-value	HR	(95% CI)	*P*-value
Age	1.04	(1.03–1.05)	<0.001	1.02	(0.99–1.05)	0.129
Age group						
65–69 years	1. 00			1.00		
70–74 years	1.17	(1.02–1.34)	0.026	0.91	(0.75–1.11)	0.345
75–79 years	1.57	(1.36–1.82)	<0.001	1.02	(0.75–1.39)	0.895
>=80 years	1.89	(1.63–2.18)	<0.001	0.89	(0.55–1.44)	0.645
Gender						
Female	1.00			1.00		
Male	0.90	(0.81–1.00)	0.055	0.96	(0.85–1.07)	0.447
Year of diagnosis						
2004–2006	1.00			1.00		
2007–2009	0.95	(0.84–1.07)	0.382	0.90	(0.80–1.03)	0.117
2010–2011	0.85	(0.75–0.98)	0.021	0.81	(0.71–0.93)	0.003
Race						
White	1.00			1.00		
Black	1.15	(0.96–1.38)	0.139	1.03	(0.85–1.24)	0.761
A.I./A.N.[∫]	0.89	(0.52–1.54)	0.680	0.87	(0.50–1.52)	0.635
Asian/P.I.[§]	0.67	(0.59–0.77)	<0.001	0.67	(0.59–0.76)	<0.001
unknown	1.47	(0.37–5.90)	0.585	1.91	(0.47–7.71)	0.363
Marital status						
Unmarried	1.00			1.00		
Married	0.82	(0.74–0.91)	0.000	0.93	(0.83–1.04)	0.211
Unknown	0.78	(0.56–1.09)	0.153	0.83	(0.60–1.17)	0.293
Stage (AJCC 6th)						
I	1.00			1.00		
II	1.06	(0.95–1.18)	0.295	1.25	(1.11–1.40)	0.000
Grade of morphology						
Well	1.00			1.00		
Moderately	0.90	(0.81–1.01)	0.080	1.14	(1.01–1.28)	0.032
Poorly	1.31	(1.13–1.52)	0.001	1.57	(1.34–1.83)	<0.001
Undifferentiated	1.10	(0.73–1.66)	0.644	1.39	(0.92–2.11)	0.121
Tumor size						
<1 cm	1.00			1.00		
>=1 and <3 cm	1.97	(1.72–2.26)	<0.001	1.66	(1.44–1.92)	<0.001
>=3 cm	1.76	(0.97–3.18)	0.063	1.23	(0.68–2.24)	0.499
Specific surgery						
None	1.00			1.00		
LD[*]	0.44	(0.38–0.51)	<0.001	0.58	(0.58–0.58)	<0.001
SR[**]	0.28	(0.24–0.33)	<0.001	0.34	(0.34–0.34)	<0.001
LR[***]	0.29	(0.25–0.35)	<0.001	0.32	(0.32–0.32)	<0.001
LT[Δ]	0.09	(0.07–0.13)	<0.001	0.12	(0.12–0.12)	<0.001
Surgery overall	0.30	(0.27–0.33)	<0.001	0.76	(0.76–0.76)	<0.001
Radiation						
None	1.00			1.00		
Yes	1.31	(1.03–1.66)	0.030	0.87	(0.68–1.11)	0.275
Chemotherapy						
None	1.00			1.00		
Yes	1.09	(0.97–1.21)	0.134	0.72	(0.64–0.81)	<0.001

(Continued)

TABLE 2 | Continued

Terms	Univariate Cox analysis			Multivariate Cox analysis		
	HR	**(95% CI)**	***P*-value**	**HR**	**(95% CI)**	***P*-value**
AFP						
Negative	1.00			1.00		
Borderline	1.06	(0.34–3.30)	0.923	1.39	(0.44–4.35)	0.576
Positive	1.54	(1.36–1.75)	<0.001	1.37	(1.20–1.57)	<0.001
Unknown	1.48	(1.29–1.71)	<0.001	1.39	(1.20–1.61)	<0.001
Fibrosis score						
1–4	1.00			1.00		
5–6	1.41	(1.12-1.76)	0.003	1.27	(1.00-1.61)	0.046
Unknown	1.71	(1.41-2.07)	<0.001	1.17	(0.96-1.43)	0.12

Univariate and multivariate analysis of CSS Cox proportional hazard ratio analysis before propensity score matching. CSS, cancer-specific survival; A.I./A.N.[∫] *American Indian/Alaska Native; Asian/P.I.*[§] *Asian/Pacific Islander; LD*, Local Destruction; SR**, Segmental Resection; LR***, Larger Resection, LT*[Δ]*, Liver Transplantation.*

TABLE 3 | Stratification analysis.

Strata	Non-surgery	Local destruction	Segmental resection	Larger resection	Liver transplantation
	***N*/reference**	***N*/HR (95% CI)**	***N*/HR (95% CI)**	***N*/HR (95% CI)**	***N*/HR (95% CI)**
Age group					
65–69 years	276	127	135	126	132
	1	0.51 (0.40–0.67)	0.3 8 (0.29–0.50)	0.33 (0.24–0.44)	0.13 (0.09–0.20)
70–74 years	273	105	127	97	37
	1	0.49 (0.37–0.65)	0.29 (0.21–0.38)	0.30 (0.22–0.41)	0.06 (0.03–0.15)
75–79 years	232	91	81	64	3
	1	0.37 (0.27–0.49)	0.23 (0.16–0.32)	0.26 (0.18–0.38)	0.11 (0.02–0.78)
>=80 years	307	58	52	47	1
	1	0.41 (0.28–0.58)	0.21 (0.13–0.32)	0.32 (0.21–0.49)	–
Tumor size					
<1 cm	864	366	369	258	173
	1	0.48 (0.41–0.56)	0.30 (0.26–0.36)	0.28 (0.23–0.35)	0.10 (0.07–0.14)
>=1 and <3 cm	212	15	25	74	0
	1	0.41 (0.22–0.77)	0.25 (0.15–0.43)	0.29 (0.21–0.41)	–
>=3 cm	12	0	1	2	0
	1	–	0.01 (0.00–17.77)	0.02 (0.00–5.17)	–
Grade of morphology					
Well	501	176	103	74	64
	1	0.42 (0.34–0.52)	0.25 (0.18–0.34)	0.23 (0.16–0.34)	0.09 (0.05–0.16)
Moderately	415	163	212	183	86
	1	0.46 (0.37–0.58)	0.27 (0.21–0.34)	0.28 (0.22–0.36)	0.09 (0.05–0.14)
Poorly	160	40	67	67	23
	1	0.45 (0.30–0.68)	0.30 (0.21–0.43)	0.29 (0.20–0.42)	0.41 (0.28–0.61)
Undifferentiated	12	2	13	10	1
	1	0.08 (0.08–0.69)	0.11 (0.03–0.35)	0.14 (0.04–0.48)	–
Stage (AJCC 6th)					
I	761	273	294	220	91
	1	0.40 (0.33–0.48)	0.25 (0.21–0.30)	0.28 (0.23–0.35)	0.09 (0.06–0.14)
II	327	108	101	114	82
	1	0.58 (0.44–0.74)	0.39 (0.29–0.52)	0.31 (0.23–0.41)	0.09 (0.06–0.15)

Cancer-specific survival comparison stratified by age group, tumor size, grade of morphology, and AJCC stage before PSM. PSM, propensity score matching; HR, hazard ratio; CI, confidence interval.

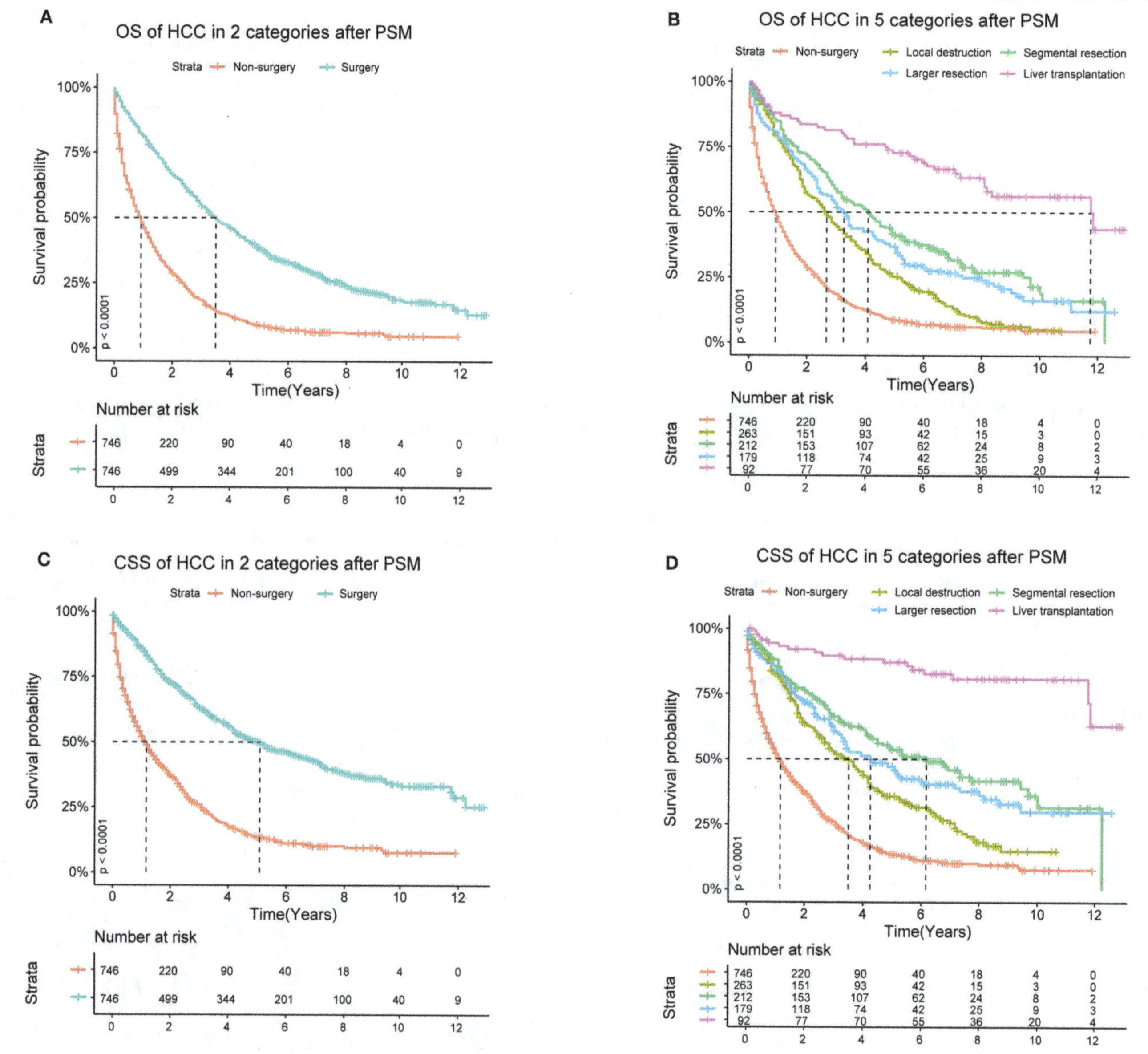

FIGURE 1 | OS (Overall Survival) and CSS (Cancer Specific Survival) analyses of HCC (Hepatocellular Carcinoma) patients in Cohort 2 after PSM (Propensity Score Matching).

are clearly demonstrated in the forest plot in **Figure 2**. In accordance with the stratification results of Cohort 1, Liver Transplantation was the best protective factor ($P < 0.001$), and Larger Resection did not show a better survival ($P < 0.001$) than did Segmental Resection.

DISCUSSION

Given the increasing population of elderly people worldwide, geriatric patients constitute a large proportion of HCC patients each year, but only a few studies have focused on the optimization of surgical treatments for them (13, 14). In our study, all of the patients who received surgical treatments, including Local Destruction, Segmental Resection, Larger Resection, and Liver Transplantation, had better survival than did the Non-surgery patients, which is consistent with the previous studies (2, 10, 12). Among the Surgery groups, Liver Transplantation was the best treatment on the condition that there were enough liver donors. Local Destruction, such as via RFA (radio-frequency ablation) or PEI (percutaneous ethanol injection), was implicated as having a worse survival rate than other surgeries, which was also reported previously (4, 15, 16). However, unexpectedly, the Larger Resection sub-group (extended liver resection, e.g., hemihepatectomy or lobectomy) was not associated with better survival than Segmental Resection (including wedge resection, usually less than a hemihepatectomy or lobectomy). Meanwhile, some authors (17) might think that RFA has good indications for HCC patients with tumor size <2 cm and no vascular

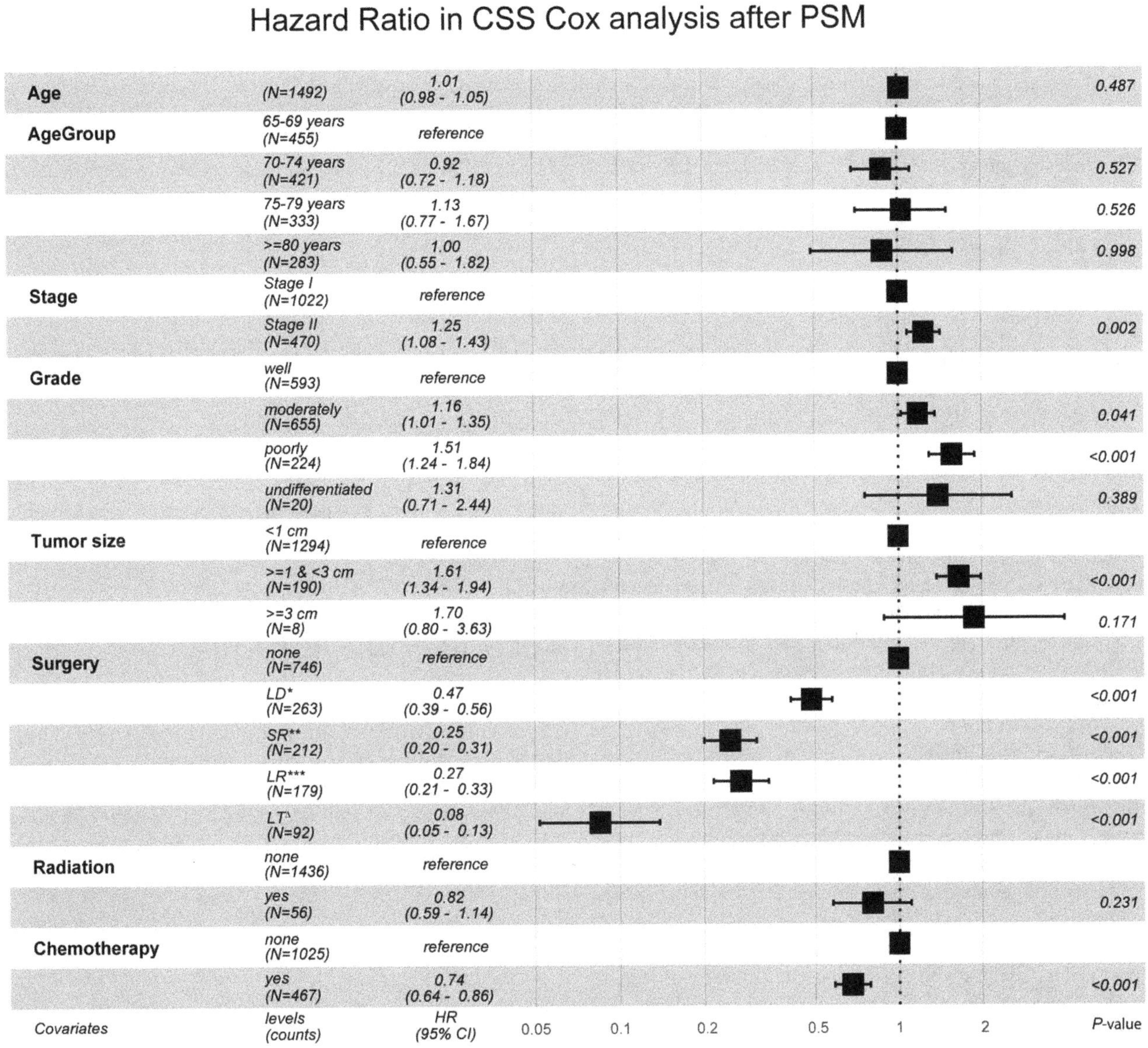

FIGURE 2 | Hazard Ratio in CSS Cox analysis after PSM. CSS, cancer specific survival; PSM, propensity score matching; LD*, Local Destruction; SR**, Segmental Resection; LR***, Larger Resection, LT$^{\Delta}$, Liver Transplantation. Global events: 968; Global *p*-value (Log-Rank): 2.8355e-90.

invasion, but this is not true in our study. We found that Local Destruction had higher HRs than did Segmental Resection, at both Stage I (level 1) and Stage II (level 2). Accordingly, in all age groups and tumor size groups, Local Destruction had higher HRs than did surgery groups (**Table 3**). Local Destruction, such as via RFA, may enable good control of local foci in the near future, but it is usually associated with higher recurrence rates and higher death rates in long-term follow-up (18). Therefore, if liver transplantation was not available, for the elderly patients with stage I–II HCC, wedge or segmental liver resection would be better choices for longer survival associated with relatively less invasiveness and a faster post-operational recovery.

In order to interrogate the significant factors that impact the survival of elderly patients with Stage I–II HCC, the precise selection of the patients is an important prerequisite, such as Age >= 65 years old, with confirmative clinical diagnosis of HCC. Those without HCC as the only primary cancer or as the first of more than one tumors and those without complete clinical data (e.g., follow-up time, morphological information) were both ruled out to make our study more convincing and rigorous. In addition, the cut-off line of the research interval was also very meaningful. Since the latest SEER data available online are always lagging behind by about 3 years and the present SEER coding system began in 2004, we chose the period 2004–2011 so that each patient in our study had the potential to help to calculate the

5 year survival rate. All of these methods were taken to ensure a more balanced and reasonable dataset, although the sample size of patients became smaller than in previous studies (2, 19).

In fact, we have collected as many variables as possible in **Table 2**, based on the available data from the SEER database. We have not screened out any variables from the UVA to MVA model, since all the possible factors and their overall effects should be considered in the end, which is much more necessary and dependable in reality. We found that Surgery, Tumor size, and Poor differentiation of morphology are the impactive factors for the post-operation survival in both the UVA and MVA of Cohort 1. Age is an influential factor in survival in UVA, but the effects are not obvious in MVA, which may be due to the sample size no being large enough. Stage is one of the key factors in MVA, and emphasis should be placed upon it in overall analyses (20).

Our study is clinical-value-oriented, and it becomes much more scientifically persuasive after stratification and PSM, based on the giant SEER database (21). Age, Tumor size, Grade of morphology, and AJCC Stage often have vital impacts on HCC patients' survival, so it was deemed necessary to perform a stratification analysis with the original data of Cohort 1. This revealed that segmental or wedge liver resection is generally a better choice for elderly patients above 69 years with Stage I–II HCC when liver transplantation is not available. This is somewhat different from some other research findings (4, 16, 22, 23). After PSM, in Cohort 2, there were no statistical differences ($P > 0.05$) between the Non-surgery and the Surgery groups in nearly all variables, so the effects of different surgeries could be more clearly compared. As shown in the forest plot, for those elderly people with stage I–II HCC, Larger Resection (extended surgery) does not show better survival than Segmental Resection does, which is consistent with the results of Cohort 1. As far as we know, this point has been reported for the first time in our study with the giant SEER dataset. It may provide some help to surgeons when they are confronted with the dilemma of how to make the best choice for geriatric patients with early-stage HCC with a poor health status when liver transplantation is unavailable.

However, there are also some drawbacks that need to be noticed. In fact, there is a lot of information that is unavailable in SEER but is closely correlated with post-operative survival, such as the details of the surgery, laboratory results, post-operational radiation, and systemic chemotherapy, as well as the performance status and severity of dysfunction of the liver or other organs (7, 16, 20, 24). Although the fibrosis score is provided, it is not sufficient to estimate the severity of cirrhosis. Also, staging information is only for the TNM system (American Joint Committee on Cancer), and there is not enough data to enable staging with the BCLC (Barcelona Clinical Liver Cancer) stage system, in which Child-Pough classification and performance status are considered (19). Besides, there also is no information about comorbidities, such as chronic obstructive pulmonary disease (COPD), coronary artery disease, and renal dysfunction (3), which are often seen in elderly patients. The specifics of chemotherapy, such as whether TACE (transarterial embolization) (25) or preoperative adjuvant chemotherapy (5) were used, is not available in SEER either. In addition, although we performed PSM to decrease the impacts of confounders and to abolish the selection bias to some degree, there are still some flaws in PSM itself (12), e.g., the smaller scale and the undermined representativeness after PSM, so the conclusions should be taken prudently. We may, in future, perhaps be able to draw on the Medicare Billing database (5, 13) for more comprehensive clinical data to make a more objective, reasonable, and convincing study of geriatric patients.

CONCLUSION

In summary, it is cautiously recommended that surgeries for elderly patients with stage I–II HCC have much better survival outcomes than non-surgical choices do, based on the limited data of SEER. Wedge or segmental liver resection has better survival than do the other surgeries (including local tumor destruction, extended liver resection, etc.) when liver transplantation is not available. More prospective randomized controlled clinical trials with a larger number of patients may be needed for further validation.

AUTHOR CONTRIBUTIONS

W-LW has access to all of the data in this study and takes responsibility for the integrity and accuracy of the data analyses. Q-QZ and W-LW: study concept and design. Q-QZ: drafting of the manuscript. Q-QZ and Z-HZ: statistical analysis. W-LW: study supervision. All authors: critical revision of the manuscript for important intellectual content, acquisition, analysis, or interpretation of data.

ACKNOWLEDGMENTS

The authors acknowledge SEER for public access to the database and Gretchen from SEER for her email replies and help.

REFERENCES

1. Torre LA, Bray F, Siegel RL, Ferlay J, Lortet-Tieulent J, Jemal A. Global cancer statistics, 2012. *CA Cancer J Clin.* (2015) 65:87–108. doi: 10.3322/caac.21262
2. Oweira H, Petrausch U, Helbling D, Schmidt J, Mannhart M, Mehrabi A, et al. Early stage hepatocellular carcinoma in the elderly: a SEER database analysis. *J Geriatr Oncol.* (2017) 8:277–83. doi: 10.1016/j.jgo.2017.03.002
3. Peters NA, Javed AA, He J, Wolfgang CL, Weiss MJ. Association of socioeconomics, surgical therapy, and survival of early stage hepatocellular carcinoma. *J Surg Res.* (2017) 210:253–60. doi: 10.1016/j.jss.2016.11.042
4. Ciccarese F, Caturelli E, Felder M, Farinati F, Frigo AC, Morisco F, et al. Survival benefit of liver resection for patients with hepatocellular carcinoma across different barcelona clinic liver cancer stages: a multicentre study. *J Hepatol.* (2014) 62:617–24. doi: 10.1016/j.jhep.2014.10.037
5. Shaya FT, Breunig IM, Seal B, Mullins CD, Chirikov V V., Hanna N. Comparative and cost effectiveness of treatment modalities for hepatocellular carcinoma in SEER-medicare. *Pharmacoeconomics.* (2014) 32:63–74. doi: 10.1007/s40273-013-0109-7

6. Hirokawa F, Hayashi M, Miyamoto Y, Asakuma M, Shimizu T, Komeda K, et al. Surgical outcomes and clinical characteristics of elderly patients undergoing curative hepatectomy for hepatocellular carcinoma. *J Gastrointest Surg.* (2013) 17:1929–37. doi: 10.1007/s11605-013-2324-0
7. Yu B, Ding Y, Liao X, Wang C, Wang B, Chen X. Radiofrequency ablation versus surgical resection in elderly patients with early-stage hepatocellular carcinoma in the era of organ shortage. *Saudi J Gastroenterol.* (2018) 24:317–25. doi: 10.4103/sjg.SJG_261_18
8. Zhang G, Li R, Zhao X, Meng S, Ye J, Zhao L. Validation of the American Joint Committee on Cancer eighth edition staging system in patients undergoing hepatectomy for hepatocellular carcinoma: a US population-based study. *J Surg Res.* (2018) 222:55–68. doi: 10.1016/j.jss.2017.09.044
9. Abdel-Rahman O. Assessment of the discriminating value of the 8th AJCC stage grouping for hepatocellular carcinoma. *HPB.* (2018) 20:41–8. doi: 10.1016/j.hpb.2017.08.017
10. Kamarajah SK. Fibrosis score impacts survival following resection for hepatocellular carcinoma (HCC): a Surveillance, end results and epidemiology (SEER) database analysis. *Asian J Surg.* (2018) 41:551–61. doi: 10.1016/j.asjsur.2018.01.001
11. Fu J, Ruan H, Zheng H, Cai C, Zhou S, Wang Q, et al. Impact of old age on resectable colorectal cancer outcomes. *PeerJ.* (2019) 7:e6350. doi: 10.7717/peerj.6350
12. Jiang Y-Q, Wang Z-X, Deng Y-N, Yang Y, Wang G-Y, Chen G-H. Efficacy of Hepatic resection vs. Radiofrequency ablation for patients With very-early-stage or early-stage hepatocellular carcinoma: a population-based study with stratification by age and tumor size. *Front Oncol.* (2019) 9:113. doi: 10.3389/fonc.2019.00113
13. Parikh ND, Marshall VD, Green M, Lawrence TS, Razumilava N, Owen D, et al. Effectiveness and cost of radiofrequency ablation and stereotactic body radiotherapy for treatment of early-stage hepatocellular carcinoma: an analysis of SEER-medicare. *J Med Imaging Radiat Oncol.* (2018) 62:673–81. doi: 10.1111/1754-9485.12754
14. Han B, Yao H, Shao L, Guo X, Han L, Romeiro FG, et al. Selection of treatment modalities for hepatocellular carcinoma at stages T1 and T2: a preliminary analysis based on the surveillance, epidemiology, and end results registry database. *J Buon.* (2018) 23:611–21.
15. Xu J, Noda C, Erickson A, Mokkarala M, Charalel R, Ramaswamy R, et al. Radiofrequency ablation vs. cryoablation for localized hepatocellular carcinoma: a propensity-matched population study. *Anticancer Res.* (2018) 38:6381–6. doi: 10.21873/anticanres.12997
16. Kim GA, Shim JH, Kim MJ, Kim SY, Won HJ, Shin YM, et al. Radiofrequency ablation as an alternative to hepatic resection for single small hepatocellular carcinomas. *Br J Surg.* (2016) 103:126–35. doi: 10.1002/bjs.9960
17. Jianyong L, Lunan Y, Dajiang L, Wentao W. Comparison of open liver resection and RFA for the treatment of solitary 3-5-cmhepatocellular carcinoma: a retrospective study. *BMC Surg.* (2019) 19:195. doi: 10.1186/s12893-019-0663-9
18. Xu XL, Liu X Di, Liang M, Luo BM. Radiofrequency ablation versus hepatic resection for small hepatocellular carcinoma: systematic review of randomized controlled trials with meta-analysis and trial sequential analysis. *Radiology.* (2018) 287:461–72. doi: 10.1148/radiol.2017162756
19. Zhao J, Mao J, Li W. Association of tumor grade with long-term survival in patients with hepatocellular carcinoma after liver transplantation. *Transplant Proc.* (2019) 51:813–9. doi: 10.1016/j.transproceed.2018.12.033
20. Sposito C, Battiston C, Facciorusso A, Mazzola M, Muscarà C, Scotti M, et al. Propensity score analysis of outcomes following laparoscopic or open liver resection for hepatocellular carcinoma. *Br J Surg.* (2016) 103:871–80. doi: 10.1002/bjs.10137
21. Zhang N, Gu J, Yin L, Wu J, Du MY, Ding K, et al. Incorporation of alpha-fetoprotein(AFP) into subclassification of BCLC C stage hepatocellular carcinoma according to a 5-year survival analysis based on the SEER database. *Oncotarget.* (2016) 7:81389–401. doi: 10.18632/oncotarget.13232
22. Lei JY, Zhong JJ, Yan LN, Zhu JQ, Wang WT, Zeng Y, et al. Response to transarterial chemoembolization as a selection criterion for resection of hepatocellular carcinomas. *Br J Surg.* (2016) 103:881–90. doi: 10.1002/bjs.9864
23. Su M, Zhao Y, Liu J. The role of definitive local treatment in metastatic hepatocellular carcinoma patients: a SEER-based study. *Medicine.* (2018) 97:e0020. doi: 10.1097/MD.0000000000010020
24. Malhotra J, Mhango G, Gomez JE, Smith C, Galsky MD, Strauss GM, et al. Adjuvant chemotherapy for elderly patients with stage I non-small-cell lung cancer ≥4 cm in size: an SEER-Medicare analysis. *Ann Oncol.* (2015) 26:768–73. doi: 10.1093/annonc/mdv008
25. Mironov O, Jaberi A, Kachura JR. Thermal ablation versus surgical resection for the treatment of stage T1 hepatocellular carcinoma in the surveillance, epidemiology, and end results database population. *J Vasc Interv Radiol.* (2017) 28:325–33. doi: 10.1016/j.jvir.2016.11.001

10

Clinical Benefit of Antiviral Agents for Hepatocellular Carcinoma Patients with Low Preoperative HBV-DNA Loads Undergoing Curative Resection

*Kai-Xuan Liu, Jian-Guo Hong, Rui Wu, Zhao-Ru Dong, Ya-Fei Yang, Yu-Chuan Yan, Chun-Cheng Yang, Lun-Jie Yan, Sheng-Yu Yao, Hai-Chao Li, Xu-Ting Zhi and Tao Li**

Department of General Surgery, Qilu Hospital, Shandong University, Jinan, China

Correspondence:
Tao Li
litao7706@163.com

Background and Aims: The clinical benefit of adjuvant antiviral therapy after curative therapy for HCC in patients with high preoperative HBV-DNA loads has been studied widely but that in patients with low preoperative HBV-DNA loads remains controversial. The purpose of this study was to determine the effect of antiviral treatment prophylaxis on HBV reactivation, overall survival (OS), and postoperative liver function in patients with low preoperative HBV-DNA levels undergoing curative resection.

Methods: A meta-analysis was conducted by searching Web of Science, PubMed, Embase, and Cochrane Library until May 2020. We used REVMAN for data analysis and completed the study under the PRISMA guidelines.

Results: Three randomized trials and seven cohort studies, comprising of 1,131 individuals, were included in the meta-analysis. Antiviral treatment significantly reduced the rate of HBV reactivation after curative treatment of HCC, with a pooled risk ratio of 0.12 (95% c.i. 0.07 to 0.21; $P < 0.00001$). The trials were consistently favorable for the antiviral group, with a pooled hazard ratio of 0.52 (95% c.i. 0.37 to 0.74; $P = 0.0002$) in respect of OS rate. However, by pooling the data from studies that reported ALT on the 30th day postoperatively, the result didn't reach statistical significance (mean difference −4.38, 95% c.i. −13.83 to 5.07; $P = 0.36$). The I^2 values of the heterogeneity test for the above three comparisons are zero.

Conclusion: Antiviral therapy during curative resection is effective in reducing HBV reactivation and improving OS rate in HCC patients with low viral load.

Keywords: hepatocellular carcinoma, HBV reactivation, antiviral therapy, prognosis, HBV-DNA load

INTRODUCTION

Hepatocellular carcinoma (HCC) is the sixth most frequent neoplasm worldwide and represents the third leading cause of cancer-related mortality (1). Surgical resection has been standard curative treatment for HCC patients with resectable tumors and unimpaired liver function (2). Unfortunately, tumor recurrence rate was very high after curative therapy with a 5-year recurrence rate of 70% (3). Currently, a major challenge encountered in HCC therapy is improving the prognosis of surgical patients. Hepatitis B virus (HBV) viral load is considered to be an important factor in predicting tumor recurrence (4), and high serum HBV-DNA levels seem to be associated with poor prognosis after the curative HCC resection (5). Liver resection can cause HBV reactivation in most HBV-related HCC patients, and HBV reactivation was related to tumor recurrence (6). However, although it has been extensively established that antiviral therapy can reduce the risk of tumor recurrence, antiviral therapy decreasing HBV reactivation has very rarely been studied.

In addition to these, previous studies have shown that antiviral therapy can reduce the risk of tumor recurrence in patients with high or low preoperative HBV-DNA loads (HBV-DNA < 2,000 IU/ml) (7, 8). However, some conflicting findings that antiviral therapy can improve outcomes in patients with low preoperative HBV-DNA loads have been reported. Huang et al., using a randomized controlled trial, suggested that antiviral group had better outcomes in the recurrence-free survival (RFS) and overall survival (OS) (8). Another study demonstrated that antiviral treatment showed a survival advantage for patients with low preoperative HBV-DNA loads (9). On the contrary, a cohort study observed antiviral treatment had no effects on improving postoperative RFS and OS (10).

Therefore, the purpose of this meta-analysis was to evaluate the effect of antiviral therapy on HBV reactivation and survival in patients with low preoperative HBV-DNA loads undergoing curative resection.

METHODS

Databases and Searches

The literature was searched by computer without language constraints, using PubMed, Web of Science, Embase, and the Cochrane Library until May 2020. The predefined search policies were combinations of the Medical Subject Heading terms: "Carcinoma, Hepatocellular," "antiviral agents," "virus activation," "Hepatectomy," "nucleotide analog," "adefovir," "entecavir," "HCC," "liver cancer," "hepatic cancer," "liver resection," "surgical resection," "radical resection," "curative resection," "hepatic resection," and free text words. Through this retrieval method, 453 articles were retrieved. A manual review of the reference list of relevant articles identified four additional studies.

Study Selection

The criteria for inclusion were: (1) randomized controlled trials (RCT), prospective or retrospective cohort studies or case-control studies that enrolled HBV-related HCC patients who received curative resection as the initial treatment and their serum HBV DNA level was <2,000 IU/ml; (2) consisting of adjuvant antiviral treatment and a control arm of placebo or no treatment after liver resection; (3) no previous antiviral therapy before surgery; (4) adequate follow-up data on HBV reactivation, postoperative liver function, and OS of HCC patients.

Data Extraction and Synthesis

Two authors (KL and JH) independently extracted the following data from the published reports: first author, country of origin, year of publication, study design, study population characteristics, number of patients AVT/non-AVT, type of antiviral agent used, cut-off value of low HBV DNA level, number of patients reactivation, hazard ratio (HR) with 95% confidence interval (CI) for OS and the value of ALT (alanine aminotransferase) at the 30th day postoperatively. In the included literature, some studies included people with both high and low viral loads, and this study only included people with low viral loads in the literature. Any disagreement between them was resolved by consensus. In this study, HBV reactivation after curative resection was considered as the primary endpoint. A consensus about the definition of HBV reactivation has been reached: it is an abrupt increase in serum HBV DNA levels by at least 1 log10 from baseline or its absolute value surpasses 10^9 copies/Ml (11). OS and the value of ALT at the 30th day postoperatively served as secondary outcome. We used Risk of Bias in Non-randomized Studies of Interventions (ROBINS-I) to assess the methodological quality of non-randomized controlled studies. The risk of bias in each included RCTs was assessed by using Cochrane risk assessment tools.

Statistical Analysis

The meta-analysis was done using the Cochrane Review Manager (RevMan, version 5.3; The Cochrane Collaboration, Copenhagen, Denmark) software. Statistical analysis for dichotomous variables time-to-event variables and continuous variables were respectively carried out using relative risk (RR), hazard ratio (HR), and mean difference (MD) as the summary statistic. A fixed effect model, the Mantel–Haenszel method, was used for homogeneous studies including dichotomous variables. Inverse variance method was used for pooling HR, MD. A value of P below 0.05 was considered statistically significant. The publication bias was evaluated by visual analysis of the funnel plots. We assessed heterogeneity by χ^2 and I^2 statistics. A fixed-effect model was used for comparison when heterogeneity was not substantial ($I^2 < 25\%$).

RESULTS

Characteristics of Studies Included in Meta-Analysis

There were 453 articles identified through the systematic search and four additional manually searched articles, which comprised 449 HCC patients receiving antiviral therapy and 682 HCC patients without antiviral therapy (**Figure 1**). The main characteristics of the studies assessed by meta-analysis are outlined in **Table 1**. The main treatment in all the included studies was surgical resection. All studies were performed in Asia, among which nine were from China (8–10, 12–16, 19), and the other one was from Republic of Korea (17). Among the reviewed studies, three were RCTs and seven were NRCTs. All included articles were published between 2012 and 2019.

The methodological features of included non-randomized controlled studies are shown in **Table 2**. Among the seven observational studies included in the meta-analysis, only one was judged to have a serious risk of confounding bias. The remaining six studies were deemed to have a moderate (n = 4) or low (n = 2) risk of bias. For the three randomized trials identified among the included studies, we had some concerns regarding the risk of bias in the random sequence generation and allocation hiding due to the design flaw of study (**Figure 2**).

Antiviral Therapy and HBV Reactivation

Nine of ten studies reported on HBV reactivation (**Figure 3**). Antiviral treatment significantly reduced the risk of HBV reactivation with a pooled risk ratio of 0.12 (95% c.i. 0.07 to 0.21); $P < 0.00001$) without statistical heterogeneity ($I^2 = 0\%$, $P = 0.97$ for $\chi 2$) in the meta-analysis.

Antiviral Therapy and Overall Survival Rate

Data were collected from three of the ten studies that reported 3-year OS. The trials were consistently favorable for the antiviral group, with a pooled hazard ratio of 0.52 (95% c.i. 0.37 to 0.74); $P = 0.0002$) without statistical heterogeneity ($I^2 = 0\%$, $P = 0.66$ for $\chi 2$) in the meta-analysis (**Figure 4**). Due to limited data available, the effect of antiviral therapy on local tumor recurrence or disease-specific survival could not be analyzed in this stud and no valid conclusions could be drawn.

Antiviral Therapy and Liver Function

Though antiviral therapy often shows an advantage in long-term liver function of patients; however, due to limited data, our study did not conduct long-term liver function analysis. According to the analysis of the included literature, the available and meaningful data were ALT values at 30 days postoperatively. Pooled data from four of the ten studies revealed that ALT levels were lower, but not statistically significant (mean difference −4.38, 95% c.i. −13.83 to 5.07; $P = 0.36$), in patients receiving antiviral therapy. There was still no heterogeneity in this group ($I^2 = 0\%$, $P = 0.92$ for $\chi 2$) (**Figure 5**). The safety of antiviral therapy was well demonstrated, and none of the included studies provided data on adverse events associated with antiviral treatment.

Publication Bias Analysis

No evidence of asymmetry was identified in funnel plots of OS and ALT. However, a funnel plot for HBV reactivation revealed a mild asymmetry, suggesting that there was publication bias (**Figure 6**).

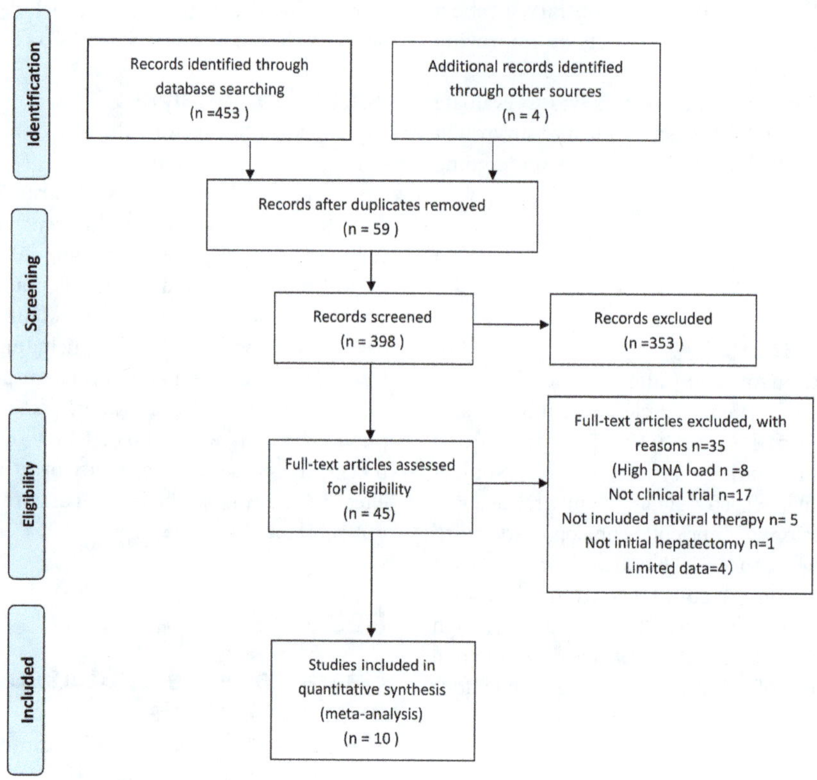

FIGURE 1 | Study flow chart of the data extraction process and selection of studies for meta-analysis.

TABLE 1 | Comparisons of the studies included for meta-analysis.

Study id	Country	No. of patients AVT/non-AVT	Study type	M/F	Type of antiviral agent used	Cut-off value of low HBV DNA (No.)	No. of reactivation	OS (HR,95% CI)	30days ALT
Chen et al. (12)	China mainland	20/54	prospective study	17/3 47/7	Entecavir	<500 IU/ml	1/20 15/54	N/A	N/A
Chen et al. (13)	China mainland	51/154	retrospective cohort study	48/3 131/ 23	Entecavir (93)* lamivudine(84) adefovir dipivoxil (13) telbivudine (2)	<2,000IU/ml	N/A	0.641 [0.215, 1.066]	N/A
Gong et al. (14)	China mainland	66/108	prospective study	58/8 92/ 16	entecavir	<500 IU/ml	2/66 30/108	N/A	35.6 ± 26.1 45.1 ± 11.8
Huang et al. (8)	China mainland	100/100	RCT	87/ 13 86/ 14	telbivudine	<2,000 IU/ml	3/100 25/100 (1year)	0.549 [0.362, 0.832]	N/A
Huang et al. (15)	China mainland	27/34	prospectively study	N/A	N/A	$<1.0 \times 10^3$ copies/ml	1/27 4/34	N/A	N/A
Huang et al. (16)	China mainland	28/29	RCT	N/A	telbivudine	$<1.0 \times 10^4$ copies/ml	1/40 14/44	N/A	22 ± 8.9 24.8 ± 8.7
Lee et al. (17)	Republic of Korea	13/20	retrospective cohort study	N/A	nucleos(t)ide analog	Undetectable, <15 IU/ml	1/13 10/20	N/A	N/A
Liu et al. (18)	China mainland	63/102	RCT	43/ 20 67/ 35	entecavir	HBV-DNA-negative	2/63 13/102	N/A	35.3 ± 16.1 37.3 ± 16.2
Xu et al. (10)	China mainland	37/37	cohort study	32/5 31/6	entecavir	<100 IU/ml	2/35 3/34	0.375 [0.168, 0.834]	N/A
Yuan et al. (19)	China mainland	44/44	cohort study	32/ 12 38/6	entecavir	<8,866 copies/ml =1,773 IU/ml	1/44 11/44	N/A	31.8 ± 22.4 43.7 ± 19.2

*Os, Overall survival; HR, Hazard Ratio; CI, Confidence Interval; ALT, Alanine aminotransferase; AVT, antiviral therapy; *The figures in brackets denote the number of patients.*

TABLE 2 | Risk of bias assessment with ROBINS-I tool.

study id	Bias due to confounding	Bias in selection of participants in to the study	Bias in measurement of interventions	Bias due to departures from intended interventions	Bias due to missing data	Bias in measurement of outcomes	Bias in selection of the reported result	Overall Risk
Chen et al. (12)	Low	Low	Low	Low	Low	Low	Low	Low
Chen et al. (13)	Moderate	Moderate	Low	Low	Low	Low	Moderate	Moderate
Gong et al. (14)	Serious	Low	Low	Low	Low	Low	Low	Serious
Huang et al. (15)	Low	Moderate	Low	Moderate	Low	Low	Moderate	Moderate
Lee et al. (17)	Low	Low	Low	Low	Low	Low	Moderate	Moderate
Xu et al. (10)	Low	Low	Low	Low	Low	Low	Low	Low
Yuan et al. (17)	Low	Moderate	Low	Low	Low	Low	Low	Moderate

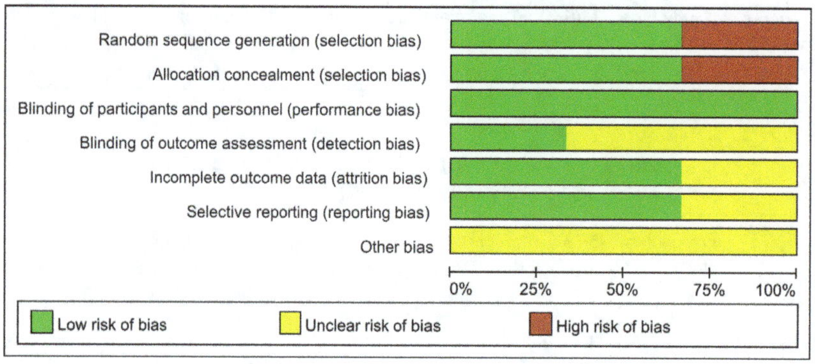

FIGURE 2 | Risk of bias graph: review authors; judgements about each risk of bias item presented as percentages across all included RCT studies.

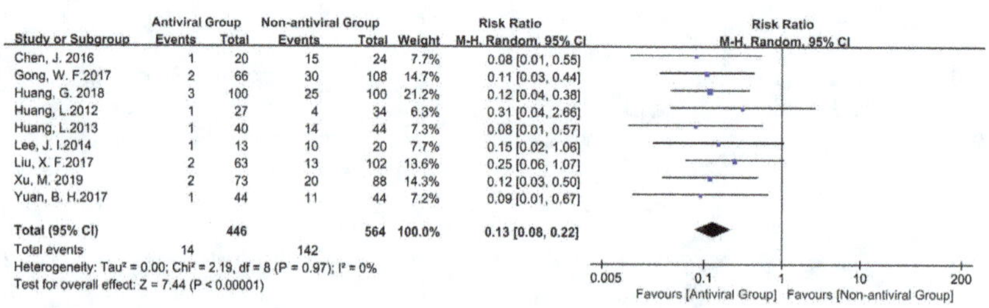

FIGURE 3 | The Forest plot to compare the effect of anti-viral treatment vs. no treatment in HBV reactivation.

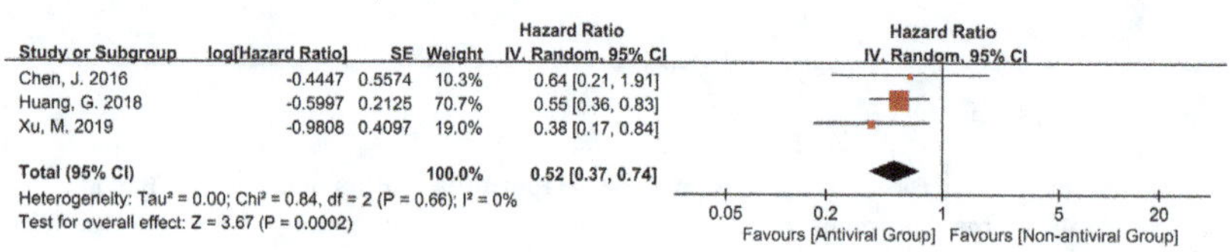

FIGURE 4 | The Forest plot to compare the effect of anti-viral treatment *vs.* no treatment in overall survival rate.

DISCUSSION

It is an urgent problem for us to improve the prognosis of liver cancer patients. Previous studies have shown that for HCC patients with preoperative high HBV-DNA loads, antiviral therapy is of great significance for preventing recurrence and improving OS (20). However, there is still uncertainty as to whether there is benefit from antiviral therapy for HCC patients with low HBV DNA load. We conducted this meta-analysis to try to answer this question.

The mechanism of HBV reactivation remains unclear. Hepatic resection induced immunosuppression may increase the risk of HBV reactivation (21), which can impair liver function (4), aggravate liver cirrhosis (22), and increase the risk of HBV-related HCC recurrence (23). However, the main therapeutic mechanism of the antiviral drug was to prevent HBV replication and then reduce HBV reactivation regardless of HBV load (24, 25). Our results showed that antiviral treatment can effectively reduce HBV reactivation in HCC patients with low preoperative HBV-DNA loads undergoing curative resection. Tseng et al. revealed that HCC risk in hepatitis e antigen negative patients with low viral loads depends on HBsAg levels, not HBV DNA levels (26). Therefore, HBsAg seroclearance is considered as a safer antiviral treatment endpoint and has good off-treatment durability (27). We did not perform subgroup analysis because there was no significant heterogeneity.

Moreover, this study demonstrates that antiviral treatment is significant in improving OS rate in low viral load patients.

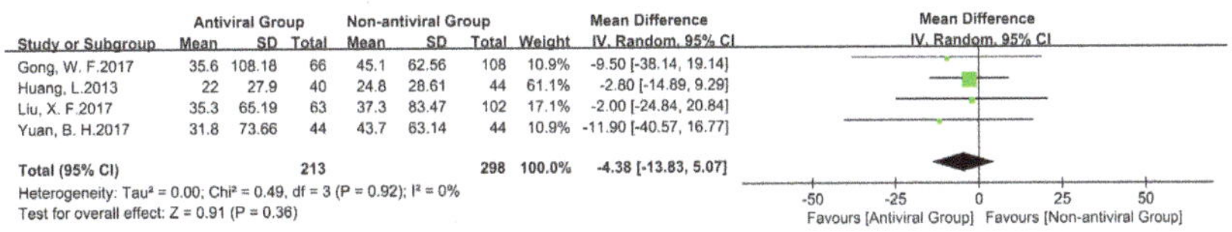

FIGURE 5 | The Forest plot to compare the effect of anti-viral treatment *vs.* no treatment in liver function.

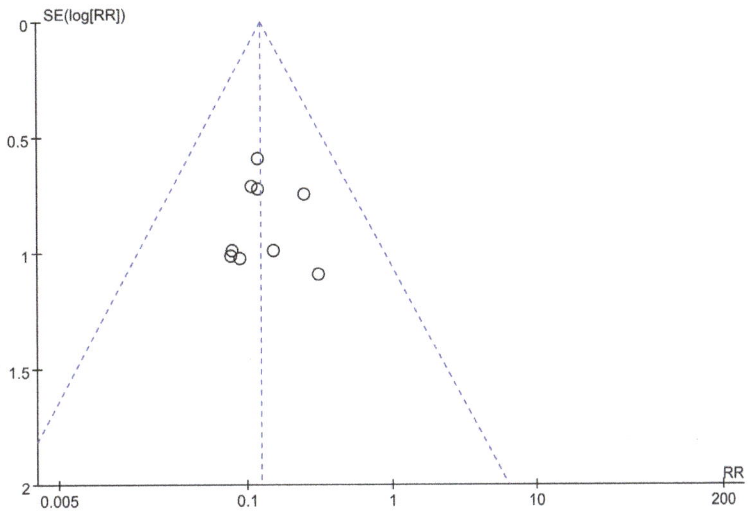

FIGURE 6 | Funnel plot for the included trials—HBV reactivation. RR, risk ratio; SE, standard error.

To strengthen the study, we restricted the meta-analysis to 3-year OS rates. All included trials have available and comparable OS rates data at that time. Though antiviral treatment has no direct antitumorous effect, it can prevent HBV reactivation, inhibit hepatitis activity, reduce inflammation in liver remnants, and reverse cirrhosis and liver dysfunction (28). The hepatitis activity in the non-tumorous liver is known to be associated with tumor recurrence after hepatectomy. Antiviral therapy can reduce HCC risks by downregulating hepatic inflammation and related nuclear signaling pathways that lead to neoplastic transformation (8). In addition, antiviral therapy can also reduce the expression of the HBx protein to levels insufficient to promote HCC development and enhance tolerance to therapy against recurrence and leads to increased OS (29).

Previous studies have revealed that antiviral therapy can significantly improve liver function in patients with HBV-related HCC (28). In the present study, there was no statistical difference in ALT level on the 30th postoperative day between antiviral groups and non-antiviral groups. During the perioperative period, surgical factors such as hepatectomy induced severe damage of liver cells, the volume of liver parenchyma resected, and clamping of hepatic vessel may play a greater role in liver function recovery. Moreover, most of patients received antiviral therapy immediately when they developed HBV reactivation, which prevented the progress of hepatitis caused by replication of virus. In fact, antiviral therapy often shows an advantage in long-term liver function of patients, especially in patients with decompensated cirrhosis (30) and the improvements became most apparent after 9 months (31). Liu et al. also revealed that the treatment group had better postoperative liver function than the control group after a 1-year follow-up (18), which suggested antiviral treatment may have the advantage in long-term prognosis.

Certain limitations must be considered when interpreting study findings. First, although we conducted an extensive literature search, only three RCTs related to this theme were included in this meta-analysis, and one of the ten studies has serious risk of bias. There is concern with lacking well-designed prospective clinical trials in the literature. More well-designed RCTs with large sample sizes of patients are required in future analysis. Second, patients were treated with variable antiviral agents, including IFN and Nucleotide Analogue, and different timing of antiviral therapy and durations also have influence on the HBV reactivation. Third, all included studies were invariably conducted in Asia. The major risk factors for HCC vary from region to region. The high HCC rates in parts of Asia largely reflect the elevated prevalence of HBV infection.

Seven genotypes (A to G) of HBV identified are associated with the disease progression and long-term outcome of HBV infection (32), and Genotypes B and C are prevalent in Asia (33). In most high risk HCC areas, such as China and South-East Asia, the key determinants are chronic HBV infection, and China alone accounting for about 50% of the total number of cases and deaths of HCC occurred worldwide (34). Therefore, it is inevitable that most HBV-related HCC studies are from Eastern countries especially from China (35). Additional studies are needed to better understand the effects of antiviral therapy on survival of HCC among other ethnic or geographic regions.

CONCLUSIONS

In conclusion, the present analysis demonstrates antiviral therapy can effectively reduce HBV reactivation and improve OS rate in patients with low viral load. Therefore, we recommend antiviral therapy for patients with HBV-associated HCC after hepatectomy without delay, regardless of the viral load.

AUTHOR CONTRIBUTIONS

Study design: K-XL, J-GH, RW, Z-RD, Y-FY, Y-CY, C-CY, L-JY, S-YY, H-CL, X-TZ, TL. Data collection: K-XL, J-GH. Data analysis: KX-L, J-GH. Writing: K-XL, TL. All authors contributed to the article and approved the submitted version.

REFERENCES

1. Forner A, Reig M, Bruix J. Hepatocellular carcinoma. *Lancet (London England)* (2018) 391:1301–14. doi: 10.1016/s0140-6736(18)30010-2
2. EASL-EORTC. EASL-EORTC clinical practice guidelines: management of hepatocellular carcinoma. *J Hepatol* (2012) 56:908–43. doi: 10.1016/j.jhep.2011.12.001
3. Ercolani G, Grazi GL, Ravaioli M, Del Gaudio M, Gardini A, Cescon M, et al. Liver resection for hepatocellular carcinoma on cirrhosis: univariate and multivariate analysis of risk factors for intrahepatic recurrence. *Ann Surg* (2003) 237:536–43. doi: 10.1097/01.Sla.0000059988.22416.F2
4. Wu JC, Huang YH, Chau GY, Su CW, Lai CR, Lee PC, et al. Risk factors for early and late recurrence in hepatitis B-related hepatocellular carcinoma. *J Hepatol* (2009) 51:890–7. doi: 10.1016/j.jhep.2009.07.009
5. Yang T, Lu JH, Zhai J, Lin C, Yang GS, Zhao RH, et al. High viral load is associated with poor overall and recurrence-free survival of hepatitis B virus-related hepatocellular carcinoma after curative resection: a prospective cohort study. *Eur J Surg Oncol* (2012) 38:683–91. doi: 10.1016/j.ejso.2012.04.010
6. Huang G, Lai ECH, Lau WY, Zhou W-p, Shen F, Pan Z-y, et al. Posthepatectomy HBV Reactivation in Hepatitis B-Related Hepatocellular Carcinoma Influences Postoperative Survival in Patients With Preoperative Low HBV-DNA Levels. *Ann Surg* (2013) 257:490–505. doi: 10.1097/SLA.0b013e318262b218
7. Huang G, Lau WY, Wang ZG, Pan ZY, Yuan SX, Shen F, et al. Antiviral therapy improves postoperative survival in patients with hepatocellular carcinoma: a randomized controlled trial. *Ann Surg* (2015) 261:56–66. doi: 10.1097/sla.0000000000000858
8. Huang G, Li PP, Lau WY, Pan ZY, Zhao LH, Wang ZG, et al. Antiviral Therapy Reduces Hepatocellular Carcinoma Recurrence in Patients With Low HBV-DNA Levels: A Randomized Controlled Trial. *Ann Surg* (2018) 268:943–54. doi: 10.1097/sla.0000000000002727
9. Liu XF, Zhang T, Tang K, Sui LL, Xu G, Liu Q. Study of Preoperative Antiviral Treatment of Patients with HCC Negative for HBV-DNA. *World J Surg Oncol* (2017) 37:4701–6. doi: 10.1186/s12957-019-1577-9
10. Xu M, Zhou Z, Xu R, Zhang H, Lin N, Zhong Y. Antiviral therapy predicts the outcomes following resection of hepatocellular carcinoma in patients negative for HBV DNA: A propensity score matching analysis. *World J Surg Oncol* (2019) 17. doi: 10.1186/s12957-019-1577-9
11. Perrillo RP, Gish R, Falck-Ytter YT. American Gastroenterological Association Institute technical review on prevention and treatment of hepatitis B virus reactivation during immunosuppressive drug therapy. *Gastroenterology* (2015) 148:221–244.e223. doi: 10.1053/j.gastro.2014.10.038
12. Chen J, Bai T, Wang XB, Xie ZB, Liu JJ, Zhang Y, et al. Factors associated with postoperative HBV reactivation in HBV related hepatocellular carcinoma patients with HBV-DNA levels less than the minimum. *Int J Clin Exp Med* (2016) 9:4533–8.
13. Chen JL, Lin XJ, Zhou Q, Shi M, Li SP, Lao XM. Association of HBV DNA replication with antiviral treatment outcomes in the patients with early-stage HBV-related hepatocellular carcinoma undergoing curative resection. *Chin J Cancer* (2016) 35. doi: 10.1186/s40880-016-0089-z
14. Gong WF, Zhong JH, Lu SD, Wang XB, Zhang QM, Ma L, et al. Effects of antiviral therapy on post-hepatectomy HBV reactivation and liver function in HBV DNA-negative patients with HBVrelated hepatocellular carcinoma. *Oncotarget* (2017) 8:15047–56. doi: 10.18632/oncotarget.14789
15. Huang L, Li J, Lau WY, Yan J, Zhou F, Liu C, et al. Perioperative reactivation of hepatitis B virus replication in patients undergoing partial hepatectomy for hepatocellular carcinoma. *J Gastroenterol Hepatol (Australia)* (2012) 27:158–64. doi: 10.1111/j.1440-1746.2011.06888.x
16. Huang L, Li J, Yan J, Sun J, Zhang X, Wu M, et al. Antiviral therapy decreases viral reactivation in patients with hepatitis B virusrelated hepatocellular carcinoma undergoing hepatectomy: a randomized controlled trial. *J Viral Hepatitis* (2013) 20:336–42. doi: 10.1111/jvh.12036
17. Lee JI, Kim JK, Chang HY, Lee JW, Kim JM, Chung HJ, et al. Impact of postoperative hepatitis B virus reactivation in hepatocellular carcinoma patients who formerly had naturally suppressed virus. *J Gastroenterol Hepatol (Australia)* (2014) 29:1019–27. doi: 10.1111/jgh.12472
18. Liu XF, Zhang T, Tang K, Sui LL, Xu G, Liu Q. Study of Preoperative Antiviral Treatment of Patients with HCC Negative for HBV-DNA. *Anticancer Res* (2017) 37:4701–6. doi: 10.21873/anticanres.11875
19. Yuan BH, Li RH, Yuan WP, Xiang BD, Zheng MH, Yang T, et al. Perioperative entecavir for patients with HBV-related hepatocellular carcinoma and low levels of viral DNA: Analysis using propensity score matching. *Oncotarget* (2017) 8:51810–6. doi: 10.18632/oncotarget.15395
20. Chan AC, Chok KS, Yuen WK, Chan SC, Poon RT, Lo CM, et al. Impact of antiviral therapy on the survival of patients after major hepatectomy for hepatitis B virus-related hepatocellular carcinoma. *Arch Surg (Chicago Ill: 1960)* (2011) 146:675–81. doi: 10.1001/archsurg.2011.125
21. Xie ZB, Zhu SL, Peng YC, Chen J, Wang XB, Ma L, et al. Postoperative hepatitis B virus reactivation and surgery-induced immunosuppression in patients with hepatitis B-related hepatocellular carcinoma. *J Surg Oncol* (2015) 112:634–42. doi: 10.1002/jso.24044
22. Wong GL, Chan HL, Mak CW, Lee SK, Ip ZM, Lam AT, et al. Entecavir treatment reduces hepatic events and deaths in chronic hepatitis B patients with liver cirrhosis. *Hepatology* (2013) 58:1537–47. doi: 10.1002/hep.26301
23. Chan SL, Wong VW, Qin S, Chan HL. Infection and Cancer: The Case of Hepatitis B. *J Clin Oncol: Off J Am Soc Clin Oncol* (2016) 34:83–90. doi: 10.1200/jco.2015.61.5724
24. Menendez-Arias L, Alvarez M, Pacheco B. Nucleoside/nucleotide analog inhibitors of hepatitis B virus polymerase: mechanism of action and resistance. *Curr Opin Virol* (2014) 8:1–9. doi: 10.1016/j.coviro.2014.04.005
25. Mesev EV, LeDesma RA, Ploss A. Decoding type I and III interferon signalling during viral infection. *Nat Microbiol* (2019) 4:914–24. doi: 10.1038/s41564-019-0421-x
26. Tseng TC, Liu CJ, Yang HC, Su TH, Wang CC, Chen CL, et al. High levels of hepatitis B surface antigen increase risk of hepatocellular carcinoma in patients with low HBV load. *Gastroenterology* (2012) 142:1140–1149 e1143; quiz e1113-1144. doi: 10.1053/j.gastro.2012.02.007
27. Kim GA, Lim YS, An J, Lee D, Shim JH, Kim KM, et al. HBsAg seroclearance after nucleoside analogue therapy in patients with chronic hepatitis B: clinical outcomes and durability. *Gut* (2014) 63:1325–32. doi: 10.1136/gutjnl-2013-305517

28. Lao XM, Luo G, Ye LT, Luo C, Shi M, Wang D, et al. Effects of antiviral therapy on hepatitis B virus reactivation and liver function after resection or chemoembolization for hepatocellular carcinoma. *Liver International: Off J Int Assoc Study Liver* (2013) 33:595–604. doi: 10.1111/liv.12112
29. Chong CC, Wong GL, Wong VW, Ip PC, Cheung YS, Wong J, et al. Antiviral therapy improves post-hepatectomy survival in patients with hepatitis B virus-related hepatocellular carcinoma: a prospective-retrospective study. *Aliment Pharmacol Ther* (2015) 41:199–208. doi: 10.1111/apt.13034
30. Chu CM, Liaw YF. Hepatitis B virus-related cirrhosis: natural history and treatment. *Semin Liver Dis* (2006) 26:142–52. doi: 10.1055/s-2006-939752
31. Villeneuve JP, Condreay LD, Willems B, Pomier-Layrargues G, Fenyves D, Bilodeau M, et al. Lamivudine treatment for decompensated cirrhosis resulting from chronic hepatitis B. *Hepatology* (2000) 31:207–10. doi: 10.1002/hep.510310130
32. Lin CL, Kao JH. Natural history of acute and chronic hepatitis B: The role of HBV genotypes and mutants. *Best Pract Res Clin Gastroenterol* (2017) 31:249–55. doi: 10.1016/j.bpg.2017.04.010
33. Kao JH, Chen DS. Global control of hepatitis B virus infection. *Lancet Infect Dis* (2002) 2:395–403. doi: 10.1016/s1473-3099(02)00315-8
34. Torre LA, Bray F, Siegel RL, Ferlay J, Lortet-Tieulent J, Jemal A. *Global cancer statistics*, 2012. *CA Cancer J Clin* (2015) 65:87–108. doi: 10.3322/caac.21262
35. Li T, Qin LX, Gong X, Zhou J, Sun HC, Qiu SJ, et al. Hepatitis B virus surface antigen-negative and hepatitis C virus antibody-negative hepatocellular carcinoma: clinical characteristics, outcome, and risk factors for early and late intrahepatic recurrence after resection. *Cancer* (2013) 119:126–35. doi: 10.1002/cncr.27697

11

Prediction of Survival and Analysis of Prognostic Factors for Patients with Combined Hepatocellular Carcinoma and Cholangiocarcinoma

Jitao Wang[1,2†], Zhi Li[3†], Yong Liao[2†], Jinlong Li[2], Hui Dong[1], Hao Peng[1], Wenjing Xu[1], Zhe Fan[1], Fengxiao Gao[2], Chengyu Liu[2], Dengxiang Liu[2] and Yewei Zhang[1,4*]*

[1] School of Medicine, Southeast University, Nanjing, China, [2] Xingtai Institute of Cancer Control, Xingtai People's Hospital, Xingtai, China, [3] Department of Infection Management, Xingtai General Hospital of North China Healthcare Group, Xingtai, China, [4] Department of Hepatobiliary and Pancreatic Surgery, The Second Affiliated Hospital of Nanjing Medical University, Nanjing, China

***Correspondence:**
Yewei Zhang
zhangyewei@njmu.edu.cn
Dengxiang Liu
rmyy666@163.com

†These authors have contributed equally to this work and share first authorship

Background: Combined hepatocellular carcinoma and cholangiocarcinoma (CHC) is an uncommon subtype of primary liver cancer. Because of limited epidemiological data, prognostic risk factors and therapeutic strategies for patients with CHC tend to be individualized. This study aimed to identify independent prognostic factors and develop a nomogram-based model for predicting the overall survival (OS) of patients with CHC.

Methods: We recruited eligible individuals from the Surveillance, Epidemiology, and End Results (SEER) database between 2004 and 2015 and randomly divided them into the training or verification cohort. Univariate and multivariate analyses were performed to identify independent variables associated with OS. Based on multivariate analysis, the nomogram was established, and its prediction performance was evaluated using the consistency index (C-index) and calibration curve.

Results: In total, 271 patients with CHC were included in our study. The median OS was 14 months, and the 1-, 3-, and 5-year OS rates were 52.3%, 27.1%, and 23.3%, respectively. In the training cohort, multivariate analysis showed that the pathological grade (hazard ratio [HR], 1.26; 95% confidence interval [CI]: 0.96–1.66), TNM stage (HR, 1.21; 95% CI: 1.02 - 1.44), and surgery (HR, 0.26; 95% CI: 0.17 - 0.40) were independent indicators of OS. The nomogram-based model related C-indexes were 0.76 (95% CI: 0.72 - 0.81) and 0.72 (95% CI: 0.66 - 0.79) in the training and validation cohorts, respectively. The calibration of the nomogram showed good consistency of 1-, 3-, and 5-year OS rates between the actual observed survival and predicted survival in both cohorts. The TNM stage (HR, 1.23; 95% CI: 1.01 - 1.49), and M stage (HR, 1.87; 95% CI: 1.14 3.05) were risk factors in the surgical treatment group. Surgical resection and liver transplantation could significantly prolong the survival, with no statistical difference observed.

Conclusions: The pathological grade, TNM stage, and surgery were independent prognostic factors for patients with CHC. We developed a nomogram model, in the form of a static nomogram or an online calculator, for predicting the OS of patients with CHC, with a good predictive performance.

Keywords: combined hepatocellular carcinoma and cholangiocarcinoma, overall survival, nomogram, prognostic factors, population-based study, Surveillance Epidemiology and End Results database

INTRODUCTION

Combined hepatocellular carcinoma and cholangiocarcinoma (CHC) is a rare tumor subtype, it accounts for only 0.4%–14.2% of primary liver malignancies, and it has characteristics of hepatocellular carcinoma (HCC) and cholangiocarcinoma (CC) (1–3). In a large population-based study, the overall incidence of CHC was 0.05 per 100,000 person-years between 2004 and 2014, and its incidence and mortality have increased in recent years (1). The number of patients diagnosed with CHC almost doubled during 2004–2007 and 2012–2015, and patients with CHC more often had advanced T3–T4 stage cancer (57.0%) based on the guidelines of the American Joint Committee on Cancer (AJCC) and had a grim prognosis (2–5). The prognosis of CHC was reported as comparable to that of ICC but was worse than that of HCC (6–10), and patients with CHC have a lower survival rate than those with both the aforementioned malignancies (11–14). Therefore, the survival and prognosis of patients with CHC remain significant concerns.

Despite progress in treatment strategies, CHC is still considered an aggressive liver cancer with a poor prognosis and negligible improvement in recent years (15, 16). The main treatments for CHC include liver resection (LR) and liver transplantation (LT). Complete LR is considered to be the first-line treatment strategy for resectable CHC; however, the median overall survival (OS) of patients with CHC who have undergone surgery was only approximately 25-35.4 months (12, 13, 17–19). LT is another surgical option that may offer the only chance for long-term survival. Although LT has a survival advantage for patients with HCC, transplantation for CHC remains controversial (3, 16, 19).

The AJCC TNM staging system is widely used to assess the severity and predict the prognosis of patients with HCC or ICC (20). Although the TNM staging system has been confirmed to be a prognostic system for CHC (2, 21), its accuracy was not as remarkable as a serological model (22). However, many studies have shown that several independent risk factors, including age (23), race (5, 9), alpha-fetoprotein (AFP) status (23), cirrhosis (4), and treatment strategies (1, 5, 9, 24–26), affect the survival and prognosis of patients with CHC. At present, some single-center studies have constructed many nomogram prediction models for CHC (22, 27–30). Furthermore, studies have recently used the Surveillance, Epidemiology, and End Results (SEER) database to describe incidence trends and clinical outcomes of patients with CHC (1, 5); however, there was a lack of a nomogram to predict long-term survival.

Thus, this study aimed to analyze potential risk factors associated with the prognosis of patients with CHC and develop and validate a prognostic nomogram to enable clinicians to make better personalized decisions for treating patients with CHC.

METHODS

Study Design and Patients

Our study collected clinical data of patients with CHC from the SEER database. The inclusion criteria of the study were patients diagnosed between 2004 and 2015, the primary tumor site was the liver, and the International Classification of Diseases for Oncology, third edition code was 8180/3: combined HCC and CC. Diagnostically confirmed cases included in our study were required to have positive histology findings. The exclusion criteria were unknown histological grade, unknown tumor size, unknown marital status at diagnosis, unknown surgical treatment, or lack of complete survival months.

Data Collection and Definition of Variables

The following clinical information was collected for further analysis: baseline demographics, including ethnicity, age at diagnosis, sex, marital status, OS, and survival status; tumor features such as tumor size, pathological grade, TNM stage [AJCC 6th edition], T stage, M stage, N stage, and treatment strategies, including surgery at the primary site, chemotherapy recode, and radiotherapy recode.

Sex was classified as male or female. Ethnicity was categorized into three race groups: Caucasian, African American, and others. Patients were classified into two groups: ≤60 years and >60 years according to the patient's age at diagnosis. Marital status at diagnosis was categorized as married, single (never married), divorced/separated, or widowed. Tumor size was classified into two groups: ≤5 cm or >5 cm. Surgical types were classified as no surgery, LR, or LT. LR included local destruction, wedge resection (or segmental resection), lobectomy, and unclear surgical type. For radiotherapy and chemotherapy, patients were classified as with, without, or unknown.

Statistical Analysis

We randomly divided all eligible patients with CHC into two groups: the training cohort (n=270) and the validation cohort (n=101).

The nomogram-based model was constructed using the training cohort and verified using the verification cohort. We identified clinical characteristics with p-values ≤0.1 in the univariate analysis and further included them in the multivariate analysis. The nomogram model was constructed with independent prognostic factors based on the multivariate Cox regression analysis (p<0.05), and the efficacy was assessed using the concordance index (C-index). Calibration plots of the nomogram-based model for 1-, 3-, and 5-year OS in the training and validation cohorts were created by comparing nomogram-predicted OS with actual observed OS. In addition, according to the optimal cut-off value of the nomogram-based model score in the training cohort, all patients with CHC were divided into two groups: low or high risk. Clinically, surgical treatment strategies are related to the tumor grade, tumor stage, and patient's clinical characteristics. The OS of patients with CHC was analyzed using the Kaplan-Meier method, and the log-rank test was used to compare the different groups. Clinical information was extracted using SEER*Stat software version 8.3.8 (www.seer.cancer.gov/seerstat). The data were analyzed using IBM SPSS Statistics 25.0 (IBM Corp., Armonk, NY, USA) and R software version 3.5.0 (The R Foundation, https://www.r-project.org/). The optimal cut-off value of the nomogram-based model score was calculated using X-Tile software version 3.6.1 (Yale University School of Medicine) (31).

Quantitative variables are expressed as median (interquartile range [IQR]) and were compared using the unpaired two-tailed Student's t-test or the Kruskal-Wallis test as appropriate. Categorical data are expressed as numbers (percentage) and were compared using the χ^2 test or the Fisher exact test as appropriate. P-values <0.05 were considered statistically significant.

RESULTS

Patient Demographics

According to the selection criteria, 271 patients (190 men; mean age, 61 years; age range, 14–88 years) were included in the final analysis (**Figure 1**). The most common race was Caucasian, accounting for 73.8% of the population. The median tumor size was 5.5 cm (IQR, 3.5–9.5 cm). Most patients presented with pathological grades III (57.2%) and II cancer (31.7%). A positive AFP status was found in 144 (53.1%) patients. Regarding treatment, most patients (161, 59.4%) underwent surgery, while 102 (37.6%) patients were administered chemotherapy, and 26 (9.6%) patients received radiotherapy. Baseline characteristics of the total, training, and validation cohorts are summarized in **Table 1**.

Survival Analysis

In the total cohort, the median OS was 14.0 months (95% confidence interval [CI]: 10.4–17.6 months), and the 1-, 3-, and 5-year OS rates were 52.3%, 27.1%, and 23.3%, respectively. The mortality rate within 1 year was 47.7% in the total cohort. Detailed information is shown in **Table 1**. Pathological grade, TNM stage, tumor size, T stage, N stage, M stage, and surgery were identified as significant indicators of OS in the univariate analysis of the training cohort (**Table 2**). Independent predictors of OS indicated in the multivariable analysis were pathological grade (hazard ratio [HR]: 1.26; 95% CI: 0.96–1.66; P=0.01), TNM stage (HR: 1.21; 95% CI: 1.02–1.44; P=0.03), and surgery (HR, 0.26; 95% CI: 0.17–0.40, P<0.01) (**Table 2**).

Nomogram for Predicting OS

A nomogram was established based on all independent prognostic variables identified in the multivariate analysis (**Figure 2**). Our nomogram was virtually displayed for predicting 1-, 3-, and 5-year OS in the training cohort and was validated in the validation cohort. The nomogram exhibited a satisfactory performance for predicting OS with C-indexes of 0.76 (95% CI: 0.72–0.81) and 0.72 (95% CI: 0.66–0.79) in the training and validation cohorts, respectively. The calibration curves for the probability of 1-, 3-, and 5-year OS manifested an optimal consistency between the actual observation and the nomogram-based model prediction in the training and validation cohorts (**Figure 3**).

By applying the optimal cut-off value of the nomogram in the training cohort, we developed a risk stratification of OS. All patients with CHC were divided into the low-risk group (≤120 points) or high-risk group (>120 points) according to the nomogram-based model score. In the total cohort, Kaplan-Meier analysis showed that the median OS values were 28.0 months (95% CI: 20.5–35.5 months) and 4.0 months (2.7–5.7 months) in the low-risk and high-risk groups, respectively (P<0.001, **Figure 4A**). In the training cohort, the median OS values were 24.0 months (95% CI: 14.0–34.0 months) and 4.0 months (2.7–5.3 months) in the low-risk and high-risk groups, respectively (P<0.001, **Figure 4B**). In the validation cohort, the median OS values were 30.0 months (95% CI: 21.3–38.7 months) and 4.0 months (1.7–6.3 months) in the low-risk and high-risk groups, respectively (P<0.001, **Figure 4C**). An online calculator based on our nomogram model for clinicians and researchers to predict the survival probability of CHC patients by simply inputting clinical characteristics was developed (https://xingtai.shinyapps.io/CHC_DynNomapp/). Using the formula based on our nomogram model, the 5-year survival probability of the 10th patient in the verification cohort was calculated to be 34%, which is close to the result of the online calculator (36%, 95% CI: 0.23-0.59), which validated the accuracy of the calculator (**Figure S1**).

Univariate and Multivariate Analyses of the Surgical Treatment Groups

The median OS values were 29 months (95% CI: 21.8–36.2 months) for patients with CHC who underwent surgical treatment (LR or LT) and 4 months (95% CI: 2.7–5.3 months) for patients with CHC who did not undergo surgical treatment (P<0.0001, **Figure 5A**). Therefore, when compared with no surgery, LR and LT significantly prolonged OS (**Figure 5B**). After excluding non-surgical patients, univariate analysis showed that the tumor size, pathological grade, TNM stage, T stage,

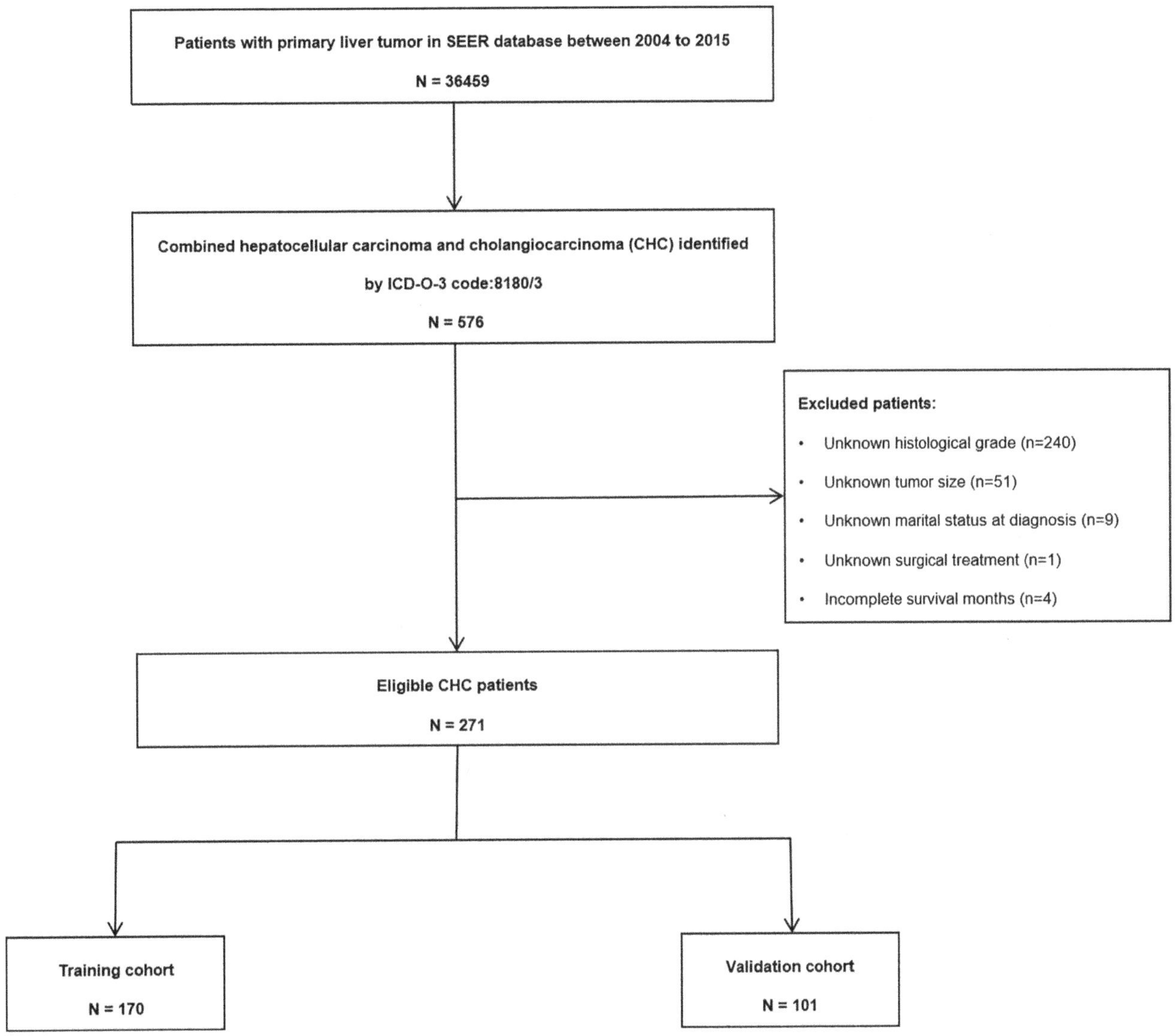

FIGURE 1 | Flow chart of the combined hepatocellular carcinoma and cholangiocarcinoma patients.

N stage, M stage, AFP status, and chemotherapy were risk factors of prognosis (P<0.1). However, in the multivariate analysis, the TNM stage (HR, 1.22; 95% CI: 1.01–1.48) and M stage (HR, 1.83; 95% CI: 1.12–2.99) alone were independent predictors of OS in the surgical treatment group (**Table 3**).

Surgical Treatment Strategies

In the surgical treatment cohort, 122 patients underwent surgical resection (including four cases of local tumor destruction and six cases of heat radiofrequency ablation) and 38 patients underwent LT. Further analysis showed that the median OS values were 13.0 months (95% CI: 7.9–18.1 months) in patients who underwent LR and 19.0 months (95% CI: 8.3–29.7 months) in patients who underwent LT; however, no significant difference was observed (P=0.34, **Figure 5C**).

Regarding clinical practice, surgeons have recommended that patients with TNM stage I+II cancer should undergo LR or LT. Therefore, in our cohort of patients with AJCC stage I+II cancer, we further analyzed the median OS of 26 patients who underwent LT, and it was estimated to be 57 months, which was longer than the median OS of 65 patients who received LR (31 months); this difference, however, was not significant (P=0.92, **Figure 5D**).

We further analyzed the difference in survival of patients with CHC who underwent different surgical strategies. Among 160 patients with CHC who underwent surgical treatment, 10 who received local destruction and nine who had an unclear surgical strategy were excluded from the final analysis. The median OS values for patients with CHC who underwent liver wedge resection, liver lobectomy, and LT were 15 months (8.3–21.7

TABLE 1 | Demographic and clinicopathologic characteristics, and overall survival of patients with combined hepatocellular carcinoma and cholangiocarcinoma.

Variables	Total cohort	Training cohort	Validation cohort
All patients	271	170	101
Year of diagnosis			
2004-2009	108 (39.8%)	73 (42.9%)	35 (34.5%)
2010-2015	163 (60.1%)	97 (57.0%)	66 (65.3%)
Gender			
Male	190 (70.1%)	114 (67.0%)	76 (75.2%)
Female	81 (29.8%)	56 (32.9%)	25 (24.7%)
Ethnicity			
Caucasian	200 (73.8%)	119 (70.0%)	81 (80.1%)
African–American	24 (8.9%)	14 (8.2%)	10 (9.9%)
Others	47 (17.3%)	37 (21.7%)	10 (9.9%)
Age at diagnosis			
≤60	129 (47.6%)	81 (47.6%)	48 (47.5%)
>60	142 (52.3%)	89 (52.3)	53 (52.4%)
Marital status			
Married	173 (63.8%)	108 (63.5%)	65 (64.3%)
Single	43 (15.9%)	25 (14.7%)	18 (17.8%)
Divorced/separated	33 (12.2%)	22 (12.9%)	11 (10.8%)
Widowed	22 (8.1%)	15 (8.8%)	7 (6.9%)
Tumor size			
≤ 5 cm	122 (45.0%)	72 (42.3%)	50 (49.5%)
> 5 cm	149 (54.9%)	98 (57.6%)	51 (50.4%)
Grade			
I	16 (5.9%)	12 (7.0%)	4 (3.9%)
II	86 (31.7%)	50 (29.4%)	36 (35.6%)
III	155 (57.1%)	98 (57.6%)	57 (56.4%)
IV	14 (5.1%)	10 (5.8%)	4 (3.9%)
TNM stage			
I	86 (31.7%)	52 (30.5%)	5 (4.9%)
II	67 (24.7%)	36 (21.1%)	34 (33.6%)
III	62 (22.8%)	41 (24.1%)	31 (30.6%)
IV	42 (15.4%)	32 (18.8%)	21 (20.7%)
Unknown stage	14 (5.1%)	9 (5.2%)	10 (9.9%)
T stage			
T1	101 (37.2%)	61 (35.8%)	40 (39.6%)
T2	83 (30.6%)	47 (27.6%)	36 (35.6%)
T3	61 (22.5%)	45 (26.4%)	16 (15.8%)
T4	22 (8.1%)	15 (8.8%)	7 (6.9%)
TX	4 (1.4%)	2 (1.1%)	2 (1.9%)
N stage			
N0	218 (80.4%)	133 (78.2%)	85 (84.1%)
N1	35 (12.9%)	23 (13.5%)	12 (11.8%)
NX	18 (6.6%)	14 (8.2%)	4 (3.9%)
M stage			
M0	215 (79.3%)	129 (75.8%)	86 (85.1%)
M1	42 (15.4%)	32 (18.8%)	10 (9.9%)
MX	14 (5.1%)	9 (5.2%)	5 (4.9%)
Surgery			
No surgery	111 (40.9%)	95 (55.8%)	35 (34.6%)
Yes	160 (59.0%)	75 (44.1%)	66 (65.3%)
Chemotherapy			
Yes	102 (37.6%)	72 (42.3%)	30 (29.7%)
No/unknown	169 (62.3%)	98 (57.6%)	71 (70.2%)
Radiation			
Yes	26 (9.5%)	17 (10.0%)	9 (8.9%)
No/unknown	245 (90.4%)	153 (90.0%)	92 (91.0%)

months), 14 months (4.1–23.9 months), and 19 months (8.3–29.7 months), respectively. There was no significant difference among the three groups (P=0.56, **Figure 5E**). The pathological grade in the transplant group was significantly different compared with those in the lobectomy group (**Table 4**). There were no significant differences in age, sex, race, marital status, T stage, N stage, M stage, and TNM stage of patients between the lobectomy group or the wedge resection group and the LT group.

DISCUSSION

In this population-based study, we identified independent prognostic factors and constructed a prognostic nomogram-based model to predict the 1-, 3-, and 5-year OS of patients with CHC. The model facilitates accurate survival prediction, high-risk patient screening, and personalized treatment. An easy-to-use online calculation application with free access was provided (https://xingtai.shinyapps.io/CHC_DynNomapp/). A patient's survival probability with 95% CI can be quickly obtained by entering three clinical characteristics.

Owing to the rarity of CHC, it is difficult to accurately assess the prognostic factors of CHC using data from a single institution. To date, few population-based studies have reported the clinical outcomes and prognostic risk factors for patients with CHC using the SEER database (1, 5, 32). However, in these studies, nearly half of the patients with CHC lacked data on the pathological grade, and there was no correlation between the pathological grade and survival of patients with CHC (1, 5), which could affect the accuracy and persuasiveness of the conclusions of the studies. More importantly, although prognostic risk factors have already been reported, previous studies did not provide a prognostic model to facilitate clinicians and patients to predict the prognosis of CHC accurately and individually (1, 5). Our study excluded patients with CHC who lacked or included uncertain important information (such as the pathological grade, tumor size, and presence of surgery) and therefore could more accurately reflect whether there are differences in survival between each group. To our knowledge, our study is the first to report that pathological grade is significantly correlated with the survival of patients with CHC, which is different from that reported in previous studies (1, 5).

In the past few decades, although the OS of patients with CHC has gradually improved, it remains to be at frustratingly poor. In our analysis, the 5-year OS rate was 23.3%, which was higher than that (10.5%) reported in a population-based study based on the SEER database conducted between 1988 and 2009 (9). This phenomenon has also been confirmed in our research. The OS of patients with CHC in 2010–2015 was better than that of patients with CHC in 2004–2009 (the 5-year survival rates were 28.3% and 19.8%, respectively); however, no significant difference was noted. The median survival in our cohort was 14 months, which was higher than that in two other large population-based studies (1, 5) (8 and 9 months); this was mainly attributed to a higher proportion of patients who underwent surgery in our cohort.

In the present study, the pathological grade, TNM stage, and surgical type were identified as independent prognostic factors, among which surgery was a particularly important factor affecting OS (2, 16, 25). The 5-year OS in patients with CHC

TABLE 2 | Univariate analysis and multivariate analysis of factors of overall survival (OS) of combined hepatocellular carcinoma and cholangiocarcinoma.

Variables	Category	Univariate analysis			Multivariate analysis		
		HR	95% CI	P value	HR	95% CI	P value
Year of diagnosis	2004-2009 */2010-2015	0.80	0.56-1.14	0.22			
Gender	Male*/Female	0.87	0.59-1.28	0.48			
Ethnicity	Caucasian*/African–American/Others	0.91	0.73-1.14	0.49			
Age at diagnosis	≤60*/>60	1.07	0.75-1.54	0.70			
Marital status	Married*/Single/(Divorced/separated)/Widowed	0.99	0.78-1.26	0.92			
Tumor size	≤ 5 cm*/>5 cm	1.48	1.02-2.14	0.04	1.02	0.68-1.51	0.94
Grade	I*/II/III/IV	1.87	1.25-2.79	<0.01	1.26	0.96-1.66	0.01
TNM stage	I*/II/III/IV/Unknown stage	2.01	1.42-2.86	<0.01	1.21	1.02-1.44	0.03
T stage	T1*/T2/T3/T4/TX	1.46	1.23-1.72	<0.01	1.16	0.95-1.43	0.12
N stage	N0*/N1/NX	1.66	1.27-2.17	<0.01	0.96	0.62-1.48	0.84
M stage	M0*/M1/MX	1.92	1.47-2.52	<0.01	1.25	0.78-2.03	0.36
Surgery	Yes*/No surgery	0.21	0.14-0.30	<0.01	0.26	0.17-0.40	<0.01
Chemotherapy	Yes*/(No/unknown)	1.13	0.78-1.62	0.52			
Radiation	Yes*/(No/unknown)	1.01	0.55-1.84	0.98			

*HR, hazard ratio; CI, confidence interval; *reference category.*

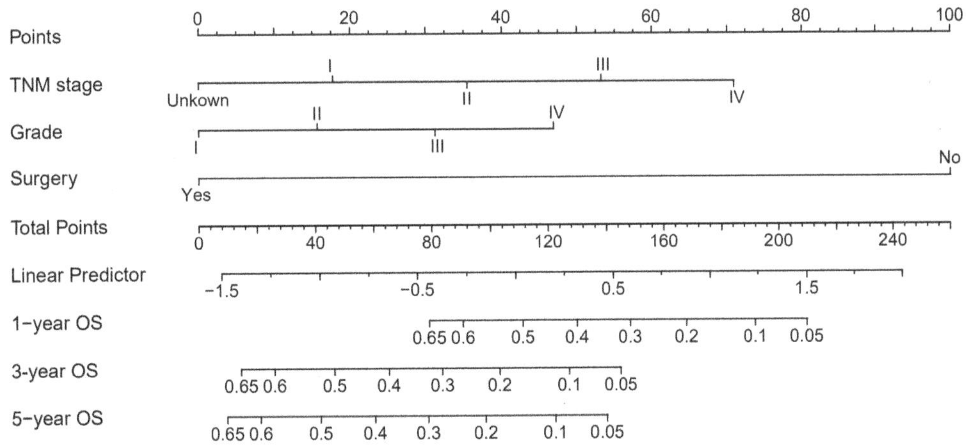

FIGURE 2 | Nomogram for predicting 1-, 3- and 5-year overall survival (OS) of combined hepatocellular cholangiocarcinoma patients.

who underwent surgery reached 28.5%, while it was only 15.6% in those who received non-surgical treatment. The pathological grade is considered to be an important prognostic indicator for many cancers, including CHC (33). The TNM staging system has been one of the most commonly used tumor staging systems and is proven to be suitable for patients with CHC (2). However, a recent study (22) showed that its predictive power may not be as good as other standards. Based on the multivariate analysis, our nomogram-based model included three important variables (pathological grade, TNM stage, and surgical type) and could accurately categorize patients with CHC into different prognostic groups.

Surgery has been the most important treatment that affects the survival of patients with CHC (1, 5, 24). To better analyze such patients, we further analyzed prognostic factors in the surgical cohort. Unlike the overall cohort, AFP status is an independent prognostic factor for patients with CHC who undergo surgery. Wang et al. also confirmed that higher serum AFP levels combined with imaging features was an independent risk factor for postoperative microvascular invasion (MVI) in patients with CHC and that patients with CHC who had MVI could have higher risks of recurrence early after surgery (34). This may suggest that in patients with CHC who undergo surgery, the AFP level should be actively monitored and evaluated.

There are some controversies about surgical strategies for patients with CHC. In the current study, patients who underwent LR and LT had significantly prolonged OS compared with those who did not undergo surgery, and they had comparable OS between the two treatment strategies. Furthermore, there was no significant difference among wedge resection, lobectomy, and LT treatment. However, the number of patients undergoing LR has increased over time, and the number of patients with CHC undergoing LR increased by 1.9 times between 2004–2009 and 2010–2015. This increase was not observed in patients with CHC who underwent LT. Between the periods of 2004–2007 and 2012–2015, the number of patients undergoing LT remained relatively

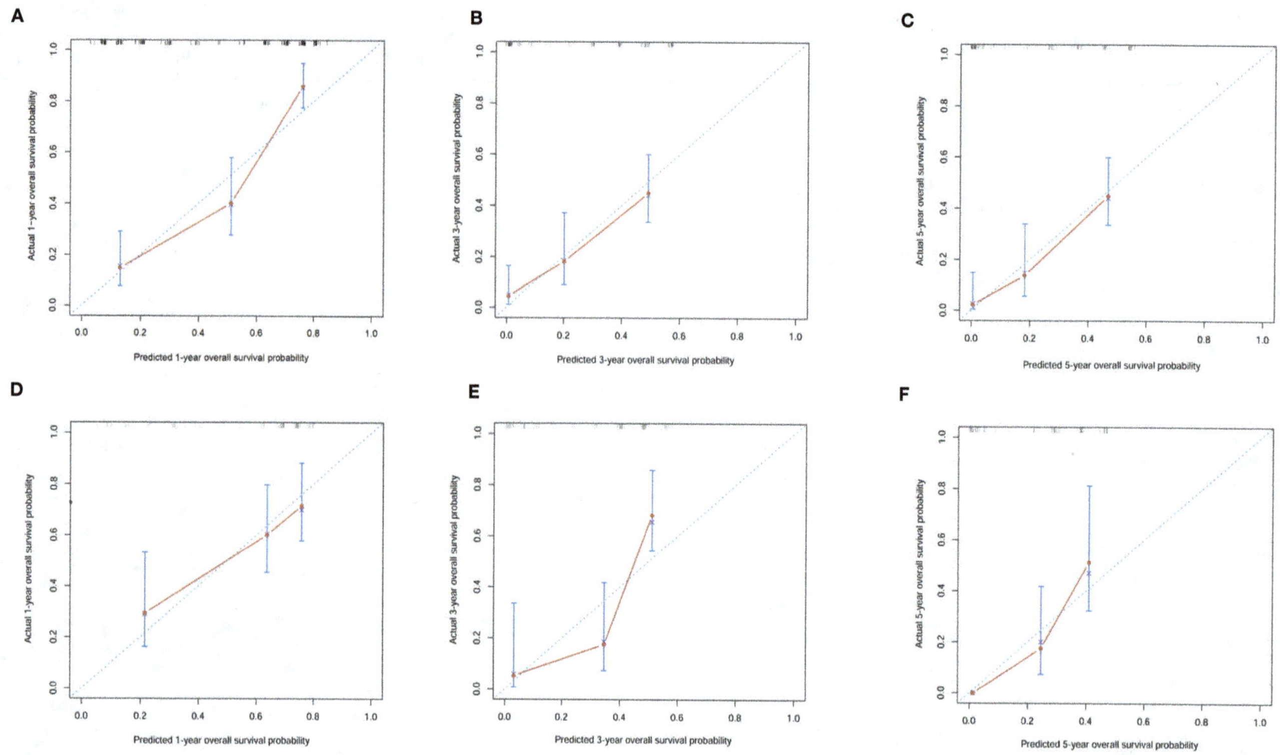

FIGURE 3 | Calibration curves for 1-, 3- and 5-year overall survival of combined hepatocellular carcinoma and cholangiocarcinoma patients in the training cohort and validation cohort. **(A)** Calibration curves for 1-year overall survival of combined hepatocellular carcinoma and cholangiocarcinoma patients in the training cohort; **(B)** Calibration curves for 3-year overall survival of combined hepatocellular carcinoma and cholangiocarcinoma patients in the training cohort; **(C)** Calibration curves for 5-year overall survival of combined hepatocellular carcinoma and cholangiocarcinoma patients in the training cohort; **(D)** Calibration curves for 1-year overall survival of combined hepatocellular carcinoma and cholangiocarcinoma patients in the validation cohort; **(E)** Calibration curves for 3-year overall survival of combined hepatocellular carcinoma and cholangiocarcinoma patients in the validation cohort; **(F)** Calibration curves for 5-year overall survival of combined hepatocellular carcinoma and cholangiocarcinoma patients in the validation cohort.

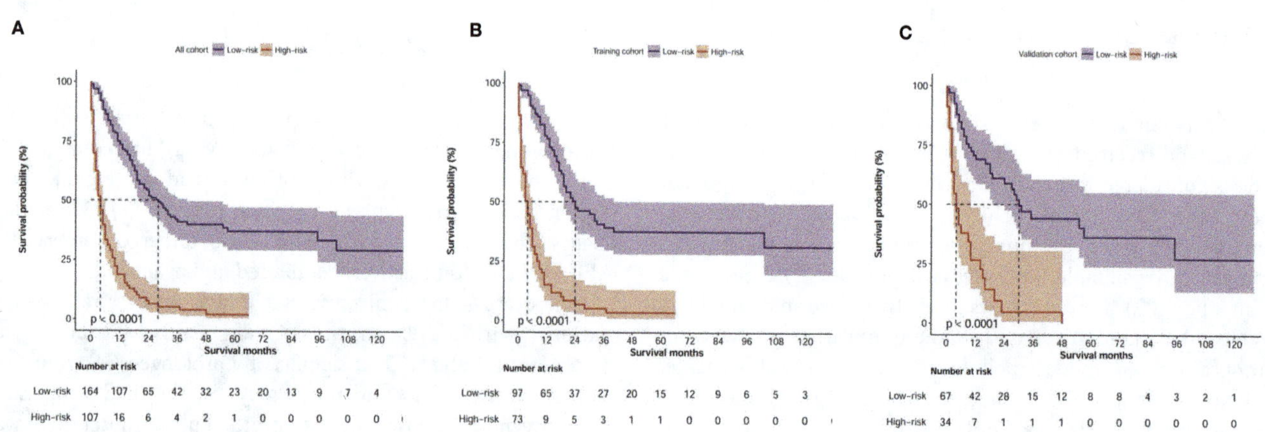

FIGURE 4 | Kaplan–Meier curves of OS for risk classification based on the nomogram scores. **(A)** In all cohort; **(B)** In the training cohort; **(C)** In the validation cohort.

stable. Groeschl et al. (32) also confirmed that although LT was another alternative treatment that resulted in better survival benefits for patients with CHC, the treatment effect was inferior to LT; this result may be related to the characteristics of CC. However, a recent multicenter retrospective study confirmed that regardless of the tumor burden, the clinical prognosis of LT was superior to that of LR in patients with CHC (24). Specifically, patients with CHC who underwent LT based on the Milan criteria

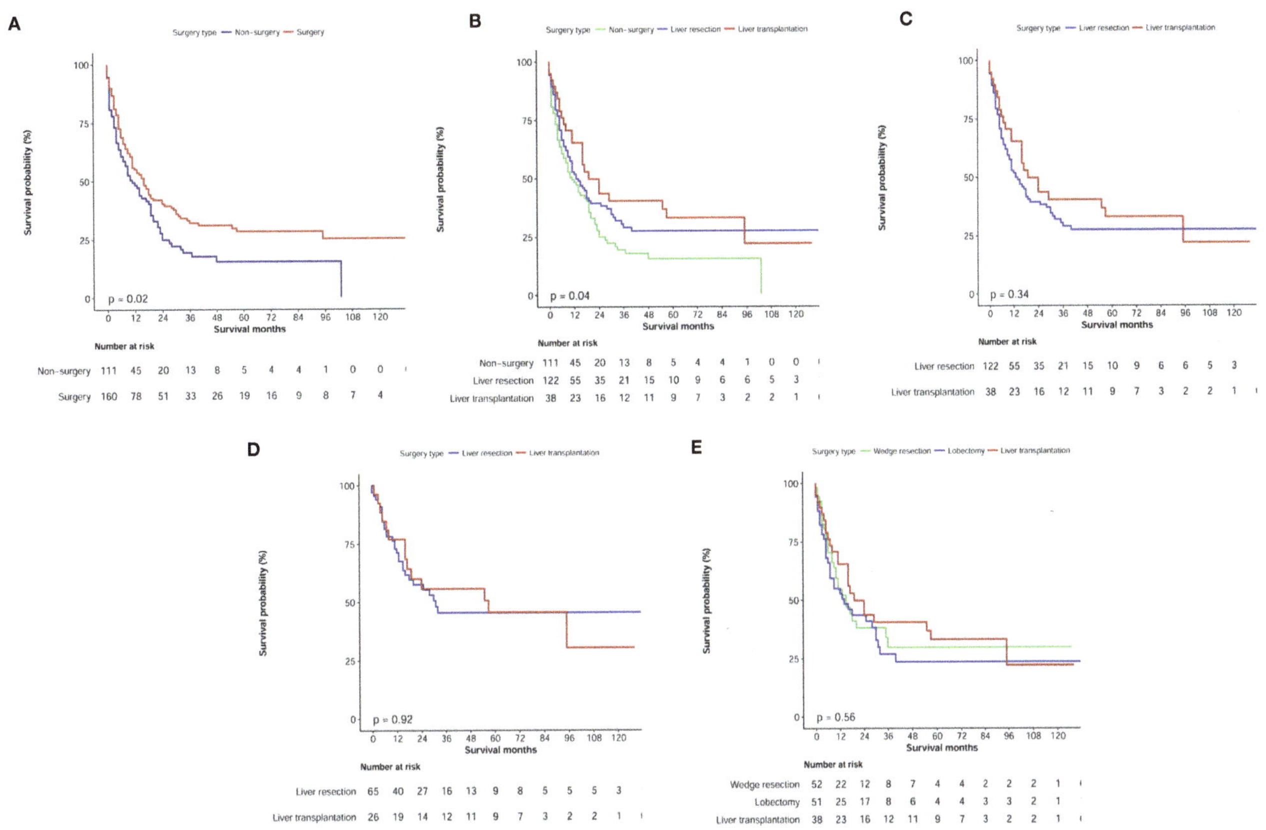

FIGURE 5 | Kaplan–Meier overall survival curves of combined hepatocellular carcinoma and cholangiocarcinoma patients with different treatment strategies. **(A, B)** Survival analysis of different surgery type; **(C)** Comparison of prognosis of patients undergoing liver resection or liver transplant before and after propensity score matching; **(D)** Comparison of prognosis of patients undergoing liver resection or liver transplant in TNM I+II stage; **(E)** Survival analysis for specific surgical strategies.

TABLE 3 | Univariate and multivariate analyses of prognostic factors of combined hepatocellular carcinoma and cholangiocarcinoma patients undergoing surgery.

Variables	Category	Univariate analysis			Multivariate analysis		
		HR	95% CI	P value	HR	95% CI	P value
Year of diagnosis	2004-2009 */2010-2015	1.02	0.69-1.51	0.93			
Gender	Male*/Female	1.11	0.73-1.69	0.64			
Ethnicity	Caucasian*/African–American/Others	1.00	0.78-1.30	0.99			
Age at diagnosis	≤60*/>60	1.09	0.85-1.40	0.50			
Marital status	Married*/Single/(Divorced/separated)/Widowed	1.17	0.89-1.55	0.27			
Tumor size	≤ 5 cm*/>5 cm	2.24	1.49-3.37	<0.01	1.52	0.96-2.40	0.07
Grade	I*/II/III/IV	1.53	1.14-2.06	<0.01	1.35	0.98-1.86	0.07
TNM stage	I*/II/III/IV/Unknown stage	1.46	1.21-1.78	<0.01	1.22	1.01-1.48	0.04
T stage	T1*/T2/T3/T4/TX	1.41	1.17-1.70	<0.01	1.02	0.82-1.28	0.86
N stage	N0*/N1/NX	2.29	1.67-3.16	<0.01	1.32	0.83-2.12	0.24
M stage	M0*/M1/MX	2.55	1.85-3.51	<0.01	1.83	1.12-2.99	0.02
Surgery type	Yes*/No surgery	0.81	0.51-1.27	0.35			
Chemotherapy	Yes*/(No/unknown)	1.59	1.07-2.36	0.02	0.95	0.60-1.48	0.81
Radiation	Yes*/(No/unknown)	1.65	0.88-3.10	0.12			

*HR, hazard ratio; CI, confidence interval; *reference category.*

had a better 5-year OS than those who underwent resection, but this was not a significant difference (70.1% and 49.7%, respectively; P=0.078). However, there was no significant difference in OS among CHC patients with tumor burden beyond University of California San Francisco (UCSF) criteria or within UCSF criteria but beyond Milan criteria. In our cohort of patients with TNM stage I+II cancer, the median OS of patients undergoing LT was longer than that of those undergoing LR (51 months and 31 months, respectively); however, there was no significant difference (P=0.92). This finding was more likely because of the statistical

TABLE 4 | The clinical characteristics of combined hepatocellular carcinoma and cholangiocarcinoma patients undergoing specific surgical strategies.

Variables	Liver transplant	Ref	Wedge resection	P value	Lobectomy	P value
All patients	38		52		51	
Year of diagnosis		Ref		0.01		0.26
2004-2009	21 (55.3%)		14 (26.9%)		22 (43.1%)	
2010-2015	17 (44.7%)		38 (73.1%)		29 (56.9%)	
Gender		Ref		0.16		0.20
Male	30 (78.9%)		34 (65.4%)		34 (66.7%)	
Female	8 (21.1%)		18 (34.6%)		17 (33.3%)	
Ethnicity		Ref		0.22		0.15
Caucasian	30 (78.9%)		36 (69.2%)		33 (64.7%)	
African-American	5 (13.2%)		5 (9.6%)		6 (11.8%)	
Others	3 (7.9%)		11 (21.2%)		12 (23.5%)	
Age at diagnosis		Ref		0.05		0.06
≤60	24 (63.2%)		22 (42.3%)		22 (43.1%)	
>60	14 (36.8%)		30 (57.7%)		29 (56.9%)	
Marital status		Ref		0.12		0.23
Married	23 (60.5%)		35 (67.3%)		30 (58.8%)	
Single	11 (28.9%)		7 (13.5%)		9 (17.6%)	
Divorced/separated	1 (2.6%)		7 (13.5%)		7 (13.7%)	
Widowed	3 (7.9%)		3 (5.8%)		5 (9.8%)	
Tumor size		Ref		0.13		0.07
≤ 5 cm	23 (60.5%)		23 (44.2%)		21 (41.2%)	
> 5 cm	15 (39.5%)		29 (55.8%)		30 (58.8%)	
Grade		Ref		0.19		0.01
I	3 (7.9%)		4 (7.7%)		0 (0.0%)	
II	17 (44.7%)		15 (28.8%)		15 (29.4%)	
III	18 (47.4%)		29 (55.8%)		29 (56.9%)	
IV	0 (0.0%)		4 (7.7%)		7 (13.7%)	
TNM stage		Ref		0.47		0.58
I	13 (34.2%)		17 (32.7%)		13 (25.5%)	
II	13 (34.2%)		10 (19.2%)		14 (27.5%)	
III	6 (15.8%)		13 (25.0%)		15 (29.4%)	
IV	4 (10.5%)		9 (17.3%)		7 (13.7%)	
Unknown stage	2 (5.3%)		3 (5.8%)		2 (3.9%)	
T stage		Ref		0.30		0.22
T1	15 (39.5%)		20 (38.5%)		15 (29.4%)	
T2	15 (39.5%)		12 (23.1%)		18 (35.3%)	
T3	5 (13.2%)		11 (21.2%)		16 (31.4%)	
T4	3 (7.9%)		7 (13.5%)		2 (3.9%)	
TX	0 (0.0%)		2 (3.8%)		0 (0.0%)	
N stage		Ref		0.69		0.20
N0	31 (81.6%)		39 (75.0%)		44 (86.3%)	
N1	6 (15.8%)		10 (19.2%)		3 (5.9%)	
NX	1 (2.6%)		3 (5.8%)		4 (7.8%)	
M stage		Ref		0.65		0.87
M0	32 (84.2%)		40 (76.9%)		42 (82.4%)	
M1	4 (10.5%)		9 (17.3%)		7 (13.7%)	
MX	2 (5.3%)		3 (5.8%)		2 (3.9%)	
Chemotherapy		Ref		0.07		0.08
Yes	9 (23.7%)		22 (42.3%)		21 (41.2%)	
No/unknown	29 (76.3%)		30 (57.7%)		30 (58.8%)	
Radiation		Ref		0.21		0.91
Yes	4 (10.5%)		2 (3.8%)		5 (9.8%)	
No/unknown	34 (89.5%)		50 (96.2%)		46 (90.2%)	

Ref, reference.

bias caused by the number of patients with CHC. Lunsford et al. confirmed that patients with CHC with low-grade, well-moderately differentiated tumors had excellent survival with a low risk for post-LT recurrence and seemed to benefit from LT (33). Therefore, doctors should remember to determine the tumor stage and pathological grade of patients with CHC before deciding surgical treatment strategies.

In this study, we constructed a nomogram-based model according to the multivariate analysis, which could categorize all patients with CHC into low-risk or high-risk prognostic subgroups. Our nomogram-based model performed well in predicting prognosis, and the C-index and calibration curves supported the survival prediction both in the training and validation groups. However, this study has some limitations. First, some important variables such as the AFP status, liver fibrosis score, health status, and underlying diseases had an excessive proportion of incomplete clinical information or were unavailable in the SEER database. Because there was no distinction between unacceptable and unknown chemotherapy/radiotherapy in the SEER database, we could not accurately analyze the effect of those variables on the survival of patients with CHC. Second, although our cohort was recruited from the SEER database, which is a high-quality, population-based cancer registry, our sample size was still relatively small owing to the rarity of CHC. Finally, although our nomogram showed good discrimination ability and a consistent calibration curve in both the training and internal verification cohorts, an external verification cohort for the nomogram-based model is still required.

CONCLUSIONS

CHC has an extremely poor prognosis, and its prognosis has not improved in recent years. Our study demonstrated that pathological grade, TNM stage, and surgery type were independent prognostic factors for patients with CHC. LR and LT significantly prolonged OS compared with non-surgical treatment. Our nomogram showed good predictive performance, and therefore, it could be used to predict the prognosis of patients with CHC, along with screening for high-risk patients. Prediction models based on static nomograms or online prediction tools (available at https://xingtai.shinyapps.io/CHC_DynNomapp/) could accurately predict the survival probability of CHC patients.

AUTHOR CONTRIBUTIONS

JW and YZ designed the study. JW and ZL provided the databases. JW, ZL, YL, JL, HD, HP, WX, ZF, FG, CL, DL, and YZ assembled and analyzed the data. JW and ZL wrote the manuscript. All authors have contributed to the article and have approved the submitted version.

ACKNOWLEDGMENTS

We would like to thank Editage (www.editage.cn) for English language editing.

REFERENCES

1. Ramai D, Ofosu A, Lai JK, Reddy M, Adler DG. Combined Hepatocellular Cholangiocarcinoma: A Population-Based Retrospective Study. *Am J Gastroenterol* (2019) 114:1496–501. doi: 10.14309/ajg.0000000000000326
2. He C, Mao Y, Wang J, Song Y, Huang X, Lin X, et al. The Predictive Value of Staging Systems and Inflammation Scores for Patients With Combined Hepatocellular Cholangiocarcinoma After Surgical Resection: A Retrospective Study. *J Gastrointest Surg* (2018) 22:1239–50. doi: 10.1007/s11605-018-3756-3
3. Wang AQ, Zheng YC, Du J, Zhu CP, Huang HC, Wang SS, et al. Combined Hepatocellular Cholangiocarcinoma: Controversies to be Addressed. *World J Gastroenterol* (2016) 22:4459–65. doi: 10.3748/wjg.v22.i18.4459
4. Zhou YM, Sui CJ, Zhang XF, Li B, Yang JM. Influence of Cirrhosis on Long-Term Prognosis After Surgery in Patients With Combined Hepatocellular-Cholangiocarcinoma. *BMC Gastroenterol* (2017) 17:25. doi: 10.1186/s12876-017-0584-y
5. Wang J, Li E, Yang H, Wu J, Lu HC, Yi C, et al. Combined Hepatocellular-Cholangiocarcinoma: A Population Level Analysis of Incidence and Mortality Trends. *World J Surg Oncol* (2019) 17:43. doi: 10.1186/s12957-019-1586-8
6. Zhao Q, Yu WL, Lu XY, Dong H, Gu YJ, Sheng X, et al. Combined Hepatocellular and Cholangiocarcinoma Originating From the Same Clone: A Pathomolecular Evidence-Based Study. *Chin J Cancer* (2016) 35:82. doi: 10.1186/s40880-016-0146-7
7. Koh KC, Lee H, Choi MS, Lee JH, Paik SW, Yoo BC, et al. Clinicopathologic Features and Prognosis of Combined Hepatocellular Cholangiocarcinoma. *Am J Surg* (2005) 189:120–5. doi: 10.1016/j.amjsurg.2004.03.018
8. Tickoo SK, Zee SY, Obiekwe S, Xiao H, Koea J, Robiou C, et al. Combined Hepatocellular-Cholangiocarcinoma: A Histopathologic, Immunohistochemical, and *In Situ* Hybridization Study. *Am J Surg Pathol* (2002) 26:989–97. doi: 10.1097/00000478-200208000-00003
9. Garancini M, Goffredo P, Pagni F, Romano F, Roman S, Sosa JA, et al. Combined Hepatocellular-Cholangiocarcinoma: A Population-Level Analysis of an Uncommon Primary Liver Tumor. *Liver Transplant* (2014) 20:952–9. doi: 10.1002/lt.23897
10. Tang Y, Wang L, Teng F, Zhang T, Zhao Y, Chen Z. The Clinical Characteristics and Prognostic Factors of Combined Hepatocellular Carcinoma and Cholangio-Carcinoma, Hepatocellular Carcinoma and Intrahepatic Cholangiocarcinoma After Surgical Resection: A Propensity Score Matching Analysis. *Int J Med Sci* (2020) 18:187–98. doi: 10.7150/ijms.50883
11. Wakizaka K, Yokoo H, Kamiyama T, Ohira M, Kato K, Fujii Y, et al. Clinical and Pathological Features of Combined Hepatocellular–Cholangiocarcinoma Compared With Other Liver Cancers. *J Gastroenterol Hepatol* (2019) 34:1074–80. doi: 10.1111/jgh.14547
12. Spolverato G, Bagante F, Tsilimigras D, Ejaz A, Cloyd J, Pawlik TM. Management and Outcomes Among Patients With Mixed Hepatocholangiocellular Carcinoma: A Population-Based Analysis. *J Surg Oncol* (2019) 119:278–87. doi: 10.1002/jso.25331
13. Jarnagin WR, Weber S, Tickoo SK, Koea JB, Obiekwe S, Fong Y, et al. Combined Hepatocellular and Cholangiocarcinoma: Demographic, Clinical, and Prognostic Factors. *Cancer* (2002) 94:2040–6. doi: 10.1002/cncr.10392
14. Lee JH, Chung GE, Yu SJ, Hwang SY, Kim JS, Kim HY, et al. Long-Term Prognosis of Combined Hepatocellular and Cholangiocarcinoma After Curative Resection Comparison With Hepatocellular Carcinoma and Cholangiocarcinoma. *J Clin Gastroenterol* (2011) 45:69–75. doi: 10.1097/MCG.0b013e3181ce5dfa
15. Gera S, Ettel M, Acosta-Gonzalez G, Xu R. Clinical Features, Histology, and Histogenesis of Combined Hepatocellular-Cholangiocarcinoma. *World J Hepatol* (2017) 9:300–9. doi: 10.4254/wjh.v9.i6.300
16. Schizas D, Mastoraki A, Routsi E, Papapanou M, Tsapralis D, Vassiliu P, et al. Combined Hepatocellular-Cholangiocarcinoma: An Update on Epidemiology, Classification, Diagnosis and Management. *Hepatobiliary Pancreat Dis Int* (2020) 19:515–23. doi: 10.1016/j.hbpd.2020.07.004
17. Chok KSH, Ng KKC, Cheung TT, Yuen WK, Poon RTP, Lo CM, et al. An Update on Long-Term Outcome of Curative Hepatic Resection for Hepatocholangiocarcinoma. *World J Surg* (2009) 33:1916–21. doi: 10.1007/s00268-009-0112-5
18. Ma KW, Cheung TT, She WH, Chok KSH, Chan ACY, Ng IOL, et al. The Effect of Wide Resection Margin in Patients With Intrahepatic Cholangiocarcinoma: A Single-Center Experience. *Med (Baltimore)* (2016) 95:e4133. doi: 10.1097/MD.0000000000004133
19. Aurélie B, Julien C, Valérie P. Combined Hepatocellular-Cholangiocarcinoma: An Update. *J Hepatol* (2021) 74:1212–24. doi: 10.1016/J.JHEP.2021.01.035
20. Benson AB, D'Angelica MI, Abbott DE, Abrams TA, Alberts SR, Saenz DA, et al. Hepatobiliary Cancers, Version 1.2017 Featured Updates to the NCCN Guidelines. *JNCCN J Natl Compr Cancer Netw* (2017) 15:563–73. doi: 10.6004/jnccn.2017.0059
21. Zhou Q, Cai H, Xu M-H, Ye Y, Li X-L, Shi G-M, et al. Do the Existing Staging Systems for Primary Liver Cancer Apply to Combined Hepatocellular Carcinoma-Intrahepatic Cholangiocarcinoma? *Hepatobiliary Pancreat Dis Int* (2021) 20:13–20. doi: 10.1016/j.hbpd.2020.10.002

22. Zhang F, Lu S, Tian M, Hu K, Chen R, Zhang B, et al. Albumin-to-Alkaline Phosphatase Ratio Is an Independent Prognostic Indicator in Combined Hepatocellular and Cholangiocarcinoma. *J Cancer* (2020) 11:5177–86. doi: 10.7150/jca.45633
23. Jiang XX, Huang XT, Huang CS, Chen LH, Liang LJ, Yin XY. Long-Term Outcome and Prognostic Factors of Combined Hepatocellular Carcinoma and Cholangiocarcinoma After Curative Resection. *Gastroenterol Rep* (2020) 8:134–42. doi: 10.1093/gastro/goaa003
24. Dageforde LA, Vachharajani N, Tabrizian P, Agopian V, Halazun K, Maynard E, et al. Multi-Center Analysis of Liver Transplantation for Combined Hepatocellular Carcinoma-Cholangiocarcinoma Liver Tumors. *J Am Coll Surg* (2021) 232:361–71. doi: 10.1016/j.jamcollsurg.2020.11.017
25. Tao CY, Liu WR, Jin L, Tang Z, Tian MX, Jiang XF, et al. Surgical Treatment of Combined Hepatocellular-Cholangiocarcinoma Is as Effective in Elderly Patients as It Is in Younger Patients: A Propensity Score Matching Analysis. *J Cancer* (2018) 9:1106–12. doi: 10.7150/jca.23921
26. Liu WR, Tian MX, Tao CY, Tang Z, Zhou YF, Song SS, et al. Adjuvant Transarterial Chemoembolization Does Not Influence Recurrence-Free or Overall Survival in Patients With Combined Hepatocellular Carcinoma and Cholangiocarcinoma After Curative Resection: A Propensity Score Matching Analysis. *BMC Cancer* (2020) 20:642. doi: 10.1186/s12885-020-07138-z
27. Wang T, Wang W, Zhang J, Yang X, Shen S, Wang W. Development and Validation of a Nomogram for Differentiating Combined Hepatocellular Cholangiocarcinoma From Intrahepatic Cholangiocarcinoma. *Front Oncol* (2020) 10:598433. doi: 10.3389/fonc.2020.598433
28. Zhang J, Wang X, Zhang L, Yao L, Xue X, Zhang S, et al. Radiomics Predict Postoperative Survival of Patients With Primary Liver Cancer With Different Pathological Types. *Ann Transl Med* (2020) 8:820–0. doi: 10.21037/atm-19-4668
29. Wang T, Yang X, Tang H, Kong J, Shen S, Qiu H, et al. Integrated Nomograms to Predict Overall Survival and Recurrence-Free Survival in Patients With Combined Hepatocellular Cholangiocarcinoma (cHCC) After Liver Resection. *Aging (Albany NY)* (2020) 12:15334–58. doi: 10.18632/aging.103577
30. He C, Zhang Y, Cai Z, Lin X. Competing Risk Analyses of Overall Survival and Cancer-Specific Survival in Patients With Combined Hepatocellular Cholangiocarcinoma After Surgery. *BMC Cancer* (2019) 19:178. doi: 10.1186/s12885-019-5398-6
31. Camp RL, Dolled-Filhart M, Rimm DL. X-Tile: A New Bio-Informatics Tool for Biomarker Assessment and Outcome-Based Cut-Point Optimization. *Clin Cancer Res* (2004) 10:7252–9. doi: 10.1158/1078-0432.CCR-04-0713
32. Groeschl RT, Turaga KK, Gamblin TC. Transplantation Versus Resection for Patients With Combined Hepatocellular Carcinoma-Cholangiocarcinoma. *J Surg Oncol* (2013) 107:608–12. doi: 10.1002/jso.23289
33. Lunsford KE, Court C, Seok Lee Y, Lu DS, Naini BV, Harlander-Locke MP, et al. Propensity-Matched Analysis of Patients With Mixed Hepatocellular-Cholangiocarcinoma and Hepatocellular Carcinoma Undergoing Liver Transplantation. *Liver Transpl* (2018) 24:1384–97. doi: 10.1002/lt.25058
34. Wang X, Wang W, Ma X, Lu X, Li S, Zeng M, et al. Combined Hepatocellular-Cholangiocarcinoma: Which Preoperative Clinical Data and Conventional MRI Characteristics Have Value for the Prediction of Microvascular Invasion and Clinical Significance? *Eur Radiol* (2020) 30:5337–47. doi: 10.1007/s00330-020-06861-2

12

Prognostic Influence of Spontaneous Tumor Rupture in Patients with Hepatocellular Carcinoma After Hepatectomy

Jiaxuan Xu[1†], Jiaze Hong[1†], Yiran Wang[1], Lingling Zhou[2], Binbin Xu[3], Yuexiu Si[4], Yujing He[1] and Yizhou Chen[5]*

[1] The Second Clinical Medical College, Zhejiang Chinese Medical University, Hangzhou, China, [2] The First Clinical Medical College, Wenzhou Medical University, Wenzhou, China, [3] Department of Nutrition, HwaMei Hospital, University of Chinese Academy of Sciences, Ningbo, China, [4] School of Basic Medical Sciences, Zhejiang Chinese Medical University, Hangzhou, China, [5] Emergency Medical Center, Ningbo Yinzhou No. 2 Hospital, Ningbo, China

***Correspondence:**
Yizhou Chen
hello666813@126.com

† These authors have contributed equally to this work and share first authorship

Objective: This study aims to comprehensively analyze the influence of spontaneous tumor rupture on the prognosis of hepatocellular carcinoma patients following hepatic resection.

Methods: We systematically searched four online electronic databases, including PubMed, Embase, Web of Science, and Cochrane Library, for eligible studies published from inception to March 2021. The main endpoints were overall survival (OS) and disease-free survival (DFS).

Results: This meta-analysis included 21 observational articles with 57,241 cases. The results revealed that spontaneous tumor rupture was associated with worse OS (hazard ratio (HR), 1.65; 95% confidence interval (CI), 1.33–2.05) and DFS (HR, 1.42; 95% CI, 1.12–1.80) in resectable hepatocellular carcinoma patients. This phenomenon was observed in most subgroups, which were classified by recorded survival time, age, country, alpha-fetoprotein (AFP) concentration, liver cirrhosis, and microvascular invasion. However, in subgroups of macrovascular invasion positive, spontaneous tumor rupture was not a risk factor for OS (HR, 1.55; 95% CI, 0.99–2.42) and DFS (HR, 1.23; 95% CI, 0.91–1.65) in hepatocellular carcinoma patients after hepatectomy. For macrovascular invasion negative, compared with non-ruptured hepatocellular carcinoma patients, ruptured hepatocellular carcinoma patients exhibited worse prognosis for OS (HR, 1.55; 95% CI, 0.99–2.42) and DFS (HR, 1.23; 95% CI, 0.91–1.65) following hepatectomy.

Conclusions: Spontaneous tumor rupture was a prognostic risk factor for hepatocellular carcinoma patients after hepatic resection. However, in macrovascular invasion patients, spontaneous tumor rupture was not a prognostic risk factor.

Keywords: hepatocellular carcinoma, spontaneous tumor rupture, hepatectomy, prognosis, meta-analysis

INTRODUCTION

Hepatocellular carcinoma (HCC), the sixth most prevalent primary neoplasm, was responsible for around 81,0000 deaths in 2015 worldwide (1, 2). Spontaneous tumor rupture (STR) of HCC is a potentially fatal complication (3). The mechanisms underlying STR remain unclear. Possible reasons include large tumor size, ischemic necrosis, and vascular compression caused by rapid tumor growth (4–6). Although the overall incidence was relatively low (3–26%), the mortality rates of ruptured HCC patients were extremely high (32–75%) in reported literature (3, 7–11). Nowadays, treating STR of HCC is challenging; the current interventions used clinically include conservative treatment, transcatheter arterial chemoembolization (TACE), and hepatic resection (12, 13). Hepatectomy, including emergent and staged (after TACE achieving hemostasis) hepatectomy, provided a better long-term prognosis than palliative treatment in ruptured HCC patients with relatively well-preserved liver functions (13).

Traditionally, STR has recognized as a terminal event of HCC, as it could lead to various symptoms, such as hemorrhagic shock, intraperitoneal hemorrhage, and metastases, and most ruptured HCC patients had portal vein tumor thrombosis (PVTT), impaired liver function, and liver cirrhosis (14–17). As a result, these advanced patients with STR were frequently unable to receive surgical treatment and were compelled to have non-surgical treatment, resulting in a worse long-term prognosis than advanced patients receiving the same therapy without STR (9, 12).

However, whether STR was a prognostic risk factor for HCC patients after hepatic resection remains unclear (18, 19). Consequently, this meta-analysis aims to evaluate the long-term prognosis of patients with or without STR following hepatectomy and explore whether STR affects the prognosis of HCC patients after surgery.

MATERIALS AND METHODS

Literature Search Strategy

This meta-analysis followed Preferred Reporting Items for Systematic Review and Meta-Analysis guidelines (20). Four online electronic databases (PubMed, Embase, Web of Science, and Cochrane Library) were searched for published literature in English from inception to March 2021. The search strategies included: ("Hepatocellular Carcinoma" OR "Hepatoma" OR "Liver Cell Carcinomas" OR "HCC") AND ("Rupture"). Furthermore, potentially eligible studies were identified through a thorough inspection from reference lists of all retrieved papers.

Abbreviations: HCC, hepatocellular carcinoma; STR, spontaneous tumor rupture; TACE, transcatheter arterial chemoembolization; PVTT, portal vein tumor thrombosis; OBSs, observational studies; OS, overall survival; DFS, disease-free survival; HR, hazard ratio; CI, confidence interval; AFP, alpha-fetoprotein; NOS, Newcastle-Ottawa scale; HBV, hepatitis B virus; HCV, hepatitis C virus; HBsAg, hepatitis B surface antigen; BCLC, Barcelona clinic liver cancer.

Inclusion Criteria

The inclusion criteria for this meta-analysis entailed: (1) Patients in experiment (ruptured HCC) and control (non-ruptured HCC) groups received hepatic resection, including emergent and staged hepatectomy. (2) The included literature is original and includes observational studies (OBSs). (3) The study evaluated the relationship between tumor rupture and prognosis. (4) The primary endpoints as overall survival (OS) or disease-free survival (DFS) were mentioned, and their hazard ratio (HR) and 95% confidence interval (CI) were obtainable or could be calculated.

Exclusion Criteria

The exclusion criteria for this meta-analysis entailed: (1) The relationship between ruptured and non-ruptured HCC in the prognosis of patients has not been explored at the same time. (2) When the duplicate publications were reviewed, the higher-quality or most updated was included. (3) The intervention for patients was not surgery but like TACE alone and palliative chemotherapy. (4) Multiple hepatic metastases, distant organ metastasis, and lymph node metastases were found in patients. (5) The tumor rupture was not spontaneous, but it was caused by trauma.

Data Extraction and Quality Evaluation

Based on pre-determined inclusion/exclusion criteria, two authors performed an independent review, extracting the following information carefully from each included study, including (1) study characteristics (author, country, and publication year), (2) patients' basic characteristics (age, gender, and number of included patients), (3) hepatic features (serum AFP, virus status, and liver cirrhosis), (4) tumor features (tumor number, size, and invasion), (5) therapeutic effect (OS and DFS, and corresponding HR and 95% CI).

The quality of incorporated OBSs was assessed using Newcastle-Ottawa Scale (NOS) that encompassed three aspects (selection of patients, comparability of groups, and evaluation of outcomes). The cumulative scores of articles less than six were considered of low-quality (21).

Statistical Analysis

The pooled HR and 95% CI for OS and DFS were calculated to estimate the relationship between tumor rupture and prognosis. Heterogeneity among included literature was assessed using I^2 statistic. For potential heterogeneity, random-effect models were employed for greater reliability. When the number of included articles in each analysis is $\geq$ 10, Egger's test based on Stata 12.0 software was conducted to evaluate publication bias (22). A sensitivity analysis was conducted to determine robustness of conclusions. *P*-value $<$ 0.05 was considered statistically significant.

RESULTS

Data Collection and Characteristics

A total of 4,285 records were initially yielded from four electronic databases using a pre-designed search strategy. After removing

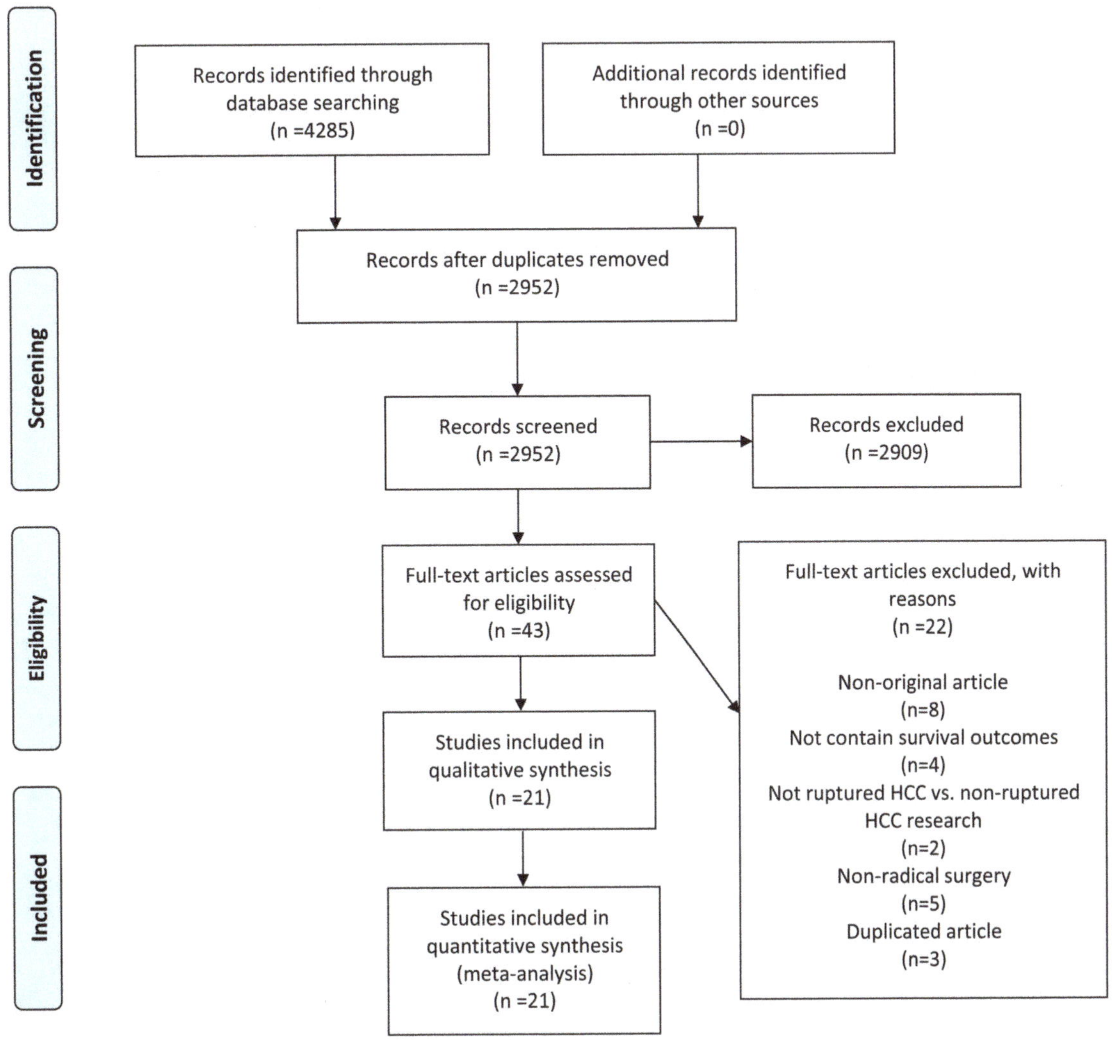

FIGURE 1 | A schematic flow for selecting the articles included in this meta-analysis.

duplicates, 2,952 records remained. Twenty-one studies (13, 18, 19, 23–40) were ultimately included following a strict screening process. The comprehensive literature review and rigorous selection process are displayed in **Figure 1**.

A total of 57,241 patients were enrolled in 21 OBSs mainly originated from Asia (19/21), followed by South America (1/21) and Europe (1/21). Eight studies simultaneously analyzed OS and DFS, ten were with OS alone, and three were only related to DFS. The detailed patients' characteristics of demographic and clinicopathological aspects are shown in **Table 1** and **Supplementary Table 1**. The quality of OBSs was assessed using NOS and assessment outcomes indicated that incorporated articles were of high quality (**Supplementary Table 2**).

Effect of STR on OS and DFS

A pooled analysis based on 18 studies including relevant OS data exhibited that STR was potentially related to a worse prognosis of ruptured HCC patients (HR, 1.65; 95% CI, 1.33–2.05) (**Figure 2**). Consistent with the pooled result of OS, pooled DFS outcomes also illustrated that ruptured HCC patients had a poorer prognosis than non-ruptured HCC patients (HR, 1.42; 95% CI, 1.12–1.80) (**Figure 3**).

Subgroup Analysis

Subgroups analyses were implemented to explore the effect of various factors on the prognosis of ruptured and non-ruptured HCC patients. We categorized the studies into 3-year OS and 5-year OS groups based on recorded survival time. For subgroups of 5-year OS, non-ruptured HCC patients obtained greater OS than ruptured HCC patients, whereas no statistical difference was found in subgroups of 3-year OS. For subgroups of patients' age $\geq$ or $<$ 60 years old, patients in China or other Asian countries, patients' AFP $\geq$ or $<$ 400 ng/mL, patients with and without liver cirrhosis, and patients' microvascular invasion positive/negative, the analysis results all indicated that STR was associated with

TABLE 1 | Characteristics of all the studies included in the meta-analysis.

Author	Country	Number of patients		AFP(ng/ml)		Liver cirrhosis (number)		Microvascular invasion (number)		Macrovascular invasion (number)	
		Rupture	Non-rupture	Rupture	Non-rupture	Rupture	Non-rupture	Rupture	Non-rupture	Rupture	Non-rupture
Aoki et al. (13)	Japan	1160	48548	510 cases≥400 504 cases<400	9,279 cases≥400 36,431 cases<400	579	26,473	NA	NA	352	5,373
Chan et al. (19)	China	84	1,254	472	91	43	750	52	583	9	102
Cheng et al. (23)	China	53	826	66.8		507		104		188	
Chua et al. (18)	Singapore	49	98	NA	NA	19	32	27	47	7	11
Fan et al. (24)	China	211		NA	NA	98		NA	NA	21	
Joliat et al. (25)	Switzerland	14	126	23	18	11	81	NA	NA	NA	NA
Kwon et al. (26)	Korea	85	186	1,2151	14,908	NA	NA	29	58	7	13
Lee et al. (27)	Korea	18	37	NA	NA	11	21	12	26	8	13
Li et al. (28)	China	89	171	138.5	73.8	73	99	0	0	NA	NA
Miyoshi et al. (29)	Japan	10	295	3 cases≥1,000 7 cases<1,000	53 cases≥1,000 242 cases<1,000	NA	NA	NA	NA	6	81
Mizuno et al. (30)	Japan	6	15	3 cases>400 3 cases<400	5 cases>400 10 cases<400	NA	NA	NA	NA	5	6
Ruan et al. (31)	China	57	57	22	20	28	NA	23	21	NA	NA
Ruiz et al. (32)	Peru	253		2,651		39		64		29	
Tanaka et al. (33)	Japan	42	42	78.8	49.5	13	14	NA	NA	2	3
Uchiyama et al. (34)	Japan	27	1,004	168 cases≥400 836 cases<400		NA	NA	NA	NA	40	
Xiao et al. (35)	China	53	181	141 cases≥400 93 cases<400		196		144		234	
Yang et al. (36)	China	143	1,090	85 cases≥400 58 cases<400	420 cases≥400 670 cases<400	NA	NA	97	668	36	172
Yeh et al. (37)	China	35	175	100 cases≥400 110 cases<400		63		NA	NA	116	
Zhang et al. (38)	China	41	446	5788.9	3947.1	24	285	NA	NA	1	48
Zhao et al. (39)	China	12	70	35 cases≥400 47 cases<400		65		19		0	0
Zhu et al. (40)	China	89	89	57 cases≥400 32 cases <400	53 cases≥400 36 cases<400	76	80	65	60	50	43

AFP, a-fetoprotein; NA, not available.

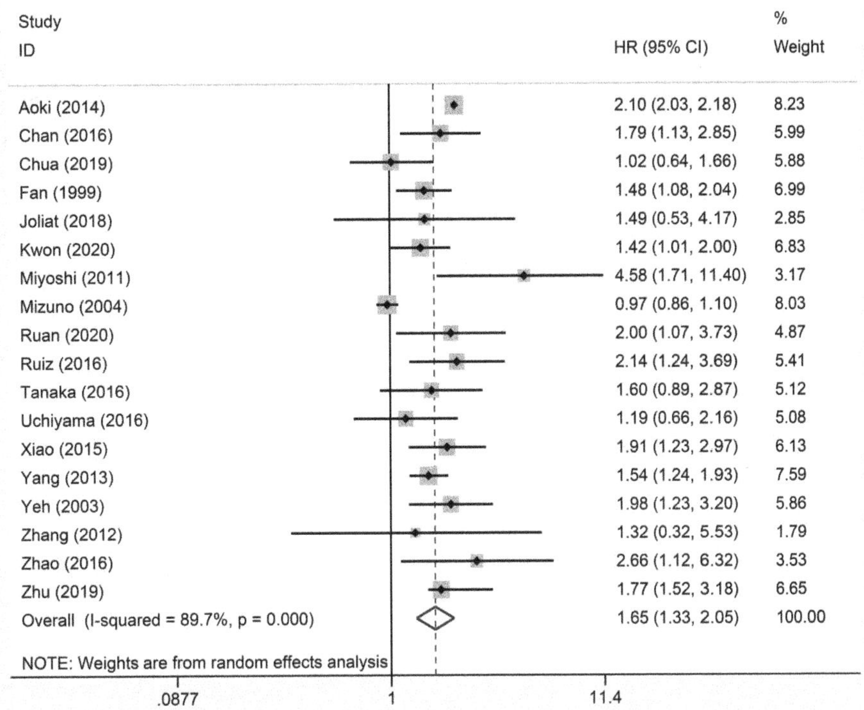

FIGURE 2 | Forest plot of OS of ruptured hepatocellular carcinoma (HCC) patients after hepatectomy ($P < 0.001$).

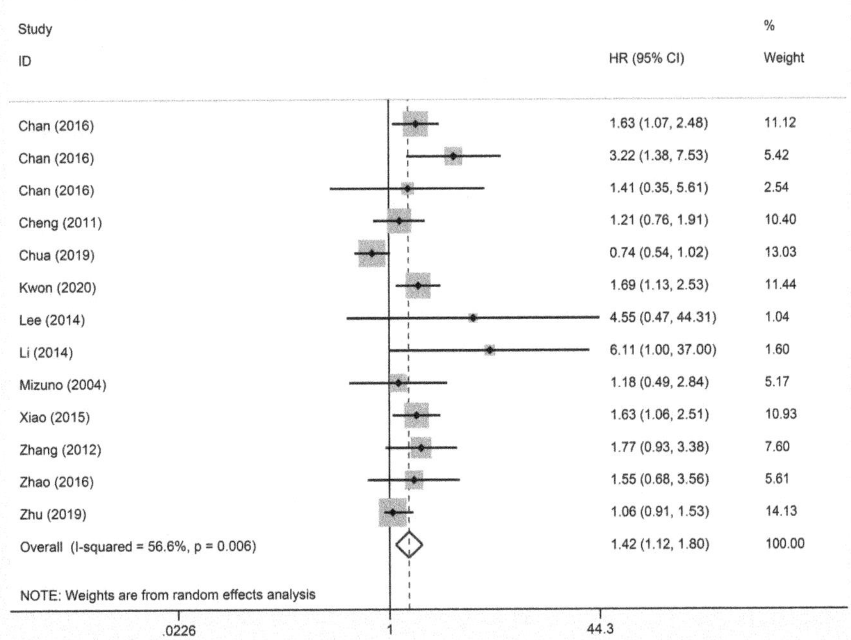

FIGURE 3 | Forest plot of DFS of ruptured hepatocellular carcinoma (HCC) patients following hepatectomy ($P = 0.004$).

TABLE 2 | Subgroup analysis of the hepatocellular carcinoma (HCC) rupture on the prognosis of patients with HCC.

	No. of studies	HR	95%CI	Heterogeneity (I^2) (%)
Overall survival (OS)				
3-year OS	3	1.87	0.80–4.39	86.4
5-year OS	15	1.68	1.46–1.94	54.8
Age ≥60 years	5	1.78	1.19–2.65	68.3
Age <60 years	11	1.66	1.47–1.88	0
China	9	1.68	1.47–1.92	0
Non-Chinese Asian countries	7	1.50	1.00–2.26	96.2
AFP≥400 ng/ml	6	1.74	1.45–2.09	0
AFP<400 ng/ml	8	1.58	1.09–2.28	95.3
Liver cirrhosis	7	2.09	2.02–2.17	0
Non-liver cirrhosis	5	1.56	1.23–1.98	26.2
Microvascular invasion positive	4	1.55	1.25–1.91	30.4
Microvascular invasion negative	5	1.74	1.40–2.17	0
Disease-free survival (DFS)				
Age <60	9	1.53	1.24–1.88	31.4
China	7	1.50	1.18–1.90	36.7
Non-Chinese Asian countries	4	1.22	0.67–2.24	74.3
AFP≥400 ng/ml	4	1.42	1.07–1.90	49.9
AFP<400 ng/ml	4	1.35	0.93–1.97	3.4
Liver cirrhosis	7	1.52	1.15–2.01	38.5
Microvascular invasion positive	4	1.11	0.74–1.65	70.6
Microvascular invasion negative	5	1.64	1.30–2.06	3.6

AFP, alpha fetoprotein; HR, hazard ratio; CI, confidence interval.

worse OS (**Table 2**). For patients with macrovascular invasion positive patients, STR had no adverse impact on ruptured HCC patients' OS compared to non-ruptured HCC patients (HR, 1.55; 95% CI, 0.99–2.42). However, in macrovascular invasion-negative patients, STR was a prognostic risk factor for HCC patients (HR, 1.67; 95% CI, 1.39–2.01) (**Figure 4**).

Nine studies were included to explore the effect of age on DFS of HCC patients. The results demonstrated that in a subgroup of age < 60 years old, ruptured HCC patients' DFS was shorter than in the control group. Although no statistical difference was observed between the two groups' DFS regarding other Asian countries, non-ruptured HCC patients achieved better DFS than ruptured HCC patients in China. When patients' AFP concentration ≥ 400 ng/mL, STR is a potential risk factor for patients' DFS. However, in patients with AFP concentration < 400 ng/mL, STR was not correlated with HCC patients' DFS. For patients with liver cirrhosis, STR was linked to worse DFS. Similar poor outcomes were also demonstrated in microvascular invasion-negative patients, but in microvascular invasion-positive patients, no significant difference in DFS was identified between the two groups (**Table 2**). For DFS of patients, STR was not a prognostic risk factor in macrovascular invasion positive patients (HR, 1.23; 95% CI, 0.91–1.65), but it was a risk factor in macrovascular invasion negative patients (HR, 1.48; 95% CI, 1.06–2.05) (**Figure 5**).

Sensitivity Analysis and Publication Bias

After omitting the included articles in sequence, sensitivity analysis results confirmed the excellent stability of HR for OS. The quantificational Egger's test was employed to evaluate publication bias, and the outcomes revealed no potential publication bias among the included articles on HR for OS ($P > 0.05$). Additionally, another sensitivity analysis was performed to verify HR robustness for DFS, resulting in reliable results. No potential publication bias was observed for HR for DFS after Egger's test ($P > 0.05$).

DISCUSSION

Most ruptured HCC patients were in advanced disease stage; among them, many patients exhibited extrahepatic metastasis, PVTT, and impaired liver function (14–17). These tended to cause them to lose the opportunity of surgery and choose conservative treatment options. Therefore, the traditional concept that STR was a prognostic risk factor for HCC patients was mostly based on receiving non-surgical treatment (9, 12, 41, 42). It is worth investigating whether STR remained a prognostic risk factor for those HCC patients undergoing liver resection. The overall findings from this meta-analysis implied that STR was a risk factor in long-term prognosis of HCC patients following hepatic resection, consistent with previous reports (19, 24, 32).

To thoroughly investigate the reasons of STR affecting long-term prognosis of HCC patients after hepatic resection, from previous literature, we inferred that potential reasons were correlated with gender, tumor size, virus status, hepatectomy style, and liver cirrhosis (13, 18, 24, 28, 37, 43–47). STR was more frequently observed in male patients from reported studies (18, 24). The literature revealed that HCC female patients exhibit a better survival rate and low recurrence rate than male patients (43). Then, it was reported that ruptured HCC patients tended to have larger tumor size than non-ruptured HCC patients, and the total tumor volume is a vital prognostic predictor, and larger HCC was associated with a worse OS and DFS (37, 44). From a nationwide survey (1160 ruptured HCC patients), Aoki et al. (13) found that hepatitis B virus (HBV)-infected patients have a higher STR incidence than hepatitis C virus (HCV)-infected patients. According to reports, long-term survival rates of HCC patients with hepatitis B surface antigen (HBsAg) positive was worse than that of HBsAg negative patients following surgery (45). Additionally, staged hepatectomy followed TACE was a prevalent surgical way for ruptured HCC patients. Hanazaki et al. (46) found that preoperative TACE would significantly increase the risk of patients' postoperative recurrence, leading to unsatisfactory long-term prognosis. Besides, numerous studies revealed that ruptured HCC patients were often accompanied by liver cirrhosis, an independent prognostic risk factor affecting prognosis of HCC patients (28, 47). For reduced liver reserve and tolerance, STR was undoubtedly a serious blow to the disease.

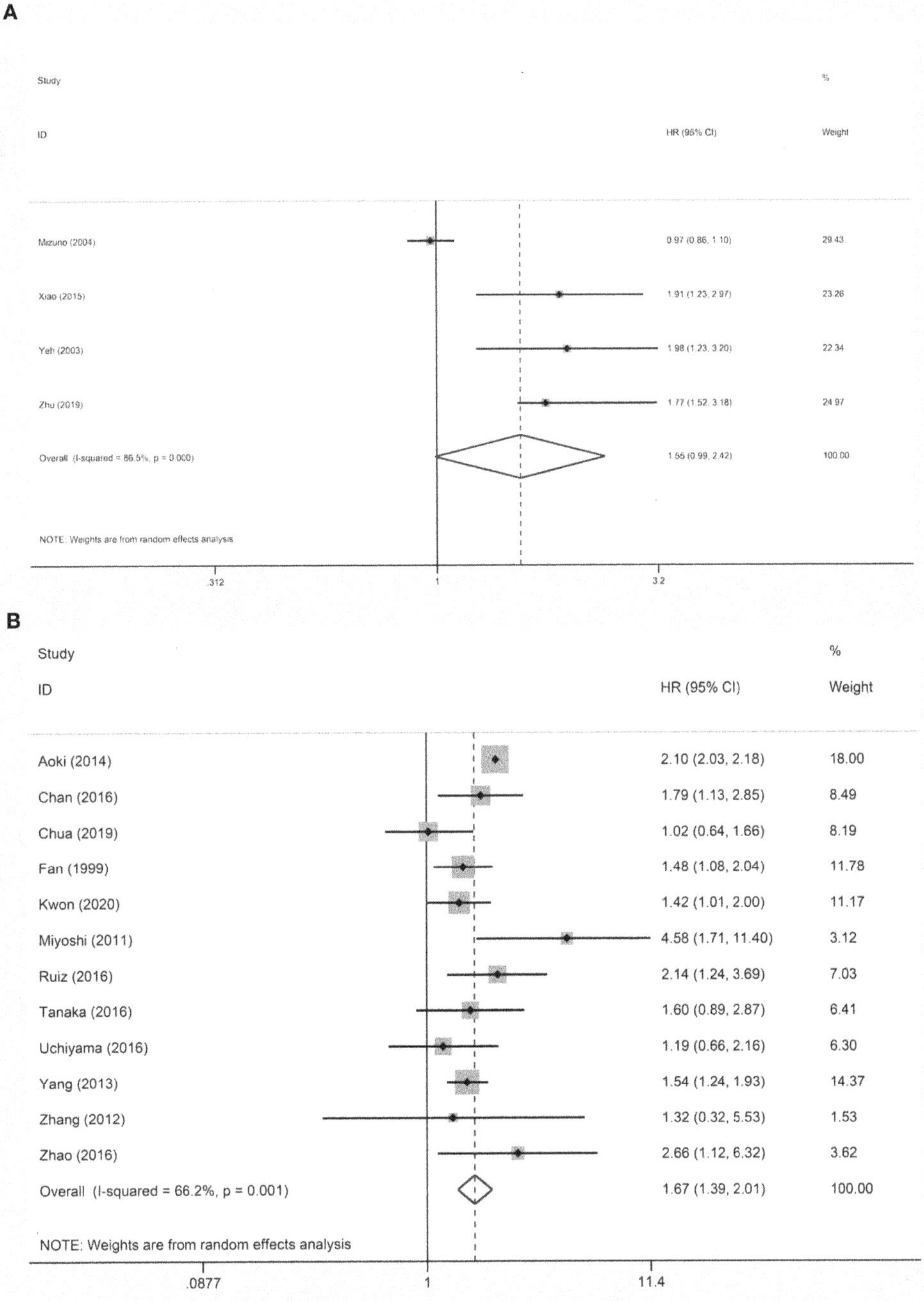

FIGURE 4 | Forest plot of OS of ruptured hepatocellular carcinoma (HCC) patients with macrovascular invasion after hepatectomy (**A**, macrovascular invasion positive, $P = 0.055$; **B**, macrovascular invasion negative, $P < 0.001$).

Due to high heterogeneity, the situations of ruptured HCC patients were complicated and diverse. We performed subgroup analyses of the prognosis of HCC patients. The analysis result of 5-year OS subgroup revealed that STR was a risk factor, but no statistical difference in survival was observed between the two groups in 3-year OS subgroup, possibly due to limited sample size (three included studies). In addition, long-term follow-up is required after hepatic resection to determine the difference in prognosis.

Our results indicated that STR was correlated with a poorer prognosis for both patients older and younger than 60 years old. There is still controversy regarding whether age affects tumor recurrence and long-term survival of HCC patients following hepatic resection. Numerous studies revealed that advanced age had no adverse effect on the prognosis of patients (48, 49).

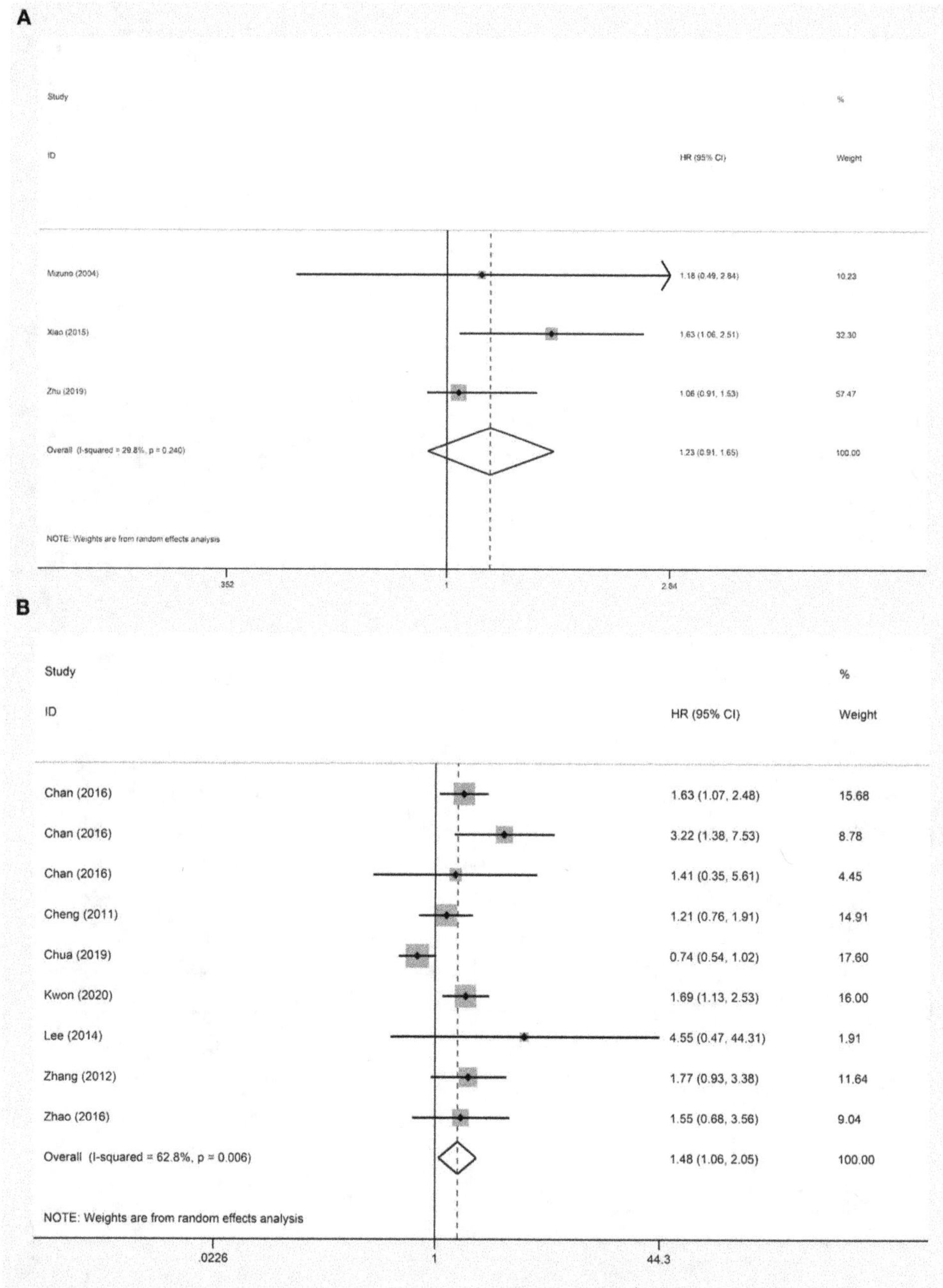

FIGURE 5 | Forest plot of DFS of ruptured hepatocellular carcinoma (HCC) patients with macrovascular invasion after hepatectomy (**A**, macrovascular invasion positive, $P = 0.170$; **B**, macrovascular invasion negative, $P = 0.021$).

Meanwhile, a previous study revealed that younger age possibly was a prognostic risk factor for HCC patients as they had more advanced tumor stage and stronger tumor aggressiveness than older HCC patients (50). However, Xu et al. found that younger HCC patients tended to have a better survival outcome regardless of tumor aggressivity (51). Moreover, our meta-analysis indicated that STR was linked to worse prognosis in China and other Asian countries. However, for other Asian countries, DFS result was not statistically different, possibly due to limited sample size. Besides, studies proved that HCV is the major etiology of HCC in Japan, whereas most Chinese HCC patients have an HBV background (52, 53). The main HBV mechanisms contributing to HCC are that HBV-DNA integrates into the host genome and induces genomic instability and insertional mutagenesis of various cancer-related genes (54). However, since HCV is an RNA virus without genes integrating into the host genome, direct cellular programming and indirect inflammatory response are possible mechanisms of inducing HCC (55). Therefore, clinicopathological characteristics and prognoses of HCC caused by different viruses may differ.

We found that STR was a risk factor regardless of subgroups with low/high serum AFP concentrations. AFP, a specific tumor marker for primary HCC, is commonly employed for early screening and diagnosis of HCC; however, its specificity and sensitivity are relatively low (56). Intriguingly, numerous investigations have discovered that several serum markers may assist in diagnosing AFP negative HCC patients (57, 58). High AFP was linked to early recurrence and poor prognosis because it promoted vascular invasion and disease progression (59). Subgroup analyses of liver cirrhosis revealed that STR was a prognostic risk factor in HCC patients with or without liver cirrhosis. Recent years have witnessed a surge in research on the risk factors for HBV-cirrhosis progressing to HCC. According to relevant literature, HBV status, antiviral drugs, and liver cirrhosis severity are potential prognostic factors (60–62).

Subgroup analysis was also used to assess the effect of microvascular invasion on prognosis. The outcomes indicated that for microvascular invasion-negative patients, ruptured HCC patients exhibited a worse prognosis than non-ruptured HCC patients. However, for microvascular invasion-positive patients, whether STR correlates with a worse prognosis remains controversial. Numerous studies have confirmed that microvascular invasion is an independent risk factor for prognosis of HCC patients undergoing hepatic resection and that occult metastases caused by microvascular invasion are a major cause of HCC recurrence following surgery (63, 64). Furthermore, numerous investigations demonstrated a substantial correlation between the existence of microvascular invasion and large tumor size, high AFP concentration, and tumor localization in segment eight (65, 66). Consequently, we speculated that, in addition to the harm caused by microvascular invasion, changes in associated clinicopathological indicators (tumor size, AFP, and tumor localization) might also cause controversies in the above results. Nowadays, it is challenging to detect microvascular invasion in preoperative imaging examination, and its diagnosis still requires validation using postoperative histopathological examination (18).

The most intriguing finding of subgroup analysis was that prognosis of ruptured HCC patients after hepatic resection was opposite depending on different macrovascular invasion status (positive/negative). STR was a significant prognostic risk factor for macrovascular invasion-negative patients; nevertheless, STR was not a prognostic risk factor in macrovascular invasion-positive patients. The possible explanation for this phenomenon is that adverse STR-related prognostic influence was overshadowed by the more harmful macrovascular invasion. In Barcelona Clinic Liver Cancer (BCLC) staging systems, macrovascular invasion HCC patients are classified as an advanced stage (67). When macrovascular invasion is present, the prognosis is extremely poor, with a median survival time of 2.7 months if left untreated (68). In addition, limited included studies in macrovascular positive-subgroup analyses (OS: 4 studies; DFS: 3 studies) might be a reason. PVTT is a prevalent type of HCC macrovascular invasion. There remain numerous controversies regarding the therapeutic options for HCC patients with PVTT. According to BCLC staging system of European and American countries, HCC patients with PVTT were classified as advanced (BCLC-C) stage, and sorafenib as a palliative treatment is recommended for these patients instead of surgery or other active methods (69). However, unlike Western countries, Asia has numerous HCC patients and various treatment methods, and because each kind of HCC is unique, PVTT is not incompatible with hepatic resection (70). Numerous doctors in Asian countries continue to use active methods like surgery to treat patients with well types and liver function, and the result revealed a favorable survival benefit than non-surgical treatment in reported literature (71, 72).

Conservative treatment, TACE, and early/delayed hepatectomy are current treatments for the management of ruptured HCC (12, 13). Conservative treatment alone is suitable for ruptured HCC patients with poor baseline or extensive metastasis (8). The advantage of TACE is its high hemostasis rate, extensive indications, and it can avoid the double blow of general anesthesia and surgery (73–75). Early surgery is suitable for patients with good baseline, and due to insufficient preoperative examinations, the recurrence rate of intrahepatic tumors after surgery is high (75). Delayed hepatectomy could reduce volume of intraoperative bleeding and blood transfusion and improve better short-and long- term prognosis of ruptured HCC patients than early hepatectomy (76). Therefore, delayed surgery (after TACE achieving hemostasis) is a better treatment option for ruptured HCC patients if they are not suitable for emergent surgery.

To the best of our knowledge, this is the first meta-analysis to assess the relationship between STR and prognosis of HCC patients following hepatic resection. Besides, various subgroup analyses were performed to investigate whether the risk effect of STR varied among various subgroups. However, this study has limitations. Firstly, the included studies were retrospective, resulting in potential risks like selection and information biases. Secondly, most populations evaluated in this study were from Asia; therefore, the conclusion does not apply to Western areas with low HCC incidence. Thirdly, since the included studies were highly heterogeneous, relevant data like postoperative recurrence and complications are fully unavailable.

CONCLUSIONS

Our study demonstrated that STR was a risk factor for long-term prognosis of HCC patients after hepatectomy. This phenomenon remained consistent in most subgroups stratified by recorded survival time, age, country, AFP concentration, liver cirrhosis, and microvascular invasion. However, STR was not associated with a worse prognosis in macrovascular invasion patients.

AUTHOR CONTRIBUTIONS

YC designed the research process. JX and JH searched the database for corresponding articles and drafted the meta-analysis. YW and LZ extracted useful information from the articles above. YH and YS used statistical software for analysis. BX polished this article. All authors had read and approved the manuscript and ensured that this was the case.

REFERENCES

1. Bray F, Ferlay J, Soerjomataram I, Siegel RL, Torre LA, Jemal A. Global cancer statistics 2018: GLOBOCAN estimates of incidence and mortality worldwide for 36 cancers in 185 countries. *CA Cancer J Clin.* (2018) 68:394-424. doi: 10.3322/caac.21492
2. Akinyemiju T, Abera S, Ahmed M, Alam N, Alemayohu MA, Allen C, et al. The Burden of primary liver cancer and underlying etiologies from 1990 to 2015 at the global, regional, and national level: results from the Global Burden of Dis ease Study (2015). *JAMA Oncol.* (2017) 3:1683-91. doi: 10.1001/jamaoncol.2017.3055
3. Lai EC, Lau WY. Spontaneous rupture of hepatocellular carcinoma: a systematic review. *Arch Surg.* (2006) 141:191-8. doi: 10.1001/archsurg.141.2.191
4. Hermann RE, David TE. Spontaneous rupture of the liver caused by hepatomas. *Surgery.* (1973) 74:715-9.
5. Castells L, Moreiras M, Quiroga S, Alvarez-Castells A, Segarra A, Esteban R, et al. Hemoperitoneum as a first manifestation of hepatocellular carcinoma in western patients with liver cirrhosis: effectiveness of emergency treatment with transcatheter arterial embolization. *Dig Dis Sci.* (2001) 46:555-62. doi: 10.1023/A:1005699132142
6. Rossetto A, Adani GL, Risaliti A, Baccarani U, Bresadola V, Lorenzin D, et al. Combined approach for spontaneous rupture of hepatocellular carcinoma. *World J Hepatol.* (2010) 2:49-51. doi: 10.4254/wjh.v2.i1.49
7. Chen MF, Hwang TL, Jeng LB, Jan YY, Wang CS. Clinical experience with hepatic resection for ruptured hepatocellular carcinoma. *Hepatogastroenterology.* (1995) 42:166-8.
8. Chen WK, Chang YT, Chung YT, Yang HR. Outcomes of emergency treatment in ruptured hepatocellular carcinoma in the ED. *Am J Emerg Med.* (2005) 23:730-6. doi: 10.1016/j.ajem.2005.02.052
9. Liu CL, Fan ST, Lo CM, Tso WK, Poon RT, Lam CM, et al. Management of spontaneous rupture of hepatocellular carcinoma: single-center experience. *J Clin Oncol.* (2001) 19:3725-32. doi: 10.1200/JCO.2001.19.17.3725
10. Ong GB, Taw JL. Spontaneous rupture of hepatocellular carcinoma. *Br Med J.* (1972) 4:146-9. doi: 10.1136/bmj.4.5833.146
11. Tan FL, Tan YM, Chung AY, Cheow PC, Chow PK, Ooi LL. Factors affecting early mortality in spontaneous rupture of hepatocellular carcinoma. *ANZ J Surg.* (2006) 76:448-52. doi: 10.1111/j.1445-2197.2006.03750.x
12. Kirikoshi H, Saito S, Yoneda M, Fujita K, Mawatari H, Uchiyama T, et al. Outcomes and factors influencing survival in cirrhotic cases with spontaneous rupture of hepatocellular carcinoma: a multicenter study. *BMC Gastroenterol.* (2009) 9:29. doi: 10.1186/1471-230X-9-29
13. Aoki T, Kokudo N, Matsuyama Y, Izumi N, Ichida T, Kudo M, et al. Prognostic impact of spontaneous tumor rupture in patients with hepatocellular carcinoma: an analysis of 1160 cases from a nationwide survey. *Ann Surg.* (2014) 259:532-42. doi: 10.1097/SLA.0b013e31828846de
14. Sonoda T, Kanematsu T, Takenaka K, Sugimachi K. Ruptured hepatocellular carcinoma evokes risk of implanted metastases. *J Surg Oncol.* (1989) 41:183-6. doi: 10.1002/jso.2930410310
15. Miyamoto M, Sudo T, Kuyama T. Spontaneous rupture of hepatocellular carcinoma: a review of 172 Japanese cases. *Am J Gastroenterol.* (1991) 86:67-71.
16. Xu HS, Yan JB. Conservative management of spontaneous ruptured hepatocellular carcinoma. *Am Surg.* (1994) 60:629-33.
17. Vergara V, Muratore A, Bouzari H, Polastri R, Ferrero A, Galatola G, et al. Spontaneous rupture of hepatocelluar carcinoma: surgical resection and long-term survival. *Eur J Surg Oncol.* (2000) 26:770-2. doi: 10.1053/ejso.2000.1001
18. Chua DW, Koh YX, Allen JC, Chan CY, Lee SY, Cheow PC, et al. Impact of spontaneous rupture on the survival outcomes after liver resection for hepatocellular carcinoma: a propensity matched analysis comparing ruptured versus non-ruptured tumors. *Eur J Surg Oncol.* (2019) 45:1652-9. doi: 10.1016/j.ejso.2019.03.044
19. Chan AC, Dai JW, Chok KS, Cheung TT, Lo CM. Prognostic influence of spontaneous tumor rupture on hepatocellular carcinoma after interval hepatectomy. *Surgery.* (2016) 159:409-17. doi: 10.1016/j.surg.2015.07.020
20. Moher D, Liberati A, Tetzlaff J, Altman DG. Preferred reporting items for systematic reviews and meta-analyses: the PRISMA statement. *PLoS Med.* (2009) 6:e1000097. doi: 10.1371/journal.pmed.1000097
21. Stang A. Critical evaluation of the Newcastle-Ottawa scale for the assessment of the quality of nonrandomized studies in meta-analyses. *Eur J Epidemiol.* (2010) 25:603-5. doi: 10.1007/s10654-010-9491-z
22. Egger M, Davey Smith G, Schneider M, Minder C. Bias in meta-analysis detected by a simple, graphical test. *BMJ.* (1997) 315:629-34. doi: 10.1136/bmj.315.7109.629
23. Cheng CH, Lee CF, Wu TH, Chan KM, Chou HS, Wu TJ, et al. Evaluation of the new AJCC staging system for resectable hepatocellular carcinoma. *World J Surg Oncol.* (2011) 9:114. doi: 10.1186/1477-7819-9-114
24. Fan ST, Ng IO, Poon RT, Lo CM, Liu CL, Wong J. Hepatectomy for hepatocellular carcinoma: the surgeon's role in long-term survival. *Arch Surg.* (1999) 134:1124-30. doi: 10.1001/archsurg.134.10.1124
25. Joliat GR, Labgaa I, Uldry E, Demartines N, Halkic N. Recurrence rate and overall survival of operated ruptured hepatocellular carcinomas. *Eur J Gastroenterol Hepatol.* (2018) 30:792-6. doi: 10.1097/MEG.0000000000001115
26. Kwon JH, Song GW, Hwang S, Kim KH, Ahn CS, Moon DB, et al. Surgical outcomes of spontaneously ruptured hepatocellular carcinoma. *J Gastrointest Surg.* (2021) 25:941-53. doi: 10.1007/s11605-020-04555-0
27. Lee HS, Choi GH, Kang DR, Han KH, Ahn SH, Kim DY, et al. Impact of spontaneous hepatocellular carcinoma rupture on recurrence pattern and long-term surgical outcomes after partial hepatectomy. *World J Surg.* (2014) 38:2070-8. doi: 10.1007/s00268-014-2502-6
28. Li J, Huang L, Liu CF, Cao J, Yan JJ, Xu F, et al. Risk factors and surgical outcomes for spontaneous rupture of BCLC stages A and B hepatocellular carcinoma: a case-control study. *World J Gastroenterol.* (2014) 20:9121-7. doi: 10.3748/wjg.v20.i27.9121
29. Miyoshi A, Kitahara K, Kohya N, Noshiro H, Miyazahi K. Outcomes of patients with spontaneous rupture of hepatocellular carcinoma. *Hepatogastroenterology.* (2011) 58:99-102.
30. Mizuno S, Yamagiwa K, Ogawa T, Tabata M, Yokoi H, Isaji S, et al. Are the results of surgical treatment of hepatocellular carcinoma poor if the tumor has spontaneously ruptured? *Scand J Gastroenterol.* (2004) 39:567-70. doi: 10.1080/00365520410005135
31. Ruan S, Shi N, Chen Z, Han H, Wang H, Jin L, et al. The role of hyperthermic intraperitoneal chemotherapy in the treatment of spontaneously ruptured hepatocellular carcinoma: a pilot study. *Ann Transl Med.* (2020) 8:1132. doi: 10.21037/atm-20-5829
32. Ruiz E, Rojas Rojas T, Berrospi F, Chávez I, Luque C, Cano L, et al. Hepatocellular carcinoma surgery outcomes in the developing world: a 20-year retrospective cohort study at the National Cancer Institute of Peru. *Heliyon.* (2016) 2:e00052. doi: 10.1016/j.heliyon.2015.e00052
33. Tanaka S, Kaibori M, Ueno M, Wada H, Hirokawa F, Nakai T, et al. Surgical Outcomes for the Ruptured Hepatocellular Carcinoma: Multicenter Analysis with a Case-Controlled Study. *J Gastrointest Surg.* (2016) 20:2021-34. doi: 10.1007/s11605-016-3280-2
34. Uchiyama H, Minagawa R, Itoh S, Kajiyama K, Harimoto N, Ikegami T, et al. Favorable outcomes of hepatectomy for ruptured hepatocellular carcinoma:

retrospective analysis of primary R0-hepatectomized patients. *Anticancer Res.* (2016) 36:379–85.

35. Xiao CZ, Wei W, Guo ZX, Li SH, Zhang YF, Wang JH, et al. A prognosis model for patients with hepatocellular carcinoma and portal vein tumor thrombus following hepatic resection. *Oncol Lett.* (2015) 10:2787–94. doi: 10.3892/ol.2015.3677
36. Yang T, Sun YF, Zhang J, Lau WY, Lai EC, Lu JH, et al. Partial hepatectomy for ruptured hepatocellular carcinoma. *Br J Surg.* (2013) 100:1071–9. doi: 10.1002/bjs.9167
37. Yeh CN, Lee WC, Chen MF. Hepatic resection and prognosis for patients with hepatocellular carcinoma larger than 10 cm: two decades of experience at Chang Gung memorial hospital. *Ann Surg Oncol.* (2003) 10:1070–6. doi: 10.1245/ASO.2003.03.072
38. Zhang XF, Wei T, Liu XM, Lv Y. Spontaneous tumor rupture and surgical prognosis of patients with hepatocellular carcinoma. *Scand J Gastroenterol.* (2012) 47:968–74. doi: 10.3109/00365521.2012.685753
39. Zhao HC, Wu RL, Liu FB, Zhao YJ, Wang GB, Zhang ZG, et al. A retrospective analysis of long term outcomes in patients undergoing hepatic resection for large (>5 cm) hepatocellular carcinoma. *HPB (Oxford).* (2016) 18:943–9. doi: 10.1016/j.hpb.2016.08.005
40. Zhu Q, Qiao G, Xu C, Yu X, Zhao J, Yu Z, et al. Conditional survival in patients with spontaneous tumor rupture of hepatocellular carcinoma after partial hepatectomy: a propensity score matching analysis. *HPB.* (2019) 21:722–30. doi: 10.1016/j.hpb.2018.10.002
41. Chearanai O, Plengvanit U, Asavanich C, Damrongsak D, Sindhvananda K, Boonyapisit S. Spontaneous rupture of primary hepatoma: report of 63 cases with particular reference to the pathogenesis and rationale treatment by hepatic artery ligation. *Cancer.* (1983) 51:1532–6.
42. Hirai K, Kawazoe Y, Yamashita K, Kumagai M, Nagata K, Kawaguchi S, et al. Transcatheter arterial embolization for spontaneous rupture of hepatocellular carcinoma. *Am J Gastroenterol.* (1986) 81:275–9.
43. Villa E, Moles A, Ferretti I, Buttafoco P, Grottola A, Del Buono M, et al. Natural history of inoperable hepatocellular carcinoma: estrogen receptors' status in the tumor is the strongest prognostic factor for survival. *Hepatology.* (2000) 32:233–8. doi: 10.1053/jhep.2000.9603
44. Goh BK, Teo JY, Chan CY, Lee SY, Jeyaraj P, Cheow PC, et al. Importance of tumor size as a prognostic factor after partial liver resection for solitary hepatocellular carcinoma: Implications on the current AJCC staging system. *J Surg Oncol.* (2016) 113:89–93. doi: 10.1002/jso.24099
45. Wu CC, Ho WL, Chen JT, Tang JS, Yeh DC, P'Eng F K. Hepatitis viral status in patients undergoing liver resection for hepatocellular carcinoma. *Br J Surg.* (1999) 86:1391–6. doi: 10.1046/j.1365-2168.1999.01272.x
46. Hanazaki K, Kajikawa S, Shimozawa N, Mihara M, Shimada K, Hiraguri M, et al. Survival and recurrence after hepatic resection of 386 consecutive patients with hepatocellular carcinoma. *J Am Coll Surg.* (2000) 191:381–8. doi: 10.1016/S1072-7515(00)00700-6
47. Taura K, Ikai I, Hatano E, Yasuchika K, Nakajima A, Tada M, et al. Influence of coexisting cirrhosis on outcomes after partial hepatic resection for hepatocellular carcinoma fulfilling the Milan criteria: an analysis of 293 patients. *Surgery.* (2007) 142:685–94. doi: 10.1016/j.surg.2007.05.009
48. Kim JM, Cho BI, Kwon CH, Joh JW, Park JB, Lee JH, et al. Hepatectomy is a reasonable option for older patients with hepatocellular carcinoma. *Am J Surg.* (2015) 209:391–7. doi: 10.1016/j.amjsurg.2013.06.010
49. Tsujita E, Utsunomiya T, Ohta M, Tagawa T, Matsuyama A, Okazaki J, et al. Outcome of repeat hepatectomy in patients with hepatocellular carcinoma aged 75 years and older. *Surgery.* (2010) 147:696–703. doi: 10.1016/j.surg.2009.10.054
50. Kim JH, Choi MS, Lee H, Kim DY, Lee JH, Koh KC, et al. Clinical features and prognosis of hepatocellular carcinoma in young patients from a hepatitis B-endemic area. *J Gastroenterol Hepatol.* (2006) 21:588–94. doi: 10.1111/j.1440-1746.2005.04127.x
51. Xu XS, Chen W, Miao RC, Zhou YY, Wang ZX, Zhang LQ, et al. Survival analysis of hepatocellular carcinoma: a comparison between young patients and aged patients. *Chin Med J.* (2015) 128:1793–800. doi: 10.4103/0366-6999.159356
52. Ukawa S, Okada E, Nakamura K, Hirata M, Nagai A, Matsuda K, et al. Characteristics of patients with liver cancer in the BioBank Japan project. *J Epidemiol.* (2017) 27:S43–8. doi: 10.1016/j.je.2016.12.007
53. Goh GB, Chang PE, Tan CK. Changing epidemiology of hepatocellular carcinoma in Asia. *Best Pract Res Clin Gastroenterol.* (2015) 29:919–28. doi: 10.1016/j.bpg.2015.09.007
54. Levrero M, Zucman-Rossi J. Mechanisms of HBV-induced hepatocellular carcinoma. *J Hepatol.* (2016) 64(1 Suppl):S84–101. doi: 10.1016/j.jhep.2016.02.021
55. Dash S, Aydin Y, Widmer KE, Nayak L. Hepatocellular carcinoma mechanisms associated with chronic HCV infection and the impact of direct-acting antiviral treatment. *J Hepatocell Carcinoma.* (2020) 7:45–76. doi: 10.2147/JHC.S221187
56. Tangkijvanich P, Anukulkarnkusol N, Suwangool P, Lertmaharit S, Hanvivatvong O, Kullavanijaya P, et al. Clinical characteristics and prognosis of hepatocellular carcinoma: analysis based on serum alpha-fetoprotein levels. *J Clin Gastroenterol.* (2000) 31:302–8. doi: 10.1097/00004836-200012000-00007
57. Shen Q, Fan J, Yang XR, Tan Y, Zhao W, Xu Y, et al. Serum DKK1 as a protein biomarker for the diagnosis of hepatocellular carcinoma: a large-scale, multicentre study. *Lancet Oncol.* (2012) 13:817–26. doi: 10.1016/S1470-2045(12)70233-4
58. Capurro M, Wanless IR, Sherman M, Deboer G, Shi W, Miyoshi E, et al. Glypican-3: a novel serum and histochemical marker for hepatocellular carcinoma. *Gastroenterology.* (2003) 125:89–97. doi: 10.1016/S0016-5085(03)00689-9
59. Peng SY, Chen WJ, Lai PL, Jeng YM, Sheu JC, Hsu HC. High alpha-fetoprotein level correlates with high stage, early recurrence and poor prognosis of hepatocellular carcinoma: significance of hepatitis virus infection, age, p53 and beta-catenin mutations. *Int J Cancer.* (2004) 112:44–50. doi: 10.1002/ijc.20279
60. Chien J, Liu J, Lee MH, Jen CL, Batrla-Utermann R, Lu SN, et al. Risk and predictors of hepatocellular carcinoma for chronic hepatitis B patients with newly developed cirrhosis. *J Gastroenterol Hepatol.* (2016) 31:1971–7. doi: 10.1111/jgh.13422
61. Bonino F, Oliveri F, Colombatto P, Brunetto MR. Impact of interferon-alpha therapy on the development of hepatocellular carcinoma in patients with liver cirrhosis: results of an international survey. *J Viral Hepat.* (1997) 4 (Suppl. 2):79–82. doi: 10.1111/j.1365-2893.1997.tb00183.x
62. Shim JJ, Oh CH, Kim JW, Lee CK, Kim BH. Liver cirrhosis stages and the incidence of hepatocellular carcinoma in chronic hepatitis B patients receiving antiviral therapy. *Scand J Gastroenterol.* (2017) 52:1029–36. doi: 10.1080/00365521.2017.1335773
63. Rodríguez-Perálvarez M, Luong TV, Andreana L, Meyer T, Dhillon AP, Burroughs AK. A systematic review of microvascular invasion in hepatocellular carcinoma: diagnostic and prognostic variability. *Ann Surg Oncol.* (2013) 20:325–39. doi: 10.1245/s10434-012-2513-1
64. Imamura H, Matsuyama Y, Tanaka E, Ohkubo T, Hasegawa K, Miyagawa S, et al. Risk factors contributing to early and late phase intrahepatic recurrence of hepatocellular carcinoma after hepatectomy. *J Hepatol.* (2003) 38:200–7. doi: 10.1016/S0168-8278(02)00360-4
65. McHugh PP, Gilbert J, Vera S, Koch A, Ranjan D, Gedaly R. Alpha-fetoprotein and tumour size are associated with microvascular invasion in explanted livers of patients undergoing transplantation with hepatocellular carcinoma. *HPB.* (2010) 12:56–61. doi: 10.1111/j.1477-2574.2009.00128.x
66. Al-Azzawi Y, Rouanet E, Hendrix RJ, Spaho L, Malik H, Devuni D, et al. Segmental Distribution of Hepatocellular Carcinoma Correlates with Microvascular Invasion in Liver Explants Undergoing Transplantation. *J Cancer Epidemiol.* (2019) 2019:8534372. doi: 10.1155/2019/8534372
67. Llovet JM, Brú C, Bruix J. Prognosis of hepatocellular carcinoma: the BCLC staging classification. *Semin Liver Dis.* (1999) 19:329–38. doi: 10.1055/s-2007-1007122
68. Llovet JM, Bustamante J, Castells A, Vilana R, Ayuso Mdel C, Sala M, et al. Natural history of untreated nonsurgical hepatocellular carcinoma: rationale for the design and evaluation of therapeutic trials. *Hepatology.* (1999) 29:62–7. doi: 10.1002/hep.510290145

69. Forner A, Reig ME, de Lope CR, Bruix J. Current strategy for staging and treatment: the BCLC update and future prospects. *Semin Liver Dis.* (2010) 30:61–74. doi: 10.1055/s-0030-1247133
70. Kudo M, Matsui O, Izumi N, Iijima H, Kadoya M, Imai Y, et al. JSH consensus-based clinical practice guidelines for the management of hepatocellular carcinoma 2014. Update by the Liver Cancer Study Group of Japan. *Liver Cancer.* (2014) 3:458–68. doi: 10.1159/000343875
71. Kokudo T, Hasegawa K, Matsuyama Y, Takayama T, Izumi N, Kadoya M, et al. Survival benefit of liver resection for hepatocellular carcinoma associated with portal vein invasion. *J Hepatol.* (2016) 65:938–43. doi: 10.1016/j.jhep.2016.05.044
72. Zhang ZY, Dong KS, Zhang EL, Zhang LW, Chen XP, Dong HH. Resection might be a meaningful choice for hepatocellular carcinoma with portal vein thrombosis: a systematic review and meta-analysis. *Medicine.* (2019) 98:e18362. doi: 10.1097/MD.0000000000018362
73. Kim JY, Lee JS, Oh DH, Yim YH, Lee HK. Transcatheter arterial chemoembolization confers survival benefit in patients with a spontaneously ruptured hepatocellular carcinoma. *Eur J Gastroenterol Hepatol.* (2012) 24:640–5. doi: 10.1097/MEG.0b013e3283524d32
74. Han XJ, Su HY, Shao HB, Xu K. Prognostic factors of spontaneously ruptured hepatocellular carcinoma. *World J Gastroenterol.* (2015) 21:7488–94. doi: 10.3748/wjg.v21.i24.7488
75. Xu X, Chen C, Liu Q, Huang X. A meta-analysis of TAE/TACE versus emergency surgery in the treatment of ruptured HCC. *Cardiovasc Intervent Radiol.* (2020) 43:1263–76. doi: 10.1007/s00270-020-02514-5
76. Zheng YJ, Li DL, Luo D, Chen XP, Zhang B, Fang C, et al. Early versus delayed hepatectomy for spontaneously ruptured hepatocellular carcinoma: a systematic review and meta-analysis. *J Invest Surg.* (2020) 1:9. doi: 10.1080/08941939.2020.1792009

13

Effect of Severity of Liver Cirrhosis on Surgical Outcomes of Hepatocellular Carcinoma After Liver Resection and Microwave Coagulation

Jiang Li[1,2], Hai-su Tao[1], Jian Li[1], Wen-qiang Wang[1], Wei-wei Sheng[3], Zhi-yong Huang[1] and Er-lei Zhang[1]*

[1] *Hepatic Surgery Center, Tongji Hospital, Tongji Medical College, Huazhong University of Science and Technology, Wuhan, China,* [2] *Hepatobiliary Surgery, The First Affiliated Hospital, College of Medicine, Shihezi University, Shihezi, China,* [3] *Department of General Surgery, People's Hospital of Wuning County, Jiujiang, China*

***Correspondence:**
Er-lei Zhang
baiyu19861104@163.com

Background: Liver resection (LR) and percutaneous microwave coagulation therapy (PMCT) are both considered as radical treatments for small hepatocellular carcinoma (HCC). However, it is still unclear whether to select LR or PMCT in HCC patients with different degrees of liver cirrhosis. The purpose of this study was to compare the efficacy of LR and PMCT in the treatment of solitary and small HCC accompanied with different degrees of liver cirrhosis.

Methods: In this study, 230 patients with solitary HCC lesions ≤ 3 cm and Child-Pugh A liver function were retrospectively reviewed. Among these patients, 122 patients underwent LR, and 108 received PMCT. The short- and long-term outcomes were compared between these two procedures. Severity of liver cirrhosis was evaluated by using clinical scoring system (CSS) as previously published. Subgroup analysis based on CSS was performed to evaluate the effect of severity of liver cirrhosis on surgical outcomes after LR and PMCT.

Results: There was no mortality within 90 days in both groups. Major complications were significantly more frequent in the LR group than in the PMCT group (18.8% *vs.* 4.6%, $p<0.001$). However, LR provided better surgical outcomes than PMCT. The 5-year overall survival (OS) rates for the LR and PMCT groups were 65.2% and 42%, respectively ($p=0.006$), and the corresponding disease-free survival (DFS) rates were 51.7% and 31.5%, respectively ($p=0.004$). Nevertheless, subgroup analysis showed that PMCT provided long-term outcomes that were similar to LR and lower surgical complications in HCC patients with CSS score≥4.

Conclusions: LR may provide better OS and DFS rates than PMCT for patients with solitary HCC lesions ≤ 3 cm and Child-Pugh A liver function irrespective of liver cirrhosis. PMCT should be viewed as the optimal treatment for solitary and small HCC with severe cirrhosis.

Keywords: liver cirrhosis, liver resection, percutaneous microwave coagulation therapy, clinical scoring system, prognosis, hepatocellular carcinoma

INTRODUCTION

Hepatocellular carcinoma (HCC) is the fifth most common malignancy in the world (1), and its incidence has been on the rise in recent years (2). Notably, HCC is increasingly detected and diagnosed at an early stage of the disease, however, the selection of optimal surgical treatments for patients with early-stage HCC remains controversial, especially for those with liver cirrhosis. Many guidelines recommend that liver resection (LR) and liver transplantation (LT) are considered as potentially curative therapies for patients with early-stage HCC (3, 4). For HCC patients with severe cirrhosis HCC and within Milan criteria, LT is widely accepted as the gold standard as it could eliminate both the tumors and cirrhotic liver which is prone to *de novo* recurrences of HCC. LT is not a conventional treatment option due to factors such as shortage of donor livers, the high associated cost and disease progression during the waiting period. Therefore, LR is still widely considered as the first option for the treatment of HCC patients without cirrhosis or Child-Pugh class A cirrhosis without portal hypertension (PH) (3, 5). In recent years, local ablations (LA), such as percutaneous microwave coagulation therapy(PMCT) and radiofrequency ablation (RFA), have been recommended as the first-line therapeutic options for patients with early-stage HCC and PMCT seems to show some advantages over RFA regarding efficacy, including better tumor control for perivascular HCCs, and better necrosis rate for cirrhotic liver (6–8). LR may sacrifice additional normal liver tissue which is critical for those with advanced liver cirrhosis, and may lead to severe surgical complications, such as liver failure (9). PMCT is easier to carry out, recovers faster, less invasive, and has a lower rate of liver decompensation in comparison with LR (10, 11). However, the degree of tumor necrosis and the necrosis range of LA are unsatisfactory. Whether LR or PMCT is an optimal option for early-stage HCC with different degrees of liver cirrhosis remains unclear.

Previous studies suggested that the prognosis of HCC depended not only on the treatment strategy and the tumor itself, but also on the underlying liver disease (12), such as chronic hepatitis or liver cirrhosis (1, 4). It has been reported that 60 to 90% of HCC patients in China have underlying liver cirrhosis (13, 14). Unsurprisingly, cirrhosis has been identified as one of the most important risk factors for the development of HCC (15), as well as one of the most important prognostic factors after surgical treatment of HCC (16). The severity of liver cirrhosis was proven to be closely related with the grade of portal hypertension (17), however, liver cirrhosis affected surgical outcomes of HCC independent of portal hypertension (18). Evaluating the status of underlying liver disease only by measuring Child-Pugh liver function and determining the "presence" or "absence" of cirrhosis is obviously unreasonable (14). Our previous studies indicated that the severity of liver cirrhosis significantly influences the short- and long-term surgical outcomes and there existed varied degrees of liver cirrhosis for HCC patients with Child-pugh A liver function and indocyanine green retention test at 15 minutes (ICG-R15) <10% (14, 18–21). Therefore, the severity of liver cirrhosis should be further sub-classified to form a reasonable surgical treatment plan with the aim of decreasing surgical complications and improving surgical outcomes (21).

Liver biopsy is considered as the gold standard for evaluating the severity of cirrhosis (22), but its invasiveness and sampling error preclude its preoperative application in HCC patients. Our previous study developed a clinical scoring system (CSS) as a non-invasive method for sub-classified the severity of liver cirrhosis in HCC patients (as described in **Table 1**) (23). The CSS exhibited high diagnostic accuracy in predicting the severity of cirrhosis, and its accuracy in predicting severe cirrhosis was 85.3%.

The purpose of this study was to compare the surgical efficacy between LR and PMCT for single HCC tumors ≤ 3cm in patients with Child-Pugh A liver function, and further explore the optimal choice of treatment for small and solitary HCC with different degrees of liver cirrhosis which was pre-operatively evaluated according to the CSS.

METHODS

This study was conducted in accordance with the Helsinki Declaration and approved by the Medical Ethics Committee of Tongji Hospital Affiliated to Huazhong University of Science and Technology. All patients gave written informed consent for post-operative data analysis. A retrospective study was conducted on patients with HCC who received curative treatment in Tongji Hospital, Huazhong University of Science and Technology from January 2008 to December 2014. Patients who met the following criteria were included in the study:

TABLE 1 | TongJi-clinical scoring model for staging liver cirrhosis.

Clinical variables	Score		
	0	1	2
Varicosity (V1)	none	F1	F2
Portal vein diameter (mm) (V2)	<12	12-14	>14
Spleen thickness (cm) (V3)	<4.0	4.0-5.0	>5.0
Platelet count(109/L) (V4)	≥100	70-100	<70
	Non/mild cirrhosis	Moderate cirrhosis	Severe cirrhosis
clinical scoring system (CSS)	0-1	2-3	≥4

1. The diagnosis of HCC was based on postoperative histopathological examination of the resected specimen or clinical diagnosis according to the American Association for the Study of the Liver Disease (AASLD) criteria (3), including AFP and/or DCP examination in combination with radiographic examination, and was confirmed by two senior physicians.
2. Single nodular HCC tumor with a maximum diameter of 3 cm. There was no portal vein thrombosis or extrahepatic metastasis.
3. Child-Pugh grade A liver function.
4. No previous surgical treatment history of HCC.

The basic information of the HCC patients and preoperative examination results were obtained from the electronic medical record system, including platelet count, aspartate aminotransferase (AST), prothrombin time (PT), albumin, total bilirubin, alpha fetoprotein (AFP), hepatitis B and hepatitis C serological detection, ultrasonography (US), computed tomography (CT), magnetic resonance imaging (MRI).

All treatments followed the clinical guidelines for the treatment of HCC at the time. The decision for LR or PMCT was made based on the disease status (such as tumor location, surgical risk, feasibility of treatment) and the patients' preferences. Surgical resection was routinely performed using an open method. PMCT was usually performed under ultrasound guidance.

Surgical Resection Procedure

Surgery was performed under general anesthesia with low central venous pressure (CVP) anesthesia (≤5 mmHg) using a right subcostal incision. We performed non-anatomical partial hepatectomy with more than 0.5 cm tumor-free margin in the cirrhotic patients. Intraoperative ultrasonography was routinely used during surgery to estimate the number, size, location, and boundary of tumors. Cavitron ultrasonic aspiration (CUSA, Valleylab Corp, USA) and Ultrasonic Scalpel (Johnson & Johnson Ltd, USA) devices were used to dissect the liver tissue. In case of accidental bleeding, the Pringle maneuver was routinely conducted, with clamping and unclamping times of 15 and 5 min, respectively.

PMCT Procedure

HCC was diagnosed by CT and MRI in line with the guidelines of the AASLD (3). PMCT was performed using ECO-100C microwave therapy instruments (ECO CO., LTD, Nanjing, China) with a frequency of 2450-MHz. The PMCT procedure was performed by a professional hepatobiliary surgeon after local anesthesia with 2% lidocaine or general inhalation anesthesia. Real-time ultrasonography (Aloka 5000, ALOKA CO., LTD, Tokyo, Japan) was used to guide and continuously monitor the entire process. After anesthesia was achieved, a 15-cm 16-guage cooling unipolar was inserted into the center of the nodule, and coagulation therapy was performed at 60-80 W output, for 8-10 min per ablation. The ablation was performed repeatedly until the tumors underwent complete necrosis as monitored using real-time ultrasonography, and the hyperechoic area overlapped the area of the tumor with a surrounding ≥1 cm safety margin. Three days later, contrast-enhanced ultrasound was used to judge whether the ablation was successfully completed. If tumor necrosis was considered to be incomplete, PMCT treatment was performed again on the nodules showing incomplete necrosis 1 week after the initial treatment. It should be noted that for a single irregular tumor with a diameter of more than 2.5 cm, a double needle beam can be directly used for ablation at the same time to achieve complete ablation.

Follow-Up and Efficacy

Liver function, alpha-fetoprotein (AFP), chest radiography and abdominal ultrasonography were routinely monitored every 2-3 months after surgery. Patients with suspected tumor recurrence or metastasis were diagnosed using CT, MR, contrast-enhanced ultrasound, or positron emission tomography (PET). The primary endpoints were overall survival (OS) and disease-free survival (DFS). OS was defined as the time between surgery and the patient's death or last follow-up. DFS was defined as the time from surgery to recurrence or distant metastasis of HCC.

Statistical Analysis

SPSS version 25.0 (IBM Corp., USA) was used to analyze the data. Continuous variables were compared using the Mann-Whitney U test, and ordinal variables were compared using Pearson's χ^2 test. Median and quartile ranges were applied to data that are not normally distributed. The Mann-Whitney U test was used to assess the significance of differences in laboratory parameters and clinical characteristics between groups. The Kaplan-Meier method was used to generate OS and DFS curves, and the log-rank test was used for comparison. The Cox proportional hazards regression model was applied to calculate the hazard ratio (HR) for survival and the 95% confidence intervals (CI) of prognostic factors for RFS or OS based on the univariate and multivariate analyses. In order to avoid collinearity, the indicators that make up the CSS were not included in the multivariate analysis. Subgroup analysis was performed to assess the effect of CSS on survival. All statistical tests were two-sided, and differences with *p*-values <0.05 were considered statistically significant.

RESULTS

Baseline Characteristics

From January 2008 to December 2014, 1022 patients received first-line treatments for HCC consisting of LR or LA. A total of 230 HCC patients who met the inclusion criteria were included in the study. Among these patients, 122 were in the LR group and 108 were in the PMCT group. All the patients had Child-Pugh class A liver function and there was no statistical difference in the baseline characteristics between the two groups. Approximately 88.3% of the patients were male, and most of them had underlying viral hepatitis B. The proportion of cirrhosis in the two groups was similar (89.3 *vs.* 92.6%, *p*= 0.393). The tumor size was also similar (median: 2.9 *vs.* 2.8 cm, *p*=0.250). **Table 2** summarizes the baseline demographic and clinical characteristics.

TABLE 2 | Patient demographic and clinical characteristics.

	All patients (n = 230)	LR (n = 122)	PMCT (n = 108)	*P*-value
Age, year	52 (45-58)	51 (44-57)	54 (48-59)	0.055
Male, %	203.0 (88.3)	111.0 (91.0)	92.0 (85.2)	0.173
HBsAg positive, %	218.0 (94.8)	115.0 (94.3)	103.0 (95.4)	0.706
Cirrhosis, %	192.0 (83.5)	109.0 (89.3)	100.0 (92.6)	0.393
A-fetoprotein, ng/ml	34.5 (6.9-225.3)	34.8 (5.9-277.2)	34.5 (7.9-148)	0.920
Tumor size, cm	2.8 (2.6-3.0)	2.9 (2.5-3.0)	2.8 (2.6-3.0)	0.250
Portal hypertension, %	74.0 (32.2)	34.0 (27.9)	40.0 (37.0)	0.137
White blood cell count, x10^9/mL	4.6 (3.4-5.5)	4.8 (3.5-5.7)	4.4 (3.3-5.3)	0.143
Alanine aminotransferase, U/L	33.0 (24.0-46.0)	31.0 (25.0-43.0)	33.0 (23.0-54.0)	0.286
Aspartate transaminase, U/L	30.0 (26.0-38.3)	29.0 (24.0-36.0)	31.0 (26.0-42.0)	0.090
Albumin, g/L	36.0 (34.9-37.9)	36.4 (35.2-38.3)	35.5 (34.8-37.3)	0.067
Serum bilirubin, mmol/L	13.5 (9.7-18.1)	13.2 (9.7-17.3)	15.0 (9.4-19.5)	0.194
PT, S	13.0 (11.4-14.1)	13.1 (11.6-14.2)	13.0 (11.4-14.1)	0.308
Presence of esophageal varices, %	80.0 (34.8)	37.0 (30.6)	43.0 (39.8)	0.383
Portal vein diameter, mm	1.2 (1.1-1.4)	1.2 (1.1-1.4)	1.2 (1.2-1.3)	0.406
Spleen thickness, cm	4.3 (3.8-4.9)	4.2 (3.7-4.9)	4.5 (3.8-5)	0.116
Platelet count, x10^9/mL	112.0 (78.8-145.3)	120.0 (83.8-155.0)	105 (72.0-131.8)	0.055

LR, liver resection; PMCT, percutaneous microwave coagulation therapy.

Long-Term Outcomes of HCC Patients Between the LR and PMCT Groups

In five of the patients who underwent PMCT, the effect was unsatisfactory at the first time, and the PMCT was performed again a week later. A total of 93 patients developed recurrence over a median follow-up period of 46.3 months. In the LR group, 89 patients developed recurrence, with a median follow-up period of 62.3 months. According to the Kaplan-Meier curve analysis, patients who received LR showed better OS and DFS than those who received PMCT. The corresponding 1-, 3-, and 5-year DFS rates were 95.4%, 74.5%, and 51.7% in the LR group, compared with 83.4%, 51.2%, and 31.5% in the PMCT group, respectively. (p=0.004, **Figure 1A**). The 1-, 3-, and 5-year OS rates were 97.2%, 91.6%, and 65.2% in the LR group, compared with 90.1%, 72.4%, and 42% in the PMCT group, respectively (p=0.006, **Figure 1B**).

Univariate and Multivariate Analyses of OS and DFS

Based on a univariate analysis, the treatment method, albumin, serum bilirubin, platelet count, portal vein diameter, spleen thickness, varicose veins, cirrhosis and CSS score were associated with DFS ($p < 0.05$, **Table 3**).

In multivariate analysis, serum bilirubin (HR=2.114, 95% CI: 1.076-4.155, $p < 0.05$), cirrhosis (HR=3.022, 95% CI:1.132-8.064, $p < 0.05$) and CSS (HR=4.570, 95% CI: 1.499-13.934, $p < 0.01$) were independent risk factors for DFS. According to the univariate analysis, the treatment method, albumin, serum bilirubin, platelet count, portal vein diameter, spleen thickness, varicose veins, cirrhosis and CSS were associated with OS ($p < 0.05$, **Table 4**). According to the multivariate analysis, independent prognostic factors for OS included serum bilirubin (HR=1.047, 95% CI: 1.005-1.091, $p < 0.05$), cirrhosis

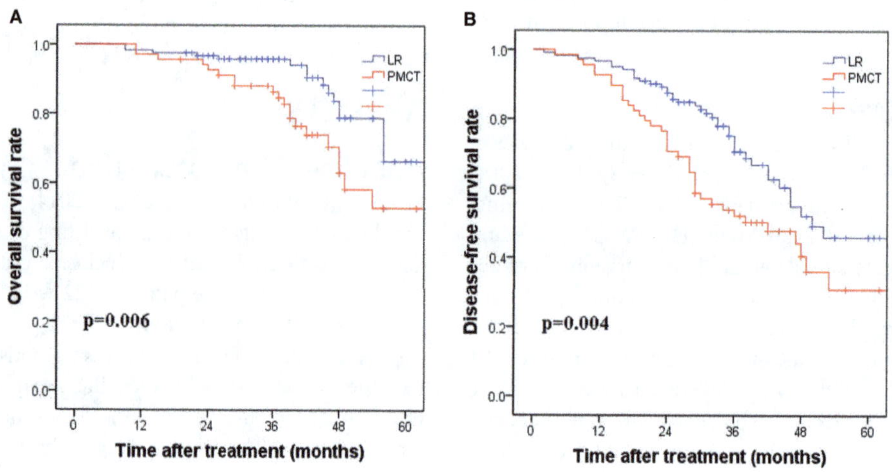

FIGURE 1 | **(A)** The corresponding 1-, 3-, and 5-year disease-free survival rates in the LR group compared with the PMCT group. (p = 0.004). **(B)** The corresponding 1-, 3-, and 5-year overall survival rates in the LR group compared with the PMCT group. (p = 0.006). LR, liver resection; PMCT, percutaneous microwave coagulation therapy.

TABLE 3 | Univariate analysis of prognostic factors of disease-free survival rate.

Factors	Univariate Cox regression		Multivariate Cox regression	
	Hazard ratio (95% CI)	*P* value	Hazard ratio (95% CI)	*P* value
Age (>50,≤50)	1.005 (0.982-1.027)	0.687		
Gender (male, female)	1.031 (0.533-1.994)	0.928		
Treatment method	0.575 (0.376-0.882)	0.011	0.747 (0.481-1.161)	0.195
HBsAg (positive, negative)	1.546 (0.633-3.773)	0.339		
AFP (>400ng/ml,≤400ng/ml)	1.185 (0.773-1.816)	0.436		
White blood cell count (≤3.5x109/mL,>3.5x109/mL)	0.742 (0.478-1.151)	0.183		
Prothrombin time (≤14.5S,>14.5S)	0.924 (0.814-1.049)	0.220		
Alanine aminotransferase (>40U/L,≤40U/L)	0.993 (0.983-1.002)	0.129		
Aspartate transaminase (>40U/L,≤40U/L)	0.997 (0.982-1.013)	0.726		
Albumin (>35g/L,≤35g/L)	0.419 (0.202-0.873)	0.020	1.238 (0.545-2.815)	0.610
Serum bilirubin (>17g/dL,≤17g/dL)	7.358 (3.775-14.342)	0.001	2.114 (1.076-4.155)	0.030
Platelet count (<100/uL, ≥100)	0.401 (0.264-0.611)	0.001		
Portal vein diameter (≤1.2cm,>1.2cm)	2.347 (1.541-3.575)	0.001		
Spleen thickness (≤4cm,>4cm)	1.656 (1.006-2.726)	0.047		
Tumor size, cm	0.819 (0.451-1.488)	0.512		
Portal hypertension (yes, no)	0.989 (0.580-1.688)	0.969		
Presence of esophageal varices (yes, no)	26.445 (9.490-73.693)	0.001		
Cirrhosis (Severe, Mild+Moderate)	17.012 (6.132-47.196)	0.001	3.022 (1.132-8.064)	0.027
CSS (≥4,<4)	2.907 (1.714-4.928)	0.001	4.570 (1.499-13.934)	0.008

TABLE 4 | Univariate analysis of prognostic factors of overall survival rate.

Factors	Univariate Cox regression		Multivariate Cox regression	
	Hazard ratio (95% CI)	*P* value	Hazard ratio (95% CI)	*P* value
Age (>50,≤50)	1.005 (0.981-1.030)	0.702		
Gender (male, female)	1.570 (0.630-3.911)	0.333		
Treatment method	0.594 (0.365-0.964)	0.035	0.814 (0.499-1.327)	0.408
HBsAg (positive, negative)	1.582 (0.638-3.923)	0.332		
AFP (>400ng/ml,≤400ng/ml)	1.199 (0.738-1.949)	0.463		
White blood cell count (≤3.5x109/mL,>3.5x109/mL)	0.936 (0.563-1.556)	0.799		
Prothrombin time (≤14.5S,>14.5S)	0.635 (0.288-1.401)	0.261		
Alanine aminotransferase (>40U/L,≤40U/L)	0.996 (0.985-1.006)	0.428		
Aspartate transaminase (>40U/L,≤40U/L)	1.000 (0.981-1.020)	0.974		
Albumin (>35g/L,≤35g/L)	0.336 (0.135-0.834)	0.019	1.059 (0.403-2.782)	0.907
Serum bilirubin (>17g/dL,≤17g/dL)	11.603 (5.019-26.825)	0.001	1.047 (1.005-1.091)	0.027
Platelet count (<100/uL,≥100)	0.990 (0.984-0.995)	0.001		
Portal vein diameter (≤1.2cm,>1.2cm)	9.100 (2.892-28.631)	0.001		
Spleen thickness (≤4cm,>4cm)	1.466 (1.139-1.885)	0.003		
Tumor size, cm	0.800 (0.404-1.588)	0.542		
Portal hypertension (yes, no)	0.989 (0.580-1.688)	0.270		
Presence of esophageal varices (yes, no)	13.328 (5.349-33.213)	0.001		
Cirrhosis (Severe, Mild+Moderate)	24.519 (9.864-60.948)	0.001	3.746 (1.221-11.495)	0.021
CSS (≥4, <4)	53.492 (13.090-218.605)	0.001	10.119 (1.706-60.026)	0.011

(HR=3.746, 95% CI: 1.221-11.495, P < 0.05) and CSS (HR=10.119, 95% CI: 1.706-60.026, $p < 0.05$).

Subgroup Analysis

Further analysis of subgroups according to the degree of cirrhosis based on CSS showed that when the CSS score ≥4, the corresponding 5-year DFS rates were 22.8% and 16.2%, respectively (p=0.818, **Figure 2A**). The 5-year OS rates for the LR group and PMCT group were 41.4% and 25.8%, respectively (p=0.3, **Figure 2B**). Thus, there were no significant differences in the DFS and OS rates between the two groups.

Complications

There was no mortality in both groups during the initial 90 days post-intervention. Hepatic hemorrhage (10/122 *vs.* 0/108) and pain (58/122 *vs.* 13/108) were significantly higher in the LR group than in the PMCT group (p<0.05). Pleural effusion (9/122 *vs.* 1/108) and ascites (15/122 *vs.* 5/108) were significantly more common in the LR group (p<0.05). Serious complications, such as liver abscess, intraperitoneal bleeding, hepatic infarction, and biliary peritonitis did not occur. Major complications were significantly more frequent in the LR group than in the PMCT group (18.8% *vs.* 4.6%, p<0.001). Among HCC patients with the CSS score ≥4, the rate of major complications was 28.4% in the

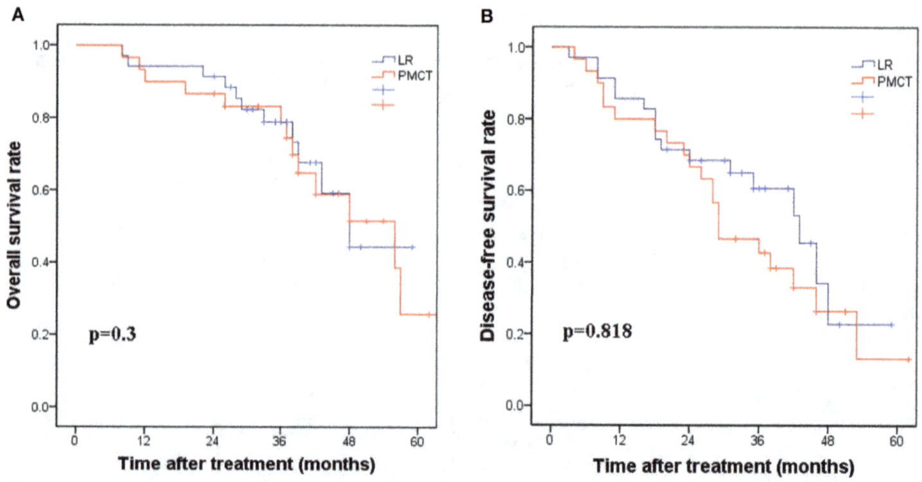

FIGURE 2 | **(A)** The corresponding 1-, 3-, and 5-year disease-free survival rates in the LR group compared with the PMCT group. (p = 0.818). **(B)** The corresponding 1-, 3-, and 5-year overall survival rates in the LR group compared with the PMCT group. (p = 0.3). LR, liver resection; PMCT, percutaneous microwave coagulation therapy.

LR group and 5.9% in the PMCT group (p=0.001, **Supplemental Figure 1**). The length of hospital stay in the LR group was greater than that in the PMCT group, and the total hospitalization cost was significantly higher than that in the PMCT group.

DISCUSSION

Nowadays, with the widely use of surveillance programs for HCC in high-risk populations, patients are increasingly diagnosed as early-stage HCC. LR and heat-based local ablations (such as RFA and PMCT) are considered to be the best curative treatments for small HCC in Western countries (10, 24). LR is the most common method in clinical practice, but the resulting tissue trauma is relatively large, and RFA is certainly less invasive. Five randomized controlled trials compared the surgical efficacy of LR and RFA, but they reported conflicting results (25–29). Of them, three randomized controlled trials showed similar survival rates between LR and RFA (25, 27, 29), but in the other two studies, LR was more favorable than RFA in terms of OS and DFS (26, 28). PMCT and RFA have been recommended as first-line therapeutic options for patients with early-stage HCC and limited liver function or severe liver cirrhosis. However, it remains unclear whether MWA is superior to RFA in terms of RFS and OS for the treatment of small and solitary HCC (30, 31). In recent years, PMCT seemed to show some advantages over RFA regarding efficacy, including better tumor control for perivascular HCCs (6), and better necrosis rate for cirrhotic liver (7). Meanwhile, PMCT can overcome the "heat sink effect" which is an obvious disadvantage of RFA (32). A Meta-Analysis of randomized controlled trials indicated a similar efficacy and safety profile between PMCT and RFA, however, distant recurrence rate was significantly lower with PMCT (RR=0.60, 0.39–0.92) in comparison with RFA (8). In China, more than 80% of HCC patients are associated with varied degrees of liver cirrhosis (14). For HCC patients with advanced liver cirrhosis, preserving adequate liver tissue is more important for surgical outcomes, therefore, the authors should consider the effect of liver cirrhosis on tumor necrosis when performed local ablation. A recent study compared the efficacy of RFA and PMCT in achieving complete response in cirrhotic patients with early and very early HCC. The results indicated that PMCT was more efficient than RFA in achieving complete response in HCC nodules with 21 to 35 mm diameter in cirrhotic liver (recurrence rates of RFA and PMCT were 31.9% *versus* 13.5%, p = 0.019) (7). Potential reasons may be that PMCT induces higher temperature around the tumor in cirrhotic liver tissues (33), and RFA may result in a cold zone easily due to the slow warming of the target area when the ablative region is restricted to perivascular tissue (6). A recent study included a total of 144 eligible patients with small (≤ 3cm) and solitary perivascular (proximity to hepatic and portal veins) HCC who underwent RFA (N=70) or PMCT (N=74) and compared the therapeutic outcomes of these two treatments (6). The results indicated that a significantly higher local tumor progression rate was observed in the RFA group than the PMCT group (5-year local tumor progression rate: RFA 24.3% *vs.* PMCT 8.4%, p=0.030) (6). As the PMCT treatment showing more superiority, in this study, we compared the efficacy of LR and PMCT in early-stage HCC patients. Many centers have adopted LR as the first-line treatment of early-stage HCC. LR can not only remove the tumor but can also remove the blood vessels and the adjacent liver tissue invaded by the tumor, thus helping prevent recurrence and metastasis in the short term. LR is also the preferred method to the treatment of tumors on the surface or margin of the liver (34). However, LR sacrifices more healthy liver tissue and leads to more surgical complications for those with severe liver cirrhosis, requiring longer hospital stay and thus incurring higher costs (29). PMCT is increasingly accepted for the treatment of early-stage HCC due to its convenient operation, less invasiveness, low postoperative liver decompensation, quick recovery and short hospital stay (35). Previous studies suggested that PMCT had comparable surgical outcomes to LR for early-stage HCC patients, with a lower incidence of complications, cheaper medical cost and shorter hospital stay (10, 33). For HCC lesions with a size <3cm, Shi et al. (36) found that PMCT had similar surgical results to LR. However, some scholars also believe that LR offers significantly better 3-year OS and 5-year DFS than PMCT (35). Moreover, larger liver tumors (including metastases) may be more suitable for LR (34), because PMCT treatment requires multiple overlapping ablations, increasing the difficulty of treatment, so that the resulting ablation margin is not as accurate as resection (36). A recent study compared the therapeutic efficacy between the robot-assisted LR and PMCT. After propensity score matching, 3-year recurrence-free survival, OS and cancer-specific survival of the patients in both groups were comparable. PMCT showed advantages of less operation time, less blood loss and lower medical cost, while LR performed better in postoperative liver function. There was no significant difference in incidence of severe complications between two groups (10). Therefore, distinguishing HCC patients who would benefit most from the two treatments will be a crucial clinical challenge in the future.

In previous studies, worse liver function, liver cirrhosis and portal hypertension were considered as important comorbidities that makes HCC patients favorable candidates for PMCT, because surgical resection may cause more blood loss and more severe complications, such as liver failure (33, 37). A study by Chong et al. (37) evaluated the surgical outcomes of HCC patients treated with LR or PMCT and the role of Albumin-Bilirubin (ALBI) score in selecting surgical modalities. Propensity scoring matching analysis according to the ALBI grade was performed. LR offered better overall and disease-free survivals in patients with ALBI grade 1 whereas PMCT provided a significantly better overall survival (p=0.025) and a trend towards better disease-free survival (p=0.39) in patients with ALBI grade 2 or 3 (37). This study suggested the liver reserve function played a crucial role in the selection of LR or PMCT for early-stage HCC patients. Our previous study indicated that LR may provide better disease-free survival and lower recurrence rates than PMCT for single HCC ≤3 cm and Child-Pugh A cirrhosis, however, PMCT may provide therapeutic effects that are similar to LR for HCC patients with portal hypertension (33). In this study, portal hypertension was defined by an indirect predictor which was less accurate. Furthermore, we did not evaluate the importance of underlying cirrhosis. The severity of liver cirrhosis played an important role in the selection of surgical modality for HCC patients (14). Obvious histological variability in the same stage of liver cirrhosis exists in the majority of HCC patients. Moreover, clinical severity and prognosis within the same histological cirrhosis vary widely, and the risk and surgical outcomes of LR may be different (38). For example, there are still some advanced cirrhosis (F4B-F4C using Laennec scoring system) for compensated cirrhosis or Child-Pugh A cirrhosis; therefore, it should be emphasized these differences to make proper surgical decisions in clinical practice. Unfortunately, it is still unclear whether LR or PMCT is the better treatment option for a single small HCC tumor with different degrees of liver cirrhosis.

In this retrospective study, we found that patients with a single HCC tumor ≤3cm and Child-Pugh class A liver function had longer DFS and OS with LR than with PMCT. At the same time, univariate and multivariate analyses also confirmed that liver cirrhosis was an independent critical risk factor for OS and DFS. In our study, about 83.5% of HCC patients had liver cirrhosis, while previous study had shown that HCC patients with liver cirrhosis had significantly worse long-term outcomes after surgical resection than patients without cirrhosis (39). It is increasingly being recognized that the presence of underlying cirrhosis is closely related to the recurrence of HCC after resection (40). Therefore, the underlying cirrhosis should be considered as a key factor affecting the surgical outcomes (14). Special attention should be paid to assessing the severity of cirrhosis before treatment decisions are made, and there are no recommendations for the treatment of single and small HCC in patients with different degrees of liver cirrhosis. In the clinical settings, the severity of liver cirrhosis may be accurately evaluated pre-operation by liver biopsy, however, the clinical feasibility of this method was severely limited owing to its invasiveness which prevented the collection of histologic information from all the HCC patients at any given time. Thus, there is an urgent need to find a non-invasive method to sub-classify liver cirrhosis that could faithfully evaluates the degrees of liver cirrhosis and that is also essential for the individualization of surgical modalities. By using several simple clinical parameters, we developed a new clinical scoring system to predict the histological severity of cirrhosis with a diagnostic accuracy of more than 80%, especially for those with severe liver cirrhosis (85.3%) (23). The preoperative evaluation of the degrees of liver cirrhosis using this non-invasive method may provide us a strong evidence for the selection of surgical treatments.

Combined with this clinical scoring system, we found that when the score ≥4, the OS and DFS between the two groups was similar. However, the occurrence of surgical complications was more frequent in the LR group than those in the PMCT group (18.8% *vs.* 4.6%, p<0.001). PMCT is a relatively less invasive procedure that preservers more liver parenchyma, has a lower cost, shorter hospital stay, and better reproducibility, with a lower risk of postoperative complications. For HCC patients with advanced liver cirrhosis, preserving adequate liver tissue is more important for surgical outcomes. LR may result in increased liver function impairment, increased risk of postoperative liver decompensation and death, and therefore higher costs and longer hospital stays due to the complicated surgical procedure and the sacrifice of more non-neoplastic liver parenchyma (25, 41). It should be pointed out that PMCT-treated HCC patients had worse clinical presentations than those treated with LR although there is no statistical difference between the two groups, therefore, PMCT should be considered as the preferred option, and priority can be given to HCC patients who were contraindicated for surgery due to age, comorbidities or background liver damage. According to the results of this study, PMCT is therefore a better treatment option for HCC patients with severe cirrhosis and tumor size ≤ 3 cm, but we should also consider factors such as the location of the tumor, the experience and proficiency of the operator when choosing PMCT.

Finally, several limitations should be considered in this study. Firstly, due to the small total sample size, the statistical power was low and there is a relatively high possibility of selection bias. Secondly, most of the patients in this study had underlying cirrhosis due to hepatitis B, which is clearly not representative of all HCC patients. Thirdly, some PMCT patients had no pathohistological results, so the well-known factors affecting prognosis such as the degree of tumor differentiation and microvascular invasion could not be analyzed. Lastly, this study was a retrospective single-center study, and multi-center clinical trials should be conducted in the later stage to provide stronger evidence and obtain more accurate results.

In conclusion, this retrospective study shows that LR provides better OS and better DFS than PMCT in patients with a single HCC ≤3cm and Child-Pugh class A liver function irrespective of liver cirrhosis. However, for those patients accompanied with severe liver cirrhosis, PMCT may provide a therapeutic effect similar to that of LR and may represent an optimal option, with less invasive, lower medical cost and complications, which should be considered as a superior option. Large number and multicenter randomized controlled trials should be performed to verify our conclusions in the future.

AUTHOR CONTRIBUTIONS

E-lZ made the concept and design. JiangL, H-sT, JianL, and W-qW acquired and analyzed the data. JiangL drafted the manuscript. E-lZ critically revised the manuscript for the final version. W-wS and JiangL conducted the statistical analysis. All authors contributed to the article and approved the submitted version.

ACKNOWLEDGMENTS

Thanks to all the staff of Hepatic Surgery Center in Tongji Hospital who contributed to the study.

REFERENCES

1. Siegel RL, Miller KD, Jemal A. Cancer Statistics, 2016. *CA Cancer J Clin* (2016) 66:7–30. doi: 10.3322/caac.21332
2. EASL. Clinical Practice Guidelines: Management of Hepatocellular Carcinoma. *J Hepatol* (2018) 69:182–236. doi: 10.1016/j.jhep.2018.03.019
3. Bruix J, Sherman M. Management of Hepatocellular Carcinoma: An Update. *Hepatology* (2011) 53:1020–2. doi: 10.1002/hep.24199
4. Llovet JM, Ducreux M, Lencioni R, Di Bisceglie AM, Galle PR, Bernardi M, et al. EASL-EORTC Clinical Practice Guidelines: Management of Hepatocellular Carcinoma. *J Hepatol* (2012) 56:908–43. doi: 10.1016/j.jhep.2011.12.001
5. Groeschl RT, Clark Gamblin T, Turaga KK. Surgical Resection in Hepatocellular Carcinoma Patients With Minimal Background Fibrosis: A Strategy in the Era of Organ Shortage. *Ann Surg Oncol* (2013) 20:2043–8. doi: 10.1245/s10434-012-2857-6
6. An C, Li WZ, Huang ZM, Yu XL, Han YZ, Liu FY, et al. Small Single Perivascular Hepatocellular Carcinoma: Comparisons of Radiofrequency Ablation and Microwave Ablation by Using Propensity Score Analysis. *Eur Radiol* (2021) 31:4764–73. doi: 10.1007/s00330-020-07571-5
7. Gaia S, Ciruolo M, Ribaldone DG, Rolle E, Migliore E, Mosso E, et al. Higher Efficiency of Percutaneous Microwave (MWA) Than Radiofrequency Ablation (RFA) in Achieving Complete Response in Cirrhotic Patients With Early Hepatocellular Carcinoma. *Curr Oncol* (2021) 28:1034–44. doi: 10.3390/curroncol28020101
8. Facciorusso A, Abd El Aziz MA, Tartaglia N, Ramai D, Mohan BP, Cotsoglou C, et al. Microwave Ablation *Versus* Radiofrequency Ablation for Treatment of Hepatocellular Carcinoma: A Meta-Analysis of Randomized Controlled Trials. *Cancers (Basel)* (2020) 12(12):3796. doi: 10.3390/cancers12123796
9. Zhou SJ, Zhang EL, Liang BY, Zhang ZY, Dong KS, Hou P, et al. Morphologic Severity of Cirrhosis Determines the Extent of Liver Resection in Patients With Hepatocellular Carcinoma and Child-Pugh Grade A Cirrhosis. *J Surg Res* (2016) 200:444–51. doi: 10.1016/j.jss.2015.08.027
10. Ding W, Yu J, Liu F, Yu X, Cheng Z, Han Z, et al. Percutaneous Microwave Ablation *Versus* Robot-Assisted Hepatectomy for Early Hepatocellular Carcinoma: A Real-World Single-Center Study. *Dig Liver Dis* (2021) S1590-8658(21)00187-0. doi: 10.1016/j.dld.2021.04.008
11. Yang G, Xiong Y, Sun J, Wang G, Li W, Tang T, et al. The Efficacy of Microwave Ablation *Versus* Liver Resection in the Treatment of Hepatocellular Carcinoma and Liver Metastases: A Systematic Review and Meta-Analysis. *Int J Surg* (2020) 77:85–93. doi: 10.1016/j.ijsu.2020.03.006
12. Liu PH, Hsu CY, Hsia CY, Lee YH, Su CW, Huang YH, et al. Prognosis of Hepatocellular Carcinoma: Assessment of Eleven Staging Systems. *J Hepatol* (2016) 64:601–8. doi: 10.1016/j.jhep.2015.10.029
13. Chen XP, Wu ZD, Huang ZY, Qiu FZ. Use of Hepatectomy and Splenectomy to Treat Hepatocellular Carcinoma With Cirrhotic Hypersplenism. *Br J Surg* (2005) 92:334–9. doi: 10.1002/bjs.4776
14. Zhang EL, Liang BY, Chen XP, Huang ZY. Severity of Liver Cirrhosis: A Key Role in the Selection of Surgical Modality for Child-Pugh A Hepatocellular Carcinoma. *World J Surg Oncol* (2015) 13:148. doi: 10.1186/s12957-015-0567-9
15. Yuen MF, Tanaka Y, Shinkai N, Poon RT, But DY, Fong DY, et al. Risk for Hepatocellular Carcinoma With Respect to Hepatitis B Virus Genotypes B/C, Specific Mutations of Enhancer II/core Promoter/Precore Regions and HBV DNA Levels. *Gut* (2008) 57:98–102. doi: 10.1136/gut.2007.119859
16. Tung-Ping Poon R, Fan ST, Wong J. Risk Factors, Prevention, and Management of Postoperative Recurrence After Resection of Hepatocellular Carcinoma. *Ann Surg* (2000) 232:10–24. doi: 10.1097/00000658-200007000-00003
17. Kim MY, Cho MY, Baik SK, Park HJ, Jeon HK, Im CK, et al. Histological Subclassification of Cirrhosis Using the Laennec Fibrosis Scoring System Correlates With Clinical Stage and Grade of Portal Hypertension. *J Hepatol* (2011) 55:1004–9. doi: 10.1016/j.jhep.2011.02.012
18. Zhang EL, Li J, Li J, Wang WQ, Gu J, Huang ZY. Sub-Classification of Cirrhosis Affects Surgical Outcomes for Early Hepatocellular Carcinoma Independent of Portal Hypertension. *Front Oncol* (2021) 11:671313. doi: 10.3389/fonc.2021.671313
19. Huang ZY, Zhang EL, Chen XP. Staging the Severity of Liver Cirrhosis and Decision of Surgical Treatment for Hepatocellular Carcinoma: Tongji Experience. *Zhonghua Wai Ke Za Zhi* (2019) 57:408–11. doi: 10.3760/cma.j.issn.0529-5815.2019.06.003
20. Dong KS, Liang BY, Zhang ZY, Zhang EL, Yang G, Xia SL, et al. Histologic Severity of Liver Cirrhosis: A Key Factor Affecting Surgical Outcomes of Hepatocellular Carcinoma in Patients With Portal Hypertension. *Asian J Surg* (2019) 42:981–9. doi: 10.1016/j.asjsur.2019.01.009
21. Huang ZY, Liang BY, Xiong M, Dong KS, Zhang ZY, Zhang EL, et al. Severity of Cirrhosis Should Determine the Operative Modality for Patients With Early Hepatocellular Carcinoma and Compensated Liver Function. *Surgery* (2016) 159:621–31. doi: 10.1016/j.surg.2015.09.002
22. Spinzi G, Terruzzi V, Minoli G. Liver Biopsy. *N Engl J Med* (2001) 344:2030. doi: 10.1056/NEJM200106283442614
23. Zhang EL, Zhang ZY, Wang SP, Xiao ZY, Gu J, Xiong M, et al. Predicting the Severity of Liver Cirrhosis Through Clinical Parameters. *J Surg Res* (2016) 204:274–81. doi: 10.1016/j.jss.2016.04.036
24. Poon RT, Fan ST, Tsang FH, Wong J. Locoregional Therapies for Hepatocellular Carcinoma: A Critical Review From the Surgeon's Perspective. *Ann Surg* (2002) 235:466–86. doi: 10.1097/00000658-200204000-00004
25. Chen MS, Li JQ, Zheng Y, Guo RP, Liang HH, Zhang YQ, et al. A Prospective Randomized Trial Comparing Percutaneous Local Ablative Therapy and

Partial Hepatectomy for Small Hepatocellular Carcinoma. *Ann Surg* (2006) 243:321–8. doi: 10.1097/01.sla.0000201480.65519.b8

26. Huang J, Yan L, Cheng Z, Wu H, Du L, Wang J, et al. A Randomized Trial Comparing Radiofrequency Ablation and Surgical Resection for HCC Conforming to the Milan Criteria. *Ann Surg* (2010) 252:903–12. doi: 10.1097/SLA.0b013e3181efc656
27. Feng K, Yan J, Li X, Xia F, Ma K, Wang S, et al. A Randomized Controlled Trial of Radiofrequency Ablation and Surgical Resection in the Treatment of Small Hepatocellular Carcinoma. *J Hepatol* (2012) 57:794–802. doi: 10.1016/j.jhep.2012.05.007
28. Liu H, Wang ZG, Fu SY, Li AJ, Pan ZY, Zhou WP, et al. Randomized Clinical Trial of Chemoembolization Plus Radiofrequency Ablation *Versus* Partial Hepatectomy for Hepatocellular Carcinoma Within the Milan Criteria. *Br J Surg* (2016) 103:348–56. doi: 10.1002/bjs.10061
29. Ng KKC, Chok KSH, Chan ACY, Cheung TT, Wong TCL, Fung JYY, et al. Randomized Clinical Trial of Hepatic Resection *Versus* Radiofrequency Ablation for Early-Stage Hepatocellular Carcinoma. *Br J Surg* (2017) 104:1775–84. doi: 10.1002/bjs.10677
30. Poulou LS, Botsa E, Thanou I, Ziakas PD, Thanos L. Percutaneous Microwave Ablation *vs* Radiofrequency Ablation in the Treatment of Hepatocellular Carcinoma. *World J Hepatol* (2015) 7:1054–63. doi: 10.4254/wjh.v7.i8.1054
31. Kamal A, Elmoety AAA, Rostom YAM, Shater MS, Lashen SA. Percutaneous Radiofrequency *Versus* Microwave Ablation for Management of Hepatocellular Carcinoma: A Randomized Controlled Trial. *J Gastrointest Oncol* (2019) 10:562–71. doi: 10.21037/jgo.2019.01.34
32. European Association for the Study of the Liver, Electronic Address eee and European Association for the Study of the L. EASL Clinical Practice Guidelines: Management of Hepatocellular Carcinoma. *J Hepatol* (2018) 69:182–236. doi: 10.1016/j.jhep.2018.03.019
33. Zhang EL, Yang F, Wu ZB, Yue CS, He TY, Li KY, et al. Therapeutic Efficacy of Percutaneous Microwave Coagulation *Versus* Liver Resection for Single Hepatocellular Carcinoma ≤3 Cm With Child-Pugh A Cirrhosis. *Eur J Surg Oncol* (2016) 42:690–7. doi: 10.1016/j.ejso.2016.02.251
34. Ryu T, Takami Y, Wada Y, Tateishi M, Matsushima H, Yoshitomi M, et al. Oncological Outcomes After Hepatic Resection and/or Surgical Microwave Ablation for Liver Metastasis From Gastric Cancer. *Asian J Surg* (2019) 42:100–5. doi: 10.1016/j.asjsur.2017.09.005
35. Glassberg MB, Ghosh S, Clymer JW, Wright GWJ, Ferko N, Amaral JF. Microwave Ablation Compared With Hepatic Resection for the Treatment of Hepatocellular Carcinoma and Liver Metastases: A Systematic Review and Meta-Analysis. *World J Surg Oncol* (2019) 17:98. doi: 10.1186/s12957-019-1632-6
36. Shi J, Sun Q, Wang Y, Jing X, Ding J, Yuan Q, et al. Comparison of Microwave Ablation and Surgical Resection for Treatment of Hepatocellular Carcinomas Conforming to Milan Criteria. *J Gastroenterol Hepatol* (2014) 29:1500–7. doi: 10.1111/jgh.12572
37. Chong CCN, Lee KF, Chu CM, Chan AWH, Wong J, Chan SL, et al. Microwave Ablation Provides Better Survival Than Liver Resection for Hepatocellular Carcinoma in Patients With Borderline Liver Function: Application of ALBI Score to Patient Selection. *HPB (Oxford)* (2018) 20:546–54. doi: 10.1016/j.hpb.2017.12.001
38. Kim SU, Jung KS, Lee S, Park JY, Kim DY, Ahn SH, et al. Histological Subclassification of Cirrhosis Can Predict Recurrence After Curative Resection of Hepatocellular Carcinoma. *Liver Int* (2014) 34:1008–17. doi: 10.1111/liv.12475
39. Taura K, Ikai I, Hatano E, Yasuchika K, Nakajima A, Tada M, et al. Influence of Coexisting Cirrhosis on Outcomes After Partial Hepatic Resection for Hepatocellular Carcinoma Fulfilling the Milan Criteria: An Analysis of 293 Patients. *Surgery* (2007) 142:685–94. doi: 10.1016/j.surg.2007.05.009
40. Sasaki K, Shindoh J, Margonis GA, Nishioka Y, Andreatos N, Sekine A, et al. Effect of Background Liver Cirrhosis on Outcomes of Hepatectomy for Hepatocellular Carcinoma. *JAMA Surg* (2017) 152:e165059. doi: 10.1001/jamasurg.2016.5059
41. Lau WY, Lai EC. The Current Role of Radiofrequency Ablation in the Management of Hepatocellular Carcinoma: A Systematic Review. *Ann Surg* (2009) 249:20–5. doi: 10.1097/SLA.0b013e31818eec29

14

Meta-Analysis of Percutaneous vs. Surgical Approaches Radiofrequency Ablation in Hepatocellular Carcinoma

Xiaozhun Huang [1†], Yibin Liu [2†], Lin Xu [1†], Teng Ma [1], Xin Yin [1], Zhangkan Huang [1], Caibin Wang [1], Zhen Huang [3], Xinyu Bi [3] and Xu Che [1,4*]*

[1] Department of Hepatobiliary Surgery, National Cancer Center/National Clinical Research Center for Cancer/Cancer Hospital and Shenzhen Hospital, Chinese Academy of Medical Sciences and Peking Union Medical College, Shenzhen, China, [2] Department of General Surgery, Longgang District Central Hospital of Shenzhen, Shenzhen, China, [3] Department of Hepatobiliary Surgery, National Cancer Center/National Clinical Research Center for Cancer/Cancer Hospital, Chinese Academy of Medical Sciences and Peking Union Medical College, Beijing, China, [4] Department of Gastrointestinal and Pancreatic Surgery, National Cancer Center/National Clinical Research Center for Cancer/Cancer Hospital, Chinese Academy of Medical Sciences and Peking Union Medical College, Beijing, China

***Correspondence:**
Xu Che
drchexu@126.com
Xinyu Bi
beexy1971@163.com

†These authors have contributed equally to this work

Background: Radiofrequency ablation (RFA) is a curative modality for hepatocellular carcinoma (HCC) patients who are not suitable for resection. It remains controversial whether a surgical or percutaneous approach is more appropriate for HCC.

Method: A search was performed on the PubMed, Web of Science, Embase, and Cochrane Library databases from the date of database inception until April 17, 2021. Studies reporting outcomes of comparisons between surgical RFA (SRFA) and percutaneous RFA (PRFA) were included in this study. The meta-analysis was performed using the Review Manager 5.3 and Stata 12.0 software.

Result: A total of 10 retrospective studies containing 12 cohorts, involving 740 patients in the PRFA group and 512 patients in the SRFA group, were selected. Although the tumor size in PRFA group was smaller than the SRFA group ($p = 0.007$), there was no significant difference in complete ablation rate between the SRFA and PRFA groups (95.63% and 97.33%, respectively; Odds ratio [OR], 0.56; 95% confidence intervals [CI], 0.26–1.24; $p = 0.15$). However, the SRFA group showed a significantly lower local tumor recurrence than the PRFA group in the sensitivity analysis (28.7% in the PRFA group and 21.79% in the SRFA group, respectively; OR, 1.84; 95% CI, 1.14–2.95; $p = 0.01$). Pooled analysis data showed that the rate of severe perioperative complications did not differ significantly between the PRFA and SRFA groups (14.28% and 12.11%, respectively; OR, 1.30; 95% CI, 0.67-2.53; $p = 0.44$). There was no significant difference in the 1-, 3-, and 5-year overall survival rates, as well as the 1- and 3-year disease-free survival (DFS) between the PRFA and SRFA groups. The 5-year DFS of the PRFA group was significantly lower than the SRFA group (hazard ratio 0.73; 95% CI 0.54–0.99).

Conclusion: Based on our meta-analysis, the surgical route was superior to PRFA in terms of local control rate. Furthermore, the surgical approach did not increase the risk of major complications.

Keywords: radiofrequency ablation, hepatocellular carcinoma, surgical, percutaneous, meta-analysis

INTRODUCTION

Radiofrequency ablation (RFA) is recognized as a curative modality for early-stage hepatocellular carcinoma (HCC), especially in patients who are not suitable for resection and liver transplantation (1–4). Although RFA for HCC can be performed using percutaneous or surgical approaches, a percutaneous approach using external ultrasonic (ETUS) is the least invasive method, with a low cost and short hospital stay (5). However, percutaneous radiofrequency ablation (PRFA) is associated with lower accuracy in cancer staging, poor accessibility in certain areas of the liver, can damage or perforate adjacent visceral organs, and cause diaphragmatic injury (6–8). These issues can be addressed using surgical radiofrequency ablation (SRFA), which is performed with open and laparoscopic approaches utilizing an intraoperative ultrasonic (IOUS) probe. It is considered a more accurate and effective method for HCC that develops in relatively inaccessible areas (9). At present, only a few studies have examined the advantages and disadvantages of percutaneous and surgical approaches. Whether SRFA is more appropriate for patients with HCC compared to PRFA remains unclear and is up for debate (10–12).

In this study, we performed a meta-analysis with inclusion and exclusion criteria to review the currently available published data comparing the safety and efficacy of these two therapeutic approaches in patients with HCC.

MATERIALS AND METHODS

The present meta-analysis was performed according to the criteria defined by the Preferred Reporting Items for Systematic Reviews and Meta-analyses statement (13).

Data Source and Search Strategy

A literature search on the PubMed, Web of Science, Embase, and Cochrane Library databases was performed to select relevant articles with no restrictions on regions starting from the date of database inception until April 17, 2021. The following keywords were searched in titles and abstracts: (hepatocellular carcinoma) AND [(radiofrequency) OR (ablation)] AND {[(open) OR (surgery) OR (laparoscopic) OR (surgical) OR (laparoscopy)] AND (percutaneous)}. All the retrieved articles were reviewed, with their reference lists manually screened to identify additional studies. When multiple reports described the same patient population, the most recent or complete report was included. The literature search was independently conducted by two researchers, and any disagreements were resolved by the adjudicating senior authors.

Inclusion and Exclusion Criteria

Studies were included in the meta-analysis when both of the following inclusion criteria were met: 1. Comparisons of postoperative and survival outcomes between PRFA and SRFA. 2. Confirmation of HCC in study patients based on clinical diagnosis. The exclusion criteria were as follows: 1. Lack of reporting or inability to calculate relevant outcomes based on available data. 2. Non-human experimental study design. 3. Publication types, other than randomized controlled trials and observational studies, such as editorials, letters to the editor, review articles, and case reports.

Data Extraction and Study Outcomes

After the removal of duplicates, the titles and abstracts of the retrieved studies were screened and sequentially excluded according to the eligibility criteria. In the event of any uncertainties after screening the titles and abstracts, the complete text was independently assessed by two investigators, and any discrepancies were resolved by consensus. The primary outcomes were complete ablation rate, postoperative complication, and recurrence rates.

Quality Assessment and Statistical Analysis

The completeness, plausibility, and integrity of the available data were reviewed before being compiled into a single database. The methodological quality of retrospective studies was assessed using the modified Newcastle–Ottawa scale (mNOS) (14, 15), which comprised three factors: patient selection, comparability of study groups, and outcome assessment. Each study was given stars based on a score of 0–9, with studies receiving eight or more stars considered as high quality. Any discrepancies were resolved by consensus. The meta-analysis was performed using the Review Manager 5.3 software (Cochrane Collaboration, Oxford, UK). The weighted mean difference (WMD) and odds ratio (OR) were used to compare continuous and dichotomous variables. All results were reported with 95% confidence intervals (CI). Statistical heterogeneity among the included studies was assessed using the chi-squared test, with a $p < 0.05$ considered significant, and heterogeneity was quantified using the I^2 statistic. In the event of significant heterogeneity among the included studies, the random-effects model was used for pooled analyses; otherwise, the fixed-effects model was used (16). Publication bias was examined using the Stata 12.0 software (Stata Corporation, College Station, TX, USA).

RESULTS

Search Results

The literature search and study selection criteria are schematically illustrated in **Figure 1**. A total of 1,399 publications were retrieved following an initial search on the biomedical databases. After reviewing the titles and/or abstracts, 519 articles were eliminated because of duplication, and 852 articles were excluded because they were deemed irrelevant for the present study. Full texts of 28 studies were reviewed: five were available as abstracts only, six were case series with inappropriate control groups, two had samples mixed with other liver malignancies, and five lacked research data. The remaining ten studies (9–12, 17–22) that evaluated the outcomes of patients with HCC using different approaches were included in the meta-analysis. Manual screening of the reference lists of these ten publications identified no additional studies. The two reviewers were in complete agreement for both the study selection and the quality assessment of trials. Two studies (11, 20) contained two sets of

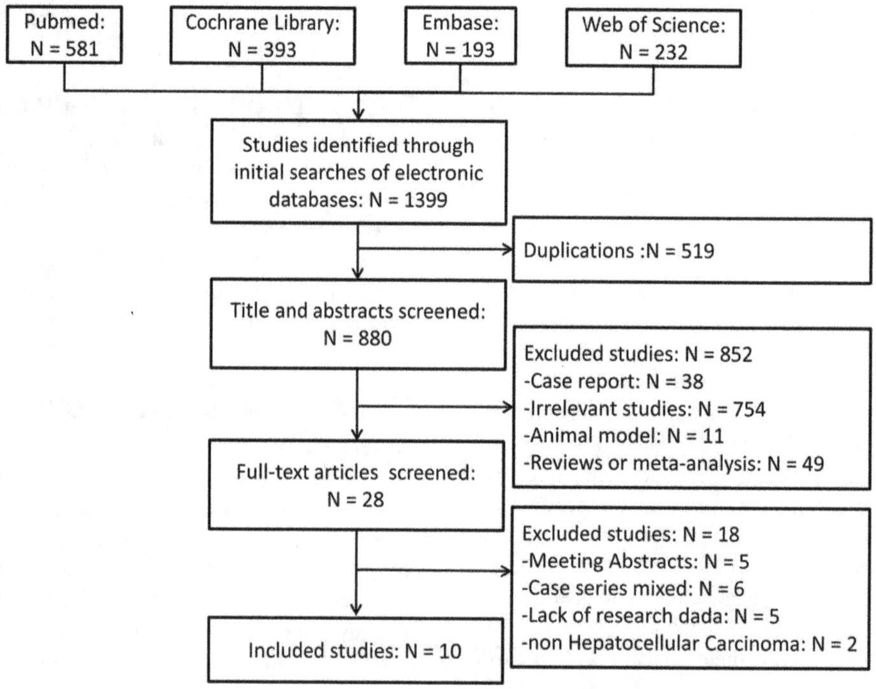

FIGURE 1 | Schematic illustration of the literature search and study-selection criteria.

TABLE 1 | Summary of characteristics of included studies.

Study	Location/year	Surgical approach	Number of patients		Number of nodules		Childs-Pugh (A: B: C)		Tumor size (cm)		Tumor number (solitary: multiple)	
			PRFA	SRFA	PRFA	SRFA	PRFA	SRFA	PRFA	SRFA	PRFA	SRFA
Eun, H. S	Korea/2017	laparoscopic	33	33	36	40	NR	NR	1.7	1.7	31:2	27:6
Chen, S	China/2018	laparoscopic	30	30	32	46	NR	NR	NR	NR	NR	NR
Khan, M. R (1)	China/2007	laparoscopic + open	92	63	110	81	87:5:0	54:8:1	1.9 ± 0.6	2.2 ± 0.6	75:17	51:12
Khan, M. R (2)	China/2007	laparoscopic + open	25	48	27	63	22:3:0	45:2:1	3.6 ± 0.4	3.9 ± 0.5	23:2	37:11
Li, J	China/2018	open	54	35	71	48	49:4:0	34:2:0	2.8 (0.8–6.0)	3.5 (0.4–5.0)	NR	NR
Hirooka, M	Japan/2009	laparoscopic	37	37	44	42	29:8:0	25:12:0	2.49 ± 0.46	2.6 ± 0.69	NR	NR
Sherif, Z	Egypt/2008	laparoscopic	30	30	36	34	6:24:0	10:20:0	NR	NR	22:8	10:20
Zhang, W (1)	China/2016	laparoscopic	77	19	175	42	74:3:0	18:1:0	2.3 ± 0.6	2.3 ± 0.6	NR	NR
Zhang, W (2)	China/2016	open	77	58	175	137	74:3:0	57:1:0	2.3 ± 0.6	2.3 ± 0.5	NR	NR
Curley, S. A	Italy/2000	laparoscopic + open	76	34	84	65	17:30:29	33:1:0	2.8 ± 0.8	4.6 ± 1.7	NR	NR
Raut, C. P	American/2005	open	140	32	190	NR	59:46:35	NR	3	NR	101:39	NR
Huang, J. W	China/2011	open	69	93	89	108	61:8:0	93:0:0	1.7 ± 1.1	1.8 ± 1.0	51:18	79:14

PRFA, percutaneous radiofrequency ablation; SRFA, surgical radiofrequency ablation; NR, not reported.

readily available independent data, which were extracted and analyzed separately.

Characteristics of the Included Studies

The characteristics of the ten studies (9–12, 17–22) included in the meta-analysis are summarized in **Table 1**. All studies were published between 2000 and 2018. The sample size in individual studies ranged from 60 to 172, for a total of 1,252 patients, consisting of 740 (59.11%) and 512 (40.89%) patients with PRFA and SRFA, respectively. The tumor size in the PRFA group was smaller than in the SRFA group ($p = 0.007$; **Supplementary Figure S1**). There was

TABLE 2 | Risk of bias using the modified Newcastle-Ottawa Scale.

Study	Selection				Comparability	Outcome			Score
	Representativeness of exposed cohort	**Selection of non-exposed cohort**	**Exposure**	**Outcome of interest not present at start**	**Comparability of PRFA vs. SRFA**	**Assessment of outcome**	**Follow-up**	**Adequacy of follow-up**	
Eun, H. S	Truly representative	Same	Surgical records	Yes	Restricted, matched	Record linkage	Yes	Complete	9⋆
Chen, S	Truly representative	Same	Surgical records	Yes	Unclear	Record linkage	Yes	Unclear	7⋆
Khan, M. R	Truly representative	Same	Surgical records	Yes	Restricted, matched	Record linkage	Yes	Complete	9⋆
Li, J	Truly representative	Same	Surgical records	Yes	Restricted, matched	Record linkage	Yes	Unclear	8⋆
Hirooka, M	Truly representative	Same	Surgical records	Yes	Not restricted, matched	Record linkage	Yes	Unclear	7⋆
Sherif, Z	Truly representative	Same	Surgical records	Yes	Restricted, matched	Record linkage	Yes	Complete	9⋆
Zhang, W	Truly representative	Same	Surgical records	Yes	Restrictions, matched	Record linkage	Yes	Complete	8⋆
Curley, S. A	Truly representative	Same	Surgical records	Yes	Unclear	Record linkage	Yes	Complete	8⋆
Raut, C. P	Truly representative	Same	Surgical records	Yes	Restrictions, matched	Record linkage	Yes	Complete	8⋆
Huang, J. W	Truly representative	Same	Surgical records	Yes	Restrictions, matched	Record linkage	Yes	Complete	9⋆

PRFA, percutaneous radiofrequency ablation; SRFA, surgical radiofrequency ablation.

Study or Subgroup	PRFA Events	PRFA Total	SRFA Events	SRFA Total	Weight	Odds Ratio M-H, Fixed, 95% CI
Curley, S. A. 2000	70	76	34	34	23.0%	0.16 [0.01, 2.87]
Eun, H. S. 2017	33	33	33	33		Not estimable
Hirooka, M. 2010	37	37	37	37		Not estimable
Huang, J. W. 2011	63	69	90	93	38.3%	0.35 [0.08, 1.45]
Khan, M. R. 2007(1)	88	92	60	63	17.8%	1.10 [0.24, 5.09]
Khan, M. R. 2007(2)	24	25	44	48	6.9%	2.18 [0.23, 20.64]
Li, J. 2018	54	54	35	35		Not estimable
Raut, C. P. 2005	134	140	32	32	14.0%	0.32 [0.02, 5.80]
Total (95% CI)		**526**		**375**	**100.0%**	**0.56 [0.26, 1.24]**
Total events	503		365			

Heterogeneity: Chi² = 3.45, df = 4 (P = 0.49); I² = 0%

Test for overall effect: Z = 1.43 (P = 0.15)

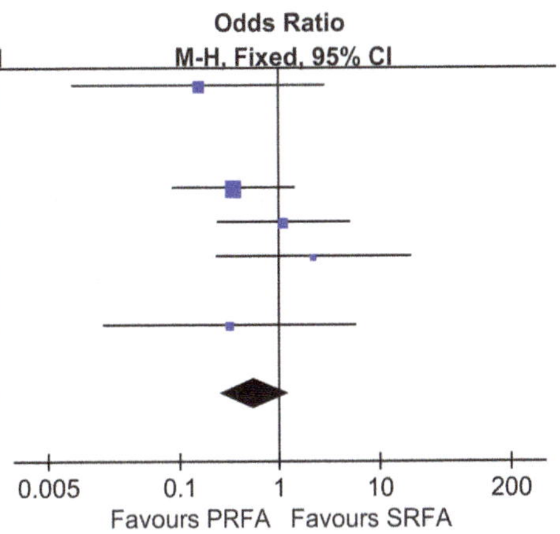

FIGURE 2 | Forest plots for complete ablation rate. Forest plot for complete ablation rate indicates no significantly between the PRFA group as compared with that in the SRFA group (95.63% and 97.33%, respectively; OR, 0.56; 95%CI, 0.26-1.24; $p = 0.15$), and no statistical heterogeneity was found ($\chi^2 = 3.45$; $p = 0.49$, $I^2 = 0\%$).

no significant difference in Child-Pugh A between the two groups ($p = 0.13$; **Supplementary Figure S2**), and the rate of chronic hepatitis B virus infection was indifferent ($p = 0.33$; **Supplementary Figure S3**). All patients in three studies (12, 17, 21) had a core biopsy of the liver cirrhosis, and 3 studies (10, 19, 20) indicated part of patients underlying cirrhosis. Two studies (9, 20) described surgical approach was offered in the dangerous circumstances: Percutaneous ablation might lead to pneumothorax or damage to the diaphragm; or tumors located near the visceral organs such as the gallbladder, colon, or stomach.

The Methodological Quality of the Included Studies

Studies were evaluated for sources of bias using the mNOS. In general, the quality of all included studies was moderate

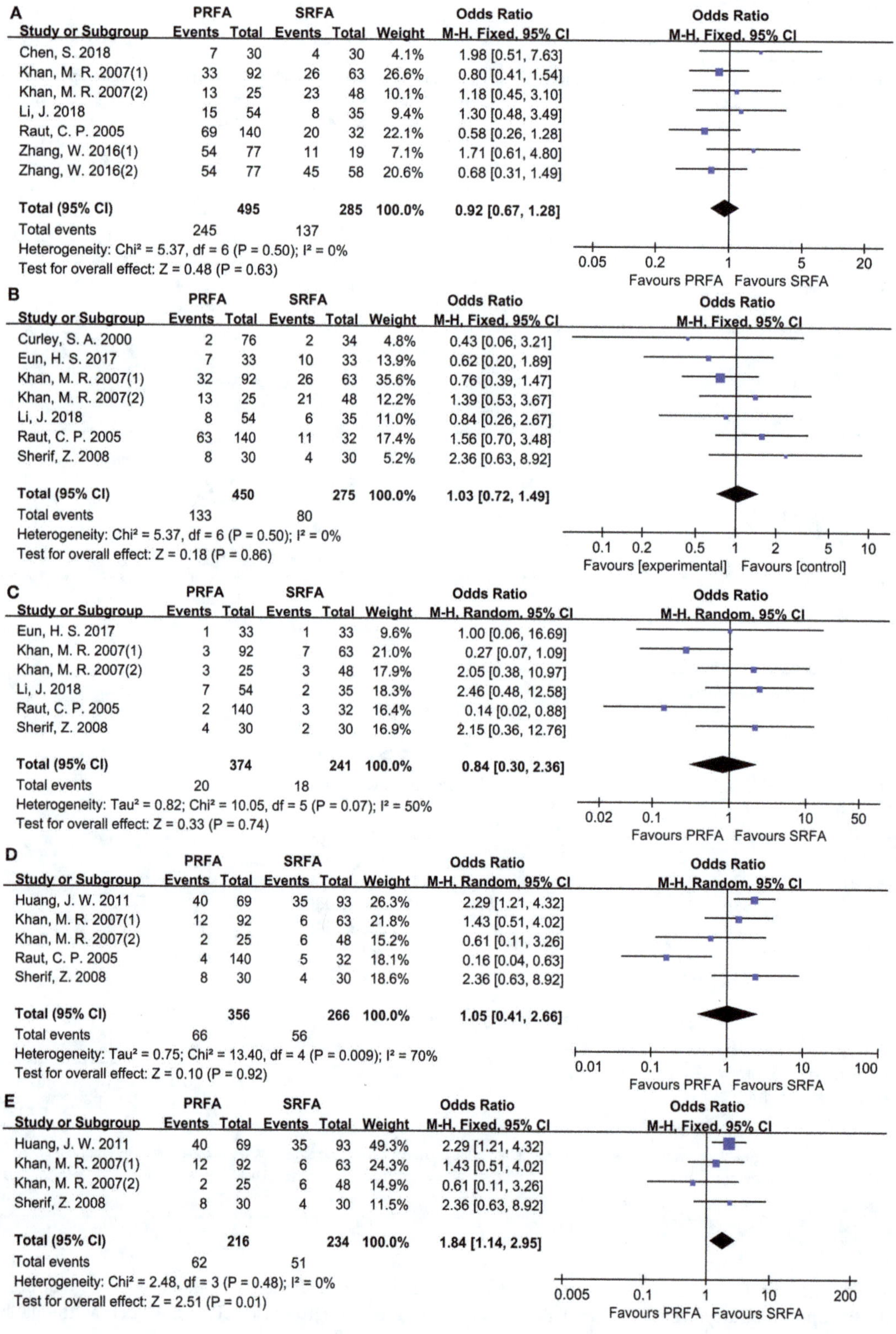

FIGURE 3 | Forest plot for tumor recurrence. **(A)** Forest plot for total recurrence indicates no significantly between the PRFA group and the SRFA group (49.49% and 48.07%, respectively; OR, 0.92; 95% CI, 0.67-1.28; $p = 0.63$). **(B)** Forest plot for intrahepatic recurrence indicates no significantly between PRFA and SRFA (29.56% and 29.09%, respectively; OR, 1.03; 95% CI, 0.72-1.49; $p = 0.86$). **(C)** Forest plot for extrahepatic metastasis indicates no significantly between PRFA and SRFA (5.35% and 7.47%, respectively; OR, 0.84; 95% CI, 0.30-2.36; $p = 0.61$). **(D)** Forest plot for local recurrence indicates no significantly between PRFA and SRFA (18.54% and 21.05%, respectively; OR, 1.05; 95% CI, 0.41-2.66; $p = 0.92$; $\chi^2 = 13.4$; $p = 0.009$, $I^2 = 70\%$). **(E)** Forest plot for sensitivity analysis of local recurrence indicates less recurrent in the SRFA group (28.7% and 21.79%, respectively; OR, 1.84; 95% CI, 1.14-2.95; $p = 0.01$; $\chi^2 = 2.48$; $p = 0.48$, $I^2 = 0\%$).

Study or Subgroup	PRFA Events	PRFA Total	SRFA Events	SRFA Total	Weight	Odds Ratio M-H, Random, 95% CI
Chen, S. 2018	2	30	0	30	3.7%	5.35 [0.25, 116.31]
Curley, S. A. 2000	10	76	4	34	11.0%	1.14 [0.33, 3.92]
Hirooka, M. 2010	0	37	0	37		Not estimable
Huang, J. W. 2011	24	69	15	93	14.5%	2.77 [1.32, 5.83]
Khan, M. R. 2007(1)	8	92	16	63	13.2%	0.28 [0.11, 0.70]
Khan, M. R. 2007(2)	6	25	5	48	10.6%	2.72 [0.74, 10.00]
Li, J. 2018	4	54	4	35	9.6%	0.62 [0.14, 2.66]
Raut, C. P. 2005	13	140	3	32	10.5%	0.99 [0.26, 3.70]
Sherif, Z. 2008	12	30	0	30	4.1%	41.22 [2.30, 737.99]
Zhang, W. 2016(1)	11	77	3	19	10.0%	0.89 [0.22, 3.56]
Zhang, W. 2016(2)	11	77	8	58	12.8%	1.04 [0.39, 2.78]
Total (95% CI)		**707**		**479**	**100.0%**	**1.30 [0.67, 2.53]**
Total events	101		58			

Heterogeneity: Tau² = 0.65; Chi² = 24.14, df = 9 (P = 0.004); I² = 63%
Test for overall effect: Z = 0.77 (P = 0.44)

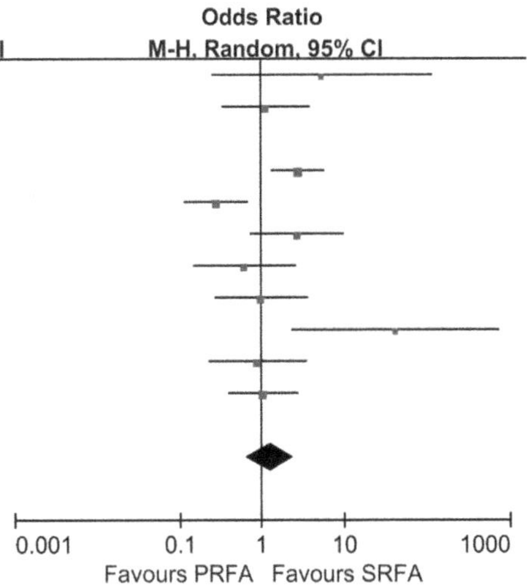

FIGURE 4 | Forest plot for severe perioperative complications. Forest plot for the rate of severe perioperative complications indicates no significantly between the PRFA group and the SRFA group (14.28% and 12.11%, respectively; OR, 1.30; 95% CI, 0.67-2.53; $p = 0.44$).

TABLE 3 | Meta-analysis results of all available studies in complication treatment related.

Postoperative outcomes	No. Cohorts	No. Patients		Heterogeneity test		Model	OR	95%CI	*P*
		PRFA	SRFA	I^2	*P*				
Internal hemorrhage	7	499	296	23	0.26	Fixed	1.73	0.80–3.73	0.16
Biliary injury	5	278	248	0	0.47	Fixed	1.54	0.53–4.42	0.42
Pain	5	402	270	38	0.17	Random	0.60	0.16–2.28	0.46
Liver abscess	4	278	248	0	0.52	Fixed	1.17	0.44–3.13	0.75
Ascites	10	670	442	23	0.23	Fixed	0.57	0.33–0.99	0.05
Organ failure	4	223	175	47	0.13	Random	1.25	0.14–10.95	0.84
Intestinal complications	3	246	140	0	0.48	Fixed	1.05	0.20–5.56	0.95
Fever	3	163	160	0	0.78	Fixed	0.57	0.31–1.05	0.07
Arrhythmia	5	387	212	9	0.41	Fixed	0.54	0.17–1.78	0.31
Atelectasis/Hydropneumothorax	4	333	177	0	0.89	Fixed	0.59	0.13–2.69	0.50
Pleural effusion	10	670	442	0	0.53	Fixed	0.61	0.33–1.09	0.10
Skin burn	4	216	234	0	0.91	Fixed	5.30	1.12–25.05	0.04

PRFA, percutaneous radiofrequency ablation; SRFA, surgical radiofrequency ablation; OR, Odds ratio; 95%CI, 95% confidence intervals.

(**Table 2**). Among the ten studies, four (17, 19, 20, 22) achieved a score of 9/9, four (10–12, 21) scored 8/9, and two (9, 18) scored 7/9. Eight studies (10–12, 17, 19–22) indicated the follow-up duration, and all studies provided intraoperative and postoperative outcomes. The methods for handling missing data were adequately described in one study (17).

Primary Outcomes

Complete Ablation Rate

When data from all included trials were pooled, seven studies (10, 12, 17–21) reported a complete ablation rate. Although the PRFA group appeared to have a lower complete ablation rate than the SRFA group, a meta-analysis using the fixed effects model revealed no significant difference in complete ablation rate between the two groups (95.63 and 97.33%, respectively; OR, 0.56; 95%CI, 0.26–1.24; $p = 0.15$), as well as no statistical heterogeneity ($\chi^2 = 3.45$; $p = 0.49$, $I^2 = 0\%$; **Figure 2**).

Tumor Recurrence

A total of seven cohorts (9–11, 20, 21) were evaluated, with 780 patients reporting overall recurrence data. According to a meta-analysis, the total recurrence in PRFA did not significantly differ from SRFA (49.49 and 48.07%, respectively; OR, 0.92; 95 CI, 0.67–1.28; $p = 0.63$; **Figure 3A**). In addition, the rate of intrahepatic recurrence between the PRFA and SRFA groups was not significantly different (29.56 and 29.09%, respectively; OR, 1.03; 95% CI, 0.72–1.49; $p = 0.86$; **Figure 3B**), and there was no statistical heterogeneity ($\chi^2 = 5.37$; $p = 0.50$, $I^2 = 0\%$). Similarly, the rate of extrahepatic metastasis in the PRFA group was not significantly different compared to the SRFA group (5.35 and 7.47%, respectively; OR, 0.84; 95% CI,

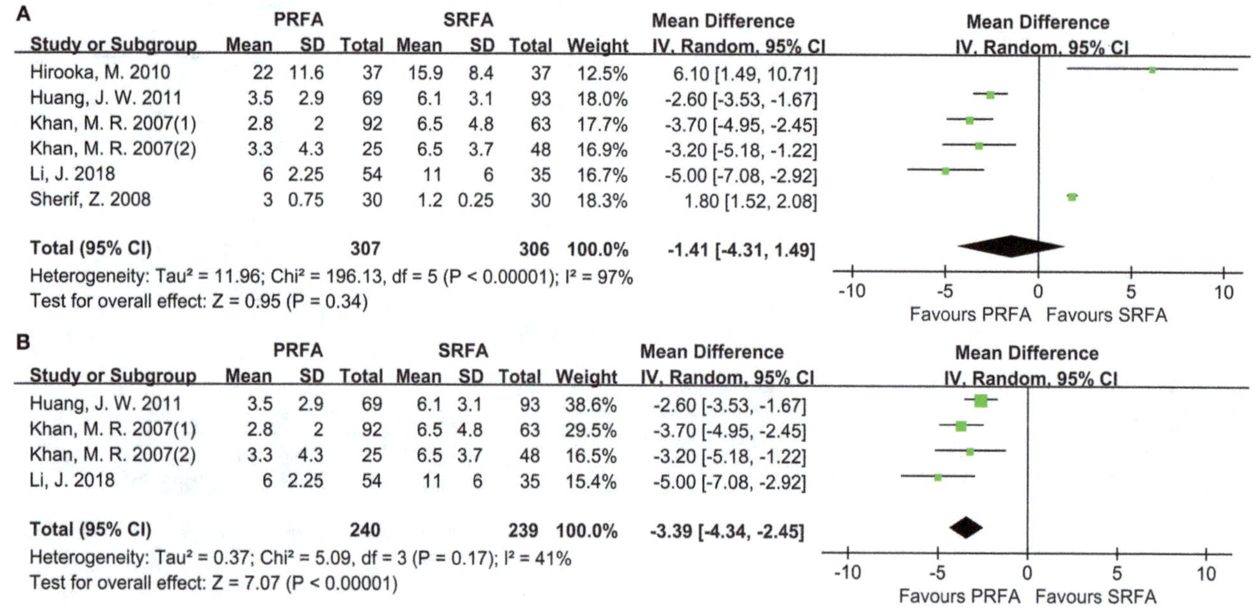

FIGURE 5 | Forest plot for length of hospital stay. **(A)** Forest plot for length of hospital stay indicates no significantly between the PRFA group and the SRFA group (WMD, 0.61 days longer in the SRFA group; 95% CI, −3.28–2.06; $p = 0.65$; ($\chi^2 = 161.19$; $p < 0.00001$, $I^2 = 97\%$). **(B)** Forest plot for sensitivity analysis of length of hospital between PRFA and open approach showed that PRFA group had a significant reduced hospital duration (WMD, 1.4 days longer in the SRFA group; 95% CI, −4.34 to −2.45; $p < 0.00001$; $\chi^2 = 5.09$; $p = 0.17$, $I^2 = 41\%$).

0.30–2.36; $p = 0.61$; **Figure 3C**). However, there was moderate heterogeneity in the data reported by the included studies ($\chi^2 = 10.05$; $p = 0.07$, $I^2 = 50\%$). The indifferent rate of complete ablation resulted in no significant difference in the rates of local recurrence between the PRFA and SRFA groups (18.54 and 21.05%, respectively; OR, 1.05; 95% CI, 0.41–2.66; $p = 0.92$; **Figure 3D**), and statistical heterogeneity was moderate ($\chi^2 = 13.40$; $p = 0.009$, $I^2 = 70\%$). A sensitivity analysis showed that there was significantly less recurrence in the SRFA group (28.7% in PRFA and 21.79% in SRFA, respectively; OR, 1.84; 95% CI, 1.14–2.95; $p = 0.01$; **Figure 3E**).

Postoperative Outcomes

According to pooled analysis data from 11 cohorts of nine included studies (9–12, 18–22), there was no significant difference in the rate of severe perioperative complications between the PRFA and SRFA groups (14.28 and 12.11%, respectively; OR, 1.30; 95% CI, 0.67–2.53; $p = 0.44$; **Figure 4**). However, there was a significant degree of heterogeneity in the data reported by the included studies ($\chi^2 = 24.14$; $p = 0.004$, $I^2 = 63\%$).

Among the various treatment-related complication (**Table 3**), internal hemorrhage rate appeared to be higher in the PRFA group, but meta-analysis revealed that it was not significantly different compared with the SRFA group. There was no difference in the rate of biliary injury, liver abscess, intestinal complications, pain, fever, arrhythmia atelectasis/hydropneumothorax, pleural effusion, and organ failure, including hepatic and renal failure, between the PRFA and SRFA groups. The rate of ascites in the PRFA group was significantly lower compared to the SRFA group (3.58% and 7.92%, respectively; OR, 0.57; 95% CI, 0.33–0.99; $p = 0.05$;), and there was heterogeneity in the data reported by the included studies ($\chi^2 = 11.72$; $p = 0.23$, $I^2 = 23\%$). Three cohorts reported that skin burn was higher in the PRFA group than in the SRFA group, with a meta-analysis showing that it was statistically significant (3.24 and 0%, respectively; OR, 5.30; 95% CI, 1.12–25.05; $p = 0.04$).

The length of hospital stay was reported by six cohorts. Although the PRFA group had a shorter hospital stay, a meta-analysis using the random-effects model found no significant difference (WMD, 1.41 days longer in the SRFA group; 95% CI, −4.31 to 1.49; $p = 0.34$; **Figure 5A**). However, there was statistical heterogeneity ($\chi^2 = 196.13$; $p < 0.00001$, $I^2 = 97\%$). A subgroup analysis revealed that the PRFA group had a significantly reduced hospital duration compared to the open approach group (WMD, 3.39 days longer in the SRFA group; 95% CI, −4.34 to −2.45; $p < 0.00001$; $\chi^2 = 5.09$; $p = 0.17$, $I^2 = 41\%$, **Figure 5B**).

Survival Analysis

Eight cohorts (9–11, 17, 20, 21) reported the 1- and 3-year overall survival (OS) rates and six cohorts (9–11, 17, 21) reported the 5-year OS rates for the PRFA and SRFA groups using hazard ratios (HR). A meta-analysis revealed that there were no significant differences in 1-, 3-, and 5-year OS rates between the PRFA and SRFA groups (**Figures 6A–C**). The HR for the 1-, 3-, and 5-year OS rates were 0.66 (95% CI 0.25–1.70), 0.75 (95% CI 0.50–1.13), and 0.79 (95% CI 0.43–1.43), respectively. The data for the 5-year timepoints revealed moderate heterogeneity ($I^2 = 61\%$, $p = 0.03$), whereas the 1- and 3-year OS rates showed no heterogeneity ($I^2 = 0\%$, $p = 0.99$ and $I^2 = 0\%$, $p = 0.49$, respectively).

Data on disease-free survival (DFS) were reported in six cohorts (11, 17, 20, 21). For the 1- and 3-year DFS, there

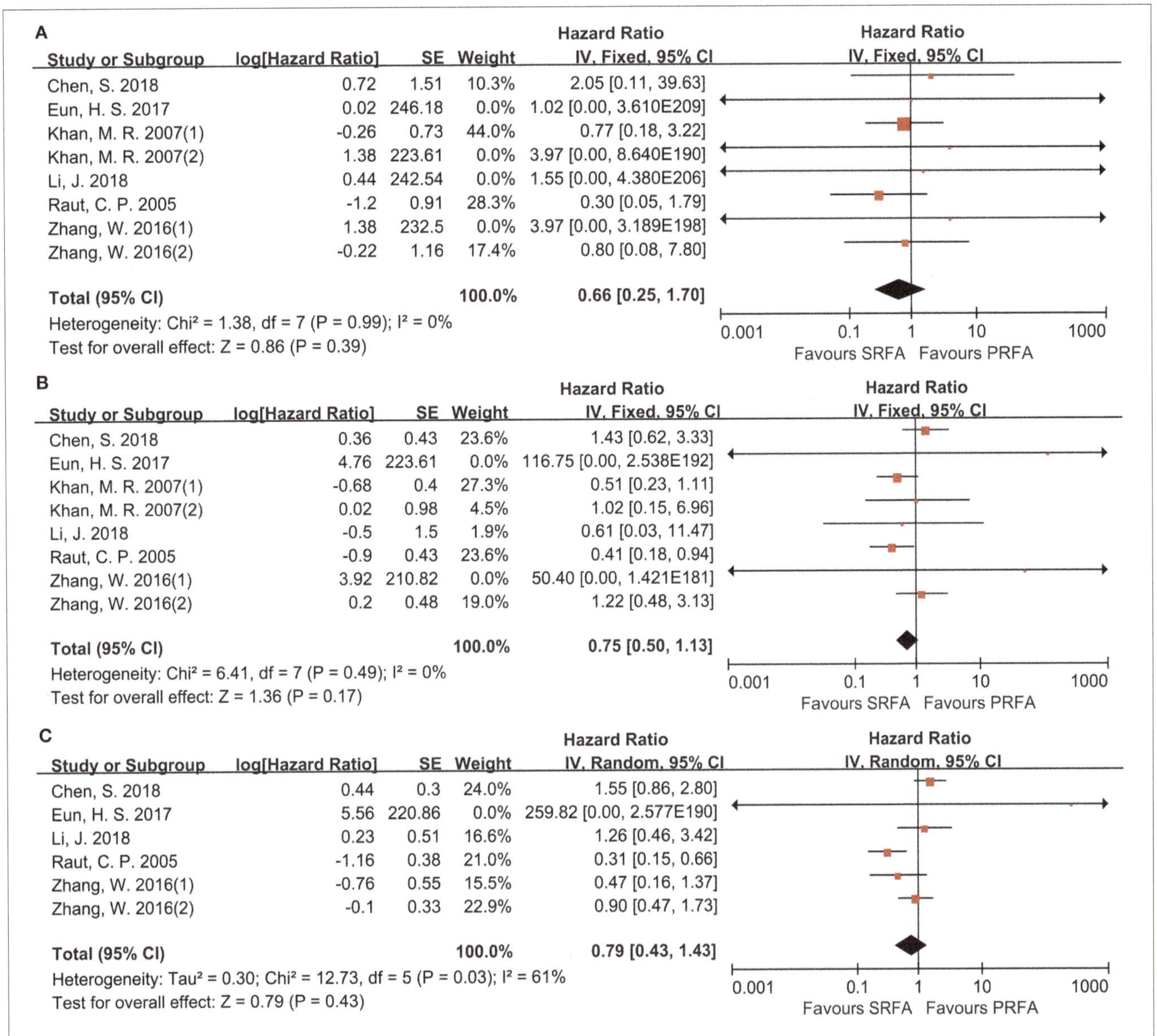

FIGURE 6 | Forest plot for OS. **(A)** Forest plot for 1-year OS indicates no significantly between the PRFA group and the SRFA group (HR, 0.66; 95% CI: 0.25–1.70). **(B)** Forest plot for 3-year OS indicates no significantly between the PRFA group and the SRFA group (HR, 0.75; 95% CI: 0.50–1.13). **(C)** Forest plot for 5-year OS indicates no significantly between the PRFA group and the SRFA group (HR, 0.79; 95% CI: 0.43–1.43)

was no difference between the PRFA and the SRFA groups (**Figures 7A,B**), with HR of 0.82 (95%CI 0.49–1.39) and 1.29 (95%CI 0.69–2.41), respectively. The 5-year DFS of the PRFA group was significantly lower than the SRFA group, with an HR of 0.73 (95%CI 0.54–0.99) and mild heterogeneity ($I^2 = 27\%$, $p = 0.25$; **Figure 7C**).

Sensitivity Analysis and Publication Bias

The sensitivity analysis included eight retrospective studies that scored eight or more stars on the mNOS. There was no significant change in complete ablation rate, complication, total recurrence, intrahepatic recurrence, and extrahepatic metastasis. For local recurrence, the degree of between-study heterogeneity significantly decreased and there was significantly less recurrence in the SRFA group.

According to the Begg's rank correlation test, there was no significant difference in publication bias in complete ablation rate ($p = 0.806$; **Figure 8A**), complication ($p = 0.917$; **Figure 8B**), total recurrence rate ($p = 0.072$; **Figure 8C**), and intrahepatic recurrence rate ($p = 0.764$; **Figure 8D**), respectively.

DISCUSSION

Radiofrequency ablation has emerged as an important alternative treatment to surgery for HCC (23). In this study, there were no significant differences in complete ablation rate, total tumor recurrence rate, and perioperative complications between the

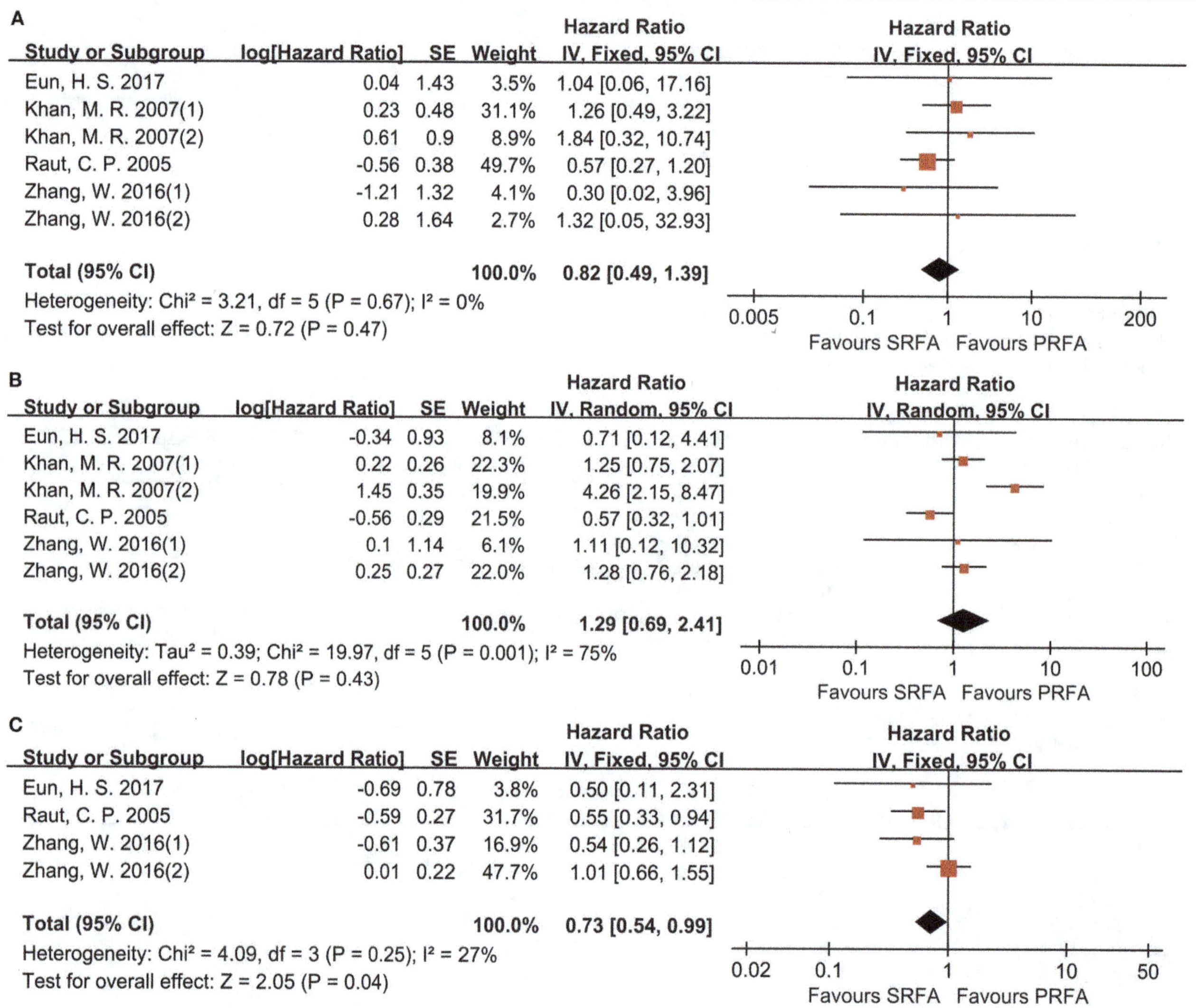

FIGURE 7 | Forest plot for DFS. **(A)** Forest plot for 1-year DFS indicates no significantly between the PRFA group and the SRFA group (HR, 0.82; 95% CI: 0.49–1.39). **(B)** Forest plot for 3-year DFS indicates no significantly between the PRFA group and the SRFA group (HR, 1.29; 95% CI: 0.69–2.41). **(C)** Forest plot for 5-year DFS indicates the PRFA group was significantly lower than the SRFA group (HR, 0.73; 95% CI: 0.54–0.99).

PRFA and SRFA groups. In the sensitivity analysis, the PRFA group had a significantly higher local recurrence rate compared to the SRFA group.

There is a consensus that tumor size is an important risk factor for local recurrence, with a meta-analysis of 34 studies revealing that maximum benefit was observed when the tumor diameter of HCC was less than 2 cm (24). A higher local recurrence rate for a larger size of HCC could be due to several factors. For large tumors, a large number of precisely calculated overlapping coagulations is necessary; statistical data showed that 14 overlapping coagulations are required to cover a 3 cm tumor and its safety margin with an electrode that produces perfect spherical coagulation of 3 cm (25). It is difficult to visualize the tumor after the first coagulation session due to the formation of a hyperechogenic microbubble cloud using ETUS and IOUS. Unfortunately, when more than one treatment session is needed to achieve complete ablation, there is a higher risk of local recurrence (26). A third factor is that larger tumors have irregular borders more frequently than small tumors, making it hard to achieve an oncologic safety margin. According to the hepatectomy principle, the required minimum length of safety margin is 5.5 and 6 mm to achieve 99% and 100% micrometastasis clearance, respectively, in surrounding the liver of HCC patients (27). In our meta-analyses, the tumor size in the PRFA group was smaller than in the SRFA group. However, the PRFA group appeared to have a lower complete ablation rate than the SRFA group, indicating that RFA through a surgical approach may achieve a more precise and complete ablation, particularly in larger tumor nodules.

The pattern of tumor recurrences, such as the total recurrence rate and extrahepatic metastasis, did not differ between PRFA and SRFA. However, sensitivity analysis revealed that the local recurrence rate was higher in the PRFA group compared to the SRFA group. Although the morbidity of malignant seeding in

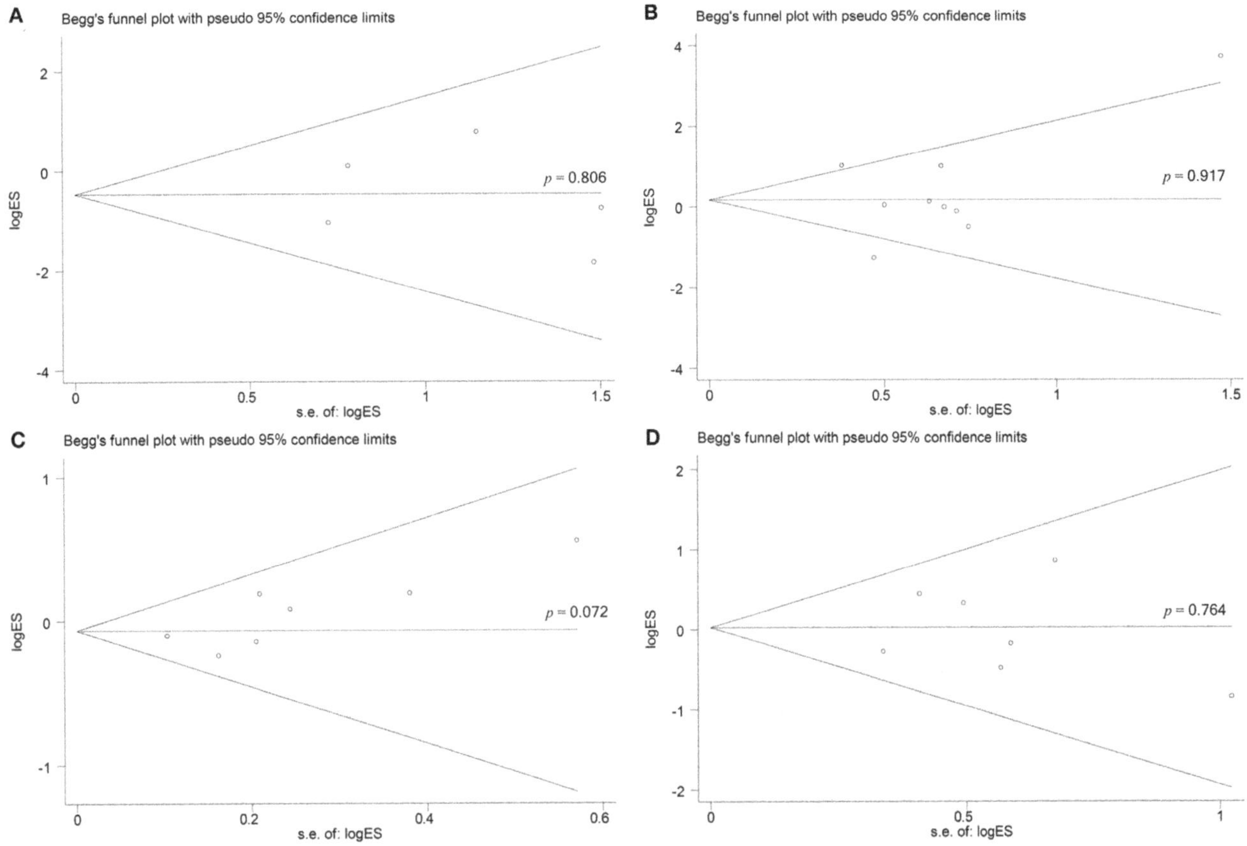

FIGURE 8 | Begg's test for does not indicate any evidence of publication bias. **(A)** Begg's funnel plot with pseudo 95% confidence limits in complete ablation rate ($p = 0.806$). **(B)** Begg's funnel plot with pseudo 95% confidence limits in complications ($p = 0.917$). **(C)** Begg's funnel plot with pseudo 95% confidence limits in total recurrence rate ($p = 0.072$). **(D)** Begg's funnel plot with pseudo 95% confidence limits in intrahepatic recurrence rate ($p = 0.764$).

the needle tract is low, two malignant seeding procedure-related cases occurred only in PRFA, making it difficult to avoid (28).

The tumor location has a significant influence on local tumor control (29). The difficulty in inserting the electrode, as well as in obtaining a sufficient ablative margin along with the liver capsule, have previously been attributed to PRFA for subcapsular tumors (30). In addition, perivascular tumor location has been identified as another risk factor for local tumor recurrence after RFA, mainly due to the insufficient ablative margin created by RFA due to the heat-sink effect (31). The surgical approach, which is different from PRFA, has several advantages: the IOUS probe is placed directly on the liver surface, without sound attenuation by the skin and subcutaneous tissue. Several studies have reported a 30% increase in tumor detection rate using intraoperative ultrasound (32–34). Improved visibility not only allows for more accurate insertion of electrodes and an increased possibility of completely covering the tumor, including its irregular margins, satellites, and safety margin but also prevents damage to organs during the procedure (35). Furthermore, the acoustic window is much wider compared to external ultrasound, which is hampered by the interposition of the ribs and bowel (36). In cases where overlapping coagulations are necessary, the surgical route allows for multiple parallel reinsertions of the electrode, which is difficult to achieve percutaneously. The open approach allows for a larger degree of freedom when inserting the electrodes at an optimal angle, with mobilization of the liver if necessary (37, 38), and ablation zone enlargement can be achieved by using the Pringle maneuver to reduce liver blood flow by 30–40% (39). Because of the pneumoperitoneum and the upward movement of the diaphragm, liver movement is minimal, allowing for precise electrode placement using the laparoscopic approach (17, 40).

The major complication rate of PRFA and SRFA remains controversial. The surgical approach is more invasive and has a significantly higher rate of postoperative ascites than PRFA. Although the incidence of more severe complications, such as bile duct injury, liver abscess, and procedure-related hemorrhage, appeared to be lower in patients than in PRFA, the results were not statistically significant. Therefore, skin burn would not occur due to the real-time visual ablation.

The advantages of PRFA include less invasiveness and a shorter hospital stay (10, 20). Interestingly, a meta-analysis found that there was no significant difference in the duration of hospital stay. However, after removing several studies using the laparoscopic approach (18, 22), it was discovered that PRFA had a shorter postoperative hospital stay than SRFA.

In the SRFA group, less recurrence may lead to a significant difference in DFS; our meta-analysis showed that the 5-year DFS of the SRFA group was significantly higher than the PRFA group. However, there was no significant difference in the 1-, 3-, and 5-year OS rates. Based on the current information, it is difficult to come up with a convincing explanation for this difference. This could be due to the difference in the follow-up treatment after radical ablation (10, 20), requiring a large sample size and more comprehensive follow-up data for follow-up evaluation, instead of the RFA approach.

This review has several limitations. First, all included studies were observational, with a lack of randomized data available, resulting in a selection bias. Second, most of the included studies were conducted over different periods and with different ablation devices. The evolving ablation technology and ultrasonic experience affected the accuracy of ablation. Third, it is difficult to compare PRFA and SRFA in terms of tumor location in the liver; for example, RFA using a surgical approach allows easy access to tumors located in the superior right lobe of the liver, which are often hard to reach percutaneously. In addition, variations in the studied populations may influence the patients' outcomes. Furthermore, the size of the cohort samples was relatively small, leading to a reduction in the quality of the conclusions, while the quality of the studies included, which were assessed using the NOS, was moderate. This is, to our knowledge, the first meta-analysis that attempted to determine the superiority of SRFA over open and laparoscopic approaches in patients with HCC. Therefore, we can reasonably conclude that SRFA provides superior local control and should be the first choice for any patient who can tolerate laparoscopy or laparotomy. Further studies with randomized trials are required to validate the results of this study.

CONCLUSION

In conclusion, based on the findings of this study, the surgical route is the preferred approach for RFA, as it resulted in a better local control rate and disease-free survival.

AUTHOR CONTRIBUTIONS

XY, CW, and ZH contributed to the screening and data collection. TM and ZH contributed to the assessment of the included article. XB and LX contributed to the data analysis. XH and YL contributed to the writing of the manuscript. XC contributed to provide expert insight into the revision of the manuscript and being as corresponding author. All authors approved the final version of the reports and contributed to the study concept, design, data interpretation, and discussion.

ACKNOWLEDGMENTS

The authors acknowledge Jianjun Zhao, MD, Ph.D work in National Cancer Center/Cancer Hospital, Chinese Academy of Medical Sciences and Peking Union Medical College, for the writing assistance and critical revision of the manuscript for important intellectual content.

REFERENCES

1. Kim YS, Lim HK, Rhim H, Lee MW, Choi D, Lee WJ, et al. Ten-year outcomes of percutaneous radiofrequency ablation as first-line therapy of early hepatocellular carcinoma: analysis of prognostic factors. *J Hepatol.* (2013) 58:89–97. doi: 10.1016/j.jhep.2012.09.020
2. Shin SW, Ahn KS, Kim SW, Kim TS, Kim YH, Kang KJ. Liver resection versus local ablation therapies for hepatocellular carcinoma within the milan criteria: A systematic review and meta-analysis. *Ann Surg.* (2021) 273:656–66. doi: 10.1097/SLA.0000000000004350
3. Forner A, Llovet JM, Bruix J. Hepatocellular carcinoma. *Lancet.* (2012) 379:1245–55. doi: 10.1016/B978-1-4377-1454-8.00080-1
4. Wu CC, Tseng CW, Tseng KC, Chen YC, Wu TW, Chang SY, et al. Radiofrequency ablation versus surgical resection for the treatment of solitary hepatocellular carcinoma 2 cm or smaller: A cohort study in Taiwan. *J Formos Med Assoc.* (2021) 120:1249–58. doi: 10.1016/j.jfma.2020.11.010
5. Zhang YH, Su B, Sun P, Li RM, Peng XC, Cai J. Percutaneous radiofrequency ablation is superior to hepatic resection in patients with small hepatocellular carcinoma. *World J Clin Cases.* (2020) 8:4380–7. doi: 10.12998/wjcc.v8.i19.4380
6. Lau WY, Leung TW, Yu SC, Ho SK. Percutaneous local ablative therapy for hepatocellular carcinoma: a review and look into the future. *Ann Surg.* (2003) 237:171–9. doi: 10.1097/01.SLA.0000048443.71734.BF
7. Curley SA, Marra P, Beaty K, Ellis LM, Vauthey JN, Abdalla EK, et al. Early and late complications after radiofrequency ablation of malignant liver tumors in 608 patients. *Ann Surg.* (2004) 239:450–8. doi: 10.1097/01.sla.0000118373.31781.f2
8. Kong WT, Zhang WW, Qiu YD, Zhou T, Qiu JL, Zhang W, et al. Major complications after radiofrequency ablation for liver tumors: analysis of 255 patients. *World J Gastroenterol.* (2009) 15:2651–6. doi: 10.3748/wjg.15.2651
9. Chen S, Wang H, Zhang W, Chen J, Lu P. Clinical application of laparoscopy-assisted and percutaneous radiofrequency ablation for hepatocellular carcinoma. *J Southern Med Univ.* (2018) 38:1147–50. doi: 10.12122/j.issn.1673-4254.2018.09.21
10. Li J, Wu H, Qian K, Zeng Y. Contrast enhanced intraoperative ultrasonography-guided radiofrequency ablation of recurrent hepatocellular carcinoma after hepatectomy through percutaneous or open approach: A retrospective cohort study. *Int J Clin Exp Med.* (2018) 11:13365–73.
11. Zhang W, Jiang L, Yan L, Yang J, Li B, Wen T, et al. Radiofrequency ablation for HCC patients with multifocal tumours meeting the Milan criteria: A single-centre experience. *Dig Liver Dis.* (2016) 48:1485–91. doi: 10.1016/j.dld.2016.07.018
12. Curley SA, Izzo F, Ellis LM, Nicolas Vauthey J, Vallone P. Radiofrequency ablation of hepatocellular cancer in 110 patients with cirrhosis. *Ann Surg.* (2000) 232:381–91. doi: 10.1097/00000658-200009000-00010
13. Moher D, Liberati A, Tetzlaff J, Altman DG. Preferred reporting items for systematic reviews and meta-analyses: the PRISMA statement. *BMJ.* (2009) 339:b2535. doi: 10.1136/bmj.b2535
14. Taggart DP, D'Amico R, Altman DG. Effect of arterial revascularisation on survival: a systematic review of studies comparing bilateral and single internal mammary arteries. *Lancet.* (2001) 358:870–5. doi: 10.1016/S0140-6736(01)06069-X
15. Stang A. Critical evaluation of the Newcastle-Ottawa scale for the assessment of the quality of nonrandomized studies in meta-analyses. *Eur J Epidemiol.* (2010) 25:603–5. doi: 10.1007/s10654-010-9491-z
16. Cumpston M, Li T, Page MJ, Chandler J, Welch VA, Higgins JPT, et al. Updated guidance for trusted systematic reviews: a new edition of the Cochrane Handbook for Systematic Reviews of Interventions. *Cochrane Database Syst Rev.* (2019) (10):ED000142. doi: 10.1002/14651858.ED000142
17. Eun HS, Lee BS, Kwon IS, Yun GY, Lee ES, Joo JS, et al. Advantages of laparoscopic radiofrequency ablation over percutaneous radiofrequency

ablation in hepatocellular carcinoma. *Dig Dis Sci.* (2017) 62:2586–600. doi: 10.1007/s10620-017-4688-6

18. Hirooka M, Kisaka Y, Uehara T, Ishida K, Kumagi T, Watanabe Y, et al. Efficacy of laparoscopic radiofrequency ablation for hepatocellular carcinoma compared to percutaneous radiofrequency ablation with artificial ascites. *Dig Endosc.* (2010) 52:278–85. doi: 10.1111/j.1443-1661.2009.00836.x
19. Huang JW, Hernandez-Alejandro R, Croome KP, Yan LN, Wu H, Chen ZY, et al. Surgical vs percutaneous radiofrequency ablation for hepatocellular carcinoma in dangerous locations. *World J Gastroenterol.* (2011) 17:123–9. doi: 10.3748/wjg.v17.i1.123
20. Khan MR, Poon RTP, Ng KK, Chan AC, Yuen J, Tung H, et al. Comparison of percutaneous and surgical approaches for radiofrequency ablation of small and medium hepatocellular carcinoma. *Arch Surg.* (2007) 142:1136–43. doi: 10.1001/archsurg.142.12.1136
21. Raut CP, Izzo F, Marra P, Ellis LM, Vauthey JN, Cremona F, et al. Significant long-term survival after radiofrequency ablation of unresectable hepatocellular carcinoma in patients with cirrhosis. *Ann Surg Oncol.* (2005) 12:616–28. doi: 10.1245/ASO.2005.06.011
22. Sherif Z, Kotb T, Yousef Y, Foda. Laparoscopic ultrasound-guided versus percutaneous radiofrequency ablation in treatment of unresectable hepatocellular carcinoma. *World J Laparosc Surg.* (2008) 1:1–12. doi: 10.5005/jp-journals-10007-1062
23. Bai X, Cui M, Yang W, Wang H, Wang S, Zhang Z, et al. The 10-year survival analysis of radiofrequency ablation for solitary hepatocellular carcinoma 5 cm or smaller: Primary versus recurrent HCC. *Radiology.* (2021) 300:458–69. doi: 10.1148/radiol.2021200153
24. Casadei Gardini A, Marisi G, Canale M, Foschi FG, Donati G, Ercolani G, et al. Radiofrequency ablation of hepatocellular carcinoma: a meta-analysis of overall survival and recurrence-free survival. *Onco Targets Ther.* (2018) 11:6555–67. doi: 10.2147/OTT.S170836
25. Dodd GD. 3rd, Frank MS, Aribandi M, Chopra S, Chintapalli KN. Radiofrequency thermal ablation: computer analysis of the size of the thermal injury created by overlapping ablations. *AJR Am J Roentgenol.* (2001) 177:777–82. doi: 10.2214/ajr.177.4.1770777
26. Adam R, Hagopian EJ, Linhares M, Krissat J, Savier E, Azoulay D, et al. A comparison of percutaneous cryosurgery and percutaneous radiofrequency for unresectable hepatic malignancies. *Arch Surg.* (2002) 137:1332–9. doi: 10.1001/archsurg.137.12.1332
27. Zhou XP, Quan ZW, Cong WM, Yang N, Zhang HB, Zhang SH, et al. Micrometastasis in surrounding liver and the minimal length of resection margin of primary liver cancer. *World J Gastroenterol.* (2007) 13:4498–503. doi: 10.3748/wjg.v13.i33.4498
28. Stigliano R, Marelli L, Yu D, Davies N, Patch D, Burroughs AK. Seeding following percutaneous diagnostic and therapeutic approaches for hepatocellular carcinoma. What is the risk and the outcome? Seeding risk for percutaneous approach of HCC Cancer. *Treat Rev.* (2007) 33:437–47. doi: 10.1016/j.ctrv.2007.04.001
29. Lee D, Kim J, Lee J, Kim J, Lee M, Rhim H, et al. Laparoscopic liver resection versus percutaneous radiofrequency ablation for small single nodular hepatocellular carcinoma: Comparison of treatment outcomes. *Liver cancer.* (2021) 10:25–37. doi: 10.1159/000510909
30. Hori T, Nagata K, Hasuike S, Onaga M, Motoda M, Moriuchi A, et al. Risk factors for the local recurrence of hepatocellular carcinoma after a single session of percutaneous radiofrequency ablation. *J Gastroenterol.* (2003) 38:977–81. doi: 10.1007/s00535-003-1181-0
31. Lee S, Kang TW, Cha DI, Song KD, Lee MW, Rhim H, et al. Radiofrequency ablation vs. surgery for perivascular hepatocellular carcinoma: Propensity score analyses of long-term outcomes. *J Hepatol.* (2018) 69:70–8. doi: 10.1016/j.jhep.2018.02.026
32. Wood TF, Rose DM, Chung M, Allegra DP, Foshag LJ, Bilchik AJ. Radiofrequency ablation of 231 unresectable hepatic tumors: indications, limitations, and complications. *Ann Surg Oncol.* (2000) 7:593–600. doi: 10.1007/BF02725339
33. Siperstein A, Garland A, Engle K, Rogers S, Berber E, Foroutani A, et al. Local recurrence after laparoscopic radiofrequency thermal ablation of hepatic tumors. *Ann Surg Oncol.* (2000) 7:106–13. doi: 10.1007/s10434-000-0106-x
34. Chung MH, Wood TF, Tsioulias GJ, Rose DM, Bilchik AJ. Laparoscopic radiofrequency ablation of unresectable hepatic malignancies. A phase 2 trial. *Surg Endosc.* (2001) 15:1020–6. doi: 10.1007/s00464-001-0026-2
35. Mulier S, Ni Y, Jamart J, Ruers T, Marchal G, Michel L. Local recurrence after hepatic radiofrequency coagulation: multivariate meta-analysis and review of contributing factors. *Ann Surg.* (2005) 242:158–71. doi: 10.1097/01.sla.0000171032.99149.fe
36. Silas AM, Kruskal JB, Kane RA. Intraoperative ultrasound. *Radiol Clin North Am.* (2001) 39:429–48. doi: 10.1016/S0033-8389(05)70290-6
37. Machi J, Uchida S, Sumida K, Limm WM, Hundahl SA, Oishi AJ, et al. Ultrasound-guided radiofrequency thermal ablation of liver tumors: percutaneous, laparoscopic, and open surgical approaches. *J Gastrointest Surg.* (2001) 5:477–89. doi: 10.1016/S1091-255X(01)80085-8
38. Rose SC, Hassanein TI, Bouvet M, Hart ME, Khanna A, Saville MW. Delivery of radiofrequency ablation probes to the targeted liver malignancy: using all the players on the field. *J Vasc Interv Radiol.* (2002) 13:1060–1. doi: 10.1016/S1051-0443(07)61875-2
39. Tungjitkusolmun S, Staelin ST, Haemmerich D, Tsai JZ, Webster JG, Lee FT, et al. Three-Dimensional finite-element analyses for radio-frequency hepatic tumor ablation. *IEEE Trans Biomed Eng.* (2002) 49:3–9. doi: 10.1109/10.972834
40. Siperstein A, Garland A, Engle K, Rogers S, Berber E, String A, et al. Laparoscopic radiofrequency ablation of primary and metastatic liver tumors. Technical considerations. *Surg Endosc.* (2000) 14:400–5. doi: 10.1007/s004640000067

15

A High Preoperative Platelet-Lymphocyte Ratio is a Negative Predictor of Survival After Liver Resection for Hepatitis B Virus-Related Hepatocellular Carcinoma

*Yun Yang†, Meng-chao Wang†, Tao Tian†, Jian Huang†, Sheng-xian Yuan, Lei Liu, Peng Zhu, Fang-ming Gu, Si-yuan Fu, Bei-ge Jiang, Fu-chen Liu, Ze-ya Pan and Wei-ping Zhou**

Eastern Hepatobiliary Surgery Hospital, Shanghai, China

Correspondence:
Wei-ping Zhou
EHPHWP@126.com

†These authors have contributed equally to this work

Objective: To evaluate the importance of preoperative blood platelet to lymphocyte ratio (PLR) in patients with hepatitis B virus (HBV)-related hepatocellular carcinoma (HCC) after liver surgery and to examine the connection with $CD8^+$ lymph cell infiltration.

Methods: Between 2009 and 2014, consecutive HCC patients who received curative liver surgery were included into this retrospective study. Baseline clinicopathological characteristics were analyzed to identify predictors of recurrence-free and overall patient survival rate after liver resection. The samples of all patients were under Tissue Microarray (TMA) construction and immunohistochemical staining for CD8+.The association of the number of CD8+T-cells in the cancer nests and peritumoral stroma with PLR level was analyzed.

Results: A total of 1,174 HBV-related HCC patients who received a liver resection without any peri-operative adjuvant therapy were enrolled into this retrospective study. Univariate and Multivariate analysis using Cox regression model showed that PLR was an independent factor affecting recurrence and overall survivals. The optimal cutoff of PLR using the receiver operating characteristic curve was 150. There were 236 patients (20.1%) who had a PLR of 150 or more. The 5-year survival rate after liver resection was 71.8% in patients with a PLR of < 150 and it was 57.2% in those with a PLR of 150 or more ($P < 0.001$). Both 5-year recurrence-free and overall survival rates in liver cancer stage A patients at Barcelona Clinic with different PLR group were also significantly different ($P = 0.007$ for recurrence and $P = 0.001$ for overall survival). Similar results were also observed in stage B patients ($P < 0.001$ for recurrence and $P = 0.033$ for overall survival). To determine the association between PLR and the severity of liver inflammation, an immuno-histological examination using $CD8^+$ staining was performed on the liver specimens of 1,174 patients. Compared with low PLR (<150) group, more $CD8^+$T-cells were found in the peritumoral tissue in high PLR (≥ 150) group.

Conclusions: PLR played as an independent factor for predicting the survival after hepatectomy for HCC patients. A high PLR was associated with an accumulation of CD8$^+$ T-cells in the peritumoral stroma.

Keywords: blood platelet-lymphocyte ratio, hepatitis B virus, hepatocellular carcinoma, prognosis, CD8$^+$ T-cell

INTRODUCTION

Inflammation has been regarded as the seventh symptom of cancer (1). Increasing evidence has shown that systemic inflammatory response (SIR) may associate with poor cancer-specific outcomes (2). The effect of SIR on carcinogenesis has been intensively studied. Current understanding suggests that SIR predisposes tumors to proliferate and metastasize through apoptosis inhibition, DNA damage, angiogenesis promotion, and tumor invasion through the upregulation of cytokines (3, 4). The presence of SIR can be determined using various markers, including c-reactive protein (CRP), absolute blood neutrophil or lymphocyte count and its ratios such as neutrophil-to-lymphocyte ratio (NLR), lymphocyte to monocyte ratio (LMR), and platelet to lymphocyte ratio (PLR). An elevation in PLR is another marker of inflammation, and has been proven to be relevant to poor clinical outcomes in different kinds of cancer patients, such as colorectal, esophageal and lung (5–7).

Recently, many researchers analyzed the impact of preoperative PLR to the survival of hepatocellular carcinoma (HCC) patients. The results of these studies are not in agreement with each other. A possible reason is that studies enrolled patients with a different pathogenesis who received discrepant treatment. Besides, a small sample size may be another reason (8–10).

In this paper, we assessed the significance of preoperative PLR in a large cohort of HCC patients with HBV infection who had undergone a potentially curative surgery and to examine the connection with CD8$^+$ lymph cell infiltration.

PATIENTS AND METHODS

Patients

This study enrolled patients with HBV-related HCC who received a liver resection carried out by one surgical team at the Eastern Hepatobiliary Surgery Hospital in Shanghai between January 2009 and June 2014. The diagnosis of HCC before surgery was relied on the diagnostic criteria for HCC according to the European Association for the Study of the Liver (EASL) (11). The pre-operative diagnosis of HCC was verified after the surgery according to the pathologic examinations. The inclusion criteria for this research were pre-operative World Health Organization (WHO) performance status of 0-1; Child-Pugh class A; no macrovascular invasion; no distant metastasis; no chemotherapy, radiotherapy, radiofrequency ablation, or percutaneous ethanol injection before liver resection; curative resection; and resected specimens confirmed as HCC on pathological result.

liver transplantation (LT) is the best treatment option for HCC patients with liver cirrhosis because it eliminates the tumor and the underlying cirrhotic tissue simultaneously. However, LT is not offered to all cirrhotic patients with HCC. In our hospital, patients within Milan criteria would be recommended to receive LT. The reasons why the patients who met the Milan criteria did not receive LT in this study were: (1) refusal to LT; (2) failure of affording the high cost of LT; (3) organ shortage; (4) concern about severe adverse effects of long term oral immunosuppressive agents after LT. In addition, previous studies indicated that overall survival of patients with Milan criteria after liver resection (LR) were comparable to those after LT (12–14). This observation may be attributable to advances in liver surgery, perioperative therapies for patients with liver cirrhosis, and the development of advanced multimodality for the recurrent lesions. Therefore, in this study, for HCC patients with cirrhosis, LR was performed instead of LT.

The definition of curative tumor resection was the complete macroscopic and microscopic removal of all tumors. The maximal diameter of liver tumor was regarded as the tumor size. The patterns of liver surgery were designed based on the lesion size, location, as wells as the residual liver volume. Remove of fewer than three couinaud liver segments was defined as minor liver resection, while remove of three or more liver segments was defined as major liver resection. The clinical staging was determined by the Barcelona Clinic Liver Cancer (BCLC) staging system (11). The histological grade of cirrhosis and inflammation in peritumor tissue was evaluated according to the Ishak classification (15). The histological grade of tumor differentiation was determined by reference to the Edmondson Steiner grading system.

All HBV-related HCC patients had a chest X-ray, ultrasonography (USG), contrast computed tomography (CT) or magnetic resonance imaging (MRI) of their liver. Laboratory blood tests were used to obtain the following: hepatitis B surface antigens (HBsAg) and HBeAg, hepatitis C virus antibody (HCV-Ab), serum alpha-Fetoprotein (AFP), carcinoembryonic antigen (CEA) and carbohydrate antigen 19-9 (CA19-9) antigens, white blood cell/neutrophil/lymphocyte/monocyte/platelet (PLT)

Abbreviations: HBV, hepatitis B virus; HCC, hepatocellular carcinoma; PLR, Platelet-Lymphocyte Ratio; SIR, systemic inflammatory response; CRP, c-reactive protein; NLR, neutrophil-to-lymphocyte ratio; LMR, lymphocyte to monocyte ratio; LT, liver transplantation; LR, liver resection; BCLC, Barcelona Clinic Liver Cancer; USG, ultrasonography; CT, computed tomography; MRI, magnetic resonance imaging; HBsAg, hepatitis B surface antigens; HBeAg hepatitis B e antigens; HCV-Ab, hepatitis C virus antibody; AFP, alpha-Fetoprotein; CEA, carcinoembryonic antigen; CA19-9 carbohydrate antigen 19-9; ALT, alanine aminotransferases; AST, aspartate aminotransferases; PT, prothrombin time; TACE, transarterial chemoembolization; PRFA, percutaneous radiofrequence ablation; PEI, percutaneous ethanol injection; TMA, tissue microarray; PSM, Propensity score matching; RFS, recurrence-free survival; OS, overall survival; SD, standard deviation; ROC curve, receiver operating characteristic curve; HR, Hazard ratio; OR, Odds ratio; 95% CI,95% Confidence Interval; AGS, antigens.

counts, serum albumin, serum total bilirubin, alanine (ALT) and aspartate (AST) aminotransferases, and prothrombin time (PT). All patients were positive for HBsAg and negative for HCV-Ab. Written informed consent was obtained from all patients. The study was approved by the Institutional Review Board of the Eastern Hepatobiliary Surgery Institute, Shanghai, China.

Follow-Up and Treatment for Tumor Recurrences

The patients were reviewed once every 3 months within the beginning 2 years, and then once every 6 months afterwards. All review procedure was conducted by hospital staff who were blinded from this research. All patients were reviewed for post-operative recurrence with regular assessment using AFP, chest x-ray and abdominal USG. A CT and (or) MRI examination were performed every 3 months after lever resection. The diagnostic criterion for HCC recurrence were the same as for pre-operative diagnosis. If recurrence was confirmed, the tumors were treated aggressively through a multimodal treatment that included re-resection, transarterial chemoembolization (TACE), percutaneous radiofrequence ablation (PRFA), and percutaneous ethanol injection (PEI). The procedure was decided by the tumor recurrence pattern, reserved liver function and general condition of the patient when the recurrence was diagnosed.

During the study period, a total of 723 patients suffered from tumor recurrence. Of 723 patients, there were 602 patients developed intrahepatic recurrence, 59 patients with extrahepatic metastasis, and 62 patients with synchronous intrahepatic and extrahepatic recurrences. Because extrahepatic metastasis is a contraindication of liver transplantation, 121 patients with extrahepatic metastasis were not recommended for liver transplantation. As described above, in our hospital, Milan criteria was used to select patients for liver transplantation. Of 602 patients with intrahepatic recurrence, only 276 patients with tumor recurrence met Milan criteria. And liver transplantation was recommended. However, they did not receive liver transplantation. The reasons why these 276 patients did not receive liver transplantation as the first treatment were due to organ shortage ($n = 73$), refusal to liver transplantation ($n = 105$) or socio-financial reasons ($n = 98$).

Tissue Microarray (TMA) and Immunohistochemical Staining

The samples of all patients were under TMA construction and immunohistochemical staining analysis as previously described (16). The primary antibodies used were mouse monoclonal anti-CD8 (1:100, Abcam). Microarrays were assessed through two-hundred times magnification under light microscopy by 2 independent observers who had no knowledge of the patient's clinicopathologic data. Any discrepancies were quickly resolved by discussion between the observers. For CD8 staining, positive cells in each 1-mm-diameter cylinder were counted and expressed as the mean value of the triplicates (cells/spot).

Propensity Score Matching (PSM)

To reduce potential biases which are inherent in retrospective studies, propensity score matching (PSM) was used. Patients with high PLR ($\geq$150) were matched with patients with low PLR (<150) using the PSM as previous description (17, 18). Covariates entered into the PSM model included hepatitis B e antigen (HbeAg), alpha-fetoprotein (AFP), aspartate aminotransferase (AST), HBV-DNA load, Ishak inflammation score, tumor diameter, tumor encapsulation, microvascular invasion, tumor number, extent of liver resection, and tumor differentiation. PSM was performed as a 1:1 matching between patients with high PLR ($\geq$150) and the low PLR (<150). The matching procedure has been described previously (19).

Statistical Analysis

Recurrence-free survival (RFS) and overall survival were used as primary endpoints. RFS was counted from the date of the operation to the date of detection of recurrence, or censored at the last known review date. Overall survival (OS) was defined as the interval between the date of operation and death. Patients clinical and follow-up data were collected from the clinical records and the hospital cancer data center. This study was censored on May 31, 2019. For individuals who followed-up before that date, a censor was applied on the last date the patient was evaluated either radiologically or clinically, and was found to have no recurrence for RFS, and on the last date the patient was known to be alive for OS.

All data were shown as the mean $\pm$ standard deviation (SD) or median (range). The characteristics of HCC cases were compared using a student two-sample unpaired t-test for continuous variables and a χ^2 test for categorical variables. Kaplan-Meier method was used to analyze RFS and OS curves. Differences between RFS and OS curves were evaluated by the log-rank test. Cox proportional hazard regression models were used to identify the independent factors of recurrence and overall survival based on the variables selected in the univariate analysis. Clinicopathological characteristics that might be associated with the number of $CD8^+$T-cells in the peritumoral stroma were evaluated by univariate logistic regression analysis, and the variables that were significant ($P < 0.05$) were subjected in the stepwise multivariate analysis. Statistical analysis was performed with SPSS 13.0 (SPSS Inc, Chicago IL).

We conducted nomograms on the results of multivariate analysis in the entire cohort and by the package of rms in R version 3.5.1 (http://www.r-project.org/). The accuracy of prediction of nomogram was quantified by the concordance index (C-index). The difference of C-index between nomograms and other predictors were compared by the rcorrp.cens in Hmisc in R (20) The prediction of survival between nomogram and other predictors was compared using ROC curve analysis. Definition of statistical significance was $P < 0.05$ in two-tailed.

RESULTS

Baseline Characteristics

During the investigation period, 1,211 patients with HBV-related HCC received a liver resection with curative intent, and they were enrolled into this study. Thirty seven patients were excluded from this study because of an early metastasis and (or) HCC recurrence within 1 month of surgery ($n = 11$), preoperative hepatic arterial chemoembolization ($n = 5$), death within 30 days of surgery due to liver failure ($n = 6$), or clinical evidence of infection or other inflammatory conditions before surgery ($n = 15$). After exclusion, 1,174 HCC patients remained for analysis (**Supplementary Figure 1**).

The background clinical characteristics of the cases are listed in **Supplementary Table 1**. The median age was 50 (range 20–70) years. 1035 (88.16%) patients were males and 139 (11.84%) females. All patients were positive for HBsAg and negative for anti-HCV. 281 (23.93%) patients were HBeAg positive, and the remaining 893 (76.07%) patients were negative for HBeAg. All patients are with a preserved liver function of Child-Pugh A grade. The median inflammation score of the patients was 6 (range 2–14), and the median fibrosis score of the patients was 4 (range 1–6). There were 552 (47.02%) patients with their HBV-DNA level ≥2,000 IU/ml. The diameters of the initial tumors ranged from 0.5 to 22 cm (median 4.9 cm). Using the BCLC staging, 695 patients (59.20%) were in BCLC stage 0 and A, 479 patients (40.80%) were in stage B. Of the 1,174 patients, there were 425 patients (36.20%) who had microvascular invasion. There were 521 (44.38%) patients who had multiple tumor nodules, and 596 (50.77%) patients who had complete tumor encapsulation. There were 230 patients received major liver resection. The tumors were well-differentiated in 245 patients (20.87%) (E-S grades I and II), and poorly differentiated in 929 patients (79.13%) (E-S grades III and IV).

The censor date of the investigation was May 31, 2019. The median follow-up time was 40.2 months (range 3.3 - 125.0 months).

Association of PLR With Clinico-Pathological Characteristics

Receiver operating characteristic (ROC) curve analysis was used to determine the cutoff value for PLR. An optimal cutoff value for PLR was 150, and this cutoff value was used to categorize between the high and the low PLR groups. The area under curve is 0.743, the specificity is 0.738, and the sensitivity is 0.710 (**Supplementary Figure 2**). 236 (20.10%) patients were categorized into the high (≥150) PLR group, and 938 (79.90%) patients were categorized into the low (<150) PLR group. **Table 1** shows the relationships of the clinico-pathological characteristics between the two groups of patients. The high PLR group had a significantly higher AFP level, higher aspartate aminotransferase value, higher Ishak inflammation score, higher viral load (≥2,000 IU/ml), larger tumor size, poorer tumor differentiation, and larger proportion of HBeAg positive patients (all $P < 0.05$), although no significant differences were found in age, gender, and Ishak fibrosis score (all $P > 0.05$). More patients received major liver resection in the high PLR group than the low PLR group ($P < 0.001$). Besides, the high PLR group had significantly more patients with multiple tumor nodules, no tumor encapsulation, and more patients with microvascular invasion than the low PLR group (all $P < 0.05$). Thus, a high PLR was associated with advanced malignant characteristics of HCC. Platelet, white blood cell and lymphocyte counts was also listed in **Table 1**, the low PLR group had a significantly lower platelet counts, and higher lymphocyte counts (all $P < 0.001$), however, the difference in white blood cell counts between two groups was not significant ($P > 0.05$).

PSM analysis created 226 pairs of patients. Baseline characteristics of the patients in the propensity matched cohort are listed in **Supplementary Table 2**. After PSM, no significant differences were found in all clinicopathological variables between the two groups ($P > 0.05$).

Correlation of PLR With Prognosis of Patients With HCC

The median follow-up of all the HCC cases was 40.2 months. The Kaplan-Meier survival curves comparing the low vs. the high PLR groups are shown in **Figures 1A,B**. The cumulative 1, 3 and 5-year recurrence-fee survival (RFS) rates of the high PLR group (≥150) were significantly lower than the low PLR group (57.30, 30.92, and 16.35%, respectively, vs. 75.71, 48.13, and 36.92%, respectively, log-rank test, $P < 0.001$). Likewise, high PLR (≥150) was negatively correlated with the cumulative 1, 3, and 5-year overall survival (OS) rates of 83.92, 59.13, and 44.92%, respectively, for the high PLR group vs. 92.51, 77.06, and 64.51%, respectively, for the low PLR group, log-rank test ($P < 0.001$).

According to the BCLC classification, 695 patients were classified into stage 0 and A. Of these patients, 95 patients are with their PLR ≥150 and 600 have low PLR (<150). The prognosis of patients with elevated PLR (≥150) are worse than those with low PLR (<150). For example, the 1, 3, and 5-year RFS rates were 63.25, 35.37, and 19.53% vs. 80.09, 51.73, and 39.21%, respectively ($P < 0.001$). Whereas, the 1, 3, and 5-year OS rates were 81.92, 61.63, and 42.45% vs. 94.73, 82.15, and 68.65%, respectively ($P < 0.001$) (**Figures 1C,D**).

Of patients in the BCLC stage B, the prognosis of cases ($n = 141$) with high lPLR (≥150) was poorer than those patients ($n = 338$) with low levels of PLR (<150). For example, the 1, 3, and 5-year RFS rates were 53.21, 29.73, and 17.11% vs. 66.51, 41.76, and 33.05%, respectively ($P < 0.001$). Whereas, the 1, 3, and 5-year OS rates were 85.71, 57.32, and 43.31% vs. 89.72, 67.65, and 56.82%, respectively ($P = 0.033$) (**Figures 1E,F**).

After PSM, the 1, 3, and 5 year RFS rates of high PLR (≥150) group were 58.52, 33.53, and 16.95%, respectively, while the corresponding figures for the patients with low PLR (<150) were 68.91, 43.32, and 34.44%, respectively. The cumulative RFS of high PLR (≥150) group was significantly lower than that of the low PLR (<150) group after PSM ($P = 0.001$). After PSM, the 1, 3, and 5 year cumulative OS rates of the patient with high PLR (≥150) were 83.81, 59.33, and 46.32%, respectively, compared with the patients with low PLR (<150) of 87.52, 66.83, and 55.37%, respectively. Thus, the OS rates of cases with high PLR (≥150) were significantly lower than those in cases with low PLR (<150) in the PSM cohort ($P = 0.032$) (**Supplementary Figures 3A,B**).

Factors Affecting Prognosis of HCC in the Total Study Population

Independent risk factors for RFS and OS were identified using cox regression analyses. Univariate regression analysis indicated that alanine and aspartate aminotransferase levels,

TABLE 1 | Comparison of Clinicopathological and Demographic Characteristics of Patients With Elevated and Low PLR.

	Low PLR(<150), *N* = 938	Elevated PLR (≥150), *N* = 236	*P*-value
Gender			
Male	831 (88.59)	204 (86.44)	0.361
Female	107 (11.41)	32 (13.56)	
Age (years)[a]	49.99 ± 10.28	50.06 ± 11.06	0.166
Liver Cirrhosis			0.486
Yes	565 (60.23)	148 (62.71)	
No	373 (39.77)	88 (37.29)	
HBeAg			0.013
Positive	210 (22.38)	71 (30.08)	
Negative	728 (77.62)	165 (65.92)	
AFP (ng/ml)			0.020
≥20	567 (60.45)	162 (68.64)	
<20	371 (39.55)	74 (31.36)	
Alanine aminotransferase (U/L)			0.152
≥40	440 (46.91)	123 (52.12)	
<40	498 (53.09)	113 (47.88)	
Aspartate aminotransferase (U/L)			<0.001
≥40	384 (40.94)	137 (58.05)	
<40	554 (59.06)	99 (41.95)	
Total bilirubin (ummol/ml)			0.646
≥17.1	341 (36.35)	82 (34.75)	
<17.1	597 (63.65)	154 (65.25)	
Albumin (g/L)			0.476
≥35	893 (95.20)	222 (94.07)	
<35	45 (4.80)	14 (5.93)	
HBV DNA (IU/ml)			0.041
≥2,000	427 (45.52)	125 (52.97)	
<2,000	511 (54.48)	111 (47.03)	
Ishak inflammation score[a]	5.12 ± 1.73	6.34 ± 2.98	0.002
Ishak fibrosis score[a]	4.73 ± 1.56	5.08 ± 1.36	0.251
Tumor diameter (cm)[a]	5.47 ± 3.67	8.64 ± 4.34	<0.001
Tumor encapsulation			<0.001
None	504 (53.73)	145 (61.02)	
Complete	434 (46.27)	91 (38.98)	
Major resection			
Yes	154 (16.41)	76 (32.20)	<0.001
No	784 (83.59)	160 (67.80)	
Microvascular invasion			0.012
Yes	323 (34.43)	102 (43.22)	
No	615 (65.57)	134 (56.78)	
Tumor number			<0.001
Single	553 (58.96)	100 (42.37)	
Multiple	385 (41.04)	136 (57.63)	
Tumor differentiation			0.001
I/II	214 (22.81)	31 (13.14)	
III/IV	724 (77.19)	205 (86.86)	
Platelet Counts (*10^9/L)	134.10 ± 56.31	231.63 ± 82.37	<0.001
White blood cell Counts (*10^9/L)	4.61 ± 1.80	4.78 ± 1.28	0.121
Lymphocyte Counts (*10^9/L)	1.61 ± 0.63	1.12 ± 0.38	<0.001

[a] *Age, Ishak inflammation score, Ishak fibrosis score, and tumor diameter are expressed as mean ± SD.*
HBeAg, hepatitis B e antigen; AFP, alpha-fetoprotein.

HBV DNA level, Ishak inflammation score, PLR, AFP, tumor encapsulation, microvascular invasion, multiple HCC, tumor differentiation, tumor size, and cirrhosis were each associated significantly with worse RFS (**Table 2**). Whereas, alanine and aspartate aminotransferase levels, albumin, HBV DNA level, PLR, AFP, tumor encapsulation, microvascular invasion, multiple HCC, tumor differentiation, and tumor size were associated with worse OS (**Table 3**). Multivariate Cox regression analysis indicated HBV DNA level ≥2,000 IU/ml (HR = 1.235; P = 0.013), Ishak inflammation score ≥3 (HR = 1.116; P = 0.035), PLR ≥150 (HR = 1.494; P < 0.001), AFP ≥20 ng/ml (HR = 1.363; P < 0.001), absence of complete tumor encapsulation (HR = 0.785; P = 0.006), microvascular invasion (HR = 1.126; P = 0.017), multiple HCC (HR = 1.216; P =0.015), and tumor size ≥5 cm (HR = 1.285; P = 0.003) were independent risk predictors of worse RFS (**Table 2**), whereas aspartate aminotransferase ≥40 U/L (HR = 1.531; P = 0.001), HBV DNA level ≥2,000 IU/ml (HR = 1.485; P = 0.001), PLR ≥150 (HR = 1.327; P = 0.017), AFP ≥20 ng/ml (HR = 1.424; P = 0.004), absence of complete tumor encapsulation (HR = 0.780; P = 0.029), and tumor size ≥5 cm (HR = 1.692; P < 0.001) were independent risk predictors of worse OS (**Table 3**).

Additional cox regression analyses was performed to assess the Independent risk factors for RFS and OS in the PSM cohort. Univariate and multivariate analyses of RFS and OS after liver surgery in the PSM cohort are indicated in **Supplementary Tables 3, 4**. On multivariate analyses, high PLR (≥150) remained independently associated with a worse RFS (HR 1.487, 95% CI 1.182–1.870; P = 0.001) and OS (HR 1.309, 95% CI 1.201–1.738; P = 0.041).

Construction Nomograms and Comparison of the Performance Between Nomograms and Predictors

The independent risk factors derived from multivariate analysis of RFS in all patients were performed to construct the RFS nomogram (**Figure 2A**). Similarly, the OS nomogram analysis were also performed (**Figure 2B**). The C-index of nomograms for RFS and OS were 0.649 (95% CI: 0.626–0.671) and 0.716 (95% CI: 0.685–0.746), respectively. Other predictors including the independent risk factors were compared with the nomograms to determine the accuracy of prediction from different models (**Supplementary Table 5**). The C-index of the nomogram for RFS was 0.649, which was statistically higher than the PLR (0.549), AFP (0.564), tumor encapsulation (0.561), tumor diameter (0.582), HBV-DNA (0.542), tumor number (0.538), ishak inflammation score (0.567) and MVI (0.559) (all P < 0.001). As for the OS, the C-index of the nomogram was 0.716, which was statistically higher than the PLR (0.559), aspartate aminotransferase (0.591), AFP (0.584), tumor encapsulation (0.591), HBV-DNA (0.569) and tumor diameter (0.635) (all P < 0.001). These data illustrated a more predication accuracy of the established nomograms than other predictors. ROC curve analyses showed the nomograms for RFS and OS both

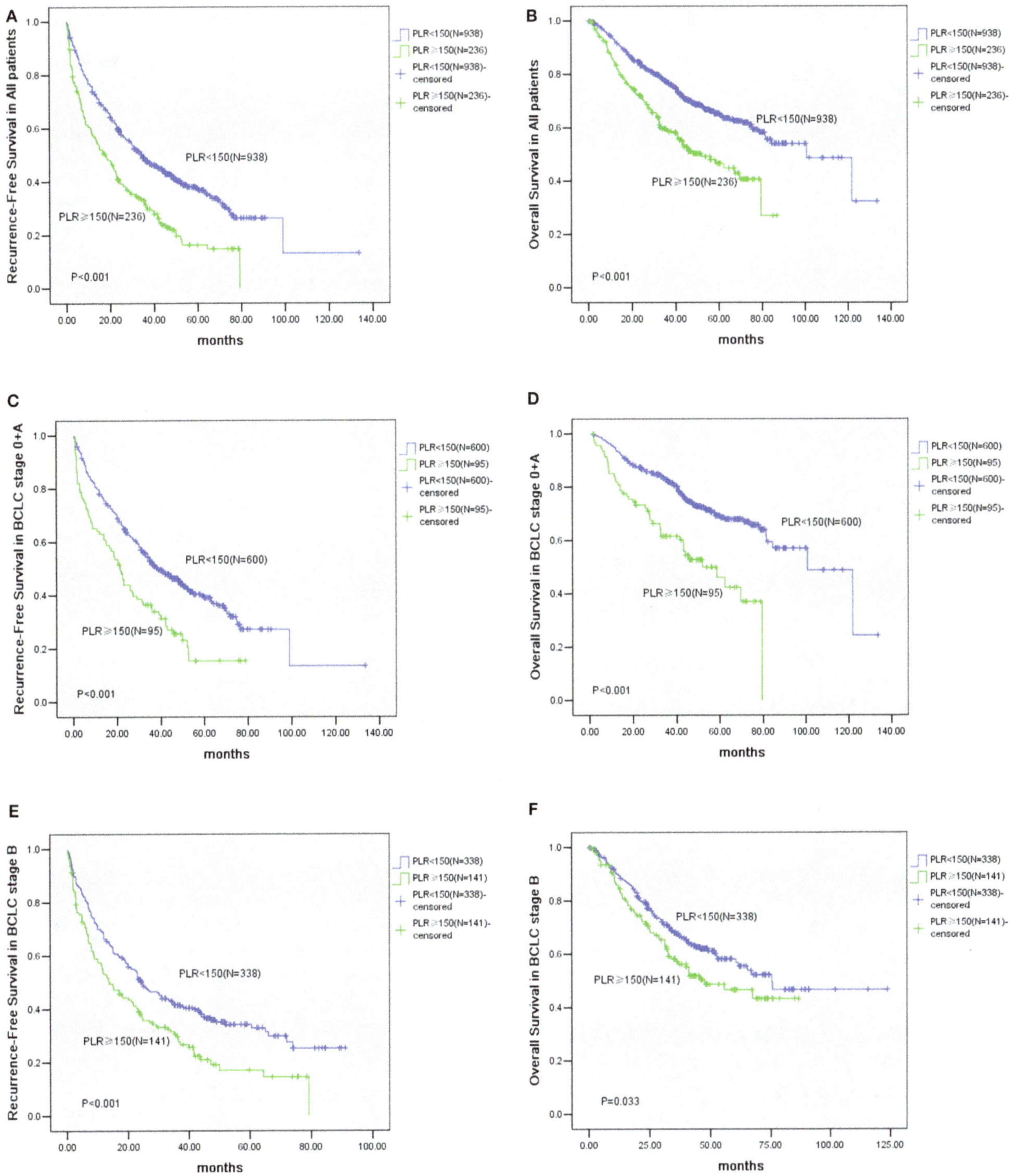

FIGURE 1 | Kaplan-Meier analysis of 1,174 Hepatocellular Carcinoma (HCC) patients and survival curves of 695 Barcelona Clinic Liver Cancer (BCLC) stage 0 + A patients and survival analysis of HCC patients in BCLC stage B. **(A)** The cumulative Recurrence-Free Survival (RFS) curve of HCC patients with high PLR (≥150) and patients with low PLR (<150) ($P < 0.001$). **(B)** The cumulative Overall Survival (OS) curve of HCC patients with high PLR (≥150) and patients with low PLR (<150) ($P < 0.001$). **(C)** The cumulative RFS curve of patients with high PLR (≥150) and patients with low PLR (<150) in BCLC stage 0 + A ($P < 0.001$). **(D)** The cumulative OS curve of patients with high PLR (≥150) and patients with low PLR (<150) in BCLC stage 0 + A ($P < 0.001$). **(E)** The cumulative Recurrence-Free Survival (RFS) curve of patients with elevated PLR (≥150) and other patients with low PLR (<150) in BCLC stage B ($P < 0.001$). **(F)** The cumulative Overall Survival (OS) curve of patients with elevated PLR (≥150) and other patients with low PLR (<150) in BCLC stage B ($P = 0.033$).

TABLE 2 | Univariate and Multivariate analysis of factors associated with Recurrence-free survival of patients with HCC.

	Hazard ratio(95%CI)	*P*-value
Univariate analysis		
Gender (male vs. female)	0.901 (0.719–1.129)	0.367
Age (year) (≤60 vs. >60)	0.848 (0.695–1.035)	0.105
Alanine aminotransferase (≥40 vs. <40 U/L)	1.212 (1.047–1.302)	0.020
Aspartate aminotransferase (≥40 vs. <40 U/L)	1.504 (1.300–1.741)	<0.001
Albumin (<35 vs. ≥35 g/L)	0.806 (0.588–1.105)	0.180
HBV DNA (≥2,000 vs. <2,000 IU/ml)	1.577 (1.564–1.883)	<0.001
Ishak inflammation score (≥3 vs. <3)	1.227 (1.156–1.345)	0.014
Ishak fibrosis score (≥3 vs. <3)	0.825 (0.731–1.267)	0.328
PLR (≥150 vs. <150)	1.747 (1.474–2.069)	<0.001
AFP (≥20 vs. <20 ng/ml)	1.649 (1.409–1.929)	<0.001
HBeAg (positive vs. negative)	1.166 (0.995–1.366)	0.058
Tumor encapsulation (yes vs. no)	0.698 (0.603–0.809)	<0.001
Major resection (yes vs. no)	1.168 (0.973–1.403)	0.096
Microvascular invasion (yes vs. no)	1.575 (1.343–1.847)	<0.001
Tumor number (multiple vs. single)	1.679 (1.377–2.048)	<0.001
Tumor differentiation (III+IV vs. I+II)	1.560 (1.281–1.899)	<0.001
Tumor diameter (≥5 vs. <5 cm)	1.644 (1.419–1.904)	<0.001
Liver cirrhosis (yes vs. no)	1.256 (1.176–1.442)	0.003
Multivariate analysis		
HBV DNA (≥2,000 vs. <2,000 IU/ml)	1.235 (1.133–1.465)	0.013
Ishak inflammation score (≥3 vs. <3)	1.116 (1.016–1.278)	0.035
PLR (≥150 vs. <150)	1.494 (1.350–1.786)	<0.001
AFP (≥20 vs. <20 ng/ml)	1.363 (1.254–1.610)	<0.001
Tumor encapsulation (yes vs. no)	0.785 (0.712–0.879)	0.006
Microvascular invasion (yes vs. no)	1.126 (1.114–1.357)	0.017
Tumor number (multiple vs. single)	1.216 (1.128–1.424)	0.015
Tumor diameter (≥5 vs. <5 cm)	1.285 (1.188–1.518)	0.003

HRs(95% CI) and P-values were calculated using univariate and multivariate Cox proportional hazard regression.
HBeAg, hepatitis B e antigen; AFP, alpha-fetoprotein.

TABLE 3 | Univariate and Multivariate analysis of factors associated with Overall survival of patients with HCC.

	Hazard ratio (95%CI)	*P*-value
Univariate analysis		
Gender (male vs. female)	0.918 (0.674–1.249)	0.585
Age (year) (≤60 vs. >60)	0.983 (0.754–1.280)	0.897
Alanine aminotransferase (≥40 vs. <40 U/L)	1.334 (1.091–1.631)	0.005
Aspartate aminotransferase (≥40 vs. <40 U/L)	2.040 (1.664–2.501)	<0.001
Albumin (≥35 vs. <35 g/L)	0.636 (0.433–0.934)	0.021
HBV DNA (≥2,000 vs. <2,000 IU/ml)	1.631 (1.292–2.058)	<0.001
Ishak inflammation score (≥3 vs. <3)	1.127 (0.786–1.635)	0.074
Ishak fibrosis score (≥3 vs. <3)	1.072 (0.821–1.782)	0.102
PLR (≥150 vs. <150)	1.891 (1.515–2.361)	<0.001
AFP (≥20 vs. <20 ng/ml)	2.073 (1.648–2.608)	<0.001
HBeAg (positive vs. negative)	1.160 (0.934–1.441)	0.180
Tumor encapsulation (yes vs. no)	0.507 (0.412–0.624)	<0.001
Major resection (yes vs. no)	1.094 (0.852–1.406)	0.481
Microvascular invasion (yes vs. no)	2.066 (1.680–2.539)	<0.001
Tumor number (multiple vs. single)	2.162 (1.680–2.781)	<0.001
Tumor differentiation (III+IV vs. I+II)	2.433 (1.758–3.366)	<0.001
Tumor diameter (≥5 vs. <5 cm)	2.628 (2.124–3.251)	<0.001
Liver cirrhosis (yes vs. no)	1.194 (0.976–1.460)	0.084
Multivariate analysis		
Aspartate aminotransferase (≥40 vs. <40 U/L)	1.531 (1.180–1.985)	0.001
HBV DNA (≥2,000 vs. <2,000 IU/ml)	1.485 (1.160–1.901)	0.001
PLR (≥150 vs. <150)	1.327 (1.053–1.674)	0.017
AFP (≥20 vs. <20 ng/ml)	1.424 (1.120–1.810)	0.004
Tumor encapsulation (yes vs. no)	0.780 (0.624–0.974)	0.029
Tumor diameter (≥5 vs. <5 cm)	1.692 (1.340–2.136)	<0.001

HRs (95% CI) and P-values were calculated using univariate and multivariate Cox proportional hazard regression.
HBeAg, hepatitis B e antigen; AFP, alpha-fetoprotein.

had a larger AUC than any other independent risk factors (**Supplementary Table 6**).

Prognostic Value of PLR for HCC Patients Survival

With respect to RFS, the C-index of PLR was 0.549, and it was significantly higher than tumor number ($P = 0.005$) (**Supplementary Table 5**). In the ROC curve analysis for RFS (**Supplementary Table 6**), there was no significantly difference between PLR and other predictors, except for tumor number. PLR had a larger AUC than tumor number ($P = 0.048$). In the multivariate analysis of RFS, the HR for PLR was the highest. We also observed that PLR had the highest specific weight in the nomogram for RFS (**Figure 2A**). Therefore, we demonstrated that PLR was the best predictor of recurrence. As for OS, The C-index of PLR was 0.559, which was the lowest among the predictors (**Supplementary Table 5**). In the ROC curve analysis for OS (**Supplementary Table 6**), PLR also had the lowest AUC value than other predictors. We also observed that PLR had the lowest specific weight in the nomogram for OS (**Figure 2B**). Thus, we combined the PLR with other predicters to identify the best predictors for OS. In the **Supplementary Table 6**, PLR combined with tumor diameter had a larger AUC than other combinations. Thus, PLR combined with tumor diameter may be the best predictor for OS.

Immunohistochemical Analysis

All of the samples of 1,174 patients were under TMA construction and immunohistochemical staining for $CD8^+$T-cells. As shown in **Figure 3A**, $CD8^+$ T-cells were present throughout the tissue samples, but they were often predominant in the peritumoral stroma rather than in the cancer nests (123.2 ± 48.6 and 19.1 ± 4.4 cells/field, respectively; $P < 0.001$; **Figures 3A,F**). When tumor infiltration by $CD8^+$ T-cells between the high and low PLR groups were compared, there was no significant difference in intratumoral $CD8^+$ T-cell counts between the two groups (18.9 ± 5.4 vs. 19.3 ± 3.3 $P = 0.845$; **Figures 3B,D,G**). However, peritumoral stroma in the high PLR group has significantly more $CD8^+$T-cells than that

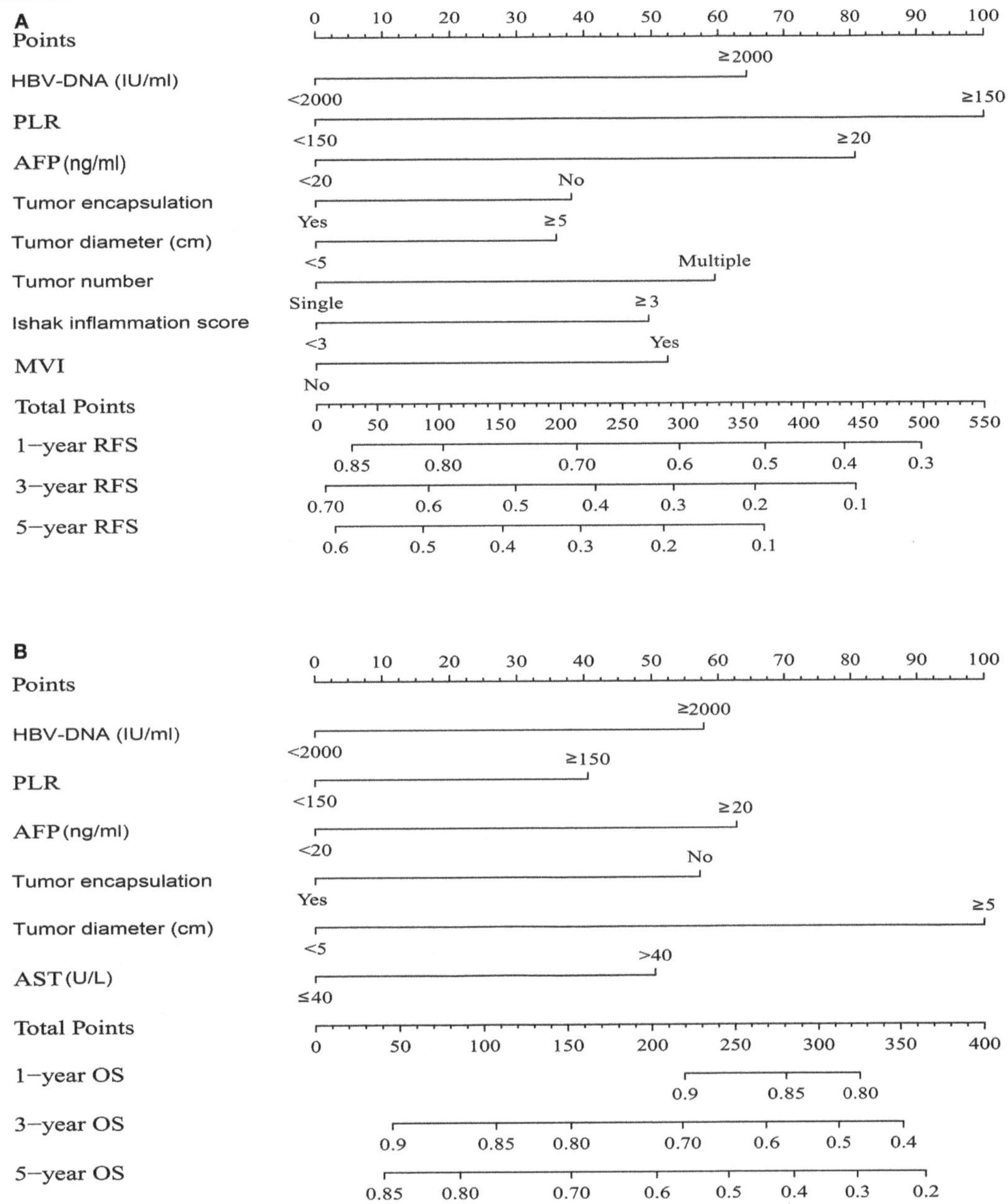

FIGURE 2 | HCC patients survival nomogram. **(A)** HCC patients survival nomogram for Recurrence-Free Survival. **(B)** HCC patients survival nomogram for Overall Survival. (To use the nomogram, individual patient's value is located on each variable axis, and a line is drawn upward to determine the number of points received for each variable value. The sum of these numbers is located on the Total Points axis, and a line is drawn downward to the survival axes to determine the likelihood of 1-, 3-, or 5-year survival).

in the low PLR group (149.7 ± 40.3 vs. 83.5 ± 29.0 $P = 0.001$; **Figures 3C,E,H**).

Association of CD8$^+$T-Cells in the Peritumoral Stroma With Clinico-Pathological Characteristics

There was no significant difference between intra tumoral CD8+ T-counts in the high PLR group and those in the low PLR group (18.9 ± 5.4 vs. 19.3 ± 3.3 $P = 0.845$; **Figures 3B,D,G**). While peritumoral stroma in the high PLR group has significantly more CD8$^+$T-cells than that in the low PLR group (149.7 ± 40.3 vs. 83.5 ± 29.0 $P = 0.001$; **Figures 3C,E,H**). Potential associations of clinicopathological factors with CD8$^+$T-cells counts in the peritumoral stroma were identified by logistic regression analysis. The median value of CD8$^+$ T-cell counts in the peritumoral stroma was chosen as the cutoff point for distinguishing high CD8$^+$ T-cell

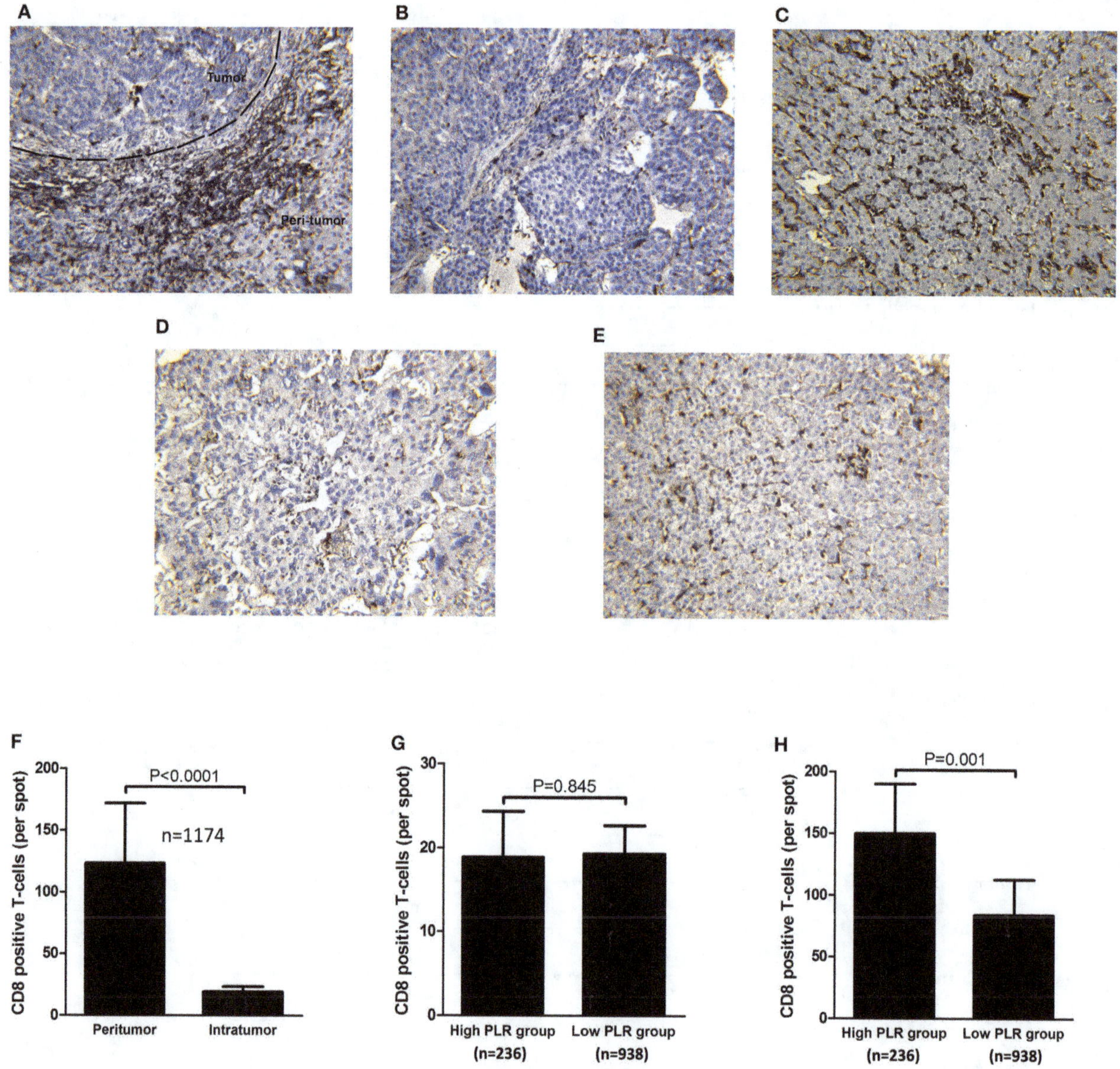

FIGURE 3 | Immunohistochemical staining of intratumoral and peritumoral CD8 from consecutive tissue microarrays and distribution of $CD8^+$ T-cells and correlations with PLR level. **(A)** Immunohistochemical staining of CD8 throughout the tissue. **(B)** Immunohistochemical staining of CD8 in HCC tissues of patients with high PLR (≥150). **(C)** Immunohistochemical staining of CD8 in tumorside tissues of patients with high PLR (≥150). **(D)** Immunohistochemical staining of CD8 in HCC tissues of patients with low PLR (<150). **(E)** Immunohistochemical staining of CD8 in tumorside tissues of patients with low PLR (<150). **(F)** $CD8^+$ T-cells were more abundant in peritumoral tissue than in tumor tissue. **(G)** There was no significant difference of intratumoral $CD8^+$ T-cell counts between patients with high PLR (≥150) and low PLR (<150). **(H)** Peritumoral $CD8^+$ T-cells were more abundant in HCC patients with high PLR (≥150) than patients with low PLR (<150).

counts cases ($N = 587$) from low $CD8^+$ T-cell counts cases (N = 587). After multivariate analysis, it was indicated that in addition to a high PLR level (≥150) (OR = 4.372; $P < 0.001$), a high Ishak inflammation score (≥3) (OR = 1.129; $P < 0.001$), cirrhosis (OR = 1.636; $P = 0.001$), and male (OR = 1.736; $P = 0.009$) was independently predictive of high $CD8^+$ T-cell counts in the peritumoral stroma (**Supplementary Table 7**).

DISCUSSION

Many recent reports have found that a high PLR is relevant to an adverse prognosis in patients with different cancer types (5–7). In this study, a high PLR is related to more advanced and multiple malignant characteristics of HCC, higher HBV DNA value, more severe liver inflammation, more advanced tumor stage, and poorer clinical outcomes of HBV-related HCC after liver resection. The Kaplan-Meier analysis of RFS and OS in these HCC patients manifested that both tumor recurrence and survival rates are different significantly between the groups of patients with high and low PLR. Multivariate analysis showed that a high PLR worked as an independent and significant risk factor for recurrence and overall survival after curative liver surgery. More importantly, a high PLR showed good accuracy in predicting long-term survival in patients with early tumors. Further analysis indicated that PLR was the best predictor of recurrence, however, for OS, PLR combined with tumor diameter may be the best predictor.

BCLC Stage A is considered as an early stage of HCC, however, some of them still have poor survival outcome. Our findings indicate that stage A patients with a high PLR have a higher cumulative recurrence rate and a lower survival rate than those patients with a low PLR. Thus, the results of this study indicate that a high PLR is a factor predicting bad prognosis in patients with early stage HCC (**Figures 1C,D**). For the BCLC stage B patients, a high PLR substantially affects the prognosis of these patients after liver resection (**Figures 1E,F**).

Previous studies have shown that relatively depleted lymphocytes impair the host immune response to malignancy (21). Previous studies have proven platelets can interact with tumor cells and promote tumor growth (22, 23). Especially for HCC, platelets could produce vascular endothelial growth factor (VEGF) (24), platelet-derived growth factor (PDGF), (25) serotonin (26), and fibroblast growth factor (FGF) and its receptors which enhance HCC growth (27). Platelets can interact with a variety of different cell types, including endothelial and dendritic cells, T-lymphocytes, neutrophils, and mononuclear phagocytes. Interestingly, aspirin can inhibit platelet activation and thus reduce HCC development (28). In Asian countries, HBV infection is the primary risk for HCC development. Chronic HBV infection can cause persistent liver damage, fibrosis, and cirrhosis. The pathogenic mechanisms of HBV-related HCC not only involve viral factors, but also host factors as well (29). A functionally inefficient $CD8^+$ T-cell response which causes a failure in virus clearance sustains a chronic necroinflammatory in liver and thus induces the carcinogenesis of HCC. During HBV infection, $CD8^+$ T-cells are significant triggers of liver immunopathology and platelets play a significant role in immune-mediated liver injury by facilitating the accumulation of virus-specific $CD8^+$ T-cells in the liver tissue. In this study, the results of immunohistochemical staining showed that the number of $CD8^+$T-cells in the peritumoral stroma was significantly higher in the high PLR group than in the low PLR group. Multivariate logistic regression analysis indicated that a high PLR level ($\geq$150), a high Ishak inflammation score, cirrhosis, and male patients was independently associated with a high $CD8^+$ T-cell counts in the peritumoral stroma. These results suggest that a high PLR level, a high Ishak inflammation score, cirrhosis, and male patient are related to the level of liver inflammation. Interestingly, liver inflammation of male HCC patients was more severe than female patients, it is associated with the level of IL-6 (30).

In mice, researchers have found platelets that exacerbate hepatitis through serotonin secretion. This causes hepatic sinusoid microcirculation failure, which can lead to delayed viral clearance and CTL-mediated liver injuries (31). It was also found that platelet depletion can reduce CTL-mediated liver damage in mice (32). Platelet activation is necessary in such mechanisms because prostaglandin E1 treatment can reverse the effect of platelet reconstitution in platelet-depleted mice and thus weaken T cell-mediated liver injuries (33). Experiments have been performed verifying aspirin and clopidogrel, which is known also as platelet activation inhibitors, as mitigating necroinflammation and antigen-specific CTL accumulation in the liver of mice (34).

However, the mechanisms of recruiting platelets into the liver and thus facilitating the hepatic accumulation of $CD8^+$ T-cells are still under covered. Research has found platelets adhere to sinusoidal hyaluronan via CD44 and circulate the $CD8^+$ arrest by docking onto platelets. These $CD8^+$ cells then propagate along liver sinusoids until hepatocellular antigens(AGS) are recognized (35). In addition, the activation-dependent expression of the platelet CD40 ligand contributes to the expansion phase of the virus-specific $CD8^+$ T-cells, resulting in their accumulation at sites of infection (36). This suggests an direct interaction between activated platelets and $CD8^+$ T-cells expressing CD40 (37, 38). Other authors have showed that the platelet CD40 ligand could potentially strengthen the virus-specific $CD8^+$ T-cell responses through an indirect way, mostly by promotion of the maturation of dendritic cells (39). Our study demonstrated that high PLR is significantly correlated with a high aspartate aminotransferase level and high Ishak inflammation scores. Immunohistochemical analysis showed that a high PLR is significantly associated with high numbers of $CD8^+$T-cells in the peritumoral stroma. Based on these observations, we reasoned that PLR reflects the severity of liver inflammation. These data provide direct evidence that PLR is an easily measurable inflammatory biomarker, and an elevated PLR is an independent predictor of survival outcome in HBV-related HCC subjects who have undertaken a liver resection.

The main limitation of this study is that this is a single institutional retrospective study, there may be potential biases in the collection of patients, so the results of this study need to be verified in further prospective studies, and relevant studies are in progress currently.

CONCLUSIONS

Platelet-to-lymphocyte ratio is a practical and easily measurable prognosis marker for HBV–related HCC patients. Elevated PLR is significantly associated with the accumulation of $CD8^+$ T-cells in peritumoral tissue. Our study indicates that PLR reflects the severity of liver inflammation.

AUTHOR CONTRIBUTIONS

YY and M-cW: data curation. TT and JH: formal analysis. W-pZ: funding acquisition and writing – original draft. S-xY, LL, PZ, and

S-yF: investigation. F-mG, B-gJ, and F-cL: methodology. Z-yP: project administration. All authors contributed to the article and approved the submitted version.

ACKNOWLEDGMENTS

My sincere appreciation also goes to the teachers and colleagues from Eastern Hepatobiliary Surgical Hospital who participated this study with great cooperation. Last but not least, I'd like to thank all my friends, especially my wife for their encouragement and support.

REFERENCES

1. Mantovani A. Cancer: inflaming metastasis. *Nature.* (2009) 457:36–7. doi: 10.1038/457036b
2. Laird BJ, Kaasa S, McMillan DC, Fallon MT, Hjermstad MJ, Fayers P, et al. Prognostic factors in patients with advanced cancer: a comparison of clinicopathological factors and the development of an inflammation-based prognostic system. *Clin Cancer Res.* (2013) 19:5456–64. doi: 10.1158/1078-0432.CCR-13-1066
3. Balkwill F, Mantovani A. Inflammation and cancer: back to Virchow? *Lancet.* (2001) 357:539–45. doi: 10.1016/S0140-6736(00)04046-0
4. Coussens LM, Werb Z. Inflammation and cancer. *Nature.* (2002) 420:860–7. doi: 10.1038/nature01322
5. Tan D, Fu Y, Su Q, Wang H. Prognostic role of platelet-lymphocyte ratio in colorectal cancer: a systematic review and meta-analysis. *Medicine.* (2016) 95:e3837. doi: 10.1097/MD.0000000000003837
6. Yodying H, Matsuda A, Miyashita M, Matsumoto S, Sakurazawa N, Yamada M, et al. Prognostic significance of neutrophil-to-lymphocyte ratio and platelet-to-lymphocyte ratio in oncologic outcomes of esophageal cancer: a systematic review and meta-analysis. *Ann Surg Oncol.* (2016) 23:646–54. doi: 10.1245/s10434-015-4869-5
7. Zhao QT, Yuan Z, Zhang H, Zhang XP, Wang HE, Wang ZK, et al. Prognostic role of platelet to lymphocyte ratio in non-small cell lung cancers: a meta-analysis including 3,720 patients. *Int J Cancer.* (2016) 139:164–70. doi: 10.1002/ijc.30060
8. Fan W, Zhang Y, Wang Y, Yao X, Yang J, Li J. Neutrophil-to-lymphocyte and platelet-to-lymphocyte ratios as predictors of survival and metastasis for recurrent hepatocellular carcinoma after transarterial chemoembolization. *PLoS ONE.* (2015) 10:e0119312. doi: 10.1371/journal.pone.0119312
9. Xue TC, Jia QA, Ge NL, Zhang BH, Wang YH, Ren ZG, et al. The platelet-to-lymphocyte ratio predicts poor survival in patients with huge hepatocellular carcinoma that received transarterial chemoembolization. *Tumour Biol.* (2015) 36:6045–51. doi: 10.1007/s13277-015-3281-x
10. Kabir T, Mohd Noor NA, Junnarkar SP, Low JK, Woon W, Shelat VG. Does preoperative platelet-lymphocyte ratio or prognostic nutritional index predict survival after surgical resection for hepatocellular carcinoma? *HPB.* (2016) 18:e709–10. doi: 10.1016/j.hpb.2016.01.128
11. Bruix J, Sherman M, Llovet JM, Beaugrand M, Lencioni R, Burroughs AK, et al. Clinical management of hepatocellular carcinoma. conclusions of the Barcelona-2000 EASL conference. European Association for the Study of the Liver. *J Hepatol.* (2001) 35:421–30. doi: 10.1016/S0168-8278(01)00130-1
12. Krenzien F, Schmelzle M, Struecker B, Raschzok N, Benzing C, Jara M, et al. Liver transplantation and liver resection for cirrhotic patients with hepatocellular carcinoma: comparison of long-term survivals. *J Gastrointest Surg.* (2018) 22:840–8. doi: 10.1007/s11605-018-3690-4
13. Shen JY, Li C, Wen TF, Yan LN, Li B, Wang WT, et al. Liver transplantation vs. surgical resection for HCC meeting the Milan criteria: a propensity score analysis. *Medicine.* (2016) 95:e5756. doi: 10.1097/MD.0000000000005756
14. Silva MF, Sapisochin G, Strasser SI, Hewa-Geeganage S, Chen J, Wigg AJ, et al. Liver resection and transplantation offer similar 5-year survival for Child-Pugh-Turcotte A HCC-patients with a single nodule up to 5 cm: a multicenter, exploratory analysis. *Eur J Surg Oncol.* (2013) 39:386–95. doi: 10.1016/j.ejso.2012.12.011
15. Ishak K, Baptista A, Bianchi L, Callea F, De Groote J, Gudat F, et al. Histological grading and staging of chronic hepatitis. *J Hepatol.* (1995) 22:696–9. doi: 10.1016/0168-8278(95)80226-6
16. Wang RY, Chen L, Chen HY, Hu L, Li L, Sun HY, et al. MUC15 inhibits dimerization of EGFR and PI3K-AKT signaling and is associated with aggressive hepatocellular carcinomas in patients. *Gastroenterology.* (2013) 145:1436–48.e1–12. doi: 10.1053/j.gastro.2013.08.009
17. Rosenbaum PR, Rubin DB. Constructing a control group using multivariate matched sampling methods that incorporate the propensity score. *Am Stat.* (1985) 39:33–8. doi: 10.1080/00031305.1985.10479383
18. Rubin DB, Thomas N. Matching using estimated propensity scores: relating theory to practice. *Biometrics.* (1996) 52:249–64. doi: 10.2307/2533160
19. Yang T, Lu JH, Lau WY, Zhang TY, Zhang H, Shen YN, et al. Perioperative blood transfusion does not influence recurrence-free and overall survivals after curative resection for hepatocellular carcinoma: a propensity score matching analysis. *J Hepatol.* (2016) 64:583–93. doi: 10.1016/j.jhep.2015.10.012
20. Wang Y, Li J, Xia Y, Gong R, Wang K, Yan Z, et al. Prognostic nomogram for intrahepatic cholangiocarcinoma after partial hepatectomy. *J Clin Oncol.* (2013) 31:1188–95. doi: 10.1200/JCO.2012.41.5984
21. Halazun KJ, Hardy MA, Rana AA, Woodland DC, Luyten EJ, Mahadev S, et al. Negative impact of neutrophil-lymphocyte ratio on outcome after liver transplantation for hepatocellular carcinoma. *Ann Surg.* (2009) 250:141–51. doi: 10.1097/SLA.0b013e3181a77e59
22. Stone RL, Nick AM, McNeish IA, Balkwill F, Han HD, Bottsford-Miller J, et al. Paraneoplastic thrombocytosis in ovarian cancer. *N Engl J Med.* (2012) 366:610–8. doi: 10.1056/NEJMoa1110352
23. Labelle M, Begum S, Hynes RO. Direct signaling between platelets and cancer cells induces an epithelial-mesenchymal-like transition and promotes metastasis. *Cancer Cell.* (2011) 20:576–90. doi: 10.1016/j.ccr.2011.09.009
24. Zhou J, Tang ZY, Fan J, Wu ZQ, Li XM, Liu YK, et al. Expression of platelet-derived endothelial cell growth factor and vascular endothelial growth factor in hepatocellular carcinoma and portal vein tumor thrombus. *J Cancer Res Clin Oncol.* (2000) 126:57–61. doi: 10.1007/s004320050009
25. Okada H, Honda M, Campbell JS, Sakai Y, Yamashita T, Takebuchi Y, et al. Acyclic retinoid targets platelet-derived growth factor signaling in the prevention of hepatic fibrosis and hepatocellular carcinoma development. *Cancer Res.* (2012) 72:4459–71. doi: 10.1158/0008-5472.CAN-12-0028
26. Soll C, Jang JH, Riener MO, Moritz W, Wild PJ, Graf R, et al. Serotonin promotes tumor growth in human hepatocellular cancer. *Hepatology.* (2010) 51:1244–54. doi: 10.1002/hep.23441
27. Gauglhofer C, Sagmeister S, Schrottmaier W, Fischer C, Rodgarkia-Dara C, Mohr T, et al. Up-regulation of the fibroblast growth factor 8 subfamily in human hepatocellular carcinoma for cell survival and neoangiogenesis. *Hepatology.* (2011) 53:854–64. doi: 10.1002/hep.24099
28. Sitia G, Iannacone M, Guidotti LG. Anti-platelet therapy in the prevention of hepatitis B virus-associated hepatocellular carcinoma. *J Hepatol.* (2013) 59:1135–8. doi: 10.1016/j.jhep.2013.05.040
29. Guidotti LG, Chisari FV. Immunobiology and pathogenesis of viral hepatitis. *Annu Rev Pathol.* (2006) 1:23–61. doi: 10.1146/annurev.pathol.1.110304.100230
30. Naugler WE, Sakurai T, Kim S, Maeda S, Kim K, Elsharkawy AM, et al. Gender disparity in liver cancer due to sex differences in MyD88-dependent IL-6 production. *Science.* (2007) 317:121–4. doi: 10.1126/science.1140485
31. Lang PA, Contaldo C, Georgiev P, El-Badry AM, Recher M, Kurrer M, et al. Aggravation of viral hepatitis by platelet-derived serotonin. *Nat Med.* (2008) 14:756–61. doi: 10.1038/nm1780
32. Guidotti LG, Iannacone M. Effector CD8 T cell trafficking within the liver. *Mol Immunol.* (2013) 55:94–9. doi: 10.1016/j.molimm.2012.10.032
33. Iannacone M, Sitia G, Isogawa M, Marchese P, Castro MG, Lowenstein PR, et al. Platelets mediate cytotoxic T lymphocyte-induced liver damage. *Nat Med.* (2005) 11:1167–9. doi: 10.1038/nm1317
34. Iannacone M, Sitia G, Guidotti LG. On the role of platelets in the pathogenesis of viral hepatitis. *J Hepatol.* (2009) 51:599–600. doi: 10.1016/j.jhep.2009.05.005

35. Guidotti LG, Inverso D, Sironi L, Di Lucia P, Fioravanti J, Ganzer L, et al. Immunosurveillance of the liver by intravascular effector CD8(+) T cells. *Cell.* (2015) 161:486–500. doi: 10.1016/j.cell.2015.03.005
36. Iannacone M, Sitia G, Isogawa M, Whitmire JK, Marchese P, Chisari FV, et al. Platelets prevent IFN-alpha/beta-induced lethal hemorrhage promoting CTL-dependent clearance of lymphocytic choriomeningitis virus. *Proc Natl Acad Sci USA.* (2008) 105:629–34. doi: 10.1073/pnas.0711200105
37. Bourgeois C, Rocha B, Tanchot C. A role for CD40 expression on CD8+ T cells in the generation of CD8+ T cell memory. *Science.* (2002) 297:2060–3. doi: 10.1126/science.1072615
38. Meunier S, Rapetti L, Beziaud L, Pontoux C, Legrand A, Tanchot C. Synergistic CD40 signaling on APCs and CD8 T cells drives efficient CD8 response and memory differentiation. *J Leukoc Biol.* (2012) 91:859–69. doi: 10.1189/jlb.0611292
39. Li N. Platelet-lymphocyte cross-talk. *J Leukoc Biol.* (2008) 83:1069–78. doi: 10.1189/jlb.0907615

16

Association of Preoperative Coagulability with Incidence and Extent of Portal Vein Tumor Thrombus and Survival Outcomes in Hepatocellular Carcinoma After Hepatectomy

Xiu-Ping Zhang [1,2†], Teng-Fei Zhou [3†], Jin-Kai Feng [1†], Zi-Yang Sun [1,4†], Zuo-Jun Zhen [5], Dong Zhou [6], Fan Zhang [7], Yi-Ren Hu [8], Cheng-Qian Zhong [9], Zhen-Hua Chen [10], Zong-Tao Chai [1], Kang Wang [1], Jie Shi [1], Wei-Xing Guo [1], Meng-Chao Wu [1], Wan Yee Lau [1,11] and Shu-Qun Cheng [1]*

[1] Department of Hepatic Surgery VI, Eastern Hepatobiliary Surgery Hospital, Second Military Medical University, Shanghai, China, [2] Faculty of Hepato-Biliary-Pancreatic Surgery, The First Medical Center of Chinese People's Liberation Army (PLA) General Hospital, Beijing, China, [3] Department of Oncology, The No. 313 Hospital of PLA, Huludao, China, [4] College of Basic Medical Sciences, Second Military Medical University, Shanghai, China, [5] Department of Hepatobiliary Surgery, Foshan First People's Hospital, Foshan, China, [6] Department of Hepatobiliary Surgery, Fujian Cancer Hospital, Fuzhou, China, [7] Department of Hepatobiliary Surgery, Affiliated Hospital of Binzhou Medical College, Binzhou, China, [8] Department of General Surgery, Wenzhou People's Hospital, Wenzhou, China, [9] Department of Hepatobiliary Surgery, LongYan First Hospital, Affiliated to Fujian Medical University, Longyan, China, [10] Department of General Surgery, Zhejiang Provincial Armed Police Corps Hospital, Hangzhou, China, [11] Faculty of Medicine, The Chinese University of Hong Kong, Hong Kong, SAR China

***Correspondence:**
Shu-Qun Cheng
chengshuqun@smmu.edu.cn*

†These authors have contributed equally to this work

Background: Occurrence of portal vein tumor thrombus (PVTT) worsens the outcomes of hepatocellular carcinoma (HCC) and imparts high economic burden on society. Patients with high risks of having hypercoagulation are more likely to experience thrombosis. Herein, we examined how preoperative international normalized ratio (INR) was related to the incidence and extent of PVTT, and associated with survival outcomes in HCC patients following R0 liver resection (LR).

Methods: Patients with HCC and PVTT were enrolled from six major hospitals in China. The overall survival (OS) and recurrence-free survival (RFS) rates of individuals with different INR levels were assessed with Cox regression analysis as well as Kaplan-Meier method.

Results: This study included 2207 HCC patients, among whom 1005 patients had concurrent PVTT. HCC patients in the Low INR group had a significantly higher incidence of PVTT and more extensive PVTT than the Normal and High INR groups ($P<0.005$). Of the 592 HCC subjects who had types I/II PVTT following R0 LR, there were 106 (17.9%),

342 (57.8%) and 144 (24.3%) patients in the High, Normal and Low INR groups, respectively. RFS and OS rates were markedly worse in patients in the Low INR group relative to those in the Normal and High INR groups (median RFS, 4.87 versus 10.77 versus 11.40 months, P<0.001; median OS, 6.30 versus 11.83 versus 12.67 months, P<0.001).

Conclusion: Preoperative INR influenced the incidence and extent of PVTT in HCC. Particularly, patients with HCC and PVTT in the Low INR group had worse postoperative prognosis relative to the High and Normal INR groups.

Keywords: hepatocellular carcinoma, portal vein tumor thrombus, international normalized ratio, liver resection, survival outcomes

INTRODUCTION

Hepatocellular carcinoma (HCC) belongs to the category of top-five leading cancers which claims many lives worldwide. It is especially prevalent in Asia and Africa due to hepatitis B virus (HBV) infection (1, 2). So far, portal vein tumor thrombus (PVTT) is estimated to develop in 44% to 62.2% in advanced HCC patients (3, 4). For cases of untreated HCC accompanied by PVTT, the reported median survival time (MST) is in the range of 2.7 to 4.0 months (1). PVTT is the bottleneck which seriously limits the survival of advanced HCC patients.

Currently, the treatment approaches for HCC with PVTT remain tremendous divergent between the east and the west. According to the established practice guidelines for the management of HCC, the recommended drug for advanced HCC with PVTT is sorafenib (3, 5). Unfortunately, this drug only leads to an MST of about 6.5 months in most patients (6–8). Giannini et al. (9) suggested that the treatment of patients with advanced HCC should be personalized instead of oral sorafenib only. Abundant clinical evidence shows that liver resection (LR) with curative intent is superior to non-surgical interventions in selected cases of advanced HCC. This is particularly the case in patients with HCC with PVTT occurring in the first-order branch of the main portal vein (MPV) or above (4, 10–12). To ease the process of selecting the optimized treatment, an EHBH-PVTT scoring system has been constructed and applied in clinical decision-making (13). Additionally, great advances in perioperative management practices and surgical techniques have increased the safety of LR in HCC complicated with PVTT.

PVTT in HCC was once named as "malignant portal vein thrombosis" because the thrombosis was regarded as cancer-related. Previous studies reported that venous embolus/thrombosis was greatly affected by the risk of plasma hypercoagulability in patients with cancer, a phenomenon caused by the host's response to cancerous cells or coagulation-promoting activity of cancer cells (14–16). High levels of plasma fibrinogen positively correlates with poor prognosis in various cancers (17). There is little evidence, however, to show the presence of a hypercoagulability state exists in HCC patients, especially in those with coexisting malignant portal vein thrombosis. International normalized ratio (INR) is a common laboratory indicator to determine the coagulation profile of an individual patient. The association of preoperative hypercoagulability with the prevalence and severity of PVTT as well as survival outcomes in patients with HCC remains unclear.

The present large-scale multicenter investigation explored the relationships between preoperative INR level and the prevalence rate and extent of PVTT, and survival outcomes of HCC post-LR.

MATERIALS AND METHODS

Patients

This study was carried out at the Eastern Hepatobiliary Surgery Hospital (EHBH), Foshan First People's Hospital (FFPH), Fujian Cancer Hospital (FCH), the Affiliated Hospital of Binzhou Medical College (AHBMC), LongYan First Hospital (LYFH), and Wenzhou People's Hospital (WPH), between January 2010 and December 2017. Study approval was obtained from the Institutional Ethics Committees of participating hospitals. Patient enrollment and other procedures followed the ethical protocols of the 1975 Declaration of Helsinki (6th revision, 2008). Each patient signed voluntarily to participate before treatment. All patients gave permission to the publication of data obtained during the investigation. These participants were categorized into three categories using preoperative INR level, hypercoagulability (Low INR group), hypocoagulability (High INR group) and normal coagulability (Normal INR group).

Diagnosis of PVTT

Eligible patients were identified based on postoperative histopathological examinations (4). The classification criteria proposed by Cheng were utilized to divide PVTT into four sub-types: I, segmental/sectoral arms of portal vein (PV); II, right or left PV; III, main portal vein (MPV); and IV, thrombus in MPV stretching towards the superior mesenteric vein (18, 19). For sub-type I and II PVTT, PVTT occurred in the first-order branch or above of the MPV, and they could be resected en bloc with the HCC in the liver.

Enrollment of Participants

All participants were enrolled based on the following criteria. HCC patients were included if they were: (I) 18–70 years old; (II) complicated with PVTT; (III) Child-Pugh score in category A or selected B (scores ≤7); (IV) initially received R0 LR and no residual tumors were present in microscopic examination based on excised samples; (V) no prior preoperative anti-cancer treatments; (VI) no distant metastases or extrahepatic spread; (VII) no macroscopic vascular invasion; (VIII) absence of coagulation-related diseases. The exclusion criteria were: (I) patients with palliative-intend tumor resection; (II) a history of other malignancies; (III) preoperative anticoagulant therapy; (IV) incomplete clinical data or lost to follow-up.

Surgical Protocols

The surgical procedures have been described in previous studies (19, 20). HCC patients with type I and II PVTT underwent curative LR en bloc with PVTT. For types III/IV PVTT, thrombectomy was carried out through an incision of the portal vein. The incision was closed after thorough flushing with normal saline after thrombectomy. The operation was performed under general anaesthesia using a right subcostal incision with a midline extension. Intraoperative ultrasonography was performed routinely to assess the number and size of lesions and the relationship of tumors to adjacent major vascular structures. The abdominal cavity was carefully searched for the extent of local disease, extrahepatic metastases and peritoneal seedings. Pringle's maneuver was applied to occlude the blood inflow of the liver with cycles of 15 minutes clamp time/5 minutes unclamped time. For types III/IV PVTT, the occlusion was done distal to the PVTT. The clamp crushing method was used for liver parenchymal transection.

Preoperative and Postoperative Investigations

Routine preoperative investigations included imaging and serological tests. Imaging examinations included abdominal ultrasonography, contrast-enhanced magnetic resonance imaging (MRI) and/or computed tomography (CT) scan of the abdomen, and plain radiography or non-contrast CT scan of the chest. All the radiological data were reviewed by two experienced radiologists. Routine preoperative laboratory investigations included complete blood counts, liver and renal function tests, hepatitis B and C serology, coagulation indexes, and serum tumor markers. The coagulability state of patients was reflected by the INR level, which was chosen from the latest examination within three days before surgery for data analysis. The criteria to define Low, Normal, and High INR were INR less than 0.80, INR in the range of 0.80–1.20, and INR higher than 1.20, respectively. Routine postoperative investigations included histopathological and immunohistochemical studies. The diagnosis of HCC and PVTT was only determined by histological examination of the resected surgical specimens. The histopathological evaluations were performed by two independent and experienced pathologists who were blinded to the study protocol.

Follow-Up and End Points

Patients were regularly followed up once every 2 to 3 months for the first year and once every 6 months thereafter, until death or dropout from the follow-up program. In addition to history-taking and physical examinations, follow-ups were conducted using laboratory tests, abdominal ultrasonography, contrast-enhanced CT or MRI. The diagnosis of disease recurrence was based on typical imaging features with or without raised serum AFP levels. Once HCC recurrence was determined, patients were actively treated. Treatment for HCC recurrence included repeat LR, radiofrequency ablation, transarterial chemoembolization (TACE) or sorafenib, depending on the general condition, the liver functional reserve and the pattern of tumor recurrence of the patients.

The primary end points of this study were recurrence-free survival (RFS) and overall survival (OS). RFS was calculated from the date of LR to the date when HCC recurrence was first diagnosed or the date of last follow-up. OS was calculated from the date of LR to the date of patient's death or the date of last follow-up.

Statistical Analysis

Continuous variables were reported as means and standard deviations (SD) or as medians and interquartile ranges (IQR). Appropriate statistical tests (the independent samples T test or Mann-Whitney U test) were used. Categorical data were reported as counts and percentages, and compared using the Chi-square test or Fisher's exact test. Univariate and multivariate analyses were conducted using the Cox proportional hazards regression model. Parameters with a P value less than 0.05 on univariate analysis were incorporated into multivariate analysis. Multivariate Cox regression analysis with a stepwise selection was performed to detect independent predictors of RFS and OS (the entry criteria for selection into the final multivariate model was $P < 0.05$). Survival curves of RFS and OS were generated using the Kaplan-Meier method and compared using the log-rank test. Median survival times and their corresponding 95% confidence intervals (CI) were reported. The data analyses were performed using the SPSS software version 24.0 (IBM Corporation, Armonk, NY, USA).

RESULTS

Patient Characteristics

This study included 2207 HCC patients at the six major cancer centers from January 2010 to December 2017 (**Figure 1**). These patients were divided into 2 groups according to whether they had PVTT (n = 1202 in the non-PVTT group; n = 1005 in the PVTT group). There were 698 patients with types I/II PVTT (592 underwent R0 LR), and 307 patients with types III/IV PVTT (86 underwent LR). The group of the 592 HCC patients with types I/II PVTT who underwent R0 LR was further divided into three groups according to preoperative INR levels (n = 106 in the High INR group; n = 342 in the Normal INR group; and n = 144 in the Low INR group). The clinicopathological features of HCC patients with types I/II PVTT who underwent R0 LR are shown in **Table 1**.

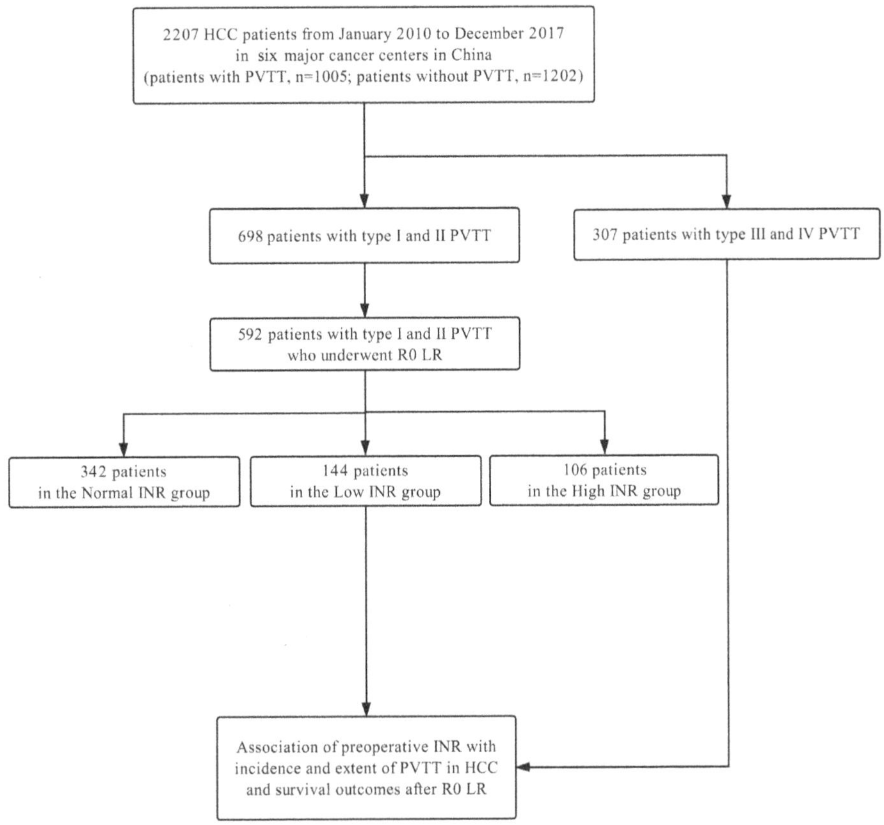

FIGURE 1 | Flowchart of patient selection for the study. HCC, hepatocellular carcinoma; PVTT, portal vein tumor thrombus; LR, liver resection; INR, international normalized ratio.

Association of Preoperative INR With Incidence and Extent of PVTT in HCC Patients

The incidence rate of PVTT was higher in HCC patients with a low INR level compared to those with a normal or high INR level (77.4% *vs* 38.2% *vs* 44.3% of patients with PVTT, in the Low, Normal and High INR groups, respectively, P<0.001) (**Figure 2A**). Of the 1202 patients who did not have PVTT, 80 patients (6.7%) were in the Low INR group, 916 patients (76.2%) in the Normal INR group, and 206 patients (17.1%) in the High INR group, respectively. Of the 1005 patients who had PVTT, 164 patients (16.3%), 567 patients (56.4%), and 274 patients (27.3%) were in the High, Normal, and Low INR groups, respectively. Notably, a low preoperative INR level was more likely to be observed in HCC patients associated with PVTT compared to those without PVTT (P<0.001) (**Figure 2B**).

Patients who had hypercoagulability in the Low INR group had more extensive PVTT (type III and IV PVTT *vs* type I and II PVTT) in comparison to the Normal and High INR groups (39.8% *vs* 28.4% *vs* 22.6% with type III and IV PVTT, 60.2% *vs* 71.6% *vs* 77.4% with type I and II PVTT in the Low, Normal and High INR groups, respectively, P<0.005) (**Figure 2C**). In other words, a significantly lower proportion of subjects with type I and II PVTT had hypercoagulability than those having type III and IV PVTT (23.6% *vs* 35.5% in the Low INR group, 58.2% *vs* 52.4% in the Normal INR group, and 18.2% *vs* 12.1% in the High INR group, respectively, P<0.005) (**Figure 2D**).

Taken together, HCC patients with hypercoagulability reflected by a low INR level had a higher incidence of PVTT and more extensive PVTT.

Independent Prognostic Factors of Survival Outcomes

Univariate and multivariate Cox regression analyses conducted on HCC patients with type I and II PVTT after R0 LR demonstrated that type of PVTT (P=0.001), INR level (P<0.001), AFP (P<0.001), tumor diameter (P=0.011), and direct bilirubin (P<0.001) to be independent predictors of OS (**Table 2**). Type of PVTT (P=0.004), INR level (P<0.001), AFP (P<0.001), tumor encapsulation (P<0.001), and aspartate aminotransferase (P=0.011) were independent predictors of RFS (**Table 3**).

Survival Analysis in 592 HCC Patients With Types I/II PVTT Among the Three Groups With Different INR Levels

The three groups of subjects with type I and II PVTT with various INR levels had markedly different RFS and OS rates

TABLE 1 | The clinicopathological features of HCC patients with types I/II PVTT who underwent R0 LR (n=592).

Variables	INR Low (N=144)	INR Normal (N=342)	INR High (N=106)	P value
PVTT				
I	55 (38.19%)	113 (33.04%)	37 (34.91%)	0.551
II	89 (61.81%)	229 (66.96%)	69 (65.09%)	
Age (years)				
<50	73 (50.69%)	203 (59.36%)	61 (57.55%)	0.210
≥50	71 (49.31%)	139 (40.64%)	45 (42.45%)	
Sex				
Male	127 (88.19%)	316 (92.40%)	98 (92.45%)	0.292
Female	17 (11.81%)	26 (7.60%)	8 (7.55%)	
Child-Pugh				
A	143 (99.31%)	335 (97.95%)	103 (97.17%)	0.431
B	1 (0.69%)	7 (2.05%)	3 (2.83%)	
HBsAg				
Positive	127 (88.19%)	309 (90.35%)	95 (89.62%)	0.775
Negative	17 (11.81%)	33 (9.65%)	11 (10.38%)	
Ascites				
Yes	15 (10.42%)	36 (10.53%)	11 (10.38%)	0.999
No	129 (89.58%)	306 (89.47%)	95 (89.62%)	
No. of tumors				
Single	120 (83.33%)	298 (87.13%)	95 (89.62%)	0.325
Multiple	24 (16.67%)	44 (12.87%)	11 (10.38%)	
Satellite nodules				
Yes	130 (90.28%)	324 (94.74%)	95 (89.62%)	0.088
No	14 (9.72%)	18 (5.26%)	11 (10.38%)	
AFP (ng/mL)				
<400	46 (31.94%)	126 (36.84%)	39 (36.79%)	0.567
≥400	98 (68.06%)	216 (63.16%)	67 (63.21%)	
Lymph node invasion				
Yes	20 (13.89%)	53 (15.50%)	14 (13.21%)	0.804
No	124 (86.11%)	289 (84.50%)	92 (86.79%)	
Tumor diameter (cm)				
<5	32 (22.22%)	58 (16.96%)	20 (18.87%)	0.394
≥5	112 (77.78%)	284 (83.04%)	86 (81.13%)	
Tumor encapsulation				
Yes	43 (29.86%)	149 (43.57%)	55 (51.89%)	**0.001**
No	101 (70.14%)	193 (56.43%)	51 (48.11%)	
Cirrhosis				
Yes	91 (63.19%)	252 (73.68%)	84 (79.25%)	**0.012**
No	53 (36.81%)	90 (26.32%)	22 (20.75%)	
TBIL (μmol/L)				
<17.1	97 (67.36%)	249 (72.81%)	69 (65.09%)	0.226
≥17.1	47 (32.64%)	93 (27.19%)	37 (34.91%)	
DBIL(μmol/L)				
<6.8	90 (62.50%)	231 (67.54%)	66 (62.26%)	0.430
≥6.8	54 (37.50%)	111 (32.46%)	40 (37.74%)	
ALB (g/L)	41.5 (40.8–42.1)	41.7 (41.3–42.1)	39.8 (38.2–41.5)	**0.004**
ALT (U/L)	55.2 (46.4–64.1)	53.8 (49.5–58.1)	53.2 (47.2–59.2)	0.921
AST (U/L)	60.3 (52.5–68.0)	56.6 (52.5–60.7)	61.8 (54.4–69.2)	0.428
GGT (U/L)	174.0 (149.6–198.2)	169.2 (153.5–184.8)	172.0 (141.8–202.2)	0.946
ALP (U/L)	121.4 (113.5–129.4)	121.1 (114.6–127.5)	121.8 (112.0–131.5)	0.993
PLT (×10^9/L)	171.8 (159.6–184.1)	166.9 (159.1–174.8)	158.3 (144.1–172.6)	0.361
CA199 (U/mL)	34.7 (27.6–41.9)	35.2 (28.1–42.2)	44.5 (24.2–64.7)	0.461

PVTT, portal vein tumor thrombus; HBsAg, hepatitis B surface antigen; AFP, α-fetoprotein; TBIL, total bilirubin; DBIL, direct bilirubin; ALB, albumin; ALT, alanine aminotransferase; AST, aspartate aminotransferase; GGT, γ-glutamyltransferase; ALP, alkaline phosphatase; PLT, platelet; CA199, carbohydrate antigen 19-9. P values in bold denote statistically significant difference.

(both P<0.001) (**Figure 3**). **Figure 3A** illustrated that the 1-, 3-, and 5-year RFS rates were significantly poorer in the Low INR group relative to those in the Normal and High INR groups (1 year, 16.9% *vs* 48.3% *vs* 53.5%; 3 years, 6.3% *vs* 19.1% *vs* 23.4%; 5 years, 0% *vs* 15.0% *vs* 20.5%; median RFS, 4.87 *vs* 10.77 *vs* 11.40 months, P<0.001). Similarly, **Figure 3B** suggested that the 1-, 3-, and 5-year OS rates of the Low INR group were markedly worse than the Normal and High INR groups (1 year, 20.1% *vs* 49.6% *vs* 50.9%; 3 years, 3.3% *vs* 22.7% *vs* 28.0%; 5 years, 1.1% *vs* 15.7% *vs* 21.2%; median OS, 6.30 *vs* 11.83 *vs* 12.67 months, P<0.001). Nevertheless, the RFS and OS rates between the Normal and High INR groups were not statistically significantly different.

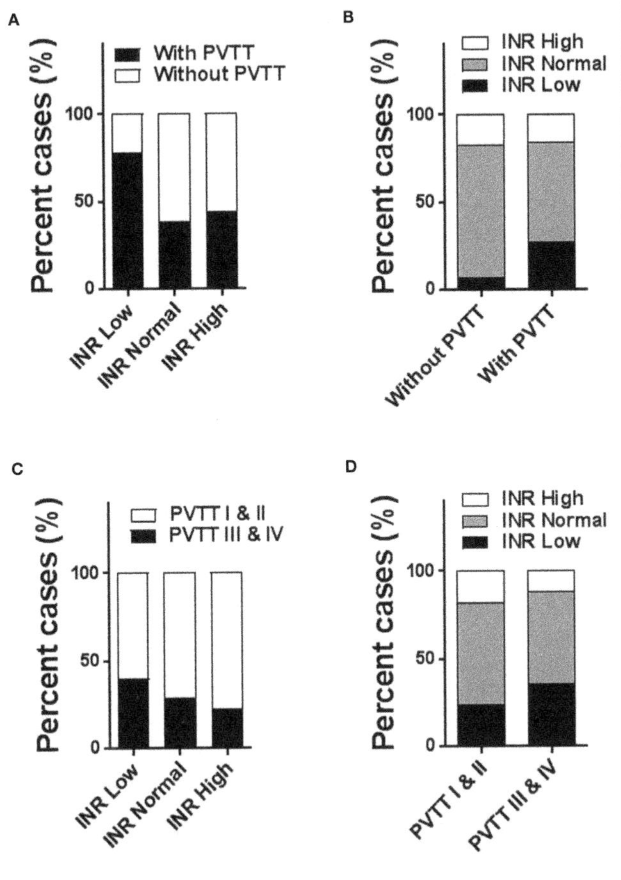

FIGURE 2 | Histogram to show the association of preoperative INR level with incidence and extent of PVTT (1005 patients with PVTT *vs* 1202 patients without PVTT; 698 patients with types I/II PVTT *vs* 307 patients with types III/IV PVTT). The incidence rates of PVTT among the Low, Normal, and High INR groups **(A)**; the distributions of INR level between patients with and without PVTT **(B)**; the incidence rates of types I/II and types III/IV PVTT among the Low, Normal, and High INR groups **(C)**; the distributions of INR level between patients with types I/II PVTT and types III/IV PVTT **(D)**. PVTT, portal vein tumor thrombus; INR, international normalized ratio.

Subgroup Analysis on Survival Outcomes for Patients With Types I/II PVTT in the Different Groups

The RFS was significantly worse in cases with low levels of INR compared to those with normal and high INR levels in type I PVTT (1 year, 19.4% *vs* 60.4% *vs* 68.6%; 3 years, 0% *vs* 19.4% *vs* 30.9%; 5 years, 0% *vs* 12.9% *vs* 30.9%, median RFS, 5.70 *vs* 16.07 months *vs* 19.50 months; P <0.001, **Supplementary Figure 1A**). Similarly, patients with type I PVTT with low levels of INR exhibited significantly poorer 1-, 3-, and 5-year OS rates than those with normal and high levels of INR (1 year, 20.0% *vs* 69.8% *vs* 70.3%; 3 years, 0% *vs* 38.6% *vs* 39.2%; 5 years, 0% *vs* 25.0% *vs* 28.0%, median OS, 5.80 *vs* 21.1 months *vs* 20.5 months; P <0.001, **Supplementary Figure 1B**). Equivalent results were obtained for survival of these three groups of HCC patients with type II PVTT after R0 LR (for RFS rates: 1 year, 15.1% *vs* 41.9% *vs* 45.3%; 3 years, 6.5% *vs* 19.9% *vs* 18.8%; 5 years, 0% *vs* 18.0% *vs* 13.4%, median RFS, 4.60 *vs* 6.80 months *vs* 7.97 months, P <0.001, **Supplementary Figure 1C**; for OS rates: 1 year, 20.2% *vs* 39.5% *vs* 40.6%; 3 years, 4.3% *vs* 16.3% *vs* 22.5%; 5 years, 1.4% *vs* 11.8% *vs* 17.9%, median OS, 6.67 *vs* 9.23 months *vs* 9.97 months; P <0.001, **Supplementary Figure 1D**).

DISCUSSION

The presence of PVTT is regarded as one of the most vital risk factors for HCC patients and always leads to unfavorable prognosis (9, 10). The available treatment for HCC complicated with PVTT is limited and the therapeutic effectiveness is not satisfactory. Owing to the great development of surgical techniques and perioperative management approaches, R0 LR operated for patients with HCC and type I and II PVTT becomes safe, and the perioperative morbidity and mortality rates have much decreased (4, 21). However, the related clinicopathological factors of PVTT occurrence largely remain to be elucidated.

To our knowledge, there is no study which focuses on determining the association between coagulation status and the incidence and extent of PVTT and survival outcomes in HCC patients. This study preliminarily investigated such an association based on a large-scale and multicenter data.

Macroscopic invasion of the main portal vein or its branches is commonly categorized to be advanced HCC (22, 23). In fact, little is known about the factors related to the occurrence and development of PVTT. A previous study reported by our laboratory revealed that HBV infection promotes PVTT development in HCC by activating and modifying the TGF-β-miR-34α-CCL22 pathway, which forms an immune-subversive micro-environment that enhances the colonization of cancerous cells in the portal vein (24). In addition, platelets were also demonstrated to regulate HCC progression and metastasis, and associated with the long-term prognosis of PVTT patients. Another study reported by our team demonstrated that preoperative thrombocytopenia independently predicted prolonged RFS and OS of individuals with HCC complicated with PVTT following hepatectomy, and high platelet counts were associated with a high rate of intrahepatic metastasis. All these add to the gathering evidence that anti-platelet drugs, such as aspirin, are potentially useful treatments for HCC with PVTT (25). A study by Gon et al. (26) indicated that liver fibrosis, AFP and extent of PVTT were independent risk factors of rapid progression of PVTT, whereas des-gamma-carboxy prothrombin (DCP), extent of PVTT and liver fibrosis were independent prognostic factors in HCC patients with PVTT.

Up to now, there is still very little evidence to demonstrate the possible relationship between coagulability state and development of PVTT in HCC patients, and the interplay between HCC cells and coagulation homeostasis is not entirely understood (27, 28). In this large-scale multicenter study, a considerably higher percentage of HCC patients with PVTT had lower INR levels relative to HCC patients without PVTT. These results indicated a

TABLE 2 | Univariate and multivariate analysis of overall survival of 592 patients with types I/ II PVTT who underwent R0 LR.

Characteristics		OS (Univariate analysis)				OS (Multivariate analysis)			
		HR	95% CI		P value	HR	95% CI		P value
PVTT	II *vs* I	1.450	1.192	1.764	<0.001	1.388	1.137	1.693	0.001
INR	Normal *vs* Low	0.602	0.517	0.700	<0.001	0.595	0.511	0.694	<0.001
Age (years)	<50 *vs* ≥50	0.951	0.793	1.141	0.591				
Sex	Male *vs* Female	0.976	0.714	1.336	0.881				
Child-Pugh	A *vs* B	0.691	0.327	1.461	0.333				
HBsAg	Positive *vs* Negative	1.008	0.748	1.358	0.960				
Ascites	Yes *vs* No	1.400	1.056	1.855	0.019				
No. of tumors	Single *vs* Multiple	0.988	0.756	1.291	0.930				
Satellite nodules	Yes *vs* No	1.172	0.830	1.654	0.367				
AFP (ng/mL)	≥400 *vs* <400	2.288	1.542	3.404	<0.001	2.476	1.653	3.719	<0.001
Lymph node invasion	Yes *vs* No	1.080	0.843	1.384	0.543				
Tumor diameter (cm)	< 5 *vs* ≥ 5	0.778	0.621	0.973	0.028	0.744	0.592	0.934	0.011
Tumor encapsulation	Yes *vs* No	0.975	0.878	1.082	0.633				
Cirrhosis	Yes *vs* No	1.262	0.828	1.896	0.277				
TBIL (μmol/L)	≥17.1 *vs* <17.1	1.194	0.983	1.450	0.074				
DBIL (μmol/L)	≥6.8 *vs* <6.8	1.380	1.145	1.663	0.001	1.796	1.371	2.353	<0.001
ALB (g/L)		0.996	0.974	1.018	0.723				
ALT (U/L)		0.999	0.997	1.001	0.289				
AST (U/L)		1.002	1.000	1.004	0.041				
GGT (U/L)		1.000	0.999	1.001	0.925				
ALP (U/L)		1.002	1.000	1.003	0.027				
PLT ($\times 10^9$/L)		1.000	0.999	1.001	0.928				
CA199 (U/mL)		1.000	0.999	1.002	0.644				

PVTT, portal vein tumor thrombus; INR, international normalized ratio; HBsAg, hepatitis B surface antigen; AFP, α-fetoprotein; TBIL, total bilirubin; DBIL, direct bilirubin; ALB, albumin; ALT, alanine aminotransferase; AST, aspartate aminotransferase; GGT, γ-glutamyltransferase; ALP, alkaline phosphatase; PLT, platelet; CA199, carbohydrate antigen 19-9.

TABLE 3 | Univariate and multivariate analysis of recurrence-free survival of 592 patients with types I/II PVTT who underwent R0 LR.

Characteristics		RFS (Univariate analysis)				RFS (Multivariate analysis)			
		HR	95% CI		P value	HR	95% CI		P value
PVTT	II *vs* I	1.406	1.146	1.726	0.001	1.351	1.100	1.660	0.004
INR	Normal *vs* Low	0.697	0.594	0.818	<0.001	0.748	0.637	0.878	<0.001
Age (years)	<50 *vs* ≥50	0.989	0.813	1.203	0.910				
Sex	Male *vs* Female	0.947	0.673	1.334	0.757				
Child-Pugh	A *vs* B	0.673	0.300	1.508	0.336				
HBsAg	Positive *vs* Negative	1.088	0.788	1.503	0.609				
Ascites	Yes *vs* No	1.221	0.895	1.665	0.208				
No. of tumors	Single *vs* Multiple	0.829	0.615	1.119	0.220				
Satellite Nodules	Yes *vs* No	1.516	1.011	2.273	0.044				
AFP (ng/mL)	≥400 *vs* <400	2.566	1.673	3.968	<0.001	2.534	1.631	3.938	<0.001
Lymph node invasion	Yes *vs* No	1.220	0.938	1.586	0.138				
Tumor diameter (cm)	<5 *vs* ≥5	0.932	0.723	1.202	0.589				
Tumor encapsulation	Yes *vs* No	0.795	0.708	0.893	<0.001	0.803	0.715	0.902	<0.001
Cirrhosis	Yes *vs* No	1.184	0.953	1.470	0.127				
TBIL (μmol/L)	≥17.1 *vs* <17.1	1.087	0.878	1.345	0.445				
DBIL (μmol/L)	≥6.8 *vs* <6.8	1.038	0.844	1.276	0.724				
ALB (g/L)		1.016	0.991	1.042	0.214				
ALT (U/L)		1.000	0.998	1.002	0.991				
AST (U/L)		1.003	1.000	1.005	0.021	1.003	1.001	1.005	0.011
GGT (U/L)		1.000	0.999	1.001	0.719				
ALP (U/L)		1.001	0.999	1.002	0.394				
PLT ($\times 10^9$/L)		1.001	0.999	1.002	0.292				
CA199 (U/mL)		0.999	0.997	1.001	0.181				

PVTT, portal vein tumor thrombus; INR, international normalized ratio; HBsAg, hepatitis B surface antigen; AFP, α-fetoprotein; TBIL, total bilirubin; DBIL, direct bilirubin; ALB, albumin; ALT, alanine aminotransferase; AST, aspartate aminotransferase; GGT, γ-glutamyltransferase; ALP, alkaline phosphatase; PLT, platelet; CA199, carbohydrate antigen 19-9.

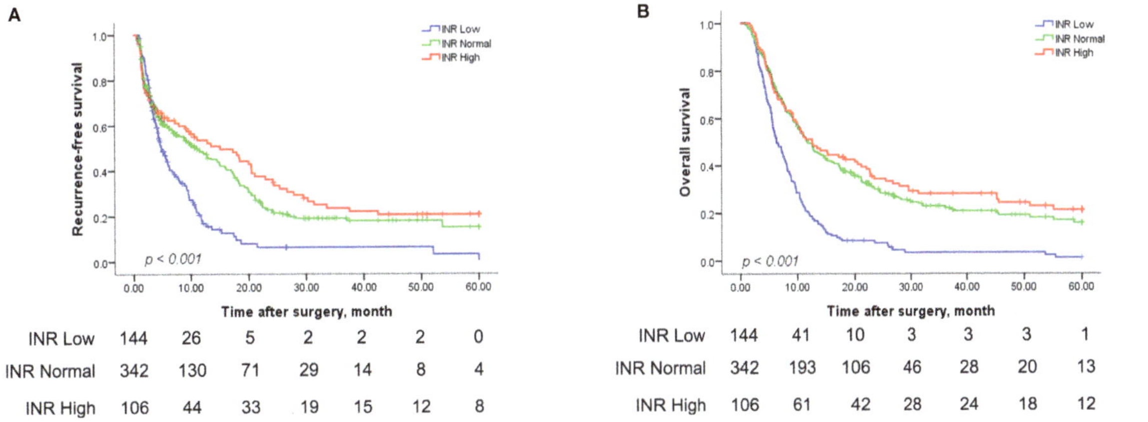

FIGURE 3 | Kaplan-Meier analysis for the RFS and OS rates in HCC patients with types I/II PVTT after R0 LR among the Low, Normal, and High INR groups. RFS for patients among the Low, Normal, and High INR groups (144 patients *vs* 342 patients *vs* 106 patients) after R0 LR **(A)** ($P < 0.001$); OS for patients among the Low, Normal, and High INR groups (144 patients *vs* 342 patients *vs* 106 patients) after R0 LR **(B)** ($P < 0.001$). INR, international normalized ratio.

close relationship between hypercoagulability and the incidence of PVTT. On the other hand, PVTT as foreign tumor masses can further promote the formation of hypercoagulability in the portal venous system. This study also showed HCC patients with types III/IV PVTT to have a significantly higher proportion of a low INR level (hypercoagulability) than those with types I/II PVTT, which suggested the potential association between coagulability status and the extent of PVTT. Hypercoagulability can increase the rate of progression of PVTT from a segmental/sectoral branch (Cheng's type I) or right/left portal vein (Cheng's type II) to the main portal vein (Cheng's type III) or the superior mesenteric vein (Cheng's type IV).

The association between preoperative coagulation state and outcomes of HCC subjects with PVTT following R0 LR has seldom been studied. In our study, HCC patients with PVTT with hypercoagulability (low INR level) had a worse prognosis compared to those with normal coagulability (normal INR level) or hypocoagulability (high INR level) after R0 LR. Patients with hypocoagulability in the High INR group exhibited comparable survival as patients with normal coagulability in the Normal INR group. On subgroup analysis, type I or type II PVTT patients with low levels of INR had poorer prognosis than those with normal or high levels of INR. On multivariate analysis, the preoperative INR level was an independent prognosis predictive factor of OS and RFS outcomes in the study population. The liver is an organ which synthesizes most coagulation factors and regulatory proteins, which play a central role in the coagulation regulation and hemostatic control. A review revealed that derangement in liver function can result in thrombotic complications, such as PVTT (15). Multiple and inter-connected mechanisms by which HCC modifies the homeostatic balance to lean toward hypercoagulability have been proposed. One study suggested that tissue factor (TF), the initiator of the coagulation process, was related to angiogenesis and invasiveness of HCC, and an elevated level of TF was an independent prognostic factor in HCC patients (29). Another study showed that circulating microparticles (MP), a population of extracellular vesicles, have the ability to induce coagulation and promote portal vein thrombosis (PVT) in patients with concomitant cirrhosis and HCC, possibly due to higher MP TF activity in these patients (30).

Several limitations of this study have to be acknowledged. First, this is a retrospective cohort study with its intrinsic bias. Nonetheless, the large sample size from six high-volume hospitals increases its reliability. Second, majority of the study participants had a history of HBV infections. Future studies involving patients with hepatitis C virus infections or alcoholism as the primary etiological factors of HCC are needed. Last, the underlying biological mechanisms between hypercoagulability and PVTT formation and progression have not been explored in this study.

In conclusion, there is a close association between preoperative INR level and the incidence and extent of PVTT in HCC patients. HCC patients with hypercoagulability in the Low INR group had a significantly higher incidence of PVTT and more extensive PVTT. HCC patients with PVTT limited to a first-order branch or above of the main portal vein in the Low INR group had worse survival outcomes than those in the Normal and High INR groups after R0 LR.

AUTHOR CONTRIBUTIONS

Conception and design: S-QC, WL, M-CW, and X-PZ. Financial support: S-QC. Provision of study materials or patients: Z-JZ, DZ, FZ, Y-RH, C-QZ, Z-TC, KW, JS, and W-XG. Collection and assembly of data: X-PZ, T-FZ, J-KF, Z-YS, and Z-HC. Data Analysis and interpretation: X-PZ, T-FZ, J-KF, and Z-YS. All authors contributed to the article and approved the submitted version.

SUPPLEMENTARY MATERIAL

Supplementary Figure 1 | Kaplan-Meier analysis for subgroup analysis of the

RFS and OS rates in HCC patients with types I/II PVTT after R0 LR among the Low, Normal, and High INR groups. RFS for patients with type I PVTT among the Low, Normal, and High INR groups (55 patients *vs* 113 patients *vs* 37 patients) after R0 LR **(A)** ($P < 0.001$); OS for patients with type I PVTT among the Low, Normal, and High INR groups (55 patients *vs* 113 patients *vs* 37 patients) after R0 LR **(B)** ($P < 0.001$); RFS for patients with type II PVTT among the Low, Normal, and High INR groups (89 patients *vs* 229 patients *vs* 69 patients) after R0 LR **(C)** ($P = 0.019$); OS for patients with type II PVTT among the Low, Normal, and High INR group (89 patients *vs* 229 patients *vs* 69 patients) after R0 LR **(D)** ($P < 0.001$). INR, international normalized ratio.

REFERENCES

1. Forner A, Llovet JM, Bruix J. Hepatocellular Carcinoma. *Lancet* (2012) 379:1245–55. doi: 10.1016/S0140-6736(11)61347-0
2. Torre LA, Bray F, Siegel RL, Ferlay J, Lortet-Tieulent J, Jemal A, et al. Global Cancer Statistics, 2012. *CA Cancer J Clin* (2015) 65:87–108. doi: 10.3322/caac.21262
3. Marrero JA, Kulik LM, Sirlin CB, Zhu AX, Finn RS, Abecassis MM, et al. Diagnosis, Staging and Management of Hepatocellular Carcinoma: 2018 Practice Guidance by the American Association for the Study of Liver Diseases. *Hepatology* (2018) 68:723–50. doi: 10.1002/hep.29913
4. Wang K, Guo WX, Chen MS, Mao YL, Sun BC, Shi J, et al. Multimodality Treatment for Hepatocellular Carcinoma With Portal Vein Tumor Thrombus: A Large-Scale, Multicenter, Propensity Matching Score Analysis. *Medicine* (2016) 95:e3015. doi: 10.1097/MD.0000000000003015
5. Bruix J, Reig M, Sherman M. Evidence-Based Diagnosis, Staging, and Treatment of Patients With Hepatocellular Carcinoma. *Gastroenterology* (2016) 150:835–53. doi: 10.1053/j.gastro.2015.12.041
6. Llovet JM, Ricci S, Mazzaferro V, Hilgard P, Gane E, Blanc JF, et al. Sorafenib in Advanced Hepatocellular Carcinoma. *N Engl J Med* (2008) 359:378–90. doi: 10.1056/NEJMoa0708857
7. Cheng AL, Kang YK, Chen Z, Tsao CJ, Qin S, Kim JS, et al. Efficacy and Safety of Sorafenib in Patients in the Asia-Pacific Region With Advanced Hepatocellular Carcinoma: A Phase III Randomised, Double-Blind, Placebo-Controlled Trial. *Lancet Oncol* (2009) 10:25–34. doi: 10.1016/S1470-2045(08)70285-7
8. Zhang XP, Wang K, Guo WX, Chen ZH, Cheng SQ. Is Sorafenib an Optimal Treatment for Hepatocellular Carcinoma With Macrovascular Invasion or Metastatic Disease? *Hepatology* (2018) 68:786. doi: 10.1002/hep.29862
9. Giannini EG, Bucci L, Garuti F, Brunacci M, Lenzi B, Valente M, et al. Patients With Advanced Hepatocellular Carcinoma Need a Personalized Management: A Lesson From Clinical Practice. *Hepatology* (2018) 67:1784–96. doi: 10.1002/hep.29668
10. Kokudo T, Hasegawa K, Matsuyama Y, Takayama T, Izumi N, Kadoya M, et al. Survival Benefit of Liver Resection for Hepatocellular Carcinoma Associated With Portal Vein Invasion. *J Hepatol* (2016) 65:938–43. doi: 10.1016/j.jhep.2016.05.044
11. Hyun MH, Lee YS, Kim JH, Lee CU, Jung YK, Seo YS, et al. Hepatic Resection Compared to Chemoembolization in Intermediate- to Advanced-Stage Hepatocellular Carcinoma: A Meta-Analysis of High-Quality Studies. *Hepatology* (2018) 68:977–93. doi: 10.1002/hep.29883
12. Cheng S, Chen M, Cai J, Sun J, Guo R, Bi X, et al. Chinese Expert Consensus on Multidisciplinary Diagnosis and Treatment of Hepatocellular Carcinoma With Portal Vein Tumor Thrombus (2018 Edition). *Liver Cancer* (2020) 9:28–40. doi: 10.1159/000503685
13. Zhang XP, Gao YZ, Chen ZH, Chen MS, Li LQ, Wen TF, et al. An Eastern Hepatobiliary Surgery Hospital/Portal Vein Tumor Thrombus Scoring System as an Aid to Decision Making on Hepatectomy for Hepatocellular Carcinoma Patients With Portal Vein Tumor Thrombus: A Multicenter Study. *Hepatology* (2019) 69:2076–90. doi: 10.1002/hep.30490
14. Falanga A, Donati MB. Pathogenesis of Thrombosis in Patients With Malignancy. *Int J Hematol* (2001) 73:137–44. doi: 10.1007/BF02981929
15. Campello E, Henderson MW, Noubouossie DF, Simioni P, Key NS. Contact System Activation and Cancer: New Insights in the Pathophysiology of Cancer-Associated Thrombosis. *Thromb Haemost* (2018) 118:251–65. doi: 10.1160/TH17-08-0596
16. Sallah S, Wan JY, Nguyen NP. Venous Thrombosis in Patients With Solid Tumors: Determination of Frequency and Characteristics. *Thromb Haemost* (2002) 87:575–9. doi: 10.1055/s-0037-1613051
17. Kinoshita A, Onoda H, Imai N, Iwaku A, Oishi M, Tanaka K, et al. Elevated Plasma Fibrinogen Levels Are Associated With a Poor Prognosis in Patients With Hepatocellular Carcinoma. *Oncology* (2013) 85:269–77. doi: 10.1159/000355502
18. Shi J, Lai EC, Li N, Guo WX, Xue J, Lau WY, et al. A New Classification for Hepatocellular Carcinoma With Portal Vein Tumor Thrombus. *J Hepatobiliary Pancreat Sci* (2011) 18:74–80. doi: 10.1007/s00534-010-0314-0
19. Shi J, Lai EC, Li N, Guo WX, Xue J, Lau WY, et al. Surgical Treatment of Hepatocellular Carcinoma With Portal Vein Tumor Thrombus. *Ann Surg Oncol* (2010) 17:2073–80. doi: 10.1245/s10434-010-0940-4
20. Sakamoto K, Nagano H. Surgical Treatment for Advanced Hepatocellular Carcinoma With Portal Vein Tumor Thrombus. *Hepatol Res* (2017) 47:957–62. doi: 10.1111/hepr.12923
21. Zhang XP, Wang K, Li N, Zhong CQ, Wei XB, Cheng YQ, et al. Survival Benefit of Hepatic Resection Versus Transarterial Chemoembolization for Hepatocellular Carcinoma With Portal Vein Tumor Thrombus: A Systematic Review and Meta-Analysis. *BMC Cancer* (2017) 17:902. doi: 10.1186/s12885-017-3895-z
22. Peng ZW, Guo RP, Zhang YJ, Lin XJ, Chen MS, Lau WY, et al. Hepatic Resection Versus Transcatheter Arterial Chemoembolization for the Treatment of Hepatocellular Carcinoma With Portal Vein Tumor Thrombus. *Cancer* (2012) 118:4725–36. doi: 10.1002/cncr.26561
23. Zhu K, Chen J, Lai L, Meng X, Zhou B, Huang W, et al. Hepatocellular Carcinoma With Portal Vein Tumor Thrombus: Treatment With Transarterial Chemoembolization Combined With Sorafenib–A Retrospective Controlled Study. *Radiology* (2014) 272:284–93. doi: 10.1148/radiol.14131946
24. Yang P, Li QJ, Feng Y, Zhang Y, Markowitz GJ, Ning S, et al. TGF-β-miR-34a-CCL22 Signaling-Induced Treg Cell Recruitment Promotes Venous Metastases of HBV-positive Hepatocellular Carcinoma. *Cancer Cell* (2012) 22:291–303. doi: 10.1016/j.ccr.2012.07.023
25. Cheng YQ, Wang K, Zhang XP, Wei XB, Jiang YB, Hu YR, et al. Thrombocytopenia: A Prognostic Factor for Hepatocellular Carcinoma Patients With Portal Vein Tumor Thrombus After Hepatectomy. *J Gastroenterol Hepatol* (2019) 34:1214–21. doi: 10.1111/jgh.14537
26. Gon H, Kido M, Tanaka M, Kinoshita H, Komatsu S, Tsugawa D, et al. Growth Velocity of the Portal Vein Tumor Thrombus Accelerated by its Progression, Alpha-Fetoprotein Level, and Liver Fibrosis Stage in Patients With Hepatocellular Carcinoma. *Surgery* (2018) 164:1014–22. doi: 10.1016/j.surg.2018.06.025
27. Zanetto A, Campello E, Spiezia L, Burra P, Simioni P, Russo FP, et al. Cancer-Associated Thrombosis in Cirrhotic Patients With Hepatocellular Carcinoma. *Cancers* (2018) 10:450. doi: 10.3390/cancers10110450
28. Zhu WL, Fan BL, Liu DL, Zhu WX. Abnormal Expression of Fibrinogen Gamma (FGG) and Plasma Level of Fibrinogen in Patients With Hepatocellular Carcinoma. *Anticancer Res* (2009) 29:2531–4.
29. Poon RT, Lau CP, Ho JW, Yu WC, Fan ST, Wong J, et al. Tissue Factor Expression Correlates With Tumor Angiogenesis and Invasiveness in Human Hepatocellular Carcinoma. *Clin Cancer Res* (2003) 9:5339–45.
30. Campello E, Zanetto A, Spiezia L, Radu CM, Gavasso S, Ferrarese A, et al. Hypercoagulability Detected by Circulating Microparticles in Patients With Hepatocellular Carcinoma and Cirrhosis. *Thromb Res* (2016) 143:118–21. doi: 10.1016/j.thromres.2016.05.021

17

Survival After Treatable Hepatocellular Carcinoma Recurrence in Liver Recipients

Cheng-Maw Ho [1], Chih-Hsin Lee [2], Ming-Chia Lee [3,4], Jun-Fu Zhang [5,6], Chin-Hua Chen [5,7,8†], Jann-Yuan Wang [9†], Rey-Heng Hu [1†] and Po-Huang Lee [1]*

[1] Department of Surgery, National Taiwan University Hospital and College of Medicine, Taipei, Taiwan, [2] Division of Pulmonary Medicine and Pulmonary Research Center, Wanfang Hospital, Taipei Medical University, Taipei, Taiwan, [3] Department of Pharmacy, New Taipei City Hospital, New Taipei City, Taiwan, [4] School of Pharmacy, College of Pharmacy, Taipei Medical University, Taipei, Taiwan, [5] Biostatistics Center, College of Management, Taipei Medical University, Taipei, Taiwan, [6] Big Data Center, Lo-Hsu Medical Foundation, Lotung Poh-Ai Hospital, Yilan, Taiwan, [7] Graduate Institute of Data Science, College of Management, Taipei Medical University, Taipei, Taiwan, [8] Department of Medical Education and Research, Wanfang Hospital, Taipei Medical University, Taipei, Taiwan, [9] Department of Internal Medicine, National Taiwan University Hospital, and College of Medicine, Taipei, Taiwan

***Correspondence:**
Jann-Yuan Wang
jywang@ntu.edu.tw

†These authors have contributed equally to this work

Background: Survival after post-transplant recurrence of HCC is dismal, and almost all treatments for recurrent HCC are off-labeled, without an extensive large-scale analysis. We aimed to delineate their post-recurrence courses and define benchmarks for comparing future treatment effectiveness.

Methods: Three national databases, including health insurance, catastrophic illness, and the cause of death, were linked for cohort establishment and data collection during the period from 2005 to 2016. Patients with HCC recurrence ≥6 months after transplant surgery and under treatment were recruited for survival analysis. Selection of treatment strategies for HCC recurrence after liver transplant was based on the same criteria for those without liver transplant.

Results: Of 2,123 liver transplant recipients, 349 developed HCC recurrence ≥6 months after liver transplant, and the median recurrence time was 17.8 months post-transplant. Within 2 years of treatment, 61% patients showed recurrence (early recurrence group), and survival in these patients was poorer than in the late recurrence group. According to a multivariable analysis, the transplant era before 2008 and radiofrequency ablation were associated with good prognosis, whereas receiving sorafenib and radiotherapy was associated with poor prognosis. The effect of transplant era became insignificant after stratification by recently receiving pretransplant transarterial chemoembolization.

Conclusion: Timing of recurrence and interventions used were associated with the outcomes of patients with post-transplant HCC recurrence. These data provide the benchmark and indicate the critical period and high-risk factors for further therapeutic trial consideration.

Keywords: hepatocellular carcinoma, liver transplantation, radiofrequency ablation, recurrence, survival

INTRODUCTION

Patients with HCC have high recurrence rates after cancer treatment (1). Although primary HCC can be cured through liver transplant under stringent criteria (2), the current trend of accommodating transplant patients through relaxing criteria and salvaging those who had recurrent HCC with multiple previous loco-regional treatments can potentially increase the pool of post-transplant recurrence tremendously in the near future (1, 3). However, guidelines for the management of HCC recurrence after liver transplantation are still lacking (3).

Currently, the management strategy of primary HCC and non-transplant setting is used for post-transplant HCC recurrence (3, 4). Thriving clinical trials on newer systemic therapies, such as target therapy and immunotherapy, which can prolong patient survival after recurrence, have always excluded transplant patients (5). Consequently, almost all transplant patients with HCC recurrence were neglected and received off-labeled cancer treatments. With the changing landscape of HCC and the approval of new systemic chemotherapeutic agents, future studies are warranted to characterize the efficacy and safety of these agents in liver transplant recipients (3).

Numerous studies have emphasized on the primary prevention of HCC recurrence (or re-recurrence) after liver transplantation (6–13) rather than on prolonging meaningful outcomes after recurrence. To address this emerging critical issue, large-scale studies are necessary but remain scant (14–16). Without a benchmark reference, institutional bias and limited overview exist in this heterogeneous population.

HCC is one of the leading causes of cancer-related mortality in Taiwan for decades, and liver transplantation is a mature surgery performed in nationwide multiple centers (17). With a longitudinal follow-up of more than 20 million patients and validated diagnoses of catastrophic illnesses, the National Health Insurance Research Database (NHIRD) provides a great platform to explore the clinical course and outcome of post-transplant recurrence.

Particularly, we aimed to illustrate the courses of post-transplant HCC recurrence by using the NHIRD as a source material and to analyze relevant prognostic factors. Additionally, this study enriches the literature and provides a benchmark reference for comparing effectiveness in future interventional analyses.

METHODS

The Institutional Review Board of National Taiwan University Hospital, Taipei, Taiwan, approved this study (NTUH REC: 201601007W). Because this was a retrospective study using an encrypted database, the institutional review board waived the need for informed consent.

Data Acquisition

Entire original data were from the following three linked national databases covering the beneficiaries of the whole population of Taiwan from 2005 to 2016: Taiwan's NHIRD, Registry for Catastrophic Illness Patient Database (RCIPD), and Cause of Death Database. Regarding HCC, the histologic confirmation or typical imaging presentation is required for registering patients in the RCIPD.

Cohort Selection

Patients with HCC who received liver transplant surgery were identified from Taiwan's NHIRD. Regardless of donor types, liver transplant surgery for HCC is reimbursed if the tumor status listed and at transplant is within the University of California San Francisco criteria (single tumor <6.5 cm, maximum of three total tumors with none >4.5 cm, and cumulative tumor size <8 cm) (1, 18, 19). Image follow-ups (every 3 to 6 months) were regularly performed for detection of recurrence. Among them, those with HCC recurrence were identified. In this study, HCC recurrence was diagnosed as having a compatible diagnostic code (International Classification of Diseases, 9th/10th Revision 155/C22) and receiving intervention, to validate the definite recurrence and to identify patients with treatable diseases. The main cohort adopted liver recipients who had recurrence ≥6 months after transplant surgery as the target population.

The date of the first intervention for treatable HCC recurrence after transplantation was defined as the index date. Interventions included hepatectomy (resection), radiofrequency ablation (RFA), transarterial chemoembolization (TACE), radiotherapy, sorafenib, and chemotherapy. The coding of interventions is detailed in the **Supplement**.

Liver transplant recipients who survived or had HCC recurrence <180 days after transplant surgery were excluded because within this period, high rejection rates, surgical complications, and infection episodes interfere in the appropriate assessment for cancer-related survival. Moreover, adjuvant systemic therapy, such as sorafenib or chemotherapy, may be administered in this period, confounding true HCC recurrence (20).

Treatment Strategies for Post-Transplant HCC Recurrence

Selection of treatment strategies for HCC recurrence after liver transplant was based on the same criteria for those without liver transplant (17, 21). Particularly for post-transplant recurrence, extensive tumor staging would be performed initially to identify the intra- and extra-hepatic involvements before treatments. Systemic therapy with sorafenib was used in patients with vascular or extrahepatic metastases. Locoregional therapies (resection, RFA, or TACE) were performed for intra-hepatic recurrence with curative intents (resection and RFA) as the priority consideration.

Since 2011, treatment decisions for patients with HCC awaiting liver transplant were audited at each center's multidisciplinary liver tumor board, attended by hepatologists, liver transplant surgeons, oncologists, and radiologists with an expertise in HCC management.

Abbreviations: ATC, anatomical therapeutic chemical; DDD, defined daily dose; ICD, International Classification of Diseases; IQR, inter-quartile range; MMF, mycophenolate mofetil; mTOR, mammalian target of rapamycin; NHIRD, National Health Insurance Research Database; RCIPD, Registry for Catastrophic Illness Patient Database; RFA, radiofrequency ablation; TACE, transarterial chemoembolization.

Pre-Claim Review of High-Priced Interventions

In Taiwan, liver transplant surgery, RFA, and sorafenib are regulated clinical treatments that need a pre-claim review process of charts and images before being implemented and reimbursed. RFA for HCC, confined within liver, is approved if the tumor number is not more than three and each tumor size is <5 cm in diameter. Sorafenib for HCC is approved if the patient has distant metastases or major vascular invasion inside the well-reserved liver.

Demographic Parameters

Demographic information, namely sex, age, monthly income, transplantation period, liver cirrhosis, and underlying comorbidity (such as diabetes mellitus, hyperlipidemia, and alcohol use), was collected, as described previously (22). Viral status, including HBV or HCV, was defined based on the prescription of antiviral medications, at least two outpatient coding, or at least one inpatient coding of the corresponding viral diagnosis within 1 year before transplantation. Reimbursement of direct-acting antiviral agents for HCV in Taiwan started since January 2017, beyond the study period (December 2016), and was therefore not included in analysis. The details of coding definitions are described in the **Supplement**.

When more than one treatment modality was used as the initial treatment (such as TACE and RFA at the same admission), the one with curative intent (resection or RFA) was prioritized and coded. Furthermore, interventions for HCC within 1 year before liver transplant surgery were collected. A minimum observation period of 3 months between local treatment and transplantation is a consensus policy required for successful downstaging of HCC (23).

Living liver donation was coded when the period of living donor surgery (procedural code: 75022B) and hospital stay overlapped with the period of liver transplant surgery and hospital stay of the recipient in the same hospital. Deceased liver donation, after brain death as only allowed by law in the studied period, was coded when liver transplant surgery and recipients' hospital stay overlapped with the date of deceased liver donation surgery (75021B).

The doses of post-transplant medications, including HBV medications (lamivudine, entecavir, and tenofovir), metformin, and immunosuppressants (tacrolimus [anatomical therapeutic chemical (ATC) code: L04AD02], cyclosporin [ATC code: L04AD01], mycophenolate mofetil [MMF]/myfortic acid [ATC code: L04AA06], sirolimus [ATC code: L04AA10], and everolimus [ATC code: L04AA18]), within 180 days after transplant surgery were calculated. Drug codes other than immunosuppressants were described previously (24).

Outcome Measurement

The patients were followed up until death, withdrawal of health insurance, or December 31, 2016. The event date was the date of death or the last follow-up date. The date of death was obtained from the Cause of Death Database. Death due to HCC was considered when the first two diagnoses on the death certificate included HCC. Overall survival and HCC-specific survival were estimated separately.

Statistical Analysis

A recent review suggested that HCC recurring >2 years after liver transplantation may host a different biological mechanism compared with early recurrence (3). Therefore, in our study, patients were stratified into two groups based on the time to recurrence, that is, recurrence within 2 years after transplantation and recurrence beyond 2 years after transplantation. In the 12-year study period, three eras (2005–2008, 2009–2012, and 2013–2016) were split even for historical comparison. Liver recipients with treatable HCC recurrence within 6 months after transplant surgery and patients with recurrence code but received no treatment were processed separately for assessment of data quality and plausibility.

Data are expressed as the mean ± standard deviation, median (interquartile range [IQR]), or number (percentage) as appropriate. Student's t test or χ^2 test was used for the intergroup comparison. The time-to-event curves were generated using the Kaplan–Meier method and compared using the log-rank test.

Cox's proportional hazard model was used for univariable and multivariable analyses. Sensitivity analysis was performed for a cohort of recipients who could be matched to one single living or deceased donor and for a subgroup of patients with primary HCC treated by upfront transplant. All statistical tests were two-sided at a significance level of 0.05, and all analyses were performed using SAS, version 9.4 (SAS Institute Inc., Cary, NC, USA).

RESULTS

Demographics

From the RCIPD and NHIRD, 2,123 patients who had HCC diagnosis and received liver transplantation in 2005–2016 were identified (**Figure 1**). The calculated post-transplant HCC recurrence rate was 24.0% (510/2123). Among them, 349 patients who developed HCC recurrence >6 months after liver transplant and were undergoing treatment were included in this study, excluding 131 patients who claimed to have recurrence within 6 months after transplantation and 30 patients who did not receive any intervention (marked in **Figure 1**).

Table 1 shows the characteristics of this cohort, which was composed of patients with an average age of 55.4 years; furthermore, 84.5% of patients were men; 90.0, 75.1, 43.0, and 22.6% had cirrhosis, HBV exposure, HCV exposure, and diabetes mellitus, respectively; and 76.2% had received living donor liver transplantation. Among 150 patients with HCV-related HCC (97 co-infected with HBV), 39 (26.0%) received pre-transplant, and 14 (9.3%) post-transplant, anti-HCV therapy. The median follow-up duration after transplantation was 33.9 months (IQR, 20.7–61.4 months) in the cohort, 24.7 months (16.6–32.6 months) in the early recurrence group, and 65.3 months (47.9–88.5 months) in the late recurrence group (P < 0.001). The

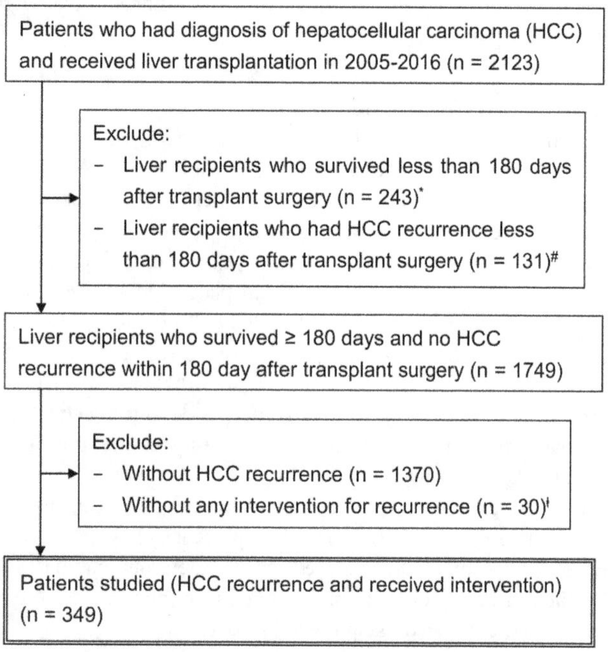

FIGURE 1 | Schematic representation of the patient selection process. *Contained patients with HCC recurrence deemed unfit or too advanced for any treatment. #Within 6 months after transplant surgery, 41 (31.3%) patients had complications (rejection, surgical complication, or sepsis) and 21 (16.0%) expired. The initial interventions included radiotherapy (n = 37), chemotherapy (n = 35), sorafenib (n = 26), transarterial chemoembolization (n = 25), and others (n = 8). However, 33 patients (25.2%) survived unusually longer than 5 years, suggesting data miscoding or adjuvant treatments, rather than true recurrence. ǂ14 (46.7%) patients had complications within 6 months after transplant surgery. Sixteen patients (53.3%) survived unusually longer than 5 years without any oncological interventions, suggesting another area of miscoding and data contamination. These patients (# and ǂ) were excluded from the main cohort for analysis because their data were highly heterogeneous and lack of confidence, and validated discrimination between true recurrence and false positivity was not possible.

median interval between transplant and post-transplant recurrence was 17.8 months (10.7–34.4 months), 11.4 months (8.3–16.5 months) in the early recurrence group, and 39.8 months (30.6–60.3 months) in the late recurrence group (P < 0.001). The distribution of patients among the three transplant eras was statistically different (P < 0.001) in terms of early and late recurrence. After 2013, nearly 41% and only 11.8% of patients in the early and late recurrence groups, respectively, received transplant surgery.

Early Post-Transplant Medications

Immunosuppressive medications majorly used for treatment within 6 months after liver transplantation were tacrolimus (94.3%) and MMF (85.7%). Mammalian target of rapamycin inhibitors (sirolimus and everolimus) was used in 14.0 and 18.6% of patients, respectively (**Table 2**). The distribution of immunosuppressive drug use and their defined daily dose were not different between early and late recurrence groups, except for MMF (171.7 ± 129.5 *vs.* 208.6 ± 159.0, P = 0.024) and everolimus (40.2 ± 93.1 *vs.* 21.3 ± 60.4, P = 0.022) (**Table S1**).

Lamivudine was used in 22.9% of patients, and its usage was higher in the late recurrence group than in the early group (30.9 *vs.* 17.8%, P = 0.007). Furthermore, lamivudine was mostly (57/80, 71.3%) prescribed in the earlier transplant period (2005–2008): 71.1% in the early recurrence group and 71.4% in the late recurrence group. By contrast, entecavir was prescribed mostly (81/102, 79.4%) in the recent era (2013–2016): 88.4% (61/69) in the early recurrence group and 60.6% (20/33) in the late recurrence group (P = 0.003).

Intervention

Only 20.3% of patients in this cohort received no interventions for HCC within 1 year before transplantation, and the late recurrence group seemed to have more of them than did the early group (25.0 *vs.* 17.4%, P = 0.084) (**Table S2**). Within 1 year before transplant surgery, 222 (63.6% in 349) received TACE and

TABLE 1 | Patient demographics.

	All recurrence (n = 349)	Recur within 2 years (n = 213)	Recur after 2 years (n = 136)	*P*-value
Survival after recurrence: months (median, IQR)	11.2 (5.7–22.3)	10.2 (5.2–19.9)	14.3 (6.6–32.6)	0.026
Age: years (mean ± SD)	55.4 ± 8.6	55.1 ± 8.7	54.1 ± 8.4	0.295
Male (n, %)	295 (84.5)	181 (85)	114 (83.8)	0.890
Cirrhosis (n, %)	314 (90.0)	189 (88.7)	125 (91.9)	0.434
Diabetes mellitus (n, %)	79 (22.6)	51 (23.9)	28 (20.6)	0.549
Hyperlipidemia (n, %)	36 (10.3)	22 (10.3)	14 (10.3)	1.000
Alcohol use (n, %)	16 (4.6)	13 (6.1)	3 (2.2)	0.151
HBV (n, %)	262 (75.1)	163 (76.5)	99 (72.8)	0.510
HBV-medication use before transplant (n, %)	173 (49.6)	104 (48.8)	69 (50.7)	0.812
HCV (n, %)	150 (43.0)	97 (45.5)	53 (39.0)	0.272
HCV-medication use before transplant (n, %)	39 (11.2)	20 (9.4)	19 (14.0)	0.250
Living donor (n, %)	266 (76.2)	163 (76.5)	103 (75.7)	0.968
Transplantation period (n, %)				< 0.001
Before 2008	112 (32.1)	55 (25.8)	57 (41.9)	
2009–2012	134 (38.4)	71 (33.3)	63 (46.3)	
After 2013	103 (29.5)	87 (40.9)	16 (11.8)	

IQR, interquartile range; SD, standard deviation.

TABLE 2 | Summary of selective medications within 6 months after transplant.

	All recurrence (n = 349)	Recur within 2 years (n = 213)	Recur after 2 years (n = 136)	*P*-value
Immunosuppressants				
Tacrolimus (n, %)	329 (94.3)	198 (93.0)	131 (96.3)	0.279
Cyclosporin (n, %)	24 (6.9)	16 (7.5)	8 (5.9)	0.712
MMF (n, %)	299 (85.7)	178 (83.6)	121 (89.0)	0.212
Sirolimus (n, %)	49 (14.0)	28 (13.1)	21 (15.4)	0.657
Everolimus (n, %)	65 (18.6)	46 (21.6)	19 (14.0)	0.100
Metformin (n, %)	84 (24.1)	51 (23.9)	33 (24.3)	1.000
HBV medication				
Lamivudine (n, %)	80 (22.9)	38 (17.8)	42 (30.9)	0.007
Entecavir (n, %)	102 (29.2)	69 (32.4)	33 (24.3)	0.132
Tenofovir (n, %)	12 (3.4)	9 (4.2)	3 (2.2)	0.479

MMF, mycophenolate mofetil.

estimated 175 (50.1%) at most used TACE as a downstaging strategy (a minimum of 3 months to observe before surgery).

For post-transplant recurrence, the number of patients who received the initial and ever-exposed treatment modalities of resection, RFA, TACE, radiotherapy, and sorafenib was 16, 22, 95, 112, and 71 and 22, 45, 151, 183, and 130, respectively (**Table 3**). Common initial treatments for HCC recurrence were radiotherapy (32.1%), TACE (27.2%), and sorafenib (20.3%). Based on reimbursement regulation for HCC treatment, the initial recurrence HCC stage was estimated to be advanced (vascular or extra-hepatic metastases) for at least 20.3% (71/349) and intrahepatic for at least 38.1% (133/349). Among the 130 (37.2%) patients exposed to sorafenib after recurrence, most (97/130, 74.6%) received other treatments in sequence or in combination. Initial treatment with sorafenib was more common in the early recurrence group than in the late recurrence group (23.0 *vs.* 16.2%, $P = 0.122$), suggesting more advanced HCC, when the first post-transplant recurrence occurred, in the early group. Consistently, sorafenib, as the only single treatment modality throughout the post-recurrence courses, was used more frequently in the early recurrence group than in the late recurrence group (12.7 *vs.* 4.4%, $P = 0.010$).

RFA was applied in 45 (12.9%) patients. Nearly half of them (22/45, 48.9%) was initial treatment, and most of them also received other treatments (37/45, 82.2%). The RFA distribution (either initial treatment or treatment exposure) between the early and late recurrence groups was not statistically significant.

Twenty-two (6.3%) patients received resection for post-transplant recurrence in this cohort, and the majority of them received it as the initial treatment (16/22, 72.7%). Over half of the patients (13/22, 59.1%) who received resection also received treatment with other modalities. The number of patients who received only resection was higher in the late recurrence group than in the early recurrence group (4.4 *vs.* 1.4%, $P = 0.096$).

Although radiotherapy is not regarded as the standard treatment for HCC, its application was more common (183, 52.4%) than that of TACE (151/349, 43.3%). Many patients who received radiotherapy (114/183, 62.3%) or TACE (104/151, 68.9%) also received other treatments in their post-recurrence courses.

TABLE 3 | Summary of HCC treatment modalities after transplantation in patients with post-transplant recurrence.

	All recurrence (n = 349)	Recur within 2Y (n = 213)	Recur after 2Y (n = 136)	*P*-value
Initial				
Hepatectomy	16 (4.6)	8 (3.8)	8 (5.9)	0.493
RFA	22 (6.3)	12 (5.6)	10 (7.4)	
TACE	95 (27.2)	53 (24.9)	42 (30.9)	
Sorafenib	71 (20.3)	49 (23.0)	22 (16.2)	
RT	112 (32.1)	70 (32.9)	42 (30.9)	
Others	33 (9.5)	21 (9.9)	12 (8.8)	
Ever exposure				
Hepatectomy only	9 (2.6)	3 (1.4)	6 (4.4)	0.024
RFA only	8 (2.3)	4 (1.9)	4 (2.9)	
TACE only	47 (13.5)	27 (12.7)	20 (14.7)	
Sorafenib only	33 (9.5)	27 (12.7)	6 (4.4)	
RT only	69 (19.8)	35 (16.4)	34 (25.0)	
Chemotherapy only	22 (6.3)	13 (6.1)	9 (6.6)	
RFA and TACE	8 (2.3)	5 (2.3)	3 (2.2)	
TACE and RT	27 (7.7)	21 (9.9)	6 (4.4)	
Sorafenib and RT	44 (12.6)	28 (13.1)	16 (11.8)	
TACE, sorafenib, and RT	16 (4.6)	6 (2.8)	10 (7.4)	
Other combinations	66 (18.9)	44 (20.7)	22 (16.2)	

RFA, radiofrequency ablation; RT, radiotherapy; TACE, transarterial chemoembolization.
Data were number (%).

Post-Recurrence Survival

The median follow-up months after recurrence was 11.2 months (5.7–22.3 months) in the cohort: 10.2 (5.2–19.9) and 14.3 (6.6–32.6) months in the early and late recurrence groups, respectively (P = 0.026). The 1-, 2-, 3-, and 4-year post-recurrence overall survival and HCC-specific survival rates were 57.0, 34.7, 24.7, and 19.0 and 66.0, 42.6, 31.9, and 27.8%, respectively. The crude survival periods were higher in the late group than in the early group (for overall, P < 0.001; for HCC-specific, P < 0.001) (**Figures 2A, B**). The early transplant era (before 2008) showed high survival rates (**Figures 2C, D**).

After stratification based on initial treatment modalities for recurrence after liver transplantation, the overall survival was statistically different (P < 0.001, **Figure 3A**). A similar pattern was observed for time to HCC-specific death (**Figure 3B**). Furthermore, **Figure 3** presents the overall survival and HCC-specific survival after individual treatment. Superior survival was observed in patients who received RFA, whereas inferior survival was observed in patients who received sorafenib or radiotherapy.

Univariable and Multivariable Analyses

The results of the univariable analysis suggested that a long interval (>2 years) between transplant and HCC recurrence and initial treatment for recurrence with RFA was significantly associated with better overall survival (**Table S3**). Moreover, these factors were significant in a multivariable analysis, with the adjusted HR of 0.57 (95% CI 0.24–0.77) for recurrence after 2 years and of 0.28 (0.12–0.63) for RFA (compared with sorafenib) (**Table 4**). Compared with the early transplant era (before 2008), while recent periods (2009–2012 and after 2013) suggested a high risk of all-cause mortality in univariable analysis, only transplant period 2009–2012 was significant in multivariable analysis (**Table 4**).

Receiving TACE within 1 year before transplant was observed more frequently in recent era after 2009 than in the early era (P = 0.002, **Table S4**). The effect of transplant era was non-significant after stratification by receiving TACE within 1 year before transplant (P = 0.124 in patients with prior TACE and P = 0.886 in those without prior TACE; **Figure S1**), suggesting the survival difference between the transplant era may be due to more frequent use of TACE as downstaging tools recently.

Consistently, the results of the multivariable analysis showed that recurrence after 2 years was associated with a long survival from HCC recurrence to HCC death (**Table S5**), and initial treatment with RFA was associated with a low risk of cancer death. Compared with the early transplant era (before 2008),

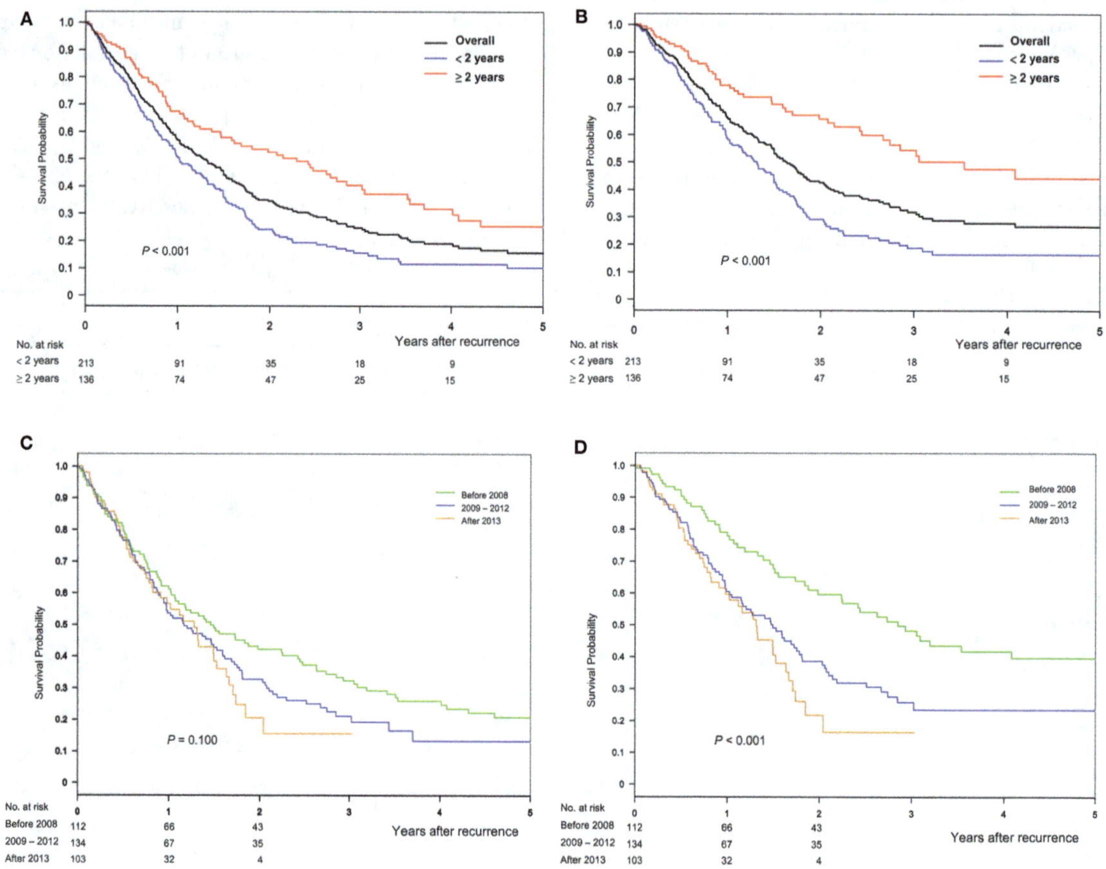

FIGURE 2 | Overall survival and HCC-specific survival after recurrence, stratified based on the timing of **(A, B)** recurrence and **(C, D)** transplant era, respectively.

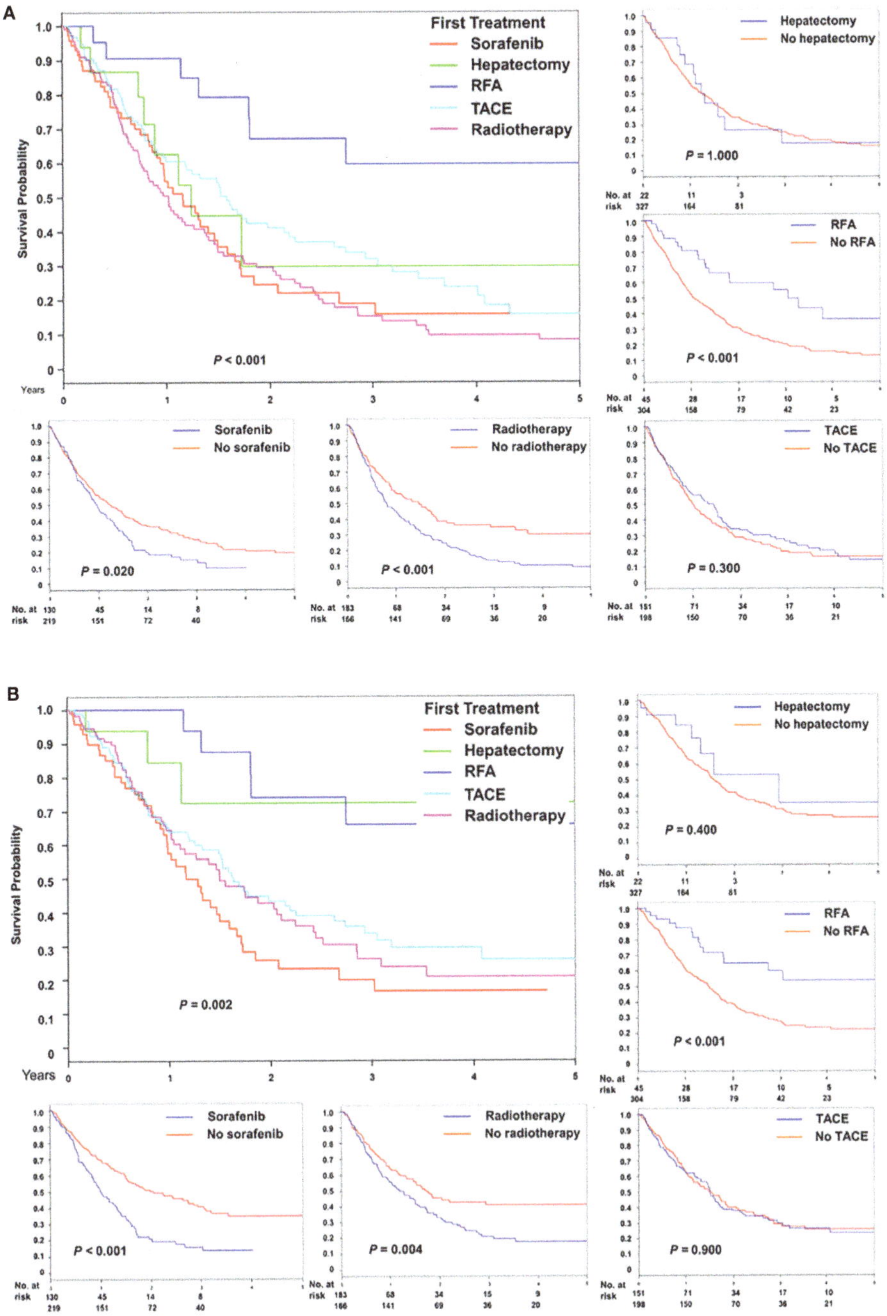

FIGURE 3 | Comparison of **(A)** overall and **(B)** HCC-specific survival after treatment for recurrence, stratified based on five initial modalities, namely sorafenib, hepatectomy, radiofrequency ablation, transarterial chemoembolization, and radiotherapy, and individual modality.

recent periods (2009–2012 and after 2013) were associated with a high risk of cancer death in both univariable and multivariable analyses.

HCV, alcohol use, and everolimus were associated with a high risk of all-cause and cancer death based on a univariable analysis but not significantly according to a multivariable analysis. Living donor appeared as a risk factor in a univariable analysis for cancer death with an HR 1.50 (1.04–2.15) but not significant in a multivariable analysis and not for all-cause death. Further sensitivity analysis with stringent donor assignment criteria showed consistent results (**Tables S6** and **S7**).

Subgroup Analysis

A total of 71 patients with primary HCC treated by upfront transplant were identified. The median follow-up month after recurrence was 15.1 months (7.1–29.5 months). Compared to the

TABLE 4 | Prognostic factors for all-cause and HCC mortality after post-transplant recurrence in multivariable analyses.

	All-cause death*	*P*-value	HCC death*	*P*-value
Recur after 2 years	0.57 (0.24–0.77)	<0.001	0.46 (0.32–0.66)	<0.001
Treatment after recurrence				
RFA *vs.* sorafenib	0.28 (0.12–0.63)	0.002	0.24 (0.07–0.81)	0.022
Transplantation periods				
2009–2012 *vs.* before 2008	1.57 (1.03–2.38)	0.036	1.96 (1.19–3.22)	0.008
After 2013 *vs.* before 2008	1.24 (0.73–2.09)	0.426	1.87 (1.01–3.45)	0.047

**Data were adjusted hazard ratios (95% confidence intervals), adjusted for male sex, HBV, HCV, cirrhosis, diabetes, hyperlipidemia, alcohol use, living donor, monthly income, post-transplant medications, and other HCC treatments (hepatectomy, transarterial chemoembolization, radiotherapy, others) after recurrence.*
RFA, radiofrequency ablation.

previously treated patients (**Figure 4A**, green curve), these patients (**Figure 4A**, blue curve) had similar post-recurrence overall survival but superior HCC-specific survival (**Figure 4B**, $P = 0.003$). In this subgroup, the HCC cancer stage met the UCSF criteria (without potentially confounded by heterogeneous original tumor status and previous treatment effects), and the survival difference between early and late recurrence was consistent with the findings on overall study population, either all-cause or HCC-related death (**Figures 4C, D**, $P < 0.001$).

DISCUSSION

Our study revealed four main findings. First, the post-recurrence survival of liver transplant recipients was time-dependent; early recurrence after liver transplant and recent transplant era were two independent risk factors for an inferior outcome. The effect of transplant era was associated with recently receiving pretransplant TACE. Second, the majority of patients (79.7%) received HCC treatments within 1 year before transplant, and TACE was the

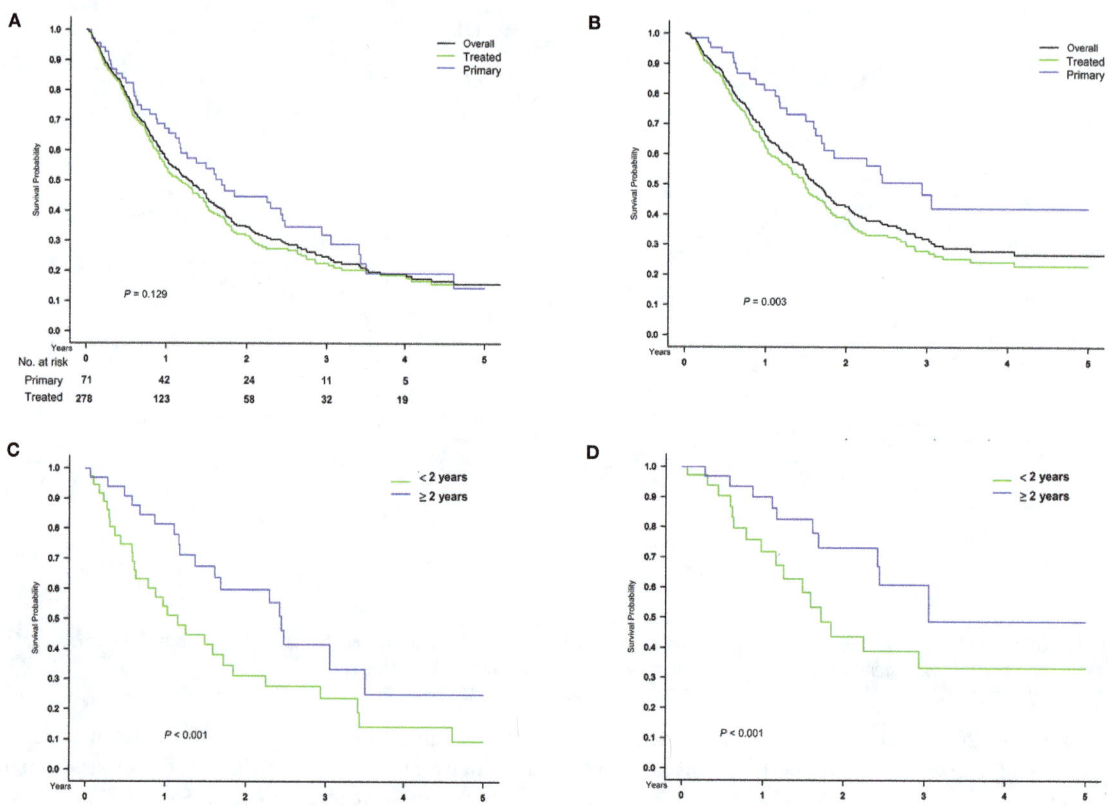

FIGURE 4 | Subgroup analysis in patients with primary HCC treated by upfront transplant. Comparison of **(A)** overall and **(B)** HCC-specific survival after treatment for recurrence, stratified based on primary and treated HCC before transplant surgery and on the timing of **(C, D)** recurrence in 71 patients with primary HCC treated by upfront transplant.

commonest application, implying a large percent of salvage liver transplant in this cohort. Third, the most common initial treatment for post-transplant recurrence was radiotherapy (32.1%), followed by TACE (27.2%) and sorafenib (20.3%). Over half of the cohort (54.0%) received only one treatment after recurrence. Lastly, when recurrence cancer stage allowed eligible interventions, RFA was associated with a superior outcome, whereas radiotherapy and sorafenib use was associated with an inferior outcome.

It is well known that disease stage is closely related to prognosis in cancer patients, and the characteristics of the transplant recipients are quite heterogeneous. Hong et al. showed, in a large South Korean single center study of 92 patients, that HCC size >5 cm at explants was associated with poor post-recurrence survival in recurrence within 6 months after transplant surgery but did not remain significant in recurrence that occurred 6 months later (16). Bodzin et al. showed that, in a largest US single center study of 106 patients, post-transplant HCC recurrence stage, rather than the primary or at transplant HCC stage, predicted post-recurrence mortality (14). The overall information for the initial primary HCC stage and definite HCC-recurrence disease stage of the patients was not available in Taiwan NHIRD. However, the heterogeneous combinations of tumor status at different stages (primary, at transplant, and post-transplant recurrence) in our large cohort would probably make the results toward the null. Moreover, our study showed the effect of recurrence timing on post-recurrence survival in a pure subgroup of patients with primary HCC treated with upfront transplant was consistent with that of the main cohort. The effect of recurrence timing on post-recurrence survival might be a robust conclusion.

The median time between transplant to HCC recurrence in our cohort, the largest one in the literature to our knowledge, was 17.8 months (IQR, 10.7–34.4 months), and 61.0% patients had recurrence within 2 years of transplantation. Consistently, peak HCC recurrence occurs within 2–3 years after transplant (3, 25, 26), and early HCC recurrence portends the worst prognosis (3, 27–29). Furthermore, a longer survival was observed in late than in early recurrence after liver resection for HCC (30). Verna et al. suggested different plausible biological mechanisms, explaining early and late post-transplant recurrence (3). Early recurrence could be due to non-detected extrahepatic metastases that may be present before transplant and as a consequence of circulating HCC clones engrafting and growing in a target organ after liver transplantation (3). Late recurrence could be due to a second unknown hit that may lead to late engrafting of HCC cells that are less in number and remained latent for a long time during the post-transplant period (3). Our data supports the statement of intense surveillance during the first 2 years after transplant (3) and justifies the urgent need for effective adjuvant therapy in this critical period. It is noteworthy that the use of mammalian target of rapamycin inhibitors early (within 6 months after transplant) in the post-transplant period did not show survival benefit in our cohort. Nonetheless, we provided the benchmark reference for future trial design and historical comparison.

HCC treatments before liver transplant can be due to several reasons: to meet transplantable criteria (downstaging tumor status), to bridge (extending waiting time), to salvage (treating transplantable HCC recurrence after other treatments), or to treat liver decompensation (non-tumor liver factor). For example, over half of our main cohort received TACE within 1 year before transplant surgery. We could not tell apart exactly the rationales of TACE treatment based solely on current databases. However, the goal of all these efforts before transplant is to increase the transplantable rates and to reduce wait-list dropout.

RFA appeared as a modality with superior comparative effectiveness in multiple dimensions of our analysis. RFA showed a comparative survival benefit in treating intrahepatic recurrence after liver resection in our previous hospital cohort (21) and another recent report (31). Because extrahepatic metastasis was observed more often in post-transplant than in postresection recurrence (1), the bias in selecting HCC-recurrent patients who were eligible for RFA is estimated to be more in the heterogeneous transplant setting. However, data on liver-directed therapy for the treatment of post-transplant HCC recurrence are lacking and limited to small case series (3). Our results contribute to the literature on the feasibility of RFA treatment for intrahepatic recurrence, which was the best determinant for the prognosis.

Initial treatment with sorafenib and its ever exposure in 20.3 and 37.2% of this cohort patients, respectively, composed a recurrence subgroup of a particular advanced stage, according to reimbursement criteria. The overall 1-year survival rate with initial treatment with sorafenib was 43.7% in our study, which was a bit lower than a pooled estimate at 63% in a meta-analysis (32). The widespread use of radiotherapy in the initial treatment for post-transplant HCC recurrence suggested bone metastasis, which is one of the most common extrahepatic sites. However, the survival benefit of radiotherapy in our study was limited. All of these highlight the therapeutic gap and warrant an investigator-initiated trial to tackle this problem.

This study is limited by the built-in shortage of no information of laboratory data (such as alpha-fetoprotein), and radiographic and pathological findings regarding tumor status in the claim database, which impedes the risk factor analysis between recurrence and non-recurrence. This might influence the analysis of post-recurrence survival. Some received pre-transplant TACE or other specific treatments probably due to the preference of transplant surgeon. This might bias the overall analysis. However, only by utilizing this large multicenter cohort, we could possibly dilute the potential bias, demonstrate the trend of the real-world nature of this heterogeneous cohort, and pave the road for tailoring potential therapeutic implications into future practice. Additionally, resection was not popular in Taiwan, and limited number of patients (n = 22) precluded a balanced assessment, although resection seems to improve cancer-specific survival.

CONCLUSION

In Taiwan, management of HCC recurrence after liver transplantation was heterogeneous. Patients with HCC recurrence within 2 years after liver transplantation had the highest mortality risk. This subgroup cohort is ideal for future interventional trial design. Our data further support the statement of intense surveillance during the early period (first

2 years) after transplant and justify the urgent need for effective adjuvant treatments in this critical period.

AUTHOR CONTRIBUTIONS

CMH and JYW made the concept and design. CMH, JYW, JFZ, and CHL acquired, analyzed, or interpreted the data. CMH drafted the manuscript. CMH, JYW, and CHC critically revised the manuscript for important intellectual content. JFZ and CHC conducted the statistical analysis. JYW obtained the funding. CHC provided administrative, technical, or material support. RHH and PHL supervised the study. All authors contributed to the article and approved the submitted version.

ACKNOWLEDGMENTS

We thank the Department of Statistics, Ministry of Health and Welfare, and National Taiwan University Health Data Research Center for providing administrative support. We thank Ms. Ching-Wen Tsai for technical assistance.

SUPPLEMENTARY MATERIAL

Supplementary Figure 1 | Overall survival after recurrence in patients receiving **(A)** and not receiving **(B)** transarterial chemoembolization (TACE) within 1 year before transplant in three transplant eras.

Supplementary Table 1 | Defined daily dose of selective medications within 6 months after transplant.

Supplementary Table 2 | Summary of HCC treatment modalities before transplantation in patients with post-transplant recurrence.

Supplementary Table 3 | Prognostic factors for all-cause mortality after post-transplant recurrence.

Supplementary Table 4 | Receiving transarterial chemoembolization (TACE) for hepatocellular carcinoma within one year before liver transplantation during three transplant era.

Supplementary Table 5 | Prognostic factors for HCC mortality after post-transplant recurrence.

Supplementary Table 6 | Prognostic factors for all-cause mortality after HCC recurrence in a sensitivity analysis of stringent donor allocation.

Supplementary Table 7 | Prognostic factors for HCC mortality after post-transplant recurrence in a sensitivity analysis of stringent donor allocation.

REFERENCES

1. Ho CM, Lee PH, Chen CL, Ho MC, Wu YM, Hu RH. Long-term outcomes after resection versus transplantation for hepatocellular carcinoma within UCSF criteria. *Ann Surg Oncol* (2012) 19:826–33. doi: 10.1245/s10434-011-1975-x
2. Mazzaferro V, Regalia E, Doci R, Andreola S, Pulvirenti A, Bozzetti F, et al. Liver transplantation for the treatment of small hepatocellular carcinomas in patients with cirrhosis. *N Engl J Med* (1996) 334:693–9. doi: 10.1056/NEJM199603143341104
3. Verna EC, Patel YA, Aggarwal A, Desai AP, Frenette C, Pillai AA, et al. Liver transplantation for hepatocellular carcinoma: Management after the transplant. *Am J Transplant* (2020) 20:333–47. doi: 10.1111/ajt.15697
4. Au KP, Chok KSH. Multidisciplinary approach for post-liver transplant recurrence of hepatocellular carcinoma: A proposed management algorithm. *World J Gastroenterol* (2018) 24:5081–94. doi: 10.3748/wjg.v24.i45.5081
5. Sanduzzi-Zamparelli M, Díaz-Gonzalez Á, Reig M. New systemic treatments in advanced hepatocellular carcinoma. *Liver Transpl* (2019) 25:311–22. doi: 10.1002/lt.25354
6. Pillai A, Couri T, Charlton M. Liver allocation policies in the USA: Past, present, and the future. *Dig Dis Sci* (2019) 64:985–92. doi: 10.1007/s10620-019-05549-y
7. Duvoux C, Roudot-Thoraval F, Decaens T, Pessione F, Badran H, Piardi T, et al. Liver transplantation for hepatocellular carcinoma: A model including alpha-fetoprotein improves the performance of Milan criteria. *Gastroenterology* (2012) 143:986–94.e983; quiz e914–985. doi: 10.1053/j.gastro.2012.05.052
8. Mazzaferro V, Sposito C, Zhou J, Pinna AD, De Carlis L, Fan J, et al. Metroticket 2.0 model for analysis of competing risks of death after liver transplantation for hepatocellular carcinoma. *Gastroenterology* (2018) 154:128–39. doi: 10.1053/j.gastro.2017.09.025
9. Toso C, Meeberg G, Hernandez-Alejandro R, Dufour JF, Marotta P, Majno P, et al. Total tumor volume and alpha-fetoprotein for selection of transplant candidates with hepatocellular carcinoma: A prospective validation. *Hepatology* (2015) 62:158–65. doi: 10.1002/hep.27787
10. Sapisochin G, Goldaracena N, Laurence JM, Dib M, Barbas A, Ghanekar A, et al. The extended Toronto criteria for liver transplantation in patients with hepatocellular carcinoma: A prospective validation study. *Hepatology* (2016) 64:2077–88. doi: 10.1002/hep.28643
11. Halazun KJ, Najjar M, Abdelmessih RM, Samstein B, Griesemer AD, Guarrera JV, et al. Recurrence after liver transplantation for hepatocellular carcinoma: A new MORAL to the story. *Ann Surg* (2017) 265:557–64. doi: 10.1097/SLA.0000000000001966
12. Sasaki K, Firl DJ, Hashimoto K, Fujiki M, Diago-Uso T, Quintini C, et al. Development and validation of the HALT-HCC score to predict mortality in liver transplant recipients with hepatocellular carcinoma: A retrospective cohort analysis. *Lancet Gastroenterol Hepatol* (2017) 2:595–603. doi: 10.1016/S2468-1253(17)30106-1
13. Halazun KJ, Tabrizian P, Najjar M, Florman S, Schwartz M, Michelassi F, et al. Is it time to abandon the Milan criteria? Results of a bicoastal US collaboration to redefine hepatocellular carcinoma liver transplantation selection policies. *Ann Surg* (2018) 268:690–9. doi: 10.1097/SLA.0000000000002964
14. Bodzin AS, Lunsford KE, Markovic D, Harlander-Locke MP, Busuttil RW, Agopian VG. Predicting mortality in patients developing recurrent hepatocellular carcinoma after liver transplantation: Impact of treatment modality and recurrence characteristics. *Ann Surg* (2017) 266:118–25. doi: 10.1097/SLA.0000000000001894
15. Lee DD, Sapisochin G, Mehta N, Gorgen A, Musto KR, Hajda H, et al. Surveillance for HCC after liver transplantation: Increased monitoring may yield aggressive treatment options and improved postrecurrence survival. *Transplantation* (2020) 104:2105–12. doi: 10.1097/TP.0000000000003117
16. Hong SK, Lee KW, Yoon KC, Kim HS, Ahn SW, Kim H, et al. Different prognostic factors and strategies for early and late recurrence after adult living donor liver transplantation for hepatocellular carcinoma. *Clin Transplant* (2019) 33:e13703. doi: 10.1111/ctr.13703
17. Surveillance group, Diagnosis group, Staging group, Surgery group, Local ablation group and TACE/TARE/HAI group, et al. Management consensus guideline for hepatocellular carcinoma: 2016 updated by the Taiwan Liver Cancer Association and the Gastroenterological Society of Taiwan. *J Formos Med Assoc* (2018) 117:381–403. doi: 110.1016/j.jfma.2017.09.007
18. Yao FY, Ferrell L, Bass NM, Watson JJ, Bacchetti P, Venook A, et al. Liver transplantation for hepatocellular carcinoma: Expansion of the tumor size limits does not adversely impact survival. *Hepatology* (2001) 33:1394–403. doi: 10.1053/jhep.2001.24563
19. Duffy JP, Vardanian A, Benjamin E, Watson M, Farmer DG, Ghobrial RM, et al. Liver transplantation criteria for hepatocellular carcinoma should be expanded: A 22-year experience with 467 patients at UCLA. *Ann Surg* (2007) 246:502–11. doi: 10.1097/SLA.0b013e318148c704

20. Duvoux C, Kiuchi T, Pestalozzi B, Busuttil R, Miksad R. What is the role of adjuvant therapy after liver transplantation for hepatocellular carcinoma? *Liver Transpl* (2011) 17 Suppl 2:S147–58. doi: 10.1002/lt.22367
21. Ho CM, Lee PH, Shau WY, Ho MC, Wu YM, Hu RH. Survival in patients with recurrent hepatocellular carcinoma after primary hepatectomy: comparative effectiveness of treatment modalities. *Surgery* (2012) 151:700–9. doi: 10.1016/j.surg.2011.12.015
22. Lee MR, Lee MC, Chang CH, Liu CJ, Chang LY, Zhang JF, et al. Use of antiplatelet agents and survival of tuberculosis patients: A population-based cohort study. *J Clin Med* (2019) 8:E923. doi: 10.3390/jcm8070923
23. Bryce K, Tsochatzis EA. Downstaging for hepatocellular cancer: harm or benefit? *Transl Gastroenterol Hepatol* (2017) 2:106. doi: 10.21037/tgh.2017.11.18
24. WHOCC. *Definition and General Considerations* (2018). Available at: https://www.whocc.no/ddd/definition_and_general_considera/#Definition (Accessed Mar 29, 2020).
25. Croome KP, Lee DD, Burns JM, Musto K, Paz D, Nguyen JH, et al. The use of donation after cardiac death allografts does not increase recurrence of hepatocellular carcinoma. *Am J Transplant* (2015) 15:2704–11. doi: 10.1111/ajt.13306
26. Azoulay D, Audureau E, Bhangui P, Belghiti J, Boillot O, Andreani P, et al. Living or brain-dead donor liver transplantation for hepatocellular carcinoma: a multicenter, western, intent-to-treat cohort study. *Ann Surg* (2017) 266:1035–44. doi: 10.1097/SLA.0000000000001986
27. Liang W, Wu L, Ling X, Ju W, Wang D, Shang Y, et al. Living donor liver transplantation versus deceased donor liver transplantation for hepatocellular carcinoma: a meta-analysis. *Liver Transpl* (2012) 18:1226–36. doi: 10.1002/lt.23490
28. Goldaracena N, Gorgen A, Doyle A, Hansen BE, Tomiyama K, Zhang W, et al. Live donor liver transplantation for patients with hepatocellular carcinoma offers increased survival vs. deceased donation. *J Hepatol* (2019) 70:666–73. doi: 10.1016/j.jhep.2018.12.029
29. Fernandez-Sevilla E, Allard MA, Selten J, Golse N, Vibert E, Sa Cunha A, et al. Recurrence of hepatocellular carcinoma after liver transplantation: Is there a place for resection? *Liver Transpl* (2017) 23:440–7. doi: 10.1002/lt.24742
30. Portolani N, Coniglio A, Ghidoni S, Giovanelli M, Benetti A, Tiberio GA, et al. Early and late recurrence after liver resection for hepatocellular carcinoma: prognostic and therapeutic implications. *Ann Surg* (2006) 243:229–35. doi: 10.1097/01.sla.0000197706.21803.a1
31. Xia Y, Li J, Liu G, Wang K, Qian G, Lu Z, et al. Long-term effects of repeat hepatectomy vs percutaneous radiofrequency ablation among patients with recurrent hepatocellular carcinoma: A randomized clinical trial. *JAMA Oncol* (2020) 6:255–63. doi: 10.1001/jamaoncol.2019.4477
32. Mancuso A, Mazzola A, Cabibbo G, Perricone G, Enea M, Galvano A, et al. Survival of patients treated with sorafenib for hepatocellular carcinoma recurrence after liver transplantation: A systematic review and meta-analysis. *Dig Liver Dis* (2015) 47:324–30. doi: 10.1016/j.dld.2015.01.001

18

Adjuvant Transarterial Chemoembolization for Barcelona Clinic Liver Cancer Stage A Hepatocellular Carcinoma After Hepatectomy

*Yue-Lin Zhang[1,2], Chun-Hui Nie[1,3], Feng Chen[4], Tan-Yang Zhou[1,2], Guan-Hui Zhou[1,2], Tong-Yin Zhu[1,2], Sheng-Qun Chen[1,3], Xin-Hua Chen[1,2], Hong-Liang Wang[1,3], Bao-Quan Wang[1,2], Zi-Niu Yu[1,2], Li Jing[1,2], Zhi-Min He[1,3] and Jun-Hui Sun[1,2,3]**

[1] Hepatobiliary and Pancreatic Interventional Treatment Center, Division of Hepatobiliary and Pancreatic Surgery, The First Affiliated Hospital, Zhejiang University School of Medicine, Hangzhou, China, [2] Zhejiang Clinical Research Center of Hepatobiliary and Pancreatic Diseases, Hangzhou, China, [3] Zhejiang Provincial Research Center for Diagnosis and Treatment of Hepatobiliary Diseases, Hangzhou, China, [4] Department of Radiology, The First Affiliated Hospital, Zhejiang University School of Medicine, Hangzhou, China

***Correspondence:**
Jun-Hui Sun
1307005@zju.edu.cn

Introduction: The care for patients with hepatocellular carcinoma (HCC) is challenging. This study is to evaluate the effect of adjuvant transarterial chemoembolization (TACE) for Barcelona Clinic Liver Cancer (BCLC) stage A HCC patients after hepatectomy.

Methods: Consecutive HCC patients with BCLC stage A, treated by hepatectomy alone (HA) or hepatectomy with TACE (HT), were retrospectively enrolled. Propensity score matching (PSM) was used to balance baseline differences. The recurrence-free survival (RFS) and overall survival (OS) were evaluated using the Kaplan-Meier. The impact of TACE on survival outcome was determined by Cox hazard regression.

Results: After PSM, 230 patients (115 HT and 115 HA) were enrolled in the analysis. The 1-, 3-, and 5-year RFS rates were 87.0, 63.5, and 50.4%, respectively, for the HT group, and 87.8, 67.0, and 58.3% for the HA group. The OS rates at 1-, 3-, and 5-year were 99.1, 93.9, and 87%, respectively, for the HT group, and 100, 92.2, and 88.7% for the HA group. No significant differences were seen in either the RFS (log-rank test, $\chi^2 = 0.891$, $p = 0.345$) or OS (log-rank test, $\chi^2 = 0.146$, $p = 0.702$) between the specific pairs of two groups. Cox regression identified that TACE was not the factor affecting RFS or OS ($p = 0.399$; HR 0.847; 95% CI 0.576–1.245 for RFS vs. $p = 0.989$; HR 0.995; 95% CI 0.471–2.100 for OS).

Conclusion: Our data indicate that TACE is not an effective intervention in the adjuvant setting for BCLC stage A HCC after hepatectomy.

Keywords: hepatocellular carcinoma, hepatectomy, recurrence, survival, transarterial chemoembolization

INTRODUCTION

Hepatocellular carcinoma (HCC) is one of the most frequently encountered malignancies globally, with the second-highest cancer-related mortality rate (1). Hepatectomy is the most widely practiced therapy, as it is a potentially curative treatment for HCC (2). However, long-term survival after hepatectomy is unsatisfactory because more than 70% tumor recur during the first 5 years (3). The prevention of tumor recurrences is the key to improve the outcome of liver resections.

The Barcelona Clinic Liver Cancer (BCLC) staging system including is widely used for HCC staging and treatment (4). Current clinical practice guidelines do not endorse any particular adjuvant therapy after hepatectomy but do recommend more and larger studies that undertake lower risks of systematic error (2, 4). Transcatheter arterial chemoembolization (TACE) has recently been reported as a postoperative adjuvant therapy for HCC patients. Previous clinical studies (5–7) showed that postoperative TACE significantly reduce tumor recurrence and improve the overall survival of patients with resectable BCLC stage B HCC or high recurrence risk (exceeding 5 cm in diameter or multiple tumors or vascular invasion) after curative liver resection. Nevertheless, none of these studies cover BCLC stage A HCC (single tumor or up to 3 tumors ≤3 cm), for which the BCLC staging system recommends surgical resection as the best option (8). The efficacy of TACE as adjuvant therapy after hepatectomy for patients with BCLC stage A HCC is not clear.

To further investigate the efficacy of TACE as adjuvant therapy after hepatectomy for patients with BCLC stage A HCC, we conducted a cohort study to follow up the survival outcome of BCLC stage A HCC who underwent hepatectomy alone or had postoperative adjuvant TACE.

MATERIALS AND METHODS

The study protocol was approved by the Ethics Committee of the First Affiliated Hospital, Zhejiang University School of Medicine, and the written informed consent was obtained from all the patients.

Patients

In this retrospective cohort study, consecutive patients with BCLC stage A HCC, who underwent curative hepatectomy, were enrolled from January 2012 to August 2014 at the First Affiliated Hospital, Zhejiang University School of Medicine. The inclusion criteria: (1) the HCC diagnosis was confirmed by pathologic examination; (2) the patients had a stage A HCC using the BCLC staging system; and (3) histologic evidence of tumor-free margins on the resected tissues (defined as the distance between the cancer tissue and resected tissue margins is 1 cm or more). The exclusion criteria: (1) an intrahepatic recurrence within 2 months after curative hepatectomy; (2) the presence of other malignant tumors; and (3) loss of patients to follow-up.

Patients were divided into two groups: (1) HCC underwent hepatectomy with adjuvant TACE (HT group) and (2) HCC underwent hepatectomy alone (HA group). Standard demographic and clinical data potentially related to recurrence and survival were collected: gender, age, hepatitis, cirrhosis, tumor characteristics, surgical margin, and pathologic results.

Adjuvant TACE

Postoperative adjuvant TACE was performed 4–6 weeks after hepatic resection, according to the Eastern Cooperative Oncology Group (ECOG) performance status and patient liver function. A 5-F angiographic catheter (Cook Inc., Bloomington, IN, United States) was introduced into the common hepatic artery through femoral artery, then hepatic angiography was performed to evaluate the arterial blood supply to the liver. 150 mg oxaliplatin (Hengrui Medicine Co., Ltd., Jiangsu, China) was slowly infused into proper hepatic artery, followed by an emulsion of 20 mg pirarubicin (Shenzhen Main Luck Pharmaceuticals Inc., Shenzhen, China) and 2–4 mL lipiodol (Lipiodol Ultrafluide, Guerbet, Aulnay-sous-Bois, France) using the microcatheter (Terumo, Tokyo, Japan). After 4–6 weeks, these patients underwent a complete assessment.

Follow-Up

All patients were followed-up every 2 to 3 months during the first year and then every 3 to 6 months after surgery until death or dropout from the follow-up (4). On the follow-up visits patients tested ECOG, liver function, serum alpha-fetoprotein (AFP), abdominal ultrasonography, and CT or MRI scan. The primary endpoint for this study was recurrence-free survival (RFS), defined as the interval from surgery to the first recurrence. Secondary endpoints were overall survival (OS), defined as the interval from surgery to the date of death.

The diagnosis of tumor recurrence or metastasis was based on cytologic/histologic evidence or non-invasive

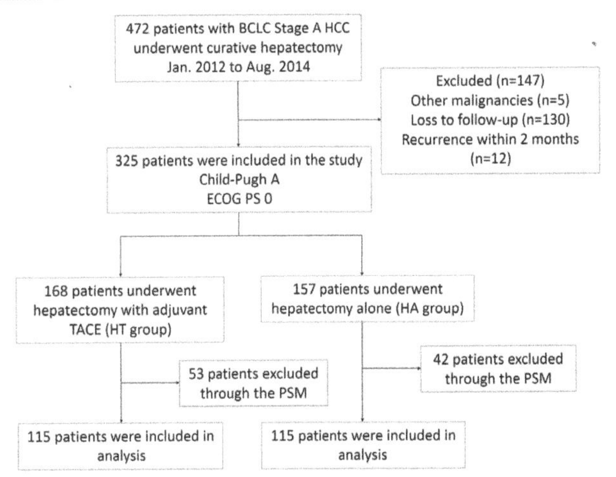

FIGURE 1 | Flow diagram for extracting eligible cases for comparison. BCLC, Barcelona Clinic Liver Cancer; HCC, hepatocellular carcinoma; TACE, transarterial chemoembolization; PSM, propensity score matching; ECOG, Eastern Cooperative Oncology Group; PS, performance status.

diagnostic by the EASL (2). Two senior radiologists independently reviewed images. If any discrepancy in CT or MRI scans, the final diagnosis was made after reviewing all clinical information. After tumor recurrence was confirmed, the patients were treated according to the practice guidelines, which included curative treatments (surgical resection, liver transplantation, or radiofrequency ablation) and/or non-curative treatments (TACE, percutaneous ethanol injection, radiotherapy, or systemic therapy) to improve survival.

Statistical Analysis

Sample sizes were computed using the RFS as the primary endpoint. Based on previous study, the 5-year RFS rate after

TABLE 1 | Baseline demographic and disease characteristics.

Variable	Before propensity score matching			After propensity score matching		
	HT group (n = 168)	HA group (n = 157)	P-value	HT group (n = 115)	HA group (n = 115)	P-value
Gender						
Male	147	125	0.055	97	99	0.710
Female	21	32		18	16	
Age, year						
≤60	120	103	0.258	78	76	0.779
>60	48	54		37	39	
HBsAg						
Positive	149	132	0.224	99	97	0.710
Negative	19	25		16	18	
HBeAg						
Positive	41	42	0.628	28	27	0.877
Negative	127	115		87	88	
HBV-DNA						
Positive	71	57	0.272	44	44	1.000
Negative	97	100		71	71	
Liver cirrhosis						
Positive	118	123	0.095	82	88	0.368
Negative	50	34		33	27	
Tumor size, cm	4.11 ± 2.24	3.10 ± 1.86	<0.001	3.55 ± 1.61	3.40 ± 2.00	0.533
Tumor number						
One	147	150	0.010	107	108	0.789
Two or Three	21	7		8	7	
Tumor capsule						
Complete	64	75	0.078	47	48	0.893
Incomplete	104	82		68	67	
Microvascular invasion						
Yes	16	11	0.411	10	9	0.811
No	152	146		105	106	
Histological differentiation						
High and/or moderate	92	107	0.013	70	68	0.788
Low	76	50		45	47	
Serum AFP, ng/mL						
≤400	122	126	0.106	91	88	0.634
>400	46	31		24	27	
Preoperative chemoembolization						
Yes	17	13	0.567	8	8	1.000
No	151	144		107	107	
Surgical margin, cm						
≥2	109	110	0.319	79	84	0.468
<2	59	47		36	31	
Operative blood loss, mL						
≤500	146	148	0.024	105	107	0.623
>500	22	9		10	8	

HT, hepatectomy with TACE; HA, hepatectomy alone; AFP, alpha-fetoprotein.

curative resection was 40% (9). We expected a 5-year RFS rate in the adjuvant TACE group of 60%. Using a two-sided test with 80% power at a significance level of 5%, the minimum sample size in each group was estimated to be 94 patients.

To eliminate potential baseline confounding factors and isolate the effects of adjuvant TACE, propensity score matching (PSM) was used to balance baseline differences and thereby simulate random group allocation. The propensity score model included all variables known to be associated with survival outcomes. A one-to-one nearest-neighbor matching without replacement was used to match patients based on the logistic regression of the propensity score within a caliper of 0.05. That is to say, one patient from the HT group could get matched with one patient from the HA group with a similar propensity score.

Quantitative data were expressed as the mean ± standard deviation or median (range), as appropriate. Categorical data between HT and HA groups were compared using the chi-square or Fisher's exact test, while quantitative data were compared using the Student's *t*-test. Survival curves in this study were analyzed using the Kaplan-Meier to measure RFS and OS and compared using the log-rank test. Multivariable Cox regression analyses were used to identify the prognostic significance of the variables to predict RFS and OS. For subgroup analyses, multiple individual Cox models were used separately from treatment comparisons for each factor. Statistical analysis of the data was performed using SPSS V.25.0 (IBM, Armonk, NY, United States) and R V.3.6.1[1] with the add-on packages survival, forestplot and survminer. A $p < 0.05$ was considered statistically significant, and all statistical tests were two-sided.

RESULTS

Patients

From January 2012 to August 2014, 472 patients with BCLC stage A HCC underwent curative hepatectomy. Among them, 147 patients were excluded due to the presence of other malignancies (5 patients), loss to follow-up evaluations (130 patients), or HCC recurrences within 2 months (12 patients). Three hundred and twenty-five patients (157 HA patients and 168 HT patients) were included in the study. Then, 95 patients (42 HA patients and 53 HT patients) were excluded using one-to-one matching of the propensity scores to balance baseline differences between two groups. Finally, 230 patients (115 HA patients and 115 HT patients) were enrolled in the analysis. All patients had a good performance status and liver function (ECOG PS 0 and Child-Pugh A). The flow diagram demonstrating the screening and grouping of participants in the study is shown in **Figure 1**.

The baseline characteristics of the patients were well-matched between the two groups after PSM. The tumor characteristics, such as the tumor size (3.40 ± 2.00 for HA and 3.55 ± 1.61 for HT), tumor number, AFP level, presence of a tumor capsule, pathologic microvascular invasion, and histologic differentiation also were similar between the two groups (**Table 1**).

[1]https://www.r-project.org

Survival

At the time of censor, 105 patients (45.7%) developed recurrence, 57 patients in the HT group, and 48 patients in the HA group, respectively. 28 patients (12.2%) had died, 15 patients in the HT group, and 13 patients in the HA group died of tumor-related causes.

In the HT group, the 1-, 3-, and 5-year RFS rates were 87.0, 63.5, and 50.4%, respectively. The corresponding figures for the HA group were 87.8, 67.0, and 58.3%, respectively. The RFS difference were not significantly in HT group compared with the HA group (log-rank test, $\chi^2 = 0.891$, $p = 0.345$, **Figure 2**). The respective 1-, 3-, and 5-year OS rates were 99.1, 93.9, and 87% for

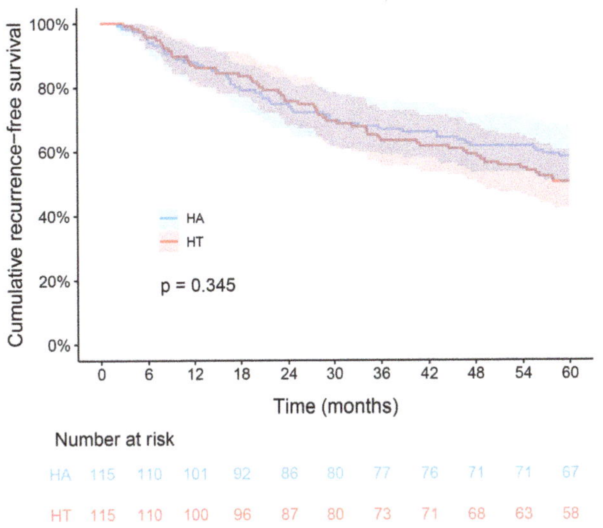

FIGURE 2 | Kaplan-Meier analysis of recurrence-free survival between HT and HA groups. HT, hepatectomy with TACE; HA, hepatectomy alone.

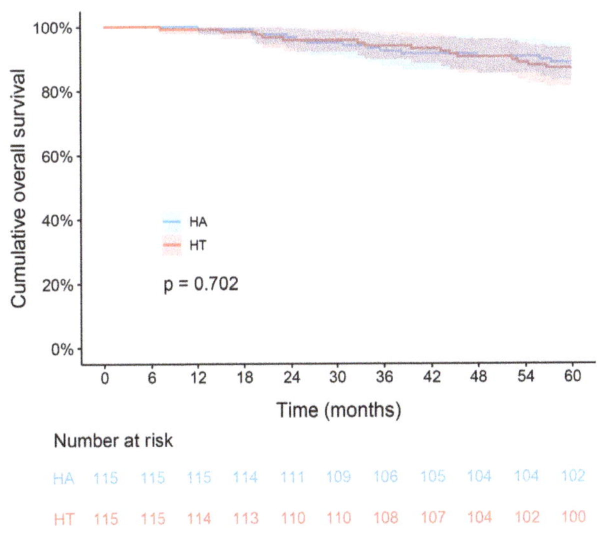

FIGURE 3 | Kaplan-Meier analysis of overall survival between HT and HA groups. HT, hepatectomy with TACE; HA, hepatectomy alone.

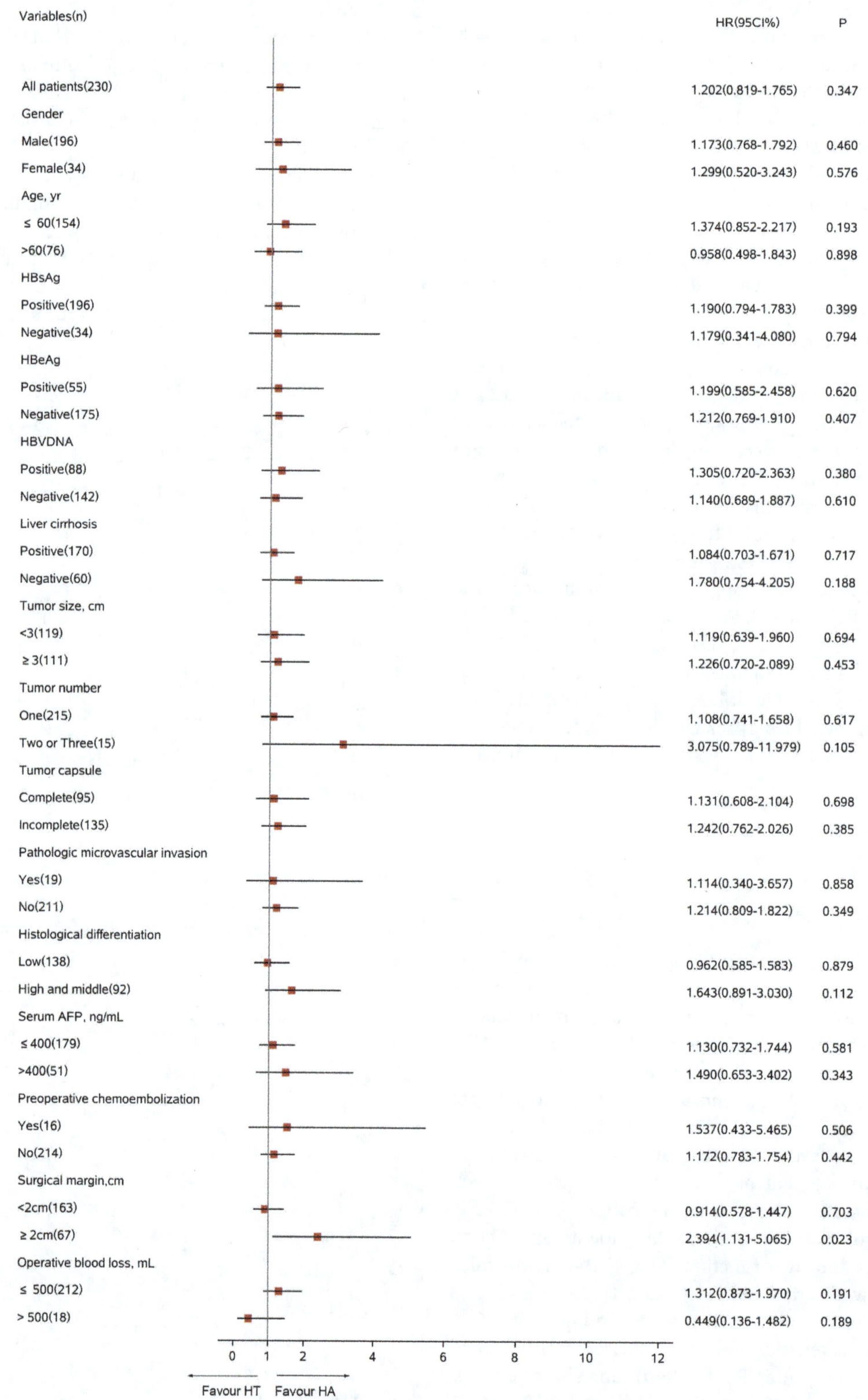

FIGURE 4 | Subgroup analysis for recurrence-free survival between HT and HA groups using Cox regression analysis. HT, hepatectomy with TACE; HA, hepatectomy alone; CI, confidence interval; HR, hazard ratio; AFP, alpha-fetoprotein.

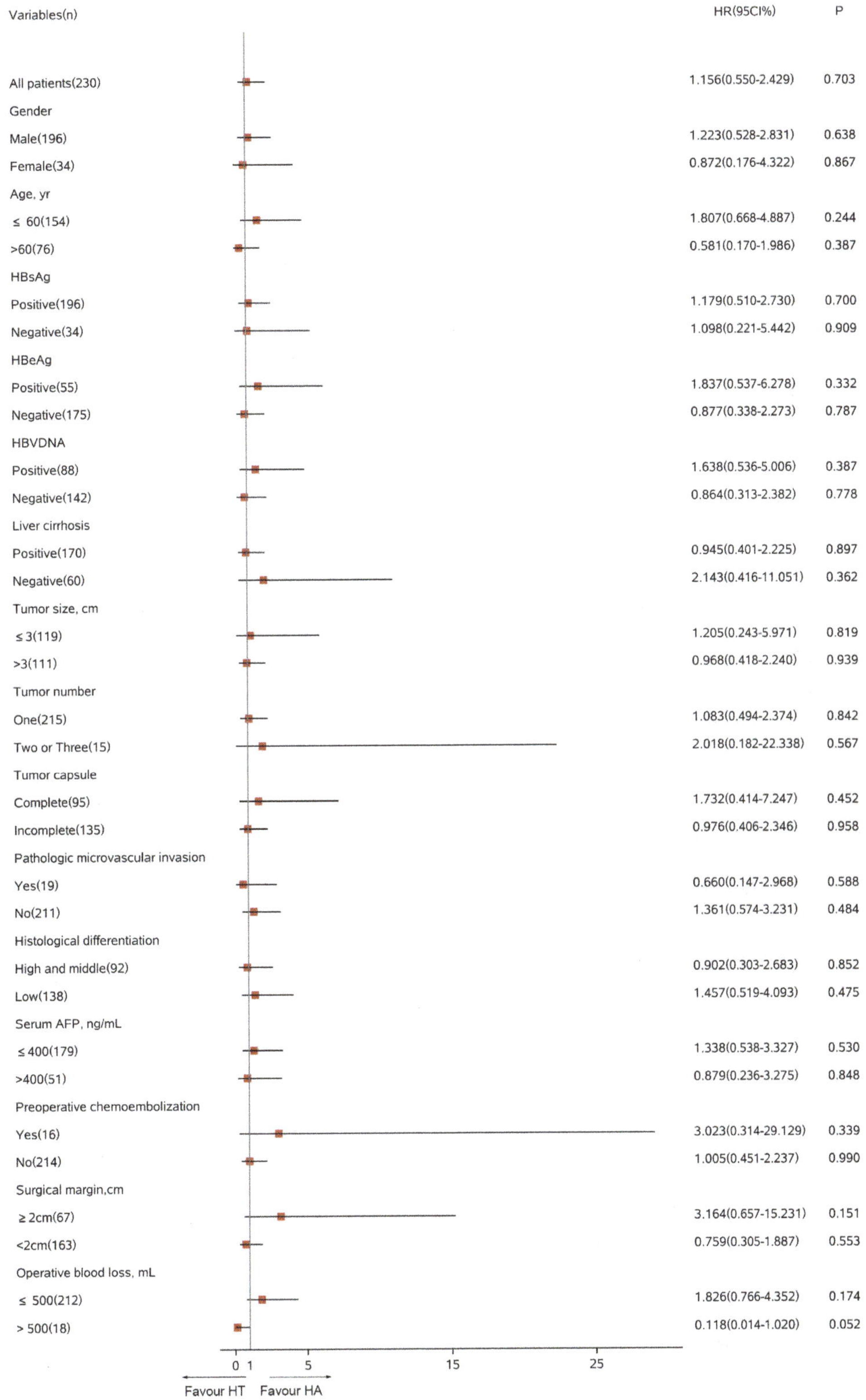

FIGURE 5 | Subgroup analysis for overall survival between HT and HA groups using Cox regression analysis. HT, hepatectomy with TACE; HA, hepatectomy alone; CI, confidence interval; HR, hazard ratio; AFP, alpha-fetoprotein.

the HT group, and 100, 92.2, and 88.7% for the HA group. The OS rates were similar between the HT and HA groups (log-rank test, $\chi^2 = 0.146$, $p = 0.702$, **Figure 3**).

In the all-exploratory subgroup analyses, adjuvant TACE did not provide a clinical benefit for RFS [hazard ratio (HR) 1.202; 95% CI 0.819–1.765; $p = 0.347$]. Despite adjuvant TACE enhanced RFS for operative blood losses >500 ml, a significant difference was not detected in the HT group compared with that of the HA group (HR 0.449; 95% CI 0.136–1.482; $p = 0.189$, **Figure 4**). Similarly, in the OS subgroup analyses, a significant benefit from adjuvant TACE was not seen in patients with the following characteristics: ages >60 years (HR 0.581; 95% CI 0.170–1.986; $p = 0.387$) and operative blood losses >500 ml (HR 0.118; 95% CI 0.014–1.020; $p = 0.052$) (**Figure 5**).

Multivariate Cox regression analysis revealed that adjuvant TACE was not the impact factor for RFS or OS ($p = 0.399$; HR 0.847; 95%CI 0.576–1.245 for RFS vs. $p = 0.989$; HR 0.995; 95% CI 0.471–2.100 for OS). Tumor size and the presence of microvascular invasion were shown to be significant OS factors (**Table 2**).

DISCUSSION

This study include a large patient cohort. One group received hepatectomy with adjuvant TACE and the other received hepatectomy alone. The result revealed that postoperative adjuvant TACE does not reduce recurrence or improve OS. Although the role of postoperative adjuvant TACE was evaluated to improve the outcomes of resected HCC in several studies, the results have been controversial. Difference in patient selection made the controversial results. A randomized controlled trial revealed that adjuvant TACE after hepatectomy markedly improved the survival outcome of Stage III A HCC patients, including a high proportion of patients with macrovascular invasion (7). However, another prospective, randomized-controlled trial failed to display a significant difference in survival between the two groups, although the main aim of this study was to look into the effect of the dose in the prevention of tumor recurrence (10). Sun et al. (11) retrospectively reported that postoperative adjuvant TACE could prolong the survival of patients with microvascular invasion with 5-year survival rates that increased to 54.0%. However, our study focused on BCLC stage A HCC (single tumor or up to 3 tumors ≤3 cm). Thus, the histopathologic factors of HCC in our study were significantly different from previous studies.

The rationale of adjuvant TACE after curative hepatectomy was to prevent intrahepatic recurrence by killing residual microscopic tumor cells in the remnant live. It can also eliminate tumor cells that might have been shed from tumor masses removed during liver surgery. Our negative results show that adjuvant TACE did not improve the outcomes of BCLC stage A HCC patients are likely related to the following factors. First, immune surveillance to control tumor recurrences and metastases could be responsible. Adjuvant TACE might have depressed host immunity against tumor progression and affected hepatocyte regeneration, resulting in poor overall or recurrence-free survival (12). Second, the recurrent tumors usually have different clones compared with those of the malignant primary tumors (13). By eliminating the subpopulation of drug-sensitive tumor cells, chemotherapy accelerate the formation of new clonal variants from the surviving subpopulation and allow cells to proliferate with higher metastatic capabilities (14).

This study revealed that tumor size and microvascular invasion were both independent prognostic factors of OS, similar to the results of previous studies (15, 16). A large tumor burden is closely associated with increased invasiveness, which was reflected in a higher incidence of microvascular invasion and poor survival (17, 18). Microvascular invasion is present in 20% of tumors 2 cm in size, 30–60% of nodules 2–5 cm in size, and up to 60–90% of nodules larger than 5 cm (19). The proportion of HCC cases with microvascular invasion was only 8.3% in our study, resulting in good long-term survival rates.

TABLE 2 | Uni- and multivariate analyses of recurrence-free survival (RFS) and overall survival (OS).

Variable	Univariate analysis		Multivariate analysis	
	χ^2 value (Log-rank)	*P*-value	HR (95% CI)	*P*-value
RFS				
Treatment (HT vs. HA)	0.891	0.345	0.847 (0.576–1.245)	0.399
Gender (female vs. male)	3.061	0.080	0.703 (0.426–1.162)	0.169
HBsAg (positive vs. negative)	3.357	0.067	0.601 (0.312–1.160)	0.129
Tumor number (two or three vs. one)	3.083	0.079	0.603 (0.311–1.168)	0.134
Pathologic microvascular invasion (yes vs. no)	3.217	0.073	0.587 (0.313–1.101)	0.097
OS				
Treatment (HT vs. HA)	0.146	0.702	0.995 (0.471–2.100)	0.989
HBeAg (positive vs. negative)	4.181	0.041	0.471 (0.220–1.009)	0.053
Tumor size, cm (>3 vs. ≤ 3)	11.698	0.001	0.320 (0.122–0.834)	0.020
Microvascular invasion (yes vs. no)	15.492	<0.001	0.299 (0.123–0.725)	0.008
Operative blood loss, mL (≤500 vs. >500)	8.827	0.003	0.416 (0.163–1.059)	0.066

HT, hepatectomy with TACE; HA, hepatectomy alone.

There are potential limitations of this study. First, it was a retrospective study with all of the inherent defects of these types of studies and is likely subject to subtle selection biases, even after PSM. Second, this is a single-center study, and the outcome is not the same as patients with BCLC stage A HCC in other countries because of demographics and the underlying causes. The multi-center randomized controlled trials involving patients with BCLC stage A HCC should examine in more detail the effects of postoperative TACE.

CONCLUSION

Transarterial chemoembolization as adjuvant treatment after hepatectomy for BCLC stage A HCC did not reduce tumor recurrences or improve the overall survival. The adjuvant setting remains an area of high unmet need in HCC management, and further research into strategies to prevent BCLC stage A HCC recurrence is needed.

AUTHOR CONTRIBUTIONS

Y-LZ and J-HS contributed to conception and design. Y-LZ, C-HN, and FC contributed to development of methodology (provided, acquired, and managed patients, etc.). Y-LZ, T-YaZ, and G-HZ contributed to analysis and interpretation of data (e.g., statistical analysis and computational analysis). Y-LZ, T-YiZ, S-QC, X-HC, H-LW, and J-HS contributed to writing, review, and/or revision of the manuscript. Y-LZ, B-QW, Z-NY, LJ, and Z-MH contributed administrative, technical, or material support (i.e., reporting or organizing the data and constructing databases). All authors contributed to the article and approved the submitted version.

ACKNOWLEDGMENTS

All authors appreciate Prof. Xinmei Chen for English proofreading.

REFERENCES

1. Maluccio M, Covey A. Recent progress in understanding, diagnosing, and treating hepatocellular carcinoma. *CA Cancer J Clin.* (2012) 62:394–9. doi: 10.3322/caac.21161
2. European Association for the Study of the Liver. EASL clinical practice guidelines: management of hepatocellular carcinoma. *J Hepatol.* (2018) 69:182–236.
3. Marubashi S, Gotoh K, Akita H, Takahashi H, Ito Y, Yano M, et al. Anatomical versus non-anatomical resection for hepatocellular carcinoma. *Br J Surg.* (2015) 102:776–84.
4. Marrero JA, Kulik LM, Sirlin CB, Zhu AX, Finn RS, Abecassis MM, et al. Diagnosis, staging, and management of hepatocellular carcinoma: 2018 practice guidance by the american association for the study of liver diseases. *Hepatology.* (2018) 68:723–50. doi: 10.1002/hep.29913
5. Dong ZR, Zhang PF, Wang CH, Zhang C, Cai JB, Shi GM, et al. Postoperative adjuvant transcatheter arterial chemoembolization for resectable multiple hepatocellular carcinoma beyond the Milan criteria: a retrospective analysis. *Am J Cancer Res.* (2014) 5:450–7.
6. Wang Z, Ren Z, Chen Y, Hu J, Yang G, Yu L, et al. Adjuvant transarterial chemoembolization for HBV-related hepatocellular carcinoma after resection: a randomized controlled study. *Clin Cancer Res.* (2018) 24:2074–81. doi: 10.1158/1078-0432.ccr-17-2899
7. Zhong C, Guo RP, Li JQ, Shi M, Wei W, Chen MS, et al. A randomized controlled trial of hepatectomy with adjuvant transcatheter arterial chemoembolization versus hepatectomy alone for Stage III A hepatocellular carcinoma. *J Cancer Res Clin Oncol.* (2009) 135:1437–45. doi: 10.1007/s00432-009-0588-2
8. Llovet JM, Bru C, Bruix J. Prognosis of hepatocellular carcinoma: the BCLC staging classification. *Semin Liver Dis.* (1999) 19:329–38. doi: 10.1055/s-2007-1007122
9. Zou H, Zhu CZ, Wang C, Wang ZS, Ma X, Han B, et al. Recurrence of barcelona clinic liver cancer stage a hepatocellular carcinoma after hepatectomy. *Am J Med Sci.* (2017) 354:262–7. doi: 10.1016/j.amjms.2017.05.014
10. Kwok PC, Lam TW, Lam PW, Tang KW, Chan SC, Hwang JS, et al. Randomized controlled trial to compare the dose of adjuvant chemotherapy after curative resection of hepatocellular carcinoma. *J Gastroenterol Hepatol.* (2003) 18:450–5. doi: 10.1046/j.1440-1746.2003.03015.x
11. Sun JJ, Wang K, Zhang CZ, Guo WX, Shi J, Cong WM, et al. Postoperative adjuvant transcatheter arterial chemoembolization after R0 hepatectomy improves outcomes of patients who have hepatocellular carcinoma with microvascular invasion. *Ann Surg Oncol.* (2016) 23:1344–51. doi: 10.1245/s10434-015-5008-z
12. Mazzola A, Costantino A, Petta S, Bartolotta TV, Raineri M, Sacco R, et al. Recurrence of hepatocellular carcinoma after liver transplantation: an update. *Future Oncol.* (2015) 11:2923–36.
13. Kwon T, Kwon OS, Cha HJ, Sung BJ. Stochastic and heterogeneous cancer cell migration: experiment and theory. *Sci Rep.* (2019) 9:16297.
14. McGranahan N, Swanton C. Clonal heterogeneity and tumor evolution: past, present, and the future. *Cell.* (2017) 168:613–28. doi: 10.1016/j.cell.2017.01.018
15. Wang H, Feng LH, Qian YW, Cao ZY, Wu MC, Cong WM. Does microvascular invasion in Barcelona Clinic Liver Cancer stage A multinodular hepatocellular carcinoma indicate early-stage behavior? *Ann Transl Med.* (2019) 7:428. doi: 10.21037/atm.2019.08.114
16. Zhang Y, Chen SW, Liu LL, Yang X, Cai SH, Yun JP. A model combining TNM stage and tumor size shows utility in predicting recurrence among patients with hepatocellular carcinoma after resection. *Cancer Manag Res.* (2018) 10:3707–15. doi: 10.2147/cmar.s175303
17. Zhang X, Li J, Shen F, Lau WY. Significance of presence of microvascular invasion in specimens obtained after surgical treatment of hepatocellular carcinoma. *J Gastroenterol Hepatol.* (2018) 33:347–54. doi: 10.1111/jgh.13843
18. Truant S, Boleslawski E, Duhamel A, Bouras AF, Louvet A, Febvay C, et al. Tumor size of hepatocellular carcinoma in noncirrhotic liver: a controversial predictive factor for outcome after resection. *Eur J Surg Oncol.* (2012) 38:1189–96. doi: 10.1016/j.ejso.2012.07.112
19. Earl TM, Chapman WC. Hepatocellular carcinoma: resection versus transplantation. *Semin Liver Dis.* (2013) 33:282–92. doi: 10.1055/s-0033-1351783

19

Meta-Analysis of Risk Factors for Bile Leakage After Hepatectomy without Biliary Reconstruction

*Ling Tan†, Fei Liu†, Zi-lin Liu and Jiang-wei Xiao**

Department of Gastrointestinal Surgery, Clinical Medical College and the First Affiliated Hospital of Chengdu Medical College, Chengdu, China

Correspondence:
Jiang-wei Xiao
xiaojiangwei2018@163.com

†These authors share first authorship

Background and Aim: The risk factors for bile leakage after hepatectomy without biliary reconstruction are controversial. This study investigated the risk factors for bile leakage after hepatectomy without biliary reconstruction.

Methods: We searched databases (Embase (Ovid), Medline (Ovid), PubMed, Cochrane Library, and Web of Science) for articles published between January 1, 2000, and May 1, 2021, to evaluate the risk factors for bile leakage after hepatectomy without biliary reconstruction.

Results: A total of 16 articles were included in this study, and the overall results showed that sex (OR: 1.21, 95% CI: 1.04–1.42), diabetes (OR: 1.21, 95% CI: 1.05–1.38), left trisectionectomy (OR: 3.53, 95% CI: 2.32–5.36), central hepatectomy (OR: 3.28, 95% CI: 2.63–4.08), extended hemihepatectomy (OR: 2.56, 95% CI: 1.55–4.22), segment I hepatectomy (OR: 2.56, 95% CI: 1.50–4.40), intraoperative blood transfusion (OR:2.40 95%CI:1.79–3.22), anatomical hepatectomy (OR: 1.70, 95% CI: 1.19–2.44) and intraoperative bleeding ≥1,000 ml (OR: 2.46, 95% CI: 2.12–2.85) were risk factors for biliary leakage. Age >75 years, cirrhosis, underlying liver disease, left hepatectomy, right hepatectomy, benign disease, Child–Pugh class A/B, and pre-operative albumin <3.5 g/dL were not risk factors for bile leakage after hepatectomy without biliary reconstruction.

Conclusion: Comprehensive research in the literature revealed that sex, diabetes, left trisectionectomy, central hepatectomy, extended hemihepatectomy, segment I hepatectomy, intraoperative blood transfusion, anatomical hepatectomy and intraoperative bleeding ≥1,000 ml were risk factors for biliary leakage.

Keywords: surgery, hepatectomy, bile leakage, risk factors, meta-analysis

INTRODUCTION

With deepening of the understanding of liver diseases and the development of hepatectomy techniques, the indications for liver resection have been continuously expanded, and the incidence of perioperative complications and mortality have been significantly reduced, but the incidence of bile leakage has not changed significantly (3.1 ∼ 28.0%) (1). Miura et al.

reported in 2016 that the biliary leakage rate of 14,970 patients who underwent more than segment I hepatectomy recorded by the Japanese National Clinical Database from 2011 to 2012 was 8.0% (2). Yamashita et al. reported in 2020 that the bile leakage rate of 10,102 patients who underwent complex hepatectomy from 2015 to 2017 was 7.2% (3). These findings show that with the development of technology, the incidence of bile leakage after hepatectomy has not been significantly reduced, and bile leakage is still a difficult clinical problem.

Bile leakage can cause severe complications such as post-operative abdominal infection and sepsis, prolong hospitalization, increase treatment costs, and even cause death (4). Studies have shown that bile leakage may inhibit liver regeneration and promote bile duct malignancies (5), thus affecting the prognosis of patients. However, the lack of standardization for the treatment of biliary leakage often delays the optimal treatment window, aggravates the patient's condition, and causes serious trauma to the patient. Clarifying the risk factors for biliary leakage, avoiding and preventing related risk factors, and minimizing the incidence of biliary leakage are particularly important after hepatectomy.

We collected relevant research reports on the risk factors for biliary leakage and further clarified the related risk factors for biliary leakage after hepatectomy without biliary reconstruction by means of meta-analysis, aiming to provide a reference for the clinical prevention and treatment of biliary leakage.

MATERIALS AND METHODS

For this systematic review, we adhered to the Meta-analysis of Observational Studies guidelines and the Reporting Items for Systematic reviews and Meta-Analysis (PRISMA) statement (6).

Search Strategy and Inclusion Criteria

A systematic search was performed based on the following databases: PubMed, Embase (Ovid), Medline (Ovid), Cochrane Library and Web of Science from January 1, 2000, to May 1, 2021. We used 'hepatectomy,' 'liver resection,' 'bile leakage,' 'biliary fistula,' 'risk factor,' and corresponding free words to search the literature in the above databases, with the language restricted to English. Literature inclusion standard: 1. literature studied the influence of different factors in the perioperative period on the occurrence of bile leakage after hepatectomy; 2. the sample size is at least 100 cases. Literature inclusion standard: 1. studies involving biliary reconstruction; 2. the sample size is less than 100 cases;3. the definition of bile leakage does not meet the ISGLS standard.

Bile Leakage Risk Factor Outcomes of Interest

The outcomes of interest included: age >75 years, sex, pre-operative albumin <3.5 g/dL, Child–Pugh class A/B, underlying liver disease, liver cirrhosis, diabetes, benign disease, intraoperative bleeding≥1,000 mL, intraoperative blood transfusion, segment I hepatectomy, left trisectionectomy, extended hemihepatectomy, central hepatectomy, left hepatectomy, right hepatectomy and anatomical hepatectomy.

Definition of Bile Leakage

This study used the International Study Group of Liver Surgery to define bile leakage (7), that is, the presence of bilirubin in the abdominal drainage or intraperitoneal fluid on or after the third day following surgery or the need for intervention due to bile collection or biliary peritonitis.

Data Extraction and Quality Assessment

First, TL and LF reviewed the titles and abstracts of all identified studies. Next, the same two reviewers independently reviewed the full texts of potentially eligible studies. If any disagreements arose, a third reviewer (LZL) was consulted, and a discussion ensued until a consensus was reached. All the data were independently extracted by TL and LF and compared for consistency. The following relevant information was extracted from all the included literature: first author, year of publication, country, journal, the number of patients, age, and surgery. The quality of the included studies was assessed using the Newcastle Ottawa Scale (NOS), with a maximum of nine points per study. Studies with a score <5 were considered low-quality studies and excluded. Publication bias was assessed by visual inspection of the symmetry of a funnel plot.

Statistical Analysis

We used the R (version 4.1.0) Meta package for meta-analysis. We calculated the odds ratios (ORs) and 95% confidence intervals (CIs) of different factors in the biliary leakage group and the non-bile leakage group after hepatectomy and the ORs and 95% CIs of multiple studies combined. The I^2 statistic was used to assess heterogeneity; $I^2 > 50\%$ was considered indicative of heterogeneity, and the random effects model is adopted, otherwise, the fixed effects model is adopted.

RESULTS

After removing duplicates, we obtained 404 publications from PubMed, Medline (Ovid), Embase (Ovid), Web of Science and Cochrane Library (**Figure 1**). A total of 16 publications (3, 8–22) and 16,051 hepatectomy patients were eligible for inclusion. **Table 1** shows the characteristics of the retrieved publications. Among the patients, 1,274 had biliary leakage, and the incidence of biliary leakage was 7.9%. The NOS scores of the nine studies ranged from 6 to 8 (**Figure 2**). The literature collected was considered qualified.

Bile Leakage Risk Factor Outcomes of Interest

Sex

Twelve (3, 8–11, 13–15, 18, 20–22) of the 16 included studies reported the influence of sex on the occurrence of bile leakage after hepatectomy. The overall outcomes showed that males had an increased incidence of bile leakage after hepatectomy (OR: 1.21, 95% CI: 1.04–1.42; $I^2 = 6\%$ $P = 0.39$), as shown in **Figure 3A**.

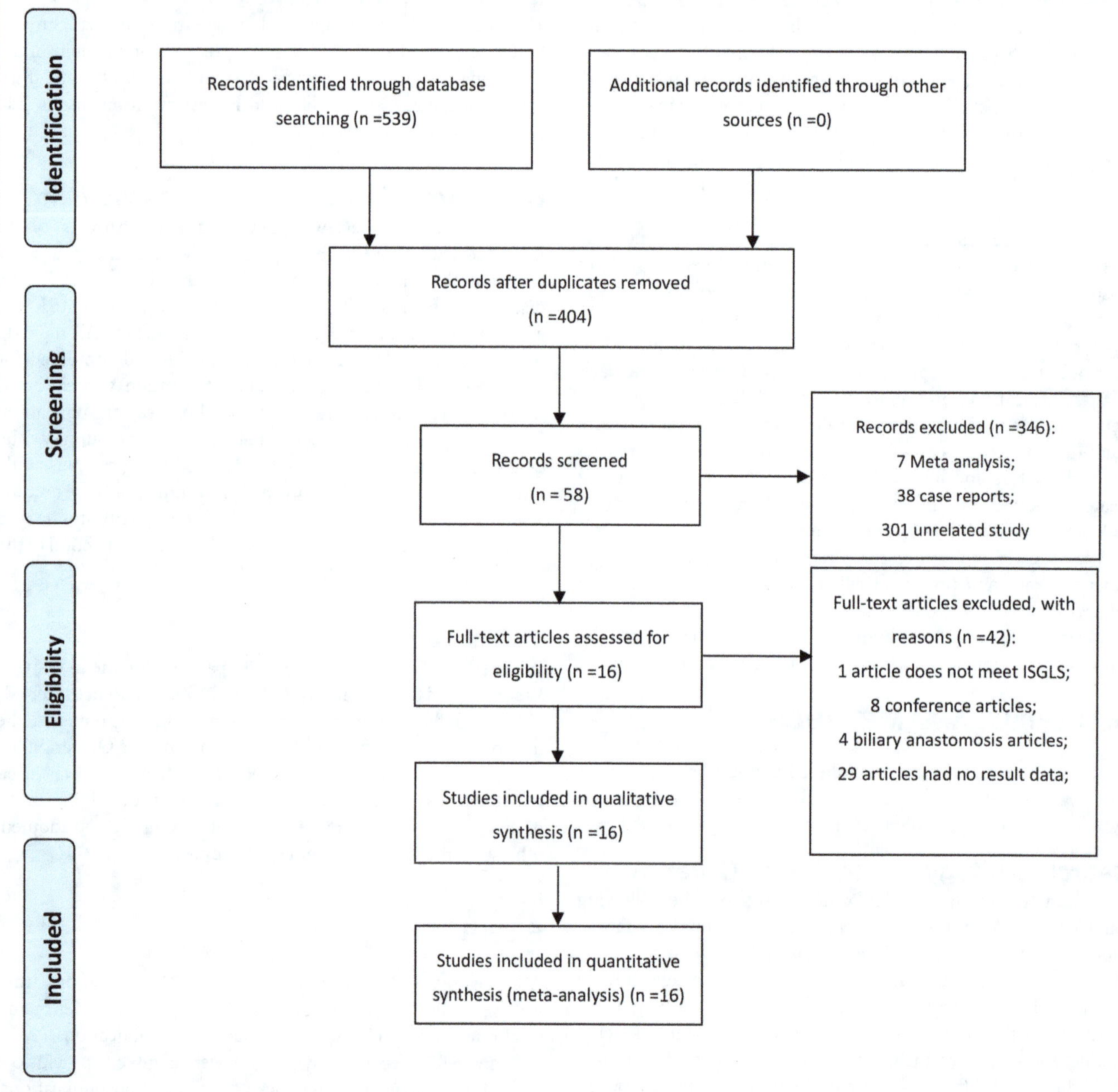

FIGURE 1 | PRISMA flow chart of search strategy and research selection.

Diabetes

Eight (3, 9, 13, 16, 18, 20–22) of the 16 included studies reported the influence of diabetes on the occurrence of bile leakage after hepatectomy. The overall outcomes showed that diabetes increased the incidence of bile leakage after hepatectomy (OR: 1.21, 95% CI: 1.05–1.38, I^2 = 0% P =0.81), as illustrated in **Figure 3B**.

Extended Hemihepatectomy

Five (8–11, 17) of the 16 included studies reported the influence of extended hemihepatectomy on the occurrence of bile leakage after hepatectomy. The overall outcomes showed that extended hemihepatectomy increased the incidence of bile leakage after hepatectomy (OR: 2.56, 95% CI: 1.55–4.22, I^2 = 40% P = 0.15), as illustrated in **Figure 3C**.

Central Hepatectomy

Six (3, 8, 9, 12, 15, 18) of the 16 included studies reported the influence of central hepatectomy on the occurrence of bile leakage after hepatectomy. The overall outcomes showed that central hepatectomy increased the incidence of bile leakage after

TABLE 1 | Characteristics of studies included in meta-analysis.

Author	Year	Journal	Country	*N*	Bile leakage rate	Age	Operation method
Yamashita, YI	2020	J Hepatobiliary Pancreat Sci	Japan	10,102	7.2%	–	Laparotomy
Sakamoto, K	2016	World J Surg	Japan	334	9.0 %	68 (32–87)	–
Sadamori, H	2013	Br J Surg	Japan	359	12.8%	–	Laparotomy
Sadamori, H	2010	J Hepatobiliary Pancreat Sci	Japan	293	12.9%	–	Laparotomy
Panaro, F	2016	Hepatobiliary Pancreat Dis Int	France	411	10.2%	–	–
Nakano, R	2018	Int J Surg	Japan	556	5.0%	69.8 ± 9.1 vs 69.9 ± 12.4	–
Nagano, Y	2003	World J Surg	Japan	313	5.4%	70.1 vs. 61.7	–
Capussotti, L	2006	Arch Surg	Italy	610	3.6%	61.65 (2–86) vs. 63.18 (49–78)	–
Cauchy, F	2016	Surg Endosc	France	223	13.5%	63.8 (24.1–86.2) vs. 62.5 (23.9–84.0)	Laparoscopic
Donadon, M	2016	World J Surg	Italy	475	8.0%	66 (23–85)	–
Erdogan, D	2008	Dig Surg	The Netherlands	234	6.8%	55.1 ± 1.0 vs. 59.2 ± 3.0	–
Guillaud, A	2013	HPB	France	1001	8.0%	64 (16–90)	Laparotomy and laparoscopic
Harimoto, N	2020	Surg Today	Japan	270	4.4%	68 (28–89)	Laparotomy
Haruki, K	2013	Langenbecks Arch Surg	Japan	105	8.6%	65.0 ± 10.0	–
Ishii, H	2011	Dig Surg	Japan	247	10.5%	63 (21–85) vs. 62 (22–81)	–
Kajiwara, T	2016	BMC Surg	Japan	518	15.6%	68 (20–84) vs 68 (44–84)	–

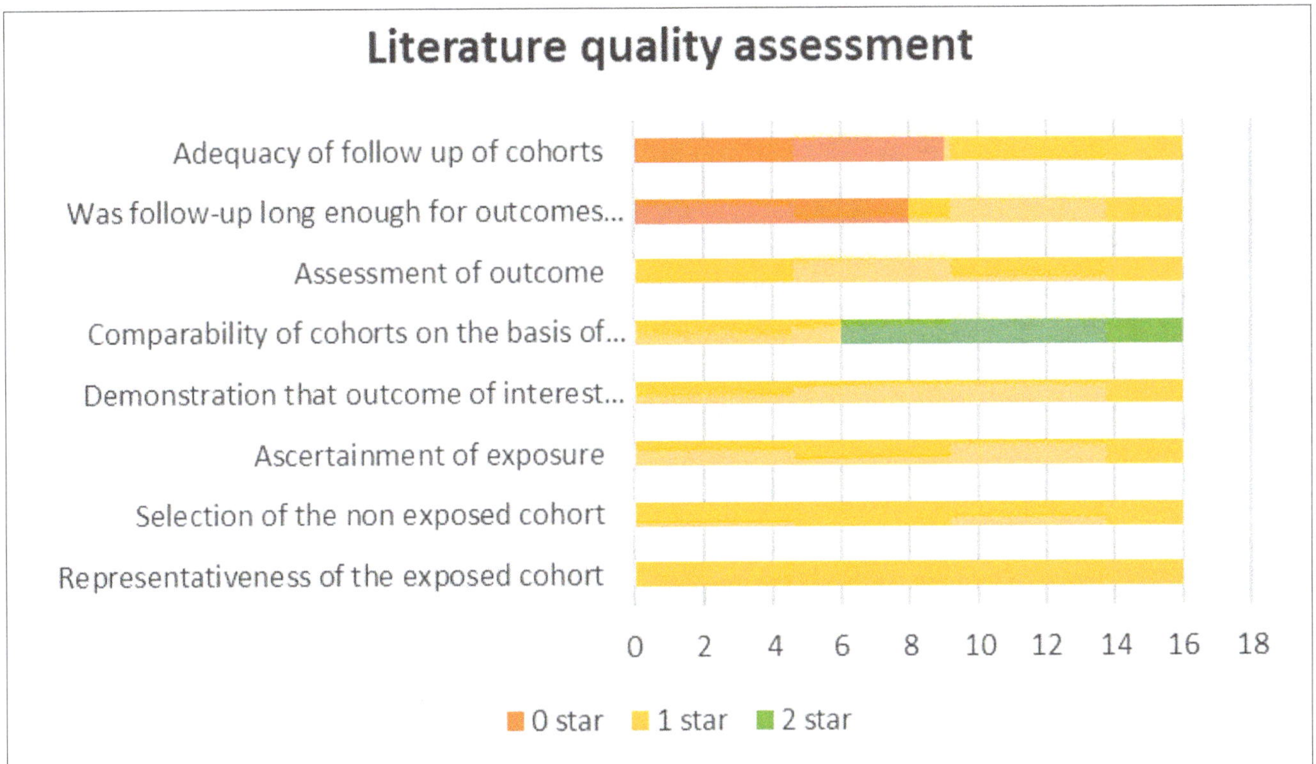

FIGURE 2 | Literature quality assessment based on the Newcastle-Ottawa Scale.

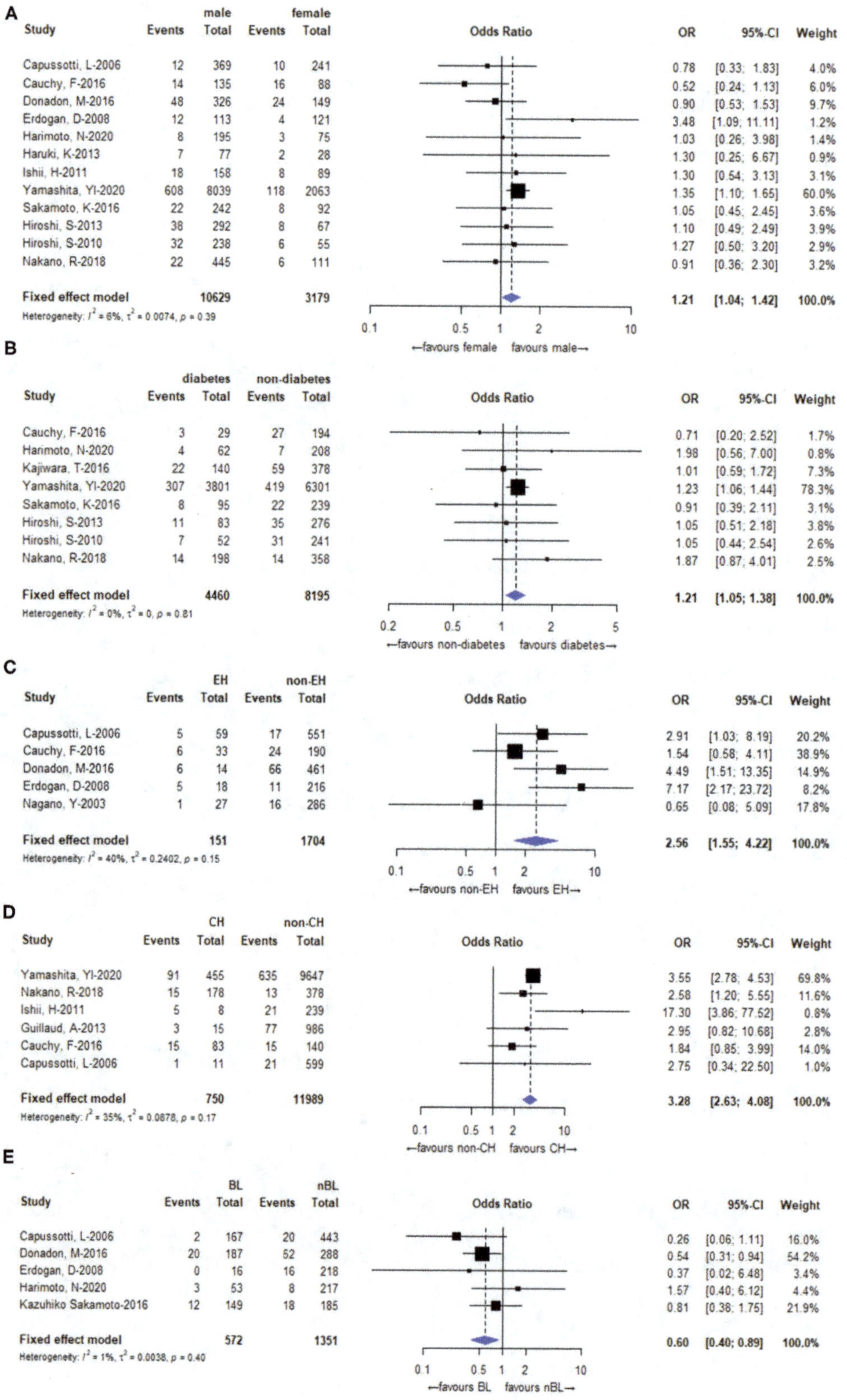

FIGURE 3 | Continued

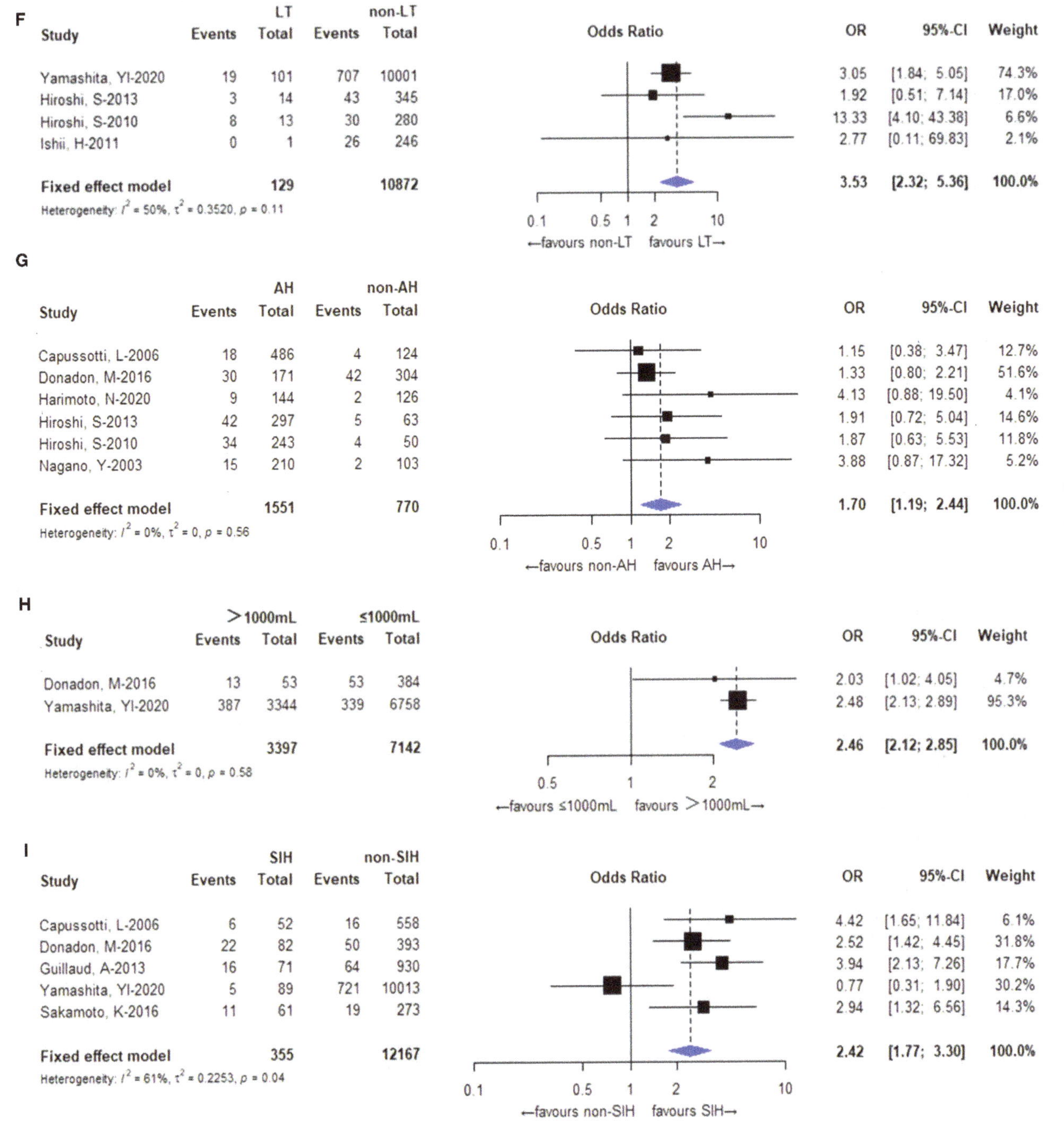

FIGURE 3 | Forest plots for the meta-analyses. **(A)** Sex; **(B)** Diabetes; **(C)** Extended hemihepatectomy (EH); **(D)** Central hepatectomy (CH); **(E)** Liver cirrhosis (LC); **(F)** Left trisectionectomy (LT); **(G)** Anatomical hepatectomy (AH); **(H)** Bleeding; **(I)** Segment I hepatectomy (SIH).

hepatectomy (OR: 3.28, 95% CI: 2.63–4.08), I^2 = 35% P =0.17), as shown in **Figure 3D**.

Liver Cirrhosis

Five (8, 10, 11, 13, 22) of the 16 included studies reported the influence of liver cirrhosis on the occurrence of bile leakage after hepatectomy. The results showed that liver cirrhosis reduced the incidence of bile leakage after hepatectomy (OR: 0.60, 95% CI: 0.40–0.89, I^2 = 1% P = 0.40), as shown in **Figure 3E**.

Left Trisectionectomy

Four (3, 15, 20, 21) of the 16 included studies reported the influence of left trisectionectomy on the occurrence of bile leakage after hepatectomy. The overall outcomes showed that left trisectionectomy increased the incidence of bile leakage after hepatectomy (OR: 3.53, 95% CI: 2.32–5.36), $I^2 = 50\%$ $P = 0.11$), as shown in **Figure 3F**.

Anatomical Hepatectomy

Six (8, 10, 13, 17, 20, 21) of the 16 included studies reported the influence of anatomical hepatectomy on the occurrence of bile leakage after hepatectomy. The overall outcomes showed that anatomical hepatectomy did not affect the occurrence of bile leakage after hepatectomy (OR: 1.70, 95% CI: 1.19–2.44, $I^2 = 0\%$ $P = 0.56$), as shown in **Figure 3G**.

Intraoperative Bleeding ≥1,000 mL

Two (3, 10) of the 16 included studies reported the influence of bleeding ≥1,000 ml on the occurrence of bile leakage after hepatectomy. The overall outcomes showed that bleeding ≥1,000 ml increased the incidence of bile leakage after hepatectomy (OR: 2.46, 95% CI: 2.12–2.85), $I^2 = 0\%$ $P = 0.58$), as shown in **Figure 3H**.

Segment I Hepatectomy

Five (3, 8, 9, 12, 22) of the 16 included studies reported the influence of segment I hepatectomy on the occurrence of bile leakage after hepatectomy. The overall outcomes showed that segment I hepatectomy increased the incidence of bile leakage after hepatectomy (OR: 2.56, 95% CI: 1.50–4.40, $I^2 = 61\%$ $P = 0.04$), as shown in **Figure 3I**.

Age>75 Years

Four (3, 8, 9, 12) of the 16 included studies reported the influence of age >75 years on the occurrence of bile leakage after hepatectomy. The overall outcomes showed that age >75 years did not affect the occurrence of bile leakage after hepatectomy (OR: 1.12, 95% CI: 0.97–1.31, $I^2 = 32\%$ $P = 0.22$), as shown in **Supplementary Figure 1A**.

Underlying Liver Disease

Nine (8, 10, 11, 13, 15, 16, 18, 20, 21) of the 16 included studies reported the influence of underlying liver disease on the occurrence of bile leakage after hepatectomy. The overall outcomes showed that underlying liver disease did not affect the occurrence of bile leakage after hepatectomy (OR: 0.91, 95% CI: 0.70–1.19, $I^2 = 0\%$ $P = 0.62$), as shown in **Supplementary Figure 1B**.

Left Hepatectomy

Six (3, 8, 11, 15, 18, 22) of the 16 included studies reported the influence of left hepatectomy on the occurrence of bile leakage after hepatectomy. The overall outcomes showed that left hepatectomy did not affect the occurrence of bile leakage after hepatectomy (OR: 0.90, 95% CI: 0.72–1.13, $I^2 = 0\%$ $P = 0.62$), as shown in **Supplementary Figure 1C**.

Right Hepatectomy

Five (8, 9, 15, 18, 22) of the 16 included studies reported the influence of right hepatectomy on the occurrence of bile leakage after hepatectomy. The overall outcomes showed that right hepatectomy did not affect the occurrence of bile leakage after hepatectomy (OR: 0.90, 95% CI: 0.72–1.13, $I^2 = 0\%$ $P = 0.62$), as shown in **Supplementary Figure 1D**.

Benign Disease

Three (8, 9, 11) of the 16 included studies reported the influence of benign disease on the occurrence of bile leakage after hepatectomy. The overall outcomes showed that benign disease did not affect the occurrence of bile leakage after hepatectomy (OR: 0.52, 95% CI: 0.22–1.26, $I^2 = 0\%$ $P = 1.00$), as shown in **Supplementary Figure 1E**.

Child-Pugh Class A/B

Six (13, 15, 16, 18, 20, 21) of the 16 included studies reported the influence of Child–Pugh class on the occurrence of bile leakage after hepatectomy. The overall outcomes showed that Child–Pugh class did not affect the occurrence of bile leakage after hepatectomy (OR: 0.68, 95% CI: 0.39–1.19, $I^2 = 27\%$ $P = 0.23$), as shown in **Supplementary Figure 1F**.

Intraoperative Blood Transfusion

Eight (9–14, 20, 21) of the 16 included studies reported the influence of intraoperative blood transfusion on the occurrence of bile leakage after hepatectomy. The overall outcomes showed that blood transfusion did not affect the occurrence of bile leakage after hepatectomy (OR: 1.57, 95% CI: 0.75–3.30, $I^2 = 84\%$ $P < 0.01$), as shown in **Supplementary Figure 1G**.

Pre-operative Albumin<3.5 g/dL

Three (3, 20, 21) of the 16 included studies reported the influence of pre-operative albumin on the occurrence of bile leakage after hepatectomy. The overall outcomes showed that pre-operative albumin <3.5 g/dL did not affect the occurrence of bile leakage after hepatectomy [OR: 0.91 (95% CI: 0.48–1.75), $I^2 = 68\%$ $P = 0.04$], as shown in **Supplementary Figure 1H**.

Sensitivity Analysis

We conducted a sensitivity analysis on heterogeneity factors (segment I hepatectomy, blood transfusion, pre-operative albumin <3.5 g/dL) and found the source of heterogeneity (as shown in **Supplementary Figure 2**). The analysis revealed the following results (as shown in **Supplementary Figure 3**): the segment I hepatectomy OR was 3.13 (2.20-4.44), and heterogeneity tests showed that the trials did not have heterogeneity ($I^2 = 0\%$; $P = 0.66$); the intraoperative blood transfusion OR was 2.40 (1.79–3.22), and heterogeneity tests showed that the trials did not have heterogeneity ($I^2 = 0\%$; $P = 0.57$); the pre-operative albumin <3.5 g/dL OR was 0.62 (0.34–1.14), and heterogeneity tests showed that the trials did not have heterogeneity ($I^2 = 0\%$; $P = 0.80$). After heterogeneity was excluded, the results for segment 1 hepatectomy and pre-operative chemotherapy were consistent with the results without heterogeneity exclusion. After excluding heterogeneity, the results showed that intraoperative blood transfusion increased the incidence of bile leakage after hepatectomy.

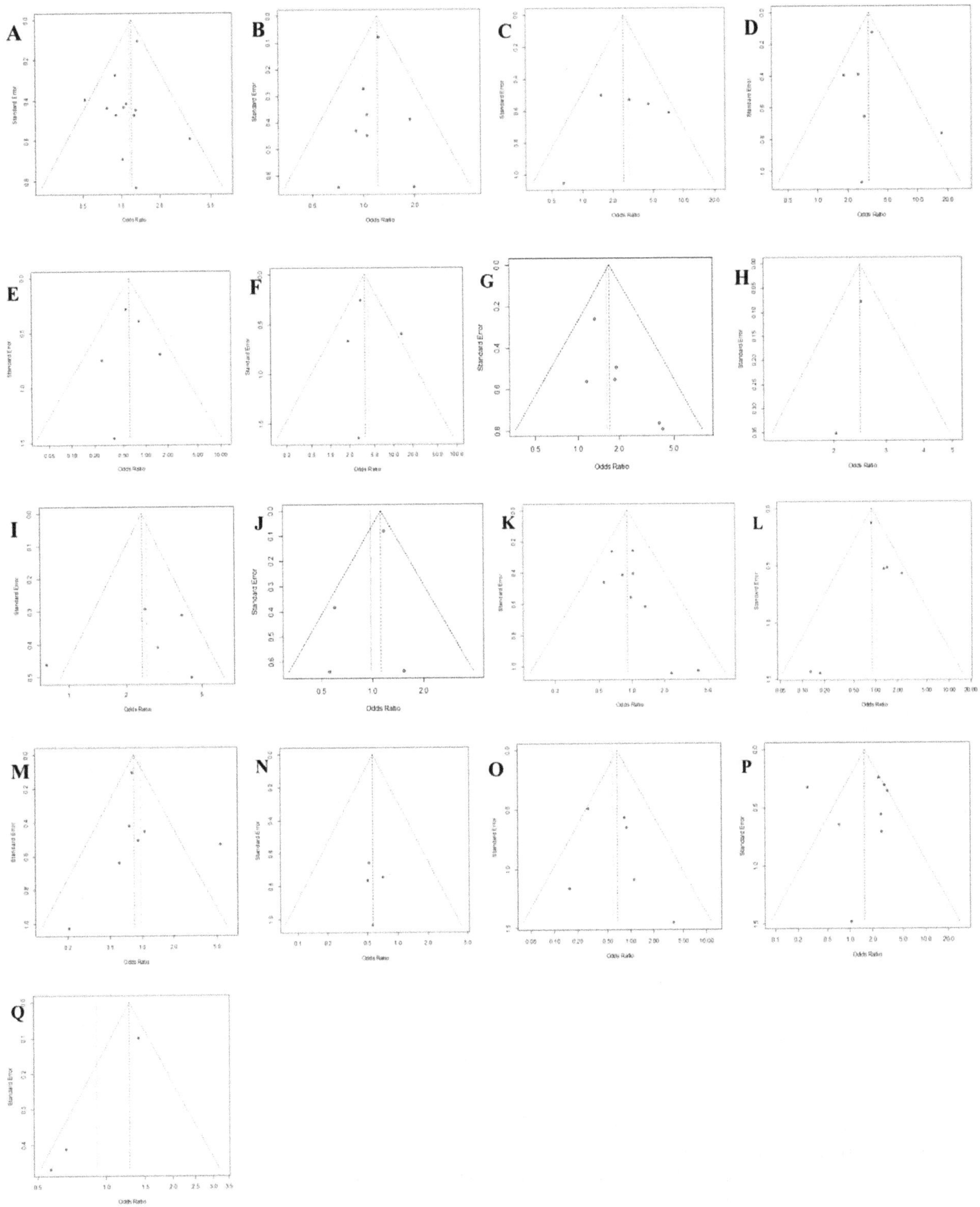

FIGURE 4 | Funnel plot of publication bias in the meta-analysis. **(A)** Sex; **(B)** Diabetes; **(C)** Extended hemihepatectomy; **(D)** Central hepatectomy; **(E)** Liver cirrhosis; **(F)** Left trisectionectomy; **(G)** Anatomical hepatectomy; **(H)** Bleeding; **(I)** Segment I hepatectomy; **(J)** Age; **(K)** Underlying liver disease; **(L)** Left hepatectomy; **(M)** Right hepatectomy; **(N)** Benign disease; **(O)** Child-Pugh class A/B; **(P)** Intraoperative blood transfusion; **(Q)** Pre-operative albumin <3.5 g/dL.

Publication Bias

Publication bias was assessed by visual examination of the symmetry of the funnel plot. Our funnel plot showed no publication bias (**Figure 4**).

DISCUSSION

Research on risk factors related to bile leakage after hepatectomy has expanded from discussions of surgical factors to the entire perioperative period. The relevant factors included in the study were patient characteristics, surgical methods and post-operative treatment (3, 8, 23). Nevertheless, the conclusions of various studies are still controversial, and maximally clarifying the related risk factors for bile leakage is very important, which will be helpful for us to prevent and reduce the occurrence of bile leakage.

Our research results show that among the risk factors for bile leakage, risk factors related to the patient are sex and diabetes, while risk factors related to surgery are left trisectionectomy, central hepatectomy, extended hemihepatectomy, segment 1 resection, intraoperative blood transfusion, anatomical hepatectomy and intraoperative bleeding >1,000 ml. However, advanced age (age >75 years), pre-operative albumin <3.5 g/dL, underlying liver disease, benign disease, hemihepatectomy, and Child–Pugh class A/B are not biliary risk factors for leakage.

Previous studies have shown that sex is a risk factor for bile leakage after hepatectomy without biliary reconstruction (3, 11). The results of our research are consistent with those of previous studies. The influence of sex hormones may be pertinent, but no relevant evidence is available at present, and further research is needed to obtain the specific influence mechanism.

Our research results fully show that diabetes is a high-risk factor for bile leakage. Diabetes is also a high-risk factor for perioperative complications. Diabetes increases the risk of post-operative infections, prolongs the hospital stay (24, 25), and even increases the mortality rate during the perioperative period (26). However, the impact of diabetes on liver resection has been controversial, especially the influence of bile leakage (26). Diabetes can cause microcirculation disorders and affect tissue healing and is generally considered an independent risk factor for bile leakage (3, 27). Research by Yamamoto et al. (28) pointed out that diabetes can damage the residual liver after hepatectomy and affect healing of the cut surface tissue, which may increase the risk of post-operative bile leakage. Therefore, reasonable blood glucose control before surgery is essential to prevent post-operative bile leakage.

Although the relationship between the type of hepatectomy and biliary leakage is not clear, previous studies mostly speculated that resection of the central segment of the liver with hilar exposure was a high-risk factor for biliary leakage (15, 17, 23, 29, 30). However, Sadamori et al. believe that the type of hepatectomy is not a risk factor for bile leakage (21). Even in the case of a large section area and exposure of the Glisson system, as long as the pre-operative liver function assessment is reasonable and surgery is meticulously performed, no bile leakage is usually observed after the operation. Our conclusions show that central hepatectomy, segment I resection, and left trisectionectomy are associated with a higher incidence of bile leakage. Due to the anatomical position, during resection of segment 1 and the central liver segment (S4, S5, S8), the main Glisson system around the hilum is easily damaged, thus causing bile leakage. Central hepatectomy involves a larger resection area, and no tissue coverage may also be one of the reasons for post-operative bile leakage (23). In previous studies, left trisectionectomy was also considered a high-risk factor for bile leakage (3, 23, 30), A large tangent area (31) and the right posterior bile duct often merge into the left bile duct, which may cause intraoperative bile duct damage and bile leakage (32). The pumping action of the right diaphragm increases the residual right hepatic bile duct pressure and increases bile leakage (33). Notably, for the more common hemihepatectomy, our results show that neither left hepatectomy nor right hepatectomy is a risk factor for bile leakage, possibly because hemihepatectomy involves less manipulation in the central area of the hepatic hilum. Therefore, resection of the central area during hepatectomy may lead to a corresponding increase in the risk of bile leakage, which must be comprehensively considered.

The choice of resection method for malignant liver tumors has always been a controversial topic. A meta-analysis by Jiao S et al. showed that anatomical hepatectomy is superior to non-anatomical hepatectomy in terms of the long-term survival rate of patients with HCC (34). Rahbari et al. (35) pointed out that anatomical hepatectomy is a risk factor for bile leakage, and given the significant adverse effects of complications after hepatectomy on the long-term prognosis of malignant liver tumors, caution is recommended when considering surgical methods. Anatomical liver resection requires too much manipulation of the Glisson ligaments, and resection of the central area of the hepatic portal region may increase the occurrence of bile leakage. However, to ensure a radical cure and a prognostic effect of the tumor, we must choose a reasonable surgical procedure based on the advantages and disadvantages. Although our results further support this view, unfortunately, we have included limited literature and insufficient evidence, and more studies are needed to further verify this conjecture in the future.

Our research indicates that intraoperative bleeding ≥1,000 ml and intraoperative blood transfusion are risk factors for post-operative bile leakage, possibly due to the combined effects of massive blood loss during hepatectomy, intraoperative hepatic blood flow obstruction, blood transfusion, etc. (36–38), which may cause and aggravate liver ischemia and reperfusion injury, affect liver function recovery, and cause bile leakage. However, the number of included studies was small, and the evidence was obviously insufficient; therefore, this result requires further confirmation.

This research found that sex, diabetes, left trisectionectomy, central hepatectomy, extended hemihepatectomy, segment I hepatectomy, intraoperative blood transfusion, anatomical hepatectomy and intraoperative bleeding ≥1,000 ml were risk factors for biliary leakage. However, this meta-analysis was mainly limited to the inclusion of only retrospective research data; retrospective research tends to introduce bias. In addition, due to the large time span of the included studies, technological development, and differences in surgical instruments, the results of the study may be biased. At the same time, due to the diversity of liver resection methods, the data in the studies are quite different, resulting in a relative lack of analysis of surgical data, which is also an obvious shortcoming of this study. We hope that more high-quality RCT results will be obtained in the future to guide our understanding of the risk factors for bile leakage.

CONCLUSION

Comprehensive research in the literature showed that male sex, diabetes, left trisectionectomy, central hepatectomy, extended hemihepatectomy, segment I hepatectomy, intraoperative blood transfusion, anatomical hepatectomy and intraoperative bleeding ≥1,000 ml were risk factors for biliary leakage.

AUTHOR CONTRIBUTIONS

LT and FL: acquisition of data, analysis and interpretation of data, drafting the article, and final approval. Z-lL: interpretation of data, revising the article, and final approval. J-wX: conception and design of the study, critical revision, and final approval. All authors contributed to the article and approved the submitted version.

ACKNOWLEDGMENTS

We are very grateful to Ni Ran for providing guidance on search strategies for this study.

REFERENCES

1. Kubo N, Shirabe K. Treatment strategy for isolated bile leakage after hepatectomy: literature review. *Ann Gastroenterol Surg.* (2020) 4:47–55. doi: 10.1002/ags3.12303
2. Miura F, Yamamoto M, Gotoh M, Konno H, Fujimoto J, Yanaga K, et al. Validation of the board certification system for expert surgeons (hepato-biliary-pancreatic field) using the data of the National Clinical Database of Japan: part 1 - Hepatectomy of more than one segment. *J Hepato Biliary Pancreat Sci.* (2016) 23:313–23. doi: 10.1002/jhbp.344
3. Yamashita Y, Yamamoto H, Miyata H, Kakeji Y, Kitagawa Y, Yamaue H, et al. Risk factors for bile leakage: latest analysis of 10 102 hepatectomies for hepatocellular carcinoma from the Japanese national clinical database. *J Hepato Biliary Pancreat Sci.* (2020) 28:556–62. doi: 10.1002/jhbp.827
4. Bednarsch J, Blüthner E, Malinowski M, Seehofer D, Pratschke J, et al. Regeneration of liver function capacity after partial liver resection is impaired in case of post-operative bile leakage. *World J Surg.* (2016) 40:2221–8. doi: 10.1007/s00268-016-3524-z
5. Braunwarth E, Primavesi F, Göbel G, Cardini B, Oberhuber R, Margreiter C, et al. Is bile leakage after hepatic resection associated with impaired long-term survival? *Eur J Surg Oncol.* (2019) 45:1077–83. doi: 10.1016/j.ejso.2019.02.021
6. Moher D, Liberati A, Tetzlaff J, Altman D. Preferred reporting items for systematic reviews and meta-analyses: the PRISMA statement. *BMJ.* (2009) 339:b2535. doi: 10.1136/bmj.b2535
7. Koch M, Garden O, Padbury R, Rahbari N, Adam R, Capussotti L, et al. Bile leakage after hepatobiliary and pancreatic surgery: a definition and grading of severity by the International Study Group of Liver Surgery. *Surgery.* (2011) 149:680–8. doi: 10.1016/j.surg.2010.12.002
8. Capussotti L, Ferrero A, Viganò L, Sgotto E, Muratore A, Polastri R. Bile leakage and liver resection: where is the risk? *Arch Surg.* (2006) 141:690–4. doi: 10.1001/archsurg.141.7.690
9. Cauchy F, Fuks D, Nomi T, Schwarz L, Belgaumkar A, Scatton O, et al. Incidence, risk factors and consequences of bile leakage following laparoscopic major hepatectomy. *Surg Endosc.* (2016) 30:3709–19. doi: 10.1007/s00464-015-4666-z
10. Donadon M, Costa G, Cimino M, Procopio F, Del Fabbro D, Palmisano A, et al. Diagnosis and management of bile leaks after hepatectomy: results of a prospective analysis of 475 hepatectomies. *World J Surg.* (2016) 40:172–81. doi: 10.1007/s00268-015-3143-0
11. Erdogan D, Busch OR, van Delden OM, Rauws EA, Gouma DJ, van Gulik TM. Incidence and management of bile leakage after partial liver resection. *Digest Surg.* (2008) 25:60–6. doi: 10.1159/000118024
12. Guillaud A, Pery C, Campillo B, Lourdais A, Sulpice L, Boudjema K. Incidence and predictive factors of clinically relevant bile leakage in the modern era of liver resections. *HPB.* (2013) 15:224–9. doi: 10.1111/j.1477-2574.2012.00580.x
13. Harimoto N, Muranushi R, Hoshino K, Yamanaka T, Hagiwara K, Ishii N, et al. Albumin-indocyanine green evaluation (ALICE) grade predicts bile leakage after hepatic resection. *Surg Today.* (2020) 50:849–54. doi: 10.1007/s00595-020-01955-2
14. Haruki K, Shiba H, Fujiwara Y, Furukawa K, Wakiyama S, Ogawa M, et al. Post-operative peripheral blood monocyte count correlates with postoperative bile leakage in patients with colorectal liver metastases after hepatic resection. *Langenbecks Arch Surg.* (2013) 398:851–5. doi: 10.1007/s00423-013-1083-4
15. Ishii H, Ochiai T, Murayama Y, Komatsu S, Shiozaki A, Kuriu Y, et al. Risk factors and management of postoperative bile leakage after hepatectomy without bilioenteric anastomosis. *Digest Surg.* (2011) 28:198–204. doi: 10.1159/000324042
16. Kajiwara T, Midorikawa Y, Yamazaki S, Higaki T, Nakayama H, Moriguchi M, et al. Clinical score to predict the risk of bile leakage after liver resection. *BMC Surg.* (2016) 16:30. doi: 10.1186/s12893-016-0147-0
17. Nagano Y, Togo S, Tanaka K, Masui H, Endo I, Sekido H, et al. Risk factors and management of bile leakage after hepatic resection. *World J Surg.* (2003) 27:695–8. doi: 10.1007/s00268-003-6907-x
18. Nakano R, Ohira M, Kobayashi T, Imaoka Y, Mashima H, Yamaguchi M, et al. Independent risk factors that predict bile leakage after hepatectomy for hepatocellular carcinoma: cohort study. *Int J Surg.* (2018) 57:1–7. doi: 10.1016/j.ijsu.2018.07.005
19. Panaro F, Hacina L, Bouyabrine H, Al-Hashmi AW, Herrero A, Navarro F. Risk factors for postoperative bile leakage: a retrospective single-center analysis of 411 hepatectomies. *Hepatobiliary Pancreat Dis. Int.* (2016) 15:81–6. doi: 10.1016/S1499-3872(15)60424-6
20. Sadamori H, Yagi T, Matsuda H, Shinoura S, Umeda Y, Yoshida R, et al. Risk factors for major morbidity after hepatectomy for hepatocellular carcinoma in 293 recent cases. *J Hepato Biliary Pancreat Sci.* (2010) 17:709–18. doi: 10.1007/s00534-010-0275-3
21. Sadamori H, Yagi T, Shinoura S, Umeda Y, Yoshida R, Satoh D, et al. Risk factors for major morbidity after liver resection for hepatocellular carcinoma. *Br J Surg.* (2013) 100:122–9. doi: 10.1002/bjs.8957
22. Sakamoto K, Tamesa T, Yukio T, Tokuhisa Y, Maeda Y, Oka M. Risk factors and managements of bile leakage after hepatectomy. *World J Surg.* (2016) 40:182–9. doi: 10.1007/s00268-015-3156-8
23. Lo C, Fan S, Liu C, Lai E, Wong J. Biliary complications after hepatic resection: risk factors, management, and outcome. *Arch Surg.* (1998) 133:156–61. doi: 10.1001/archsurg.133.2.156
24. Bagdade J, Stewart M, Walters E. Impaired granulocyte adherence. A reversible defect in host defense in patients with poorly controlled diabetes. *Diabetes.* (1978) 27:677–81. doi: 10.2337/diabetes.27.6.677
25. Li Q, Wang Y, Ma T, Lv Y, Wu R. Clinical outcomes of patients with and without diabetes mellitus after hepatectomy: a systematic review and meta-analysis. *PLoS ONE.* (2017) 12:e0171129. doi: 10.1371/journal.pone.0171129

26. Inoue Y, Suzuki Y, Yokohama K, Ohama H, Tsuchimoto Y, Asai A, et al. Diabetes mellitus does not influence results of hepatectomy in hepatocellular carcinoma: case control study. *Contempor Oncol.* (2020) 24:211–5. doi: 10.5114/wo.2020.102825
27. Fischer A, Fuchs J, Stravodimos C, Hinz U, Billeter A, Büchler M, et al. Influence of diabetes on short-term outcome after major hepatectomy: an underestimated risk? *BMC Surg.* (2020) 20:305. doi: 10.1186/s12893-020-00971-w
28. Yamamoto K, Takada Y, Fujimoto Y, Haga H, Oike F, Kobayashi N, et al. Nonalcoholic steatohepatitis in donors for living donor liver transplantation. *Transplantation.* (2007) 83:257–62. doi: 10.1097/01.tp.0000250671.06456.3f
29. Hong J, Zhang X, Luo R, Cai X. The clinical risk factors associated with postoperative bile leakage after hepatectomy: a meta-analysis. *Minerva Med.* (2016) 107:39–53.
30. Tanaka S, Hirohashi K, Tanaka H, Shuto T, Lee S, Kubo S, et al. Incidence and management of bile leakage after hepatic resection for malignant hepatic tumors. *J Am Coll Surg.* (2002) 195:484–9. doi: 10.1016/S1072-7515(02)01288-7
31. Ito A, Ebata T, Yokoyama Y, Igami T, Mizuno T, Yamaguchi J, et al. Ethanol ablation for refractory bile leakage after complex hepatectomy. *Br J Surg.* (2018) 105:1036–43. doi: 10.1002/bjs.10801
32. Mizumoto R, Suzuki H. Surgical anatomy of the hepatic hilum with special reference to the caudate lobe. *World J Surg.* (1988) 12:2–10. doi: 10.1007/BF01658479
33. Paquet J, Dziri C, Hay J, Fingerhut A, Zeitoun G, Suc B, et al. Prevention of deep abdominal complications with omentoplasty on the raw surface after hepatic resection. The French Associations for Surgical Research. *Am J Surg.* (2000) 179:103–9. doi: 10.1016/S0002-9610(00)00277-4
34. Jiao S, Li G, Zhang D, Xu Y, Liu J, Li G. Anatomic versus non-anatomic resection for hepatocellular carcinoma, do we have an answer? A meta-analysis. *Int J Surg.* (2020) 80:243–55. doi: 10.1016/j.ijsu.2020.05.008
35. Rahbari NN, Elbers H, Koch M, Kirchberg J, Dutlu M, Mehrabi A, et al. Bilirubin level in the drainage fluid is an early and independent predictor of clinically relevant bile leakage after hepatic resection. *Surgery.* (2012) 152:821–31. doi: 10.1016/j.surg.2012.03.012
36. Peralta C, Jiménez-Castro M, Gracia-Sancho JJJoh. Hepatic ischemia and reperfusion injury: effects on the liver sinusoidal milieu. *J Hepatol.* (2013) 59:1094–106. doi: 10.1016/j.jhep.2013.06.017
37. Fu P, Li W. Nitric oxide in liver ischemia-reperfusion injury. In: Muriel P, editor. *Liver Pathophysiology.* Vol. 8. Boston, MA: Academic Press (2017). p. 125–7. doi: 10.1016/B978-0-12-804274-8.00008-4
38. Glanemann M, Vollmar B, Nussler A, Schaefer T, Neuhaus P, Menger M. Ischemic preconditioning protects from hepatic ischemia/reperfusion-injury by preservation of microcirculation and mitochondrial redox-state. *J Hepatol.* (2003) 38:59–66. doi: 10.1016/S0168-8278(02)00327-6

20

Sub-Classification of Cirrhosis Affects Surgical Outcomes for Early Hepatocellular Carcinoma Independent of Portal Hypertension

*Er-lei Zhang, Jiang Li, Jian Li, Wen-qiang Wang, Jin Gu and Zhi-yong Huang**

Hepatic Surgery Center, Tongji Hospital, Tongji Medical College, Huazhong University of Science and Technology, Wuhan, China

Correspondence:
Zhi-yong Huang
huangzy@tjh.tjmu.edu.cn

Severity of liver cirrhosis is distinct from clinical portal hypertension because there exist different degrees of liver cirrhosis in hepatocellular carcinoma (HCC) patients without significant clinical portal hypertension. Whether severity of cirrhosis affects surgical outcomes for HCC patients in absence of portal hypertension or not remains unclear. This study aims to analyze the effect of cirrhotic severity on surgical outcomes for HCC patients with hepatitis B virus (HBV) infection in absence of portal hypertension. This retrospective study enrolled 166 patients who underwent curative resection for a single HCC ≤5 cm in absence of portal hypertension between February 2011 and December 2013. Liver cirrhosis was sub-classified into no/mild (no/F4A) and moderate/severe (F4B/F4C) according to the Laennec scoring system. The surgical outcomes and complications were analyzed. The surgical mortality was zero in this study. Major complications were apparently higher in the F4B/F4C group than in the no/F4A group (17.0% vs 7.4%, p <0.001). The 1-year, 3-year and 5-year overall survival (OS) rates were 98.5, 88.1 and 80%, respectively, in the no/F4A group, which were significantly higher than those in the F4B/F4C group (98.0, 69.2 and 54.7%, p = 0.001). Microscopic vascular invasion, absence of tumor capsule and severity of liver cirrhosis were independent risk factors of surgical outcomes for HCC patients without portal hypertension. In conclusion, severity of liver cirrhosis affected surgical outcomes for early-stage HCC patients independent of portal hypertension.

Keywords: cirrhosis, histological, hepatocellular carcinoma, Laennec staging, portal hypertension, liver resection

INTRODUCTION

Hepatocellular carcinoma (HCC) is the fifth most common cancer worldwide and the second most common cause of cancer mortality (1). In China, more than four fifths of HCC patients have presented with varied degrees of liver cirrhosis (2). For the past ten years, due to active surveillance programs, the detection of early-stage HCC has increased, therefore, the number of HCC patients who are suitable for curative treatment has consequently increased. Together with local ablation (LA) and liver transplantation (LT), liver resection (LR) is considered as the first-line treatment for small HCC patients with relatively good liver function, which offers a chance of cure and long-term surgical outcomes. However, the factors affecting surgical outcomes for early-stage HCC concomitant with liver cirrhosis remain a major concern. It should be noted that the prognosis of HCC patients was influenced not only by the tumor status but also underlying liver cirrhosis. In addition, tumor recurrence remains a major issue in clinical management of HCC and the cumulative risk of recurrence during the first five years after LR is still high (3, 4). The high risk of recurrence after curative-intent LR is attributable to the following two patterns: recurrence derived from residual micro-metastases and *de novo* recurrence due to the underlying liver cirrhosis (5, 6). Tumor recurrence is associated with the different degrees of underlying liver cirrhosis (7) and the annual incidence of HCC in patients with liver cirrhosis has been reported to range between 2.5 and 6.6% (8–10). The cumulative incidence of recurrence owing to *de novo* carcinogenesis would result in significant differences in surgical outcomes between patients with liver cirrhosis versus those with normal liver (11, 12). Moreover, liver cirrhosis is a dynamic process and the severity and clinical prognosis vary greatly, even among HCC patients within the same histological degree of cirrhosis (10, 13, 14). It needs to further reveal the impact of histological sub-classification of cirrhosis on surgical outcomes after LR for HCC patients.

The Laennec scoring system histologically subdivided liver cirrhosis into three stages (F4A, F4B and F4C) according to the thickness of the fibrous septa and size of the nodules (15). Studies reported that histological sub-classification of liver cirrhosis using the Laennec scoring system could predict late recurrence in HCC patients after curative resection, and it was obviously correlated with grade of portal hypertension but not the same disease (15, 16). However, there exist an obvious heterogeneity within cirrhosis even in HCC patients without significant portal hypertension, and the importance of cirrhotic severity in clinical practice should be further validated in this circumstance.

More and more surgeons have realized the key role of cirrhotic severity in surgical modalities and long-term outcomes (10, 16–18). The present study aimed to elucidate whether histological sub-classification of liver cirrhosis affected surgical outcomes of the early-stage HCC patients in absence of significant portal hypertension.

MATERIALS AND METHODS

Patients

From February 2011 to December 2013, 1,187 patients underwent liver resection (LR) for the first time in the Hepatic Surgery Center at Tongji Hospital of Tongji Medical College, Huazhong University of Science and Technology. HCC was diagnosed based on cyto-histological evidence from excised specimens. Demographic characteristics, laboratory parameters, imageological and histological results of all the selected patients were all collected. Portal hypertension was indirectly diagnosed according to the following criteria: esophageal varices by endoscopy or total platelet count <100,000/ml combined with splenomegaly (19). A total of 166 patients met the following inclusion criteria:

1. Early-stage HCC (solitary lesions less than 5 cm) with HBV infection.
2. No portal vein tumor thrombus or extra-hepatic metastases.
3. Child–Pugh A liver functions and absence of portal hypertension.
4. No previous treatments for HCC.
5. Patients with no severe comorbidities that cannot tolerate surgery.

Figure S1 shows a flow diagram of enrolled HCC patients in the present study.

Surgical Treatment

LR was carried out in patients who satisfied the surgical indication with central venous pressure (CVP) less than 5mmHg using a right sub-costal incision. Intra-operative ultrasound was routinely performed to confirm tumor location and satellite nodules, as well as assess the vascular anatomy of the liver. We performed all the hepatectomies with R0 resection. The Cavitron Ultrasonic Aspiration (CUSA, Valleylab Corp, USA) and Harmonic scalpel (Johnson & Johnson Ltd, USA) were used to transect liver parenchyma. Pringle's maneuver was performed intermittently, each time for less than 15 min, with an interval of 5 min aiming to minimize peri-operative blood loss.

Histological Evaluation of Liver Specimens

Histological evaluation of liver specimens was carried out by two experienced pathologists blinded to clinical information according to the Laennec scoring system (15). The samples were re-examined to analyze for discrepancies and a consensus was reached when the two pathologists get the inconsistent results. Liver cirrhosis was evaluated in non-cancerous tissues and was scored on four scales depending on the Laennec scoring system: F0–F3: no cirrhosis; F4A: mild cirrhosis (most septa are thin, allowing only one broad septum); F4B: moderate cirrhosis (at least two broad septa); F4C: severe cirrhosis (more than one very broad septum or many micro-nodules). According to the comparison between the thickness of fibrous septa and the nodule size, "broad septum" was defined as septal thickness being thinner than nodule size, and when the septal thickness is thicker than nodule size, "very broad septum" was diagnosed (15, 20).

Follow-Up and Efficacy

For HCC patients with chronic HBV infection, Adefovir Dipivoxil 10 mg or Entecavir 0.5 mg was orally administered daily when the pre-operative HBV DNA was positive. All patients were continuously followed up follow up every 2 months during the first 6 months after operation or 3 months thereafter. Surveillance for HCC included serum alpha-fetoprotein (AFP) level, chest radiography and abdominal ultrasonographic examination. Postoperative enhanced Computed Tomography (CT) or Magnetic Resonance Imaging (MRI) scans were performed every three months if necessary.

HCC recurrence was diagnosed on the basis of the two consistent imaging examinations or the combination of increased AFP and one imaging result with consistent radiologic features of HCC. LR was performed when recurrence occurred if it was suitable for surgery according to the same criteria with the first surgical resection. If the patients were not suitable for LR, transarterial chemoembolization (TACE), local ablation or systemic therapy were applied. The overall survival (OS) was calculated from the day of operation to final follow-up or death. The disease-free survival (DFS) was calculated from the date of operation to the date when recurrence/metastasis was diagnosed.

Statistical Analysis

Clinico-pathological parameters were expressed as frequencies and percentages for qualitative variables and mean ± SD or median (range) for continuous variables. Significance of differences between the groups were evaluated using Student's t-test. Descriptive variables were analyzed with $\chi 2$ or Fisher's exact test as appropriate. Surgical outcomes were estimated using the Kaplan–Meier curve and the log-rank test was used to compare the survival rates among all the groups. All significant predictors of OS and DFS in univariate and multivariate analysis were analyzed in cox proportional hazards regression model. All the risk factors that were significant (p <0.05) for the prediction of long-term outcomes in an univariate analysis were selected for further multivariate analysis. The 95% confidence intervals (95% CIs) and hazard ratios (HRs) were calculated. All tests were two-tailed and 0.05 was intended to be statistically significant. Statistical analysis was performed using SPSS19.0 (SPSS Inc., Chicago, IL, USA).

TABLE 1 | Clinical characteristics and demographics of 166 patients with a solitary hepatocellular carcinoma.

Variables	Value
Age (years)	49.0 ± 10.5 (22–76)
Sex (Male : Female)	148 (89.2): 18 (10.8)
HBV-DNA (IU/L)	
>2,000	70 (42.2%)
≤2,000	96 (57.8%)
ALT (U/L)	37.1 ± 18.4 (9–99)
AST (U/L)	33.0 ± 13.5 (12–89)
Total bilirubin (umol/L)	13 ± 3.8
INR	1.1 ± 0.1
Albumin (g/L)	40.6 ± 4.0
Platelet count (×10^9/L)	126.6 ± 51.8
AFP (ng/ml)	
>400 (n, %)	52 (31.3)
≤400 (n, %)	114 (68.7)
ICGR-15 (%)	5.2 ± 3.6
Spleen thickness (cm)	3.9 ± 0.7
Tumor size (cm)	3.9 ± 0.9
>3 (n, %)	105 (63.3)
≤3 (n, %)	61 (36.7)
Anatomic resection (n, %)	36 (21.7)
Capsule (n, %)	112 (67.5)
Tumor differentiation (n, %)	
Well	40 (24.1)
Moderate	88 (53.0)
Poor	38 (22.9)
Microscopic vascular invasion (n,%)	
Yes	18 (10.8)
No	148 (89.2)
Laennec fibrosis stage (n, %)	
F0–F3	22 (13.2)
F4A	46 (27.7)
F4B	65 (39.2)
F4C	33 (19.9)

RESULTS

Patients

A total of 166 patients were enrolled in the present study according to the including criteria. Baseline characteristics of all the included HCC patients were described in **Table 1**. Based on the Laennec scoring system, the proportion of no cirrhosis, mild cirrhosis (F4A), moderate cirrhosis (F4B) and severe cirrhosis (F4C) were 13.2% (n = 22), 27.7% (n = 46), 39.2% (n = 65) and 19.9% (n = 33), respectively. The proportion of patients with microvascular invasion and poor histological grades were 10.8 and 22.9%, respectively. One hundred and twelve (67.5%) tumors had integrated capsule.

Mortality and Complications

There was no surgical-related mortality in this study. Major complications occurred in 12% of the patients (n = 20). Depending on the histological severity of liver cirrhosis, we divided all the patients into two groups: no/F4A group (n = 68) and F4B/4C group (n = 98). The surgical complications between the two groups were compared. Major complications were apparently higher in the F4B/F4C group (n = 15) than the no/F4A group (n = 5) (15.3% vs 7.4%, p <0.001). Surgical complications and perioperative details of patients in both groups shows in **Table S1**. All the above complications were recovered with conservative therapy while in hospital.

Recurrence and Treatment

HCC recurrence was found in 88 patients during the follow-up period. The 1-, 3-, 5-year recurrence rates were 11.4, 34.9, 50.6%, respectively. We further subdivided the patients into the no/F4A group (n = 68) and the F4B/4C group (n = 98) according to the Laennec scoring system. Clinico-pathological characteristics showed no significant difference between the two groups except from types of resection (as shown in **Table S2**). Subgroup analysis suggested that the recurrence rates of HCC patients in the F4B/4C group were significantly higher than those in the no/F4A group, the corresponding 1-, 3-, 5-year recurrence rates were 14.3, 42.9, 60.2% versus 7.4, 23.5, 36.8%, respectively (p <0.001). Late-stage recurrence rates (>2 years) were still significantly higher in the F4B/4C group compared with those in the no/F4A group (65/98 vs16/68, p <0.001).

For the 88 patients with tumor recurrences, 38 patients were treated with Percutaneous Microwave Coagulation (PMCT); 10 patients performed with the second LR; 24 patients received trans-arterial chemotherapy and embolization (TACE); 10 patients were treated with the combination therapy of PMCT and TACE; six patients received TACE combined with systemic therapy (summarized in **Table S3**).

Survival

During a median of 47.7 months (interquartile range: 16.7–83.6 months) of follow-up, 58 patients (34.9%) were dead. The 1-, 3-, 5-year OS rates were 98.2, 77.2, 65.8% and the corresponding DFS rates were 88.6, 64.0, 40.9% (**Figures 1A, B**). According to the Laennec scoring system, liver cirrhosis was histologically sub-classified into four groups: no cirrhosis (n = 22), mild cirrhosis (F4A, n = 46), moderate cirrhosis (F4B, n = 65), severe cirrhosis (F4C, n = 33). Subgroup analysis indicated that the OS and DFS rates differed significantly among the four groups (**Tables 2** and **S4**). Surgical outcomes decreased significantly with the increasing degrees of liver cirrhosis (as shown in **Figures S2A, B,** p <0.001). We further found that the 1-, 3-, 5-year OS rates were 98.5, 88.1, 80% for patients in the no/F4A group and 98.0, 69.2, 54.7% for patients in the F4B/4C group, respectively (**Figure 2A,** p = 0.001). The corresponding DFS rates for the two groups were 92.6, 76.3, 57.1% and 85.7, 55.0, 28.8%, respectively (**Figure 2B,** p = 0.001).

Univariate and multivariate cox regression analyses identified that no microscopic vascular invasion (MVI), no capsule and F4B/4C cirrhosis were independent risk factors of long-term outcomes (OS and DFS), as shown in **Tables 3** and **4**.

DISCUSSION

Most histological scoring systems of fibrosis regarded cirrhosis as the end stage. In the past few years, increasing evidence indicated that there existed an obvious histological difference within cirrhosis, and liver cirrhosis should be further sub-classified based on its histological severity (10, 14, 15, 17, 18, 20). The BCLC guideline advocated that LR was recommended only for HCC patients without clinical portal hypertension and with normal total bilirubin levels. Histological sub-classification of liver cirrhosis is tightly correlated with the grade of clinical portal hypertension but not the same disease (15). For those HCC patients without portal hypertension, the importance of the underlying severity of liver cirrhosis should be further emphasized. Actually, most of HCC patients arise from varied degrees of liver cirrhosis in China (2). It is essential to enlighten on the value of histological sub-classification of cirrhosis in predicting potential surgical outcomes of HCC and individualize therapy. Till date, the role of the severity of liver cirrhosis in affecting the surgical outcomes for HCC patients without significant portal hypertension remains unclear. In this study, we aimed to analyze the effect of cirrhotic severity on surgical outcomes for HBV-related HCC patients in absence of portal hypertension.

Current guidelines recommended LR as the first-line treatment for a single HCC with Child–Pugh A liver function, normal serum bilirubin without clinically significant portal hypertension. And it was expected to be able to give a chance for better long-term OS and DFS (21). A meta-analysis and review indicated that portal hypertension had an adverse impact on short- and long-term outcomes for HCC patients undergoing partial hepatectomy (22). Meanwhile, liver cirrhosis was considered as one of the most important risk factors for surgical outcomes in HCC patients (3, 16, 23, 24). In the present study, the 5-year OS and DFS in HCC patients with liver cirrhosis are 63.2 and 38.1%, whereas 82.7 and 59.8% for those without liver cirrhosis. Furthermore, the results suggested that surgical outcomes decreased significantly with the increasing degrees of liver cirrhosis. A study from Kim et al. (9) showed that histological sub-classification of liver cirrhosis according to the

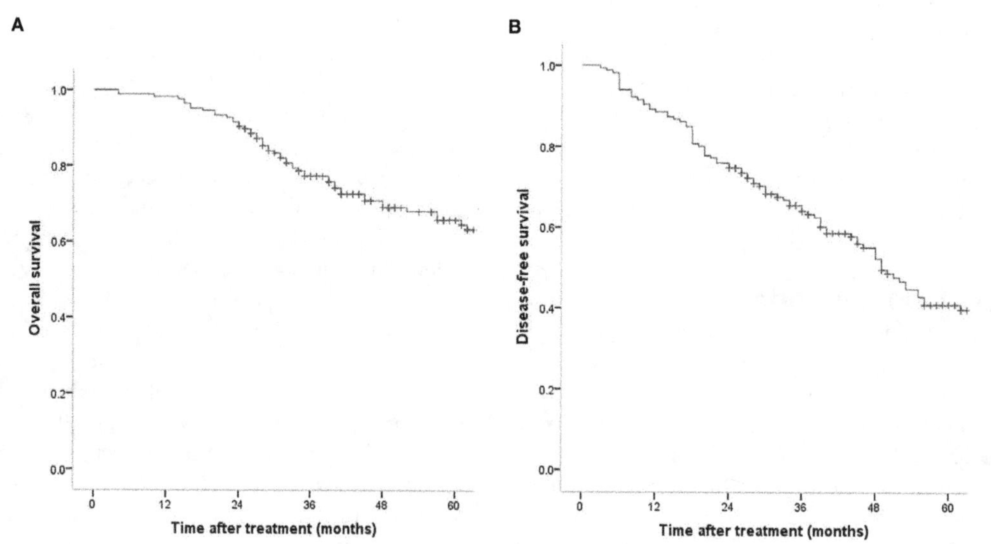

FIGURE 1 | Overall survival **(A)** and disease-free survival **(B)** in the whole study population who underwent liver resection.

TABLE 2 | Comparison of the overall and disease-free survival among the HCC patients with different degrees of liver cirrhosis.

	1-year (%)	3-year (%)	5-year (%)	*P*-value
Overall survival				
F0–F3 vs.F4A–4C (22/144)	100/97.9	90.2/75.3	82.7/63.2	0.044
F0–F4A vs.F4B–4C (68/98)	98.5/98.0	88.1/69.2	80.0/54.7	0.001
F0–F4B vs.F4C (133/33)	98.5/97	81.2/61.1	72.1/38.9	0.02
F0–F3 vs.F4A (22/46)	100/97.8	90.2/87.0	82.7/78.7	0.381
F4A vs.F4B (46/65)	97.8/98.5	87.0/73.4	78.7/63.0	0.081
F4B vs.F4C (65/33)	98.5/97	73.4/61.6	63.0/38.9	0.09
Disease-free survival				
F0–F3 vs.F4A–4C (22/144)	95.5/87.5	81.6/61.4	59.8/38.1	0.051
F0–F4A vs.F4B–4C (68/98)	92.6/85.7	76.3/55.0	57.1/28.8	0.001
F0–F4B vs.F4C (133/33)	91.7/75.8	70.7/36.5	46.1/18.9	<0.001
F0–F3 vs.F4A (22/46)	95.5/91.3	81.6/73.9	59.8/55.9	0.532
F4A vs.F4B (46/65)	91.3/90.8	73.9/64.5	55.9/33.6	0.082
F4B vs.F4C (65/33)	90.8/75.8	64.5/36.5	33.6/18.9	0.018

Laennec scoring system was a significant predictor of late recurrence in HBV-induced HCC patients after surgical resection. However, due to the small study population and short follow-up period, the results might be unconvincing. Our subgroup analysis showed that the 5-year OS and DFS were 54.7 and 28.8% in HCC patients with moderate or severe liver cirrhosis, which was significantly better than the results in our previous study (45 and 25%) (17). This was probably because of the fact that we excluded the cases with clinical significant portal hypertension in this study. Accordingly, the surgical outcomes were relatively good. Our results suggested that the severity of cirrhosis was inversely correlated with surgical prognosis of HCC patients even in those HCC patients without clinical portal hypertension. Moreover, cox-regression analysis suggested that F4B/4C stage was an independent risk factor for tumor recurrence and long-term outcomes after surgical resection. The mechanism of tumor recurrences which are prone to occurring in cirrhotic liver remains unclear. The poor surgical outcomes associated with liver cirrhosis have been hypothesized by previous studies. Hepatitis-induced repeated inflammation and cellular necrosis might led to hepatocyte proliferation and increase random gene mutations, which would accelerate the carcinogenesis of HCC (25, 26).

Perioperative mortality was not observed in the present study. Major complications were significantly higher for patients in the F4B/F4C group than those in the no/F4A group (17.0% vs 7.4%, p <0.001). The results seemed to be consistent with the aforementioned confirmed correlation among histological sub-classification of cirrhosis and clinical stages of portal hypertension which could reflect reserve liver function (15). HCC recurrence was found in more than half of patients who underwent curative surgical resection during the follow-up period. Subgroup analysis indicated that tumor recurrence was more frequent in the F4B/4C group than in the no/F4A group. Tumor recurrence over 2 years was believed to be *de novo* new tumor and coexistence of moderate or severe liver cirrhosis were

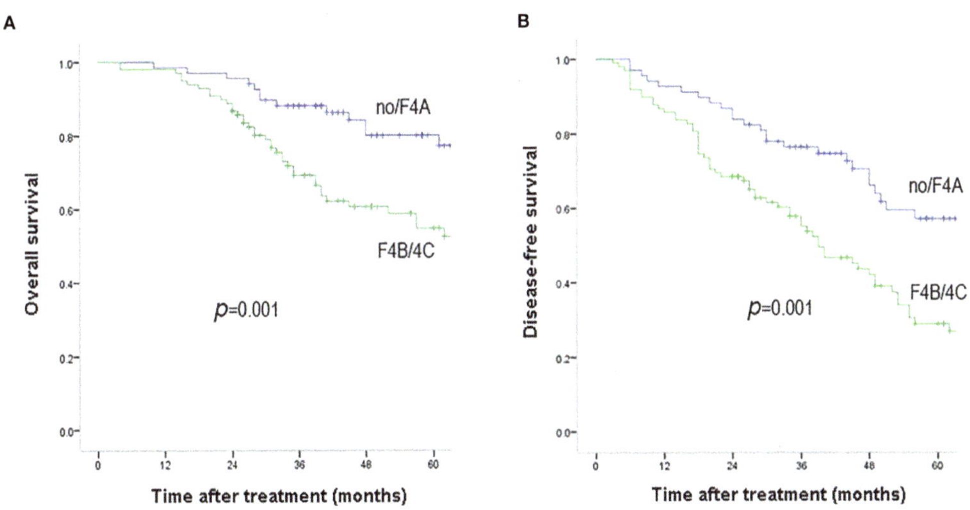

FIGURE 2 | Overall survival **(A)** and disease-free survival **(B)** outcomes of HCC patients with F4B/F4C and no/F4A. Overall survival and disease-free survival rates were significantly better in patients with no/F4A than those with F4B/4C (P = 0.001).

TABLE 3 | Univariate and multivariate analysis of the relative risk of overall survival.

Variables	OS				
	Comparison	Univariate HR (95% CI)	*p*-value	MultivariateHR (95% CI)	*P*-value
Age (years)	>50 vs ≤50	0.857 (0.508,1.447)	0.564		
Sex	Male vs Female	0.972 (0.417, 2.266)	0.947		
HBV-DNA (IU/L)	>2,000 vs ≤2,000	1.001 (0.591,1.697)	0.996		
ALT (U/L)	>35 vs ≤35	1.579 (0.941,2.651)	0.084		
AST (U/L)	>35 vs ≤35	1.444 (0.850,2.453)	0.174		
Total bilirubin (umol/L))	>17 vs ≤17	0.980 (0.493,1.947)	0.955		
INR	>1.2 vs ≤1.2	1.884 (0.891,3.983)	0.097		
Albumin (g/L)	>35 vs ≤35	0.708 (0.303,1.652)	0.424		
Platelet count (×109/L)	>100 vs ≤100	0.779 (0.449,1.352)	0.374		
AFP (ng/ml)	>400vs ≤400	1.595 (0.941,2.703)	0.083		
ICGR-15 (%)	>10 vs ≤10	0.920 (0.332,2.546)	0.872		
Spleen thickness (cm)	>4 vs ≤4	1.310 (0.776,2.212)	0.311		
Tumor size (cm)	>3 vs ≤3	1.153 (0.670,1.982)	0.607		
Anatomic resection	Yes vs No	0.899 (0.484,1.671)	0.737		
MVI	Yes vs No	3.003 (1.664,5.417)	<0.001	2.652 (1.298,5.419)	0.007
Capsule	Yes vs No	0.447 (0.264,0.758)	0.003	0.419 (0.245,0.715)	0.001
Tumor differentiation	Poor vs well and moderate	2.214 (1.046,4.688)	0.038	1.973 (0.891,4.367)	0.094
Laennec fibrosis stage	Moderate/severe vs no/mild	2.256 (1.417,4.626)	0.002	2.145 (1.156,3.980)	0.016

more likely relapse (27). Theoretically, anatomic resection was effective for eradication of the intrahepatic metastases of HCC though portal vein system and thus decreased tumor recurrence (28). However, most HCC patients with moderate or severe liver cirrhosis were not suitable for major anatomic resection owing to their impaired hepatic reserve function. Only thirty-six HCC patients (21.7%) underwent anatomic LR and mostly performed in patients with no or mild liver cirrhosis. We also found that late recurrence was more frequent in the F4B/4C group than those in the no/F4A group (66.3% vs 23.5%, p <0.001), which was consistent with the results of previous studies (16, 27).

Some studies illustrated that tumor size was one of the most important risk factors for surgical outcomes in HCC patients for the reason that increasing tumor size was associated with the presence of microscopic vascular invasion (MVI) (4, 21). However, in the present study, the results showed that tumor size was not associated with worse prognosis in HCC patients with lesions ≤5 cm, which was inconsistent with the results from the previous studies. The most plausible explanation for this inconsistence was the small sample size and HCC patients with portal hypertension were excluded in our study.

It is widely known that MVI and absence of tumor capsule are strongly related to survival and recurrence after LR for HCC patients (4, 6, 29). Previous studies reported that the rates of MVI incidence ranged from 15 to 33% (16, 30–32) in excised HCC which is higher than our current finding of 10.8%. Nagano et al. (33) demonstrated that tumors larger than 7 cm, single nodular type tumors without regular tumor capsule were associated with

TABLE 4 | Univariate and multivariate analysis of the relative risk of disease-free survival.

Variables	DFS				
	Comparison	Univariate HR (95% CI)	*p*-value	MultivariateHR (95% CI)	*p*-value
Age (years)	>50 vs ≤50	0.923 (0.606, 1.406)	0.709		
Sex	Male vs Female	0.706 (0.374, 1.330)	0.281		
HBV-DNA (IU/L)	>2,000 vs ≤2,000	1.378 (0.904,2.101)	0.136		
ALT (U/L)	>35 vs ≤35	1.064 (0.699,1.619)	0.771		
AST (U/L))	>35 vs ≤35	1.152 (0.743,1.785)	0.527		
Total bilirubin (umol/L))	>17 vs ≤17	0.944 (0.539,1.652)	0.839		
INR	>1.2 vs ≤1.2	1.577 (0.789,3.155)	0.198		
Albumin (g/L)	>35 vs ≤35	0.934 (0.450,1.935)	0.853		
Platelet count (×109/L)	>100 vs ≤100	0.826 (0.526,1.296)	0.406		
AFP (ng/ml)	>400vs ≤400	1.558 (1.007,2.410)	0.046	1.492 (0.942, 2.364)	0.088
ICGR-15 (%)	>10 vs ≤10	1.421 (0.685,2.946)	0.345		
Spleen thickness (cm)	>4 vs ≤4	1.421 (0.930,2.171)	0.104		
Tumor size (cm)	>3 vs ≤3	1.552 (0.980,2.455)	0.060		
Anatomic resection	Yes vs No	0.845 (0.508,1.404)	0.515		
MVI	Yes vs No	3.003 (1.664,5.417)	<0.001	3.163 (1.658,6.032)	<0.001
Capsule	Yes vs No	0.466 (0.302,0.717)	0.001	0.387 (0.248,0.603)	<0.001
Tumor differentiation	Poor vs well/moderate	2.223 (1.204,4.104)	0.011	1.915 (0.991,3.699)	0.053
Laennec fibrosis stage	Moderate/severe vs no/mild	2.130 (1.351,3.358)	0.001	1.928 (1.187,3.134)	0.008

an increased risk of MVI. Small tumor size in the present study may be responsible for the relative lower MVI incidence. Our findings showed that MVI was an important risk factor for predicting the long-term outcomes of HCC patients who underwent LR, which was consistent with previous study (4). Sumie et al. (34) recognized the impact of MVI on surgical outcomes and sought for a model to predict patients who were at an increased risk for having MVI. They hoped that its ability to predict the likelihood of MVI would be helpful to decide the appropriate treatment modalities. The underlying mechanism of MVI and absence of tumor capsule adversely affecting surgical outcomes remain unclear. A study suggested that the portal vein acted as an efferent vessel for tumor cells and it also was the path for tumor cell infiltration or expansion. Tumor cells invaded efferent vessels and then extended beyond the capsule to the portal vein branches (35). However, the number of patients with MVI in this study was only eighteen patients and fifty-four patients in absence of tumor capsule. Multi-center studies are necessary to establish the confirmative role of MVI and absence of tumor capsule for HCC recurrence after LR.

There are still several limitations in our study. At first, small study population of HCC patients and retrospective study might increase selection bias and weaken the statistical strength. Furthermore, because preoperative hepatic venous pressure gradient (HVPG) was not routinely measured in our center before April 2018, portal hypertension was indirectly defined as presence of esophageal varices or a platelet count <100,000/ml combined with splenomegaly. The accuracy decreased accordingly. Thirdly, routine antiviral treatment for HBV after LR may slow down the progression of liver cirrhosis, and the status of cirrhotic severity after LR during the follow-up period could not be accurately assessed due to the fact that liver biopsies could not be performed repeatedly in clinical settings. Multi-center studies with large sample should be carried out to provide stronger evidence to get more convincing results. Fourthly, although the present study showed the clinical importance of cirrhotic severity, it is of no use to choose suitable candidates for LR or predict surgical complications due to histological evaluation obtained after LR. Thus, preoperative prediction of severity of cirrhosis using non-invasive methods is urgent to be investigated. Finally, MVI-positive was reported to be an important risk of intrahepatic metastatic after curative liver resection, therefore, systemic therapy might improve recurrence and long-term outcomes for this subgroup of HCC patients (36). However, eighteen HCC with MVI-positive did not receive systemic therapy after surgical resection at that time.

CONCLUSION

In summary, results from the present study emphasized the importance of histological severity of liver cirrhosis in surgical outcomes for HCC patients. Microscopic vascular invasion, absence of tumor capsule and severity of liver cirrhosis were independent risk factors of surgical outcomes for early HCC patients without portal hypertension. Histological severity of liver cirrhosis affected surgical outcomes of early-stage HCC patients independently of portal hypertension and gave useful prognostic information that aided in the optimal management of early-stage HCC patients in absence of portal hypertension.

AUTHOR CONTRIBUTIONS

E-lZ and Z-yH made the concept and design. JiangL, JianL, W-qW, and JG acquired and analyzed the data. E-lZ drafted the manuscript. Z-yH critically revised the manuscript for the final version. E-lZ and JiangL conducted the statistical analysis. All authors contributed to the article and approved the submitted version.

ACKNOWLEDGMENTS

Thanks to all the staff of Hepatic Surgery Center in Tongji Hospital who contributed to the study.

SUPPLEMENTARY MATERIAL

Supplementary Figure 1 | The flow chart of the present study.

Supplementary Figure 2 | Overall survival **(A)** and disease-free survival **(B)** outcomes of HCC patients with different degrees of liver cirrhosis according to the Laennec scoring system (*P* < 0.001).

REFERENCES

1. Sung H, Ferlay J, Siegel RL, Laversanne M, Soerjomataram I, Jemal A, et al. Global Cancer Statistics 2020: GLOBOCAN Estimates of Incidence and Mortality Worldwide for 36 Cancers in 185 Countries. *CA Cancer J Clin* (2021) 71:209–49. doi: 10.3322/caac.21660
2. Zhang B, Zhang B, Zhang Z, Huang Z, Chen Y, Chen M, et al. 42,573 Cases of Hepatectomy in China: A Multicenter Retrospective Investigation. *Sci China Life Sci* (2018) 61:660–70. doi: 10.1007/s11427-017-9259-9
3. Sasaki K, Shindoh J, Margonis GA, Nishioka Y, Andreatos N, Sekine A, et al. Effect of Background Liver Cirrhosis on Outcomes of Hepatectomy for Hepatocellular Carcinoma. *JAMA Surg* (2017) 152:e165059. doi: 10.1001/jamasurg.2016.5059
4. Zhu Q, Yuan B, Qiao GL, Yan JJ, Li Y, Duan R, et al. Prognostic Factors for Survival After Hepatic Resection of Early Hepatocellular Carcinoma in HBV-related Cirrhotic Patients. *Clin Res Hepatol Gastroenterol* (2016) 40:418–27. doi: 10.1016/j.clinre.2015.12.007
5. Cucchetti A, Piscaglia F, Caturelli E, Benvegnu L, Vivarelli M, Ercolani G, et al. Comparison of Recurrence of Hepatocellular Carcinoma After Resection in Patients With Cirrhosis to its Occurrence in a Surveilled Cirrhotic Population. *Ann Surg Oncol* (2009) 16:413–22. doi: 10.1245/s10434-008-0232-4
6. Cheng Z, Yang P, Qu S, Zhou J, Yang J, Yang X, et al. Risk Factors and Management for Early and Late Intrahepatic Recurrence of Solitary Hepatocellular Carcinoma After Curative Resection. *HPB (Oxford)* (2015) 17:422–7. doi: 10.1111/hpb.12367
7. Oliveri RS, Wetterslev J, Gluud C. Hepatocellular Carcinoma. *Lancet* (2012) 380:470. doi: 10.1016/S0140-6736(12)61285-9
8. Flemming JA, Yang JD, Vittinghoff E, Kim WR, Terrault NA. Risk Prediction of Hepatocellular Carcinoma in Patients With Cirrhosis: The ADRESS-HCC Risk Model. *Cancer* (2014) 120:3485–93. doi: 10.1002/cncr.28832
9. Jung KS, Kim SU, Ahn SH, Park YN, Kim DY, Park JY, et al. Risk Assessment of Hepatitis B Virus-Related Hepatocellular Carcinoma Development Using Liver Stiffness Measurement (Fibroscan). *Hepatology* (2011) 53:885–94. doi: 10.1002/hep.24121

10. Kim G, Lee SS, Baik SK, Cho YZ, Kim MY, Kwon SO, et al. The Need for Histological Subclassification of Cirrhosis: A Systematic Review and Meta-Analysis. *Liver Int* (2016) 36:847–55. doi: 10.1111/liv.12923
11. Taura K, Ikai I, Hatano E, Yasuchika K, Nakajima A, Tada M, et al. Influence of Coexisting Cirrhosis on Outcomes After Partial Hepatic Resection for Hepatocellular Carcinoma Fulfilling the Milan Criteria: An Analysis of 293 Patients. *Surgery* (2007) 142:685–94. doi: 10.1016/j.surg.2007.05.009
12. Suh SW, Choi YS. Influence of Liver Fibrosis on Prognosis After Surgical Resection for Resectable Single Hepatocellular Carcinoma. *ANZ J Surg* (2018) 89:211–5. doi: 10.1111/ans.14732
13. de Franchis R. Evolving Consensus in Portal Hypertension. Report of the Baveno IV Consensus Workshop on Methodology of Diagnosis and Therapy in Portal Hypertension. *J Hepatol* (2005) 43:167–76. doi: 10.1016/j.jhep.2005.05.009
14. Garcia-Tsao G, Friedman S, Iredale J, Pinzani M. Now There are Many (Stages) Where Before There was One: In Search of a Pathophysiological Classification of Cirrhosis. *Hepatology* (2010) 51:1445–9. doi: 10.1002/hep.23478
15. Kim MY, Cho MY, Baik SK, Park HJ, Jeon HK, Im CK, et al. Histological Subclassification of Cirrhosis Using the Laennec Fibrosis Scoring System Correlates With Clinical Stage and Grade of Portal Hypertension. *J Hepatol* (2011) 55:1004–9. doi: 10.1016/j.jhep.2011.02.012
16. Kim SU, Jung KS, Lee S, Park JY, Kim DY, Ahn SH, et al. Histological Subclassification of Cirrhosis can Predict Recurrence After Curative Resection of Hepatocellular Carcinoma. *Liver Int* (2014) 34:1008–17. doi: 10.1111/liv.12475
17. Huang ZY, Liang BY, Xiong M, Dong KS, Zhang ZY, Zhang EL, et al. Severity of Cirrhosis Should Determine the Operative Modality for Patients With Early Hepatocellular Carcinoma and Compensated Liver Function. *Surgery* (2016) 159:621–31. doi: 10.1016/j.surg.2015.09.002
18. Zhang EL, Liang BY, Chen XP, Huang ZY. Severity of Liver Cirrhosis: A Key Role in the Selection of Surgical Modality for Child-Pugh A Hepatocellular Carcinoma. *World J Surg Oncol* (2015) 13:148. doi: 10.1186/s12957-015-0567-9
19. Zhang EL, Yang F, Wu ZB, Yue CS, He TY, Li KY, et al. Therapeutic Efficacy of Percutaneous Microwave Coagulation Versus Liver Resection for Single Hepatocellular Carcinoma <3 Cm With Child-Pugh A Cirrhosis. *Eur J Surg Oncol* (2016) 42:690–7. doi: 10.1016/j.ejso.2016.02.251
20. Zhang EL, Zhang ZY, Wang SP, Xiao ZY, Gu J, Xiong M, et al. Predicting the Severity of Liver Cirrhosis Through Clinical Parameters. *J Surg Res* (2016) 204:274–81. doi: 10.1016/j.jss.2016.04.036
21. Roayaie S, Jibara G, Tabrizian P, Park JW, Yang J, Yan L, et al. The Role of Hepatic Resection in the Treatment of Hepatocellular Cancer. *Hepatology* (2015) 62:440–51. doi: 10.1002/hep.27745
22. Liu J, Zhang H, Xia Y, Yang T, Gao Y, Li J, et al. Impact of Clinically Significant Portal Hypertension on Outcomes After Partial Hepatectomy for Hepatocellular Carcinoma: A Systematic Review and Meta-Analysis. *HPB (Oxford)* (2018) 21:1–13. doi: 10.1016/j.hpb.2018.07.005
23. Lee HW, Choi GH, Kim DY, Park YN, Kim KS, Choi JS, et al. Less Fibrotic Burden Differently Affects the Long-Term Outcomes of Hepatocellular Carcinoma After Curative Resection. *Oncology* (2017) 93:224–32. doi: 10.1159/000477173
24. Shrager B, Jibara G, Schwartz M, Roayaie S. Resection of Hepatocellular Carcinoma Without Cirrhosis. *Ann Surg* (2012) 255:1135–43. doi: 10.1097/SLA.0b013e31823e70a3
25. Liu P, Yang JM, Niu WY, Kan T, Xie F, Li DQ, et al. Prognostic Factors in the Surgical Treatment of Caudate Lobe Hepatocellular Carcinoma. *World J Gastroenterol* (2010) 16:1123–8. doi: 10.3748/wjg.v16.i9.1123
26. Barreto SG, Brooke-Smith M, Dolan P, Wilson TG, Padbury RT, Chen JW. Cirrhosis and Microvascular Invasion Predict Outcomes in Hepatocellular Carcinoma. *ANZ J Surg* (2013) 83:331–5. doi: 10.1111/j.1445-2197.2012.06196.x
27. Huang ZY, Liang BY, Xiong M, Zhan DQ, Wei S, Wang GP, et al. Long-Term Outcomes of Repeat Hepatic Resection in Patients With Recurrent Hepatocellular Carcinoma and Analysis of Recurrent Types and Their Prognosis: A Single-Center Experience in China. *Ann Surg Oncol* (2012) 19:2515–25. doi: 10.1245/s10434-012-2269-7
28. Hasegawa K, Kokudo N, Imamura H, Matsuyama Y, Aoki T, Minagawa M, et al. Prognostic Impact of Anatomic Resection for Hepatocellular Carcinoma. *Ann Surg* (2005) 242:252–9. doi: 10.1097/01.sla.0000171307.37401.db
29. Ikai I, Arii S, Kojiro M, Ichida T, Makuuchi M, Matsuyama Y, et al. Reevaluation of Prognostic Factors for Survival After Liver Resection in Patients With Hepatocellular Carcinoma in a Japanese Nationwide Survey. *Cancer* (2004) 101:796–802. doi: 10.1002/cncr.20426
30. Shimada S, Kamiyama T, Yokoo H, Orimo T, Wakayama K, Einama T, et al. Clinicopathological Characteristics of Hepatocellular Carcinoma With Microscopic Portal Venous Invasion and the Role of Anatomical Liver Resection in These Cases. *World J Surg* (2017) 41:2087–94. doi: 10.1007/s00268-017-3964-0
31. Shirabe K, Kajiyama K, Harimoto N, Masumoto H, Fukuya T, Ooya M, et al. Prognosis of Hepatocellular Carcinoma Accompanied by Microscopic Portal Vein Invasion. *World J Gastroenterol* (2009) 15:2632–7. doi: 10.3748/wjg.15.2632
32. Wang H, Wu MC, Cong WM. Microvascular Invasion Predicts a Poor Prognosis of Solitary Hepatocellular Carcinoma Up to 2 Cm Based on Propensity Score Matching Analysis. *Hepatol Res* (2018) 49:344–54. doi: 10.1111/hepr.13241
33. Nagano Y, Shimada H, Takeda K, Ueda M, Matsuo K, Tanaka K, et al. Predictive Factors of Microvascular Invasion in Patients With Hepatocellular Carcinoma Larger Than 5 Cm. *World J Surg* (2008) 32:2218–22. doi: 10.1007/s00268-008-9585-x
34. Sumie S, Kuromatsu R, Okuda K, Ando E, Takata A, Fukushima N, et al. Microvascular Invasion in Patients With Hepatocellular Carcinoma and its Predictable Clinicopathological Factors. *Ann Surg Oncol* (2008) 15:1375–82. doi: 10.1245/s10434-008-9846-9
35. Mitsunobu M, Toyosaka A, Oriyama T, Okamoto E, Nakao N. Intrahepatic Metastases in Hepatocellular Carcinoma: The Role of the Portal Vein as an Efferent Vessel. *Clin Exp Metastasis* (1996) 14:520–9. doi: 10.1007/BF00115112
36. Erstad DJ, Tanabe KK. Prognostic and Therapeutic Implications of Microvascular Invasion in Hepatocellular Carcinoma. *Ann Surg Oncol* (2019) 26:1474–93. doi: 10.1245/s10434-019-07227-9

21

Thoracoscopic Ablation of Critically Located Liver Tumors: A Safety and Efficacy Cohort Study

*Umberto Cillo[1], Michele Finotti[1], Chiara Di Renzo[1], Alessandro Vitale[1], Giacomo Zanus[1], Enrico Gringeri[1], Alessandra Bertacco[1], Marina Polacco[1] and Francesco D'Amico[1,2]**

[1] *Department of Surgery, Oncology and Gastroenterology, Hepatobiliary Surgery and Liver Transplantation, Padova University, Padova, Italy,* [2] *Department of Surgery, Immunology and Transplantation Unit, Yale University, New Haven, CT, United States*

Correspondence:
Francesco D'Amico
drdamico@hotmail.com

Background: Liver resection represents the first curative treatment to treat primary and secondary hepatic tumors. Thoracoscopic liver ablation is a viable and minimally invasive alternative treatment, especially for patients with previous multiple abdominal surgeries. The aim of the study was to evaluate the safety and efficacy of thoracoscopic ablation for liver tumors.

Methods: Retrospective analysis of a prospective database of patients with liver tumors, treated with thoracoscopic trans-diagrammatic ablation (MWA or RFA) at our institution from 2012 to 2018. The primary endpoint was post-operative mortality at 30 days, while secondary endpoints were morbidity and efficacy of ablation (i.e., response rate evaluated according to mRECIST criteria, and overall patient survival). Patient demographics, operational characteristics, and complications were recorded.

Results: A total of 13 nodules were treated in 10 patients with a median age of 65.5 years. Post-operative mortality was 0%, and overall morbidity was 40% (Clavien-Dindo I complications 30%, II 0%, III 10%, IV 0%). Complete radiological response was obtained in 83.3% of nodules at 3 months. After a median follow-up of 20.95 months, the local tumor progression rate was 30%, with an intra-segmental-recurrence of 30%, and an intra-hepatic-recurrence of 30%. The overall 1-, 2-, and 3-years survival rates were 80%, 58%, and 58%.

Conclusion: Thoracoscopic trans-diaphragmatic ablation proved to be a safe and effective way to treat liver tumors when abdominal approach is not feasible. Considering the low morbidity, it is a viable option to treat patients with recurrent disease and/or previous multiple abdominal surgeries.

Keywords: hepatocellular carcinoma, colon rectal liver metastases, microwave ablation, minimal invasive treatments, thoracoscopic liver ablation, trans-diaphragmatic approach

INTRODUCTION

Liver resection represents the first curative indication to treat primary and secondary hepatic tumors (1). However, surgical excision is not always feasible. Liver resection in patients with numerous comorbidities, poor liver function due to cirrhosis, and/or multiple previous surgeries, is associated with higher mortality and morbidity (2).

As alternative therapies, minimally invasive treatments, such as laparoscopic or percutaneous RadioFrequency (RFA) and MicroWave (MWA) ablation, have been gaining interest (3).

Loco regional treatments are considered safe and effective in the treatment of HCC and liver metastases (4). However, for hepatic tumors located beneath the diaphragm and/or in the hepatic dome (segments 7, 8, and 4A), or in patients with multiple previous abdominal surgeries, conventional laparoscopic or percutaneous approaches are demanding, due to the difficulties related to tumor identification.

In this scenario, a trans-thoracic and/or a thoracoscopic ablation has been proposed.

Most clinical data of trans-thoracic/thoracoscopic liver tumor ablation are based on experience with RFA and have short follow-ups (5). The use of MWA to treat liver tumors is less investigated despite several theoretical advantages compared to RFA. MWA ablation, with a shorter operative time, allows a larger ablation area and higher temperature. Moreover, MWA ablation is not affected by the so-called heat-sink effect and multiple probes can be used at the same time (6–9).

We describe, to the best of our knowledge, the largest series of hepatic tumors treated with a thoracoscopic approach with RFA or MWA ablation, in terms of specific safety and efficacy endpoints. Moreover, we report a detailed literature review on this specific field.

MATERIALS AND METHODS

Patients

A retrospective analysis conducted on a longitudinal, prospectively collected database of identified patients with liver tumors treated with thoracoscopic trans-diaphragmatic ablation (RFA or MWA) from January 2012 to March 2018 at the Hepato-Biliary Surgery and Liver Transplantation at Padua University Hospital. No IRB approval was needed for this study.

The inclusion criteria were as follows:

1) Ineligibility for liver resection due to: critical position near major hepatic structures (hepatic veins), insufficient future liver remnant after resection, and/or poor liver function (Child score B/C)
2) Nodules critically approachable with abdominal ablation (open, laparoscopic, or percutaneous) due to previous abdominal surgery (multiple laparotomies) or due to location in the hepatic dome (Sg.s VII; VII; IVA)
3) Permissive respiratory function
4) No extra hepatic disease
5) Hepatocellular carcinoma (HCC) <5 cm, intrahepatic cholangiocarcinoma (iCCA) and ColoRectal Liver Metastases (CRLMs) <3 cm.

Previous thoracic surgery was not an absolute contraindication to the procedure.

To reduce confounding factors, nodules previously treated with other loco regional therapies were excluded from the analysis.

Pre- and Post-Surgical Evaluation

Once the diagnosis of liver tumors was suspected, a complete staging of the disease was done as follows:

1. CT/MRI scan of chest/abdomen and pelvis.
2. PET-CT was performed in clinical suspect of extra hepatic disease.
3. Laboratory tests: blood chemistry, hepatic, renal, coagulation function, and tumor biomarkers (CA125, CA19-9, CA 15-3, CEA).

After hospital discharge, all patients were followed up at the outpatient clinic with physical examinations, biochemical liver function tests, tumor markers, CT, and/or MRI at 1 month and then repeated every 3 months for the first 2 years.

Surgical Procedure

The main goal of minimally invasive thermal ablation (RFA or MWA) is to destroy the malignant cells using heat without damaging adjacent vital structures. MWA were performed using a 2.45-MHz generator (AMICA-GEN, © 2020 H.S. Hospital Service S.p.A., Aprilia, Italy) delivering energy through a 14- or 16-gauge internally cooled coaxial antenna (AMICA PROBE, © 2020 H.S. Hospital Service S.p.A, Aprilia, Italy), featuring a miniaturized quarter wave impedance transformer (referred to as a mini choke) for reflected wave confinement, as previously reported (3). The radiofrequency (RF) ablation techniques were performed using a Cool-tip™RFA (Medtronic, Minneapolis, MN, USA).

The surgical procedures were performed with a thoracoscopic trans-diaphragmatic approach; the patient was placed in a left lateral and mild anti-Trendelenburg position, in consideration of the location of nodules in the right hepatic dome. Double-lumen tube intubation was necessary in order to exclude right lung ventilation during the procedures. Usually, two or three trocars were placed in the fifth and sixth intercostal space, for optic and US evaluation. Under vision of the diaphragm, triangulating the liver nodules across the diaphragm with US, we positioned the MW/RFA needle with an approach trans-thoracic through the diaphragm (**Figure 1**).

Study Endpoints

Primary Endpoint

1. Safety of thoracoscopic trans-diaphragmatic ablation: post-operative mortality at 30 days.

Abbreviations: CRLM, Colon Rectal Liver Metastases; CR, Complete Response; DFS, disease free survival; EHR, ExtraHepatic Recurrence; HCC, HepatoCellular Carcinoma; IHR, IntraHepatic Recurrence; ISR, Intra Segmental Recurrence; LTP, Local Tumor Progression; MWA, microwave thermal ablation; OS, Overall Survival; RFA, Radiofrequency Ablation.

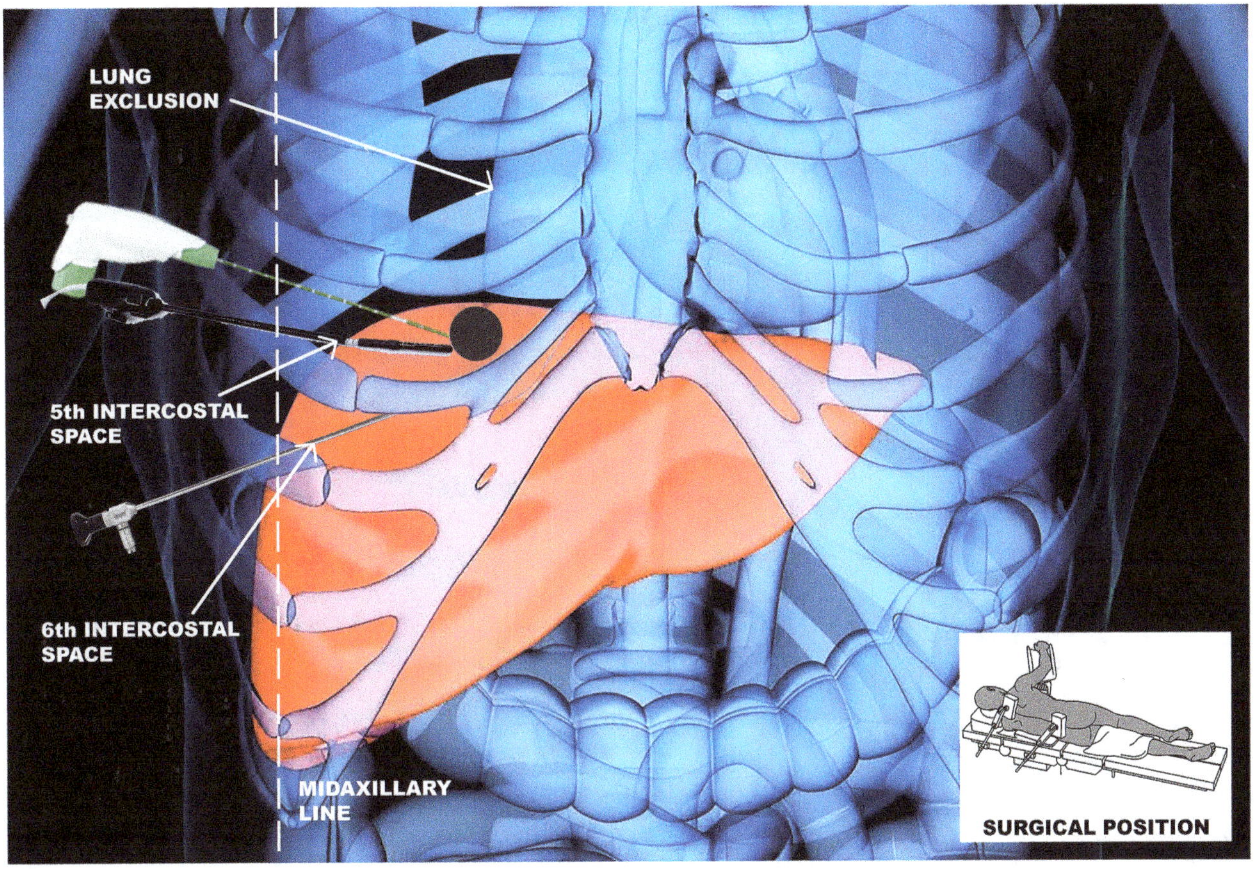

FIGURE 1 | The surgical procedure with a thoracoscopic trans-diaphragmatic approach to perform tumor ablation at the liver dome.

Secondary Endpoints

1. Morbidity profile (according to the Clavien-Dindo classification) (7); days of hospitalization; total operative time; ICU long of stay.
2. Radiological response rate: Local tumor progression (LTP), Intra-segmental recurrence (ISR), and intrahepatic recurrence (IHR) rates (m-RECIST Criteria)
3. Overall Survival (OS)
4. Disease-free rate and Overall recurrence rate.

Response Rate Evaluation

Local tumor progression (LTP) was defined as the persistence of active, enhancing tissue within or adjacent (2 cm) to the ablation site (4).

Intra-segmental recurrence was defined as the occurrence of tumor nodules in the same liver segment where ablation had been performed (4), but distant from the ablation site.

Intrahepatic recurrence (IHR) was defined as the appearance of tumor nodules in other liver segments (apart from any LTP or ISR) (4).

To evaluate the effectiveness of the ablative technique, a CT or MRI abdomen with contrast were performed at 3 months using modified-RECIST (m-RECIST) criteria. Two different and independent radiologists evaluated the imaging. M-RECIST criteria were used to evaluate treatment efficacy (8).

Statistical Analysis

Values for continuous variables are presented as medians (ranges). Values for categorical-nominal variables are presented as frequencies (%).

The length of the follow-up after thoracoscopic trans-diaphragmatic ablation was calculated from the date of the operation to the date of HCC recurrence (for disease-free survival analysis), the patient's death (for survival analysis), or the latest follow-up. The last follow-up date considered was 31 December 2019. The length of follow-up and survival were expressed as median (range). Overall survival curves were calculated using the Kaplan–Meier technique and compared with the log-rank test. A $P < 0.05$ was considered to indicate statistical significance. All statistical calculations were performed using jmp Version 9.0 2010 (SAS Institute, Inc., Cary, NC, USA).

Characteristics of Patients and Procedures

From January 2012 to March 2018, a total of 10 consecutive thoracoscopic ablation procedures on 10 patients were performed in our institution.

TABLE 1 | Characteristics of patients and previous treatments.

Variables		
Age	Median 65.5 years (range 59–74)	
Sex	Males: 9	
	Females: 1	
Type of primary tumor	HCC: 8 iCCA: 4 CRLM: 1	
Number of nodules	Median 1 (range 1–3)	1 nodule: 8 patients 2 nodules: 1 patient 3 nodules: 1 patient
Tumor size	Median 21 mm (range 4–46) HCC: median 20.5 mm (range 10–46) iCCA: median 14.7 mm (range 4–25) CRLM: 25 mm	
Approach	Thoracoscopic ablation	
Location of the nodules	S8: 6 nodules	
	S7: 6 nodules	
	S4: 1 nodules	
Previous surgery	100% (10 patients)	
Type of previous surgery	Thermal ablation	70%
	Liver resection	80%
	Liver Transplant	20%
	Lung resection	10%
Other procedures	TACE (30%), hemicolectomy (10%)	

HCC, hepatocellular carcinoma; iCCA, intra-hepatic cholangiocarcinoma; CRLM, colorectal liver metastasis; S, segment; TACE, trans-arterial chemoembolization.

TABLE 2 | Characteristics of procedures and complications.

Variables	MWA 8 patients	RFA2 patients
Time of ablation (minutes)	Median 8 min (range 5–15 min)	Median 24 min*
Power (Watt)	Median 40 Watt (range 40–60 Watt)	Median 100 Watt*
Length of operation (minutes)	Median 85 min (range 40–225 min)	Median 143 min (range 120–165 min)
Post-operative length (days)	Median 6 days (range 3–20)	Median 9 days (range 6–11)
Complications Clavien-Dindo classification	MWA 8 patients	RFA 2 patients
C-D I: 3 patients (30%)	C-D I: 2 Pleural effusion, subcutaneous emphysema and PNX	C-D I: 1 Pleural effusion
C-D II: 0	C-D II: 0	C-D II: 0
C-D III: 1 patients (10%)	C-D III: 1 Biliary fistula requiring explorative laparotomy	C-D III: 0
C-D IV: 0	C-D IV: 0	C-D IV: 0
C-D V: 0	C-D V: 0	C-D V: 0

**The 2 RFA have 24 min time of ablation and 100 W power. MWA, microwave ablation; RFA, radiofrequency ablation; C-D, Clavien Dindo; PNX, pneumothorax.*

TABLE 3 | Response rate evaluation.

Variable	13 nodules
Overall recurrence rate	40%
• LTP rate	30%
• ISR rate	30%
• IHR rate	30%
• EHR rate	30%
Disease free rate	60%

LTP, local tumor progression; ISR, intra-segmental recurrence; IHR, intra-hepatic recurrence; EHR, extra-hepatic recurrence.

A total of 13 liver tumors were ablated. Eight HCC nodules in seven cirrhotic patients, four iCCA nodules in two patients, and one CRLMs nodule in one patient were treated (**Table 1**). Two nodules were ablated with RFA and 11 with MWA ablation technique.

Median age was 65.5 years (range 59–74 years) with nine males and one female.

All patients received at least one abdominal surgery before our procedure (**Table 1**). Most patients had been through multiple laparotomies, especially for liver resection, thermal ablation, or liver transplantation. To note, one patient had previous thoracoscopic surgery for a biopsy of a nodule in the right apex, with a condition of minimal adhesion in the right chest, not precluding the procedure.

RESULTS

Median tumor size was 21 mm (range 4–46 mm). A single nodule was treated in 80% of the procedures, while multiple nodules (range 1–3) were treated in 20% of the procedures. Most nodules were in the liver segments seven and eight (90.9%). The median total operating time was 120 min (range 40–225 min) and the mean ablation time per nodule was 8 min (range 3–24 min) at a median power of 40 Watt (range 40–60 Watt) for MWA and 100 Watt for RFA. The characteristics of procedures and their complications are described in **Table 2**.

Safety

Regarding the primary endpoint of this study, we did not observe any intra or post-operative death (**Table 2**). All patients positioned a chest drainage that was removed on post-operative day 3. The median hospital stay was 7 days (range 3–20 days), and no patient required ICU stay. The overall morbidity rate according to Clavien-Dindo classification (**Table 2**) was 40%, with grade I complications occurring in 30% of patients, and grade III in 10% (one patient). The most common complication was a mild pleural effusion (Clavien Dindo I) occurring in three patients and probably related to a thermal-ablation inflammation of the diaphragm, associated with other low-risk complications: pneumothorax <2 cm in one patient and subcutaneous emphysema in one patient. Only one patient

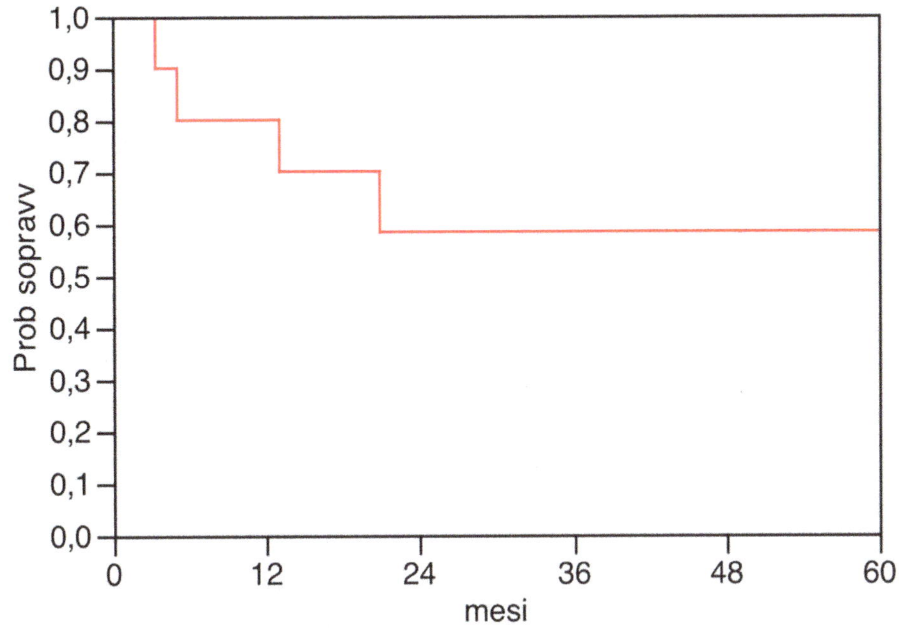

FIGURE 2 | Overall survival after thoracoscopic thermal ablation in 10 patients.

TABLE 4 | Morbidity, mortality, and recurrence after thoracoscopic liver ablation: review of the literature and our experience.

References and year	*N* of patients	Type	Mean *n.* nodules	Mean size (mm)	Mean LOS (days)	PO mortality (%)	Morbidity ≥ III (%)	FU (months)	LTP (%)	IHR (%)	3 y OS (%)
Yamashita et al. (22) '98	6	4 HCC 2 CRLM	MWA	1	11–22	10.5	0	0	4–23	0	0	–
Ishikawa et al. (23) '01	9	HCC	• 8 MWA 1 RFA	1	17.2	–	0	11	25	22–56	–	–
Lee et al. (24) '04	3	1 CCA 1 CRLM 1 metastatic melanoma	RFA	2	40	7	0	0	8	0–67	–	–
Kurokohchi et al. (25) '06	6	HCC	RFA	–	10–25	–	–	–	6.6	0	–	–
Padua experience Present series 20	10	7 HCC 2 iCCA 1 CRLMs	2 RFA 8 MWA	1 (1–3)	21 (4–46)	7	0	10%	20.95 (3.37–94.97)	30%	30%	58%

required a laparotomic surgical revision due to a post-operative biliary fistula that prolonged post-operative stay (20 days) that was treated by closing the needle track in the liver with a laparotomic approach. We did not observe any grade IV complications.

Efficacy

According to mRECIST classification, a complete radiological response was achieved in 83.3 and 62.5% of the nodules, respectively, at 3 months and 1 year.

After a median follow-up of 20.95 months (range 3.37–94.97), the overall disease-free survival rate was 60%, the LTP was 30%, the ISR was 30%, the IHR of 30%, and the EHR was 30% (**Table 3**). The overall survival at 1, 2, and 3 years was 80, 58, and 58%, respectively (**Figure 2**). Median survival was not reached.

DISCUSSION

Surgical resection is the gold standard to treat resectable liver tumors. The benefit in terms of overall survival after complete resection is well-recognized and established. However, liver resection is not always feasible, often due to patient comorbidities, disease stage, and/or poor liver function (10).

Loco regional treatments, such RFA and MWA, have been considered possible alternative therapies (11). Recently, in unresectable liver tumors (especially HCC and CRLM), national and international guidelines considered local therapies as a practicable alternative to resection (4).

For liver tumors located in the hepatic dome, a lateral thoracic approach has been proposed (thoracotomy, thoracoscopy, or trans-thoracic percutaneous). Thoracotomy is usually indicated in case of liver resection, but it is an invasive procedure not always feasible in fragile patients. Trans-thoracic percutaneous, US or CT guided, has been shown to be effective and safe (12, 13). However, tumors located in difficult positions can be challenging to detect with a percutaneous approach, and risk related to the induce pneumothorax (especially in patient with previous thoracic surgery) and air embolism secondary to lung penetration have been described (14). A combined approach has been proposed, using an abdominal laparoscopic approach plus trans-thoracic percutaneous. However, in case of patients with previous multiple abdominal surgeries, the combined approach is not always safe and possible (15).

In the present study we considered the thoracoscopic approach as the best-balanced alternative between the thoracotomy and trans-thoracic percutaneous approach, especially for patients fit for a loco regional treatment, but not for open surgery, and with multiple previous abdominal surgeries. We preferred the use of MWA, associated with some theoretical advantages compared to RFA (6), despite the lack of definitive evidence supporting one or the other.

Our series underlines the indication of minimally invasive treatment in patients with high risk of morbidity and mortality: the median age of the patients was 65.5 years old. All patients had previous abdominal surgeries and liver treatments, especially liver resections or open liver ablations. One patient was treated for a recurrent HCC after liver transplantation, since the absence of adjuvant therapy to prevent tumor recurrence in this specific setting is well-known (16).

It is important to emphasize that this cohort of patients would not be fit for other procedures, due to their comorbidity and previous surgical therapies. The thoracoscopic approach allowed a potentially radical therapeutic chance with no mortality and low morbidity.

Indeed, despite this high-risk patient selection, the overall intra and peri-operative mortality was 0 and the overall morbidity was 40%; most complications (30%) were minor (grade I), and only one patient had grade III complications.

In several observational studies, complications after MWA ranged between 0 and 54% (17–21).

Factors associated with the safety of the minimally invasive approach were the short operative time (median of 120 min), the possibility to treat more than one nodule in the same procedure, and the relatively rare occurrence of severe complications after surgery (only one patient had a Dindo Clavien 3).

Comparable with the literature, in our series the most common complications were pleural effusion, pneumothorax, and subcutaneous emphysema. Diaphragmatic hernia due to heat injury, a possible fatal complication, did not occur.

The first series of thoracoscopic liver ablation was described in 1998 by Yamashita et al. (22) (**Table 4**). Six HCC nodules were treated with MWA technique, with low morbidity and mortality. This study, even if LTP, IHR, and EHR had not been described in detail, showed that the thoracoscopic approach is a viable option to treat liver tumors in the hepatic dome, especially in patients with poor liver function.

In 2001, Ishikawa et al. treated nine HCC nodules with good outcome: only one patient had major pleural bleeding (23).

Lee at al. In 2004 reported zero mortality and morbidity in three patients treated with a RFA thoracoscopic approach. In the follow-up, one patient was lost and the other two patients died of progressive metastatic disease at 8 and 20 months, respectively (24).

Thoracoscopic ablation with RFA associated with ethanol injection has been proposed: Kurokohchi et al. treated six HCC patients with no local recurrence, but a short follow-up was described (6.6 months) (25).

Recently, only case reports with thoracoscopic RFA have been reported (26, 27).

The thoracoscopic approach has also been evaluated in association with other procedures.

A combined laparoscopic abdominal liver resection and thoracoscopic ablation have been proposed, according to the tumor liver location. The laparoscopic approach allowed for better parenchymal and vascular control during the liver thoracoscopic resection and/or ablation, with low post-operative complications (15, 28, 29).

This type of technique can be used to minimize the invasiveness of open liver resection, but the laparoscopic abdominal approach is not always feasible in patients with poor liver function and multiple previous surgeries.

Fujiwara et al. evaluated the safety and efficacy of CT-guided RFA ablation for sub diaphragmatic HCC (14). The procedure was proposed with an induced artificial pneumothorax to reduce the risk of lung penetration related to percutaneous approach. This technique achieved good results in term of ablation with low complications. However, the limitations of the percutaneous approach persisted and patients with previous thoracic surgeries would not be suitable for this procedure.

Limitations

Our study has a number of limitations. First, even though it is based on a prospectically collected dataset, it is a retrospective study. Second, the low number of procedures limits the possibility to draw definitive conclusions. The process of patient superselection justifies such a low numerosity in the present study and in the previous ones. In this sense, the thoracoscopic tool may represent a "niche" therapy to increase the armamentarium aimed at potential radicality. On this perspective, however, we have to stress that enrolled patients had only palliative solutions as therapeutic alternatives. Third, series inhomogeneity including HCC, CCA, and CRLM may act as a confounding factor, in particular in the interpretation of data related to prevalence of complete ablation and disease-free survival. Finally, two different ablation techniques have been used in treating liver nodules: MWA and RFA.

All the above-mentioned limitations prompt the need to carry out further prospective multicenter studies including an adequate number of homogeneously stratified patients.

To the best to our knowledge, we described the largest series of thoracoscopic liver tumors' ablation with MWA or RFA. For the first time, local tumor progression and OS are described in detail with the longest follow-up in literature (**Table 4**).

The present series supports the use of minimally invasive thoracoscopic ablation as a viable alternative treatment for liver tumor, to implement the therapeutic armamentarium of critically located liver tumors. The procedure was associated with a good local tumor control and with low risk of peri- and post-procedural complication. In patients with high comorbidities and previous multiple abdominal surgeries, the treatment was safe and enabled the opportunity to achieve oncologic radicality. Patient selection is a crucial step for thoracoscopic ablation: our series reveals that tumor dimension and liver function have been associated with overall survival, disease-free rate, and complete nodules response at 1 year.

In the thoracoscopic approach, compared to percutaneous treatment, hepatic dome lesion can be better recognized; an extended intra operative liver ultrasound can be easily performed and an optimal visualization and control of the thermal ablation procedure can be achieved, especially for lesions in critical locations and/or lesions near the heart or diaphragm.

AUTHOR CONTRIBUTIONS

UC and FD'A: conceptualization, methodology, writing—review, and editing. MF: data curation and writing—original draft. CDR: data curation. AV: data curation, validation, review, and editing. GZ, EG, AB, and MP: validation. All authors have read and agreed to the published version of the manuscript.

REFERENCES

1. Glassberg MB, Ghosh S, Clymer JW, Wright GWJ, Ferko N, Amaral JF. Microwave ablation compared with hepatic resection for the treatment of hepatocellular carcinoma and liver metastases: a systematic review and meta-analysis. *World J Surg Oncol.* (2019) 17:98. doi: 10.1186/s12957-019-1632-6
2. Vega EA, Kutlu OC, Joechle K, De La Cruz N, Ko D, Conrad C. Preoperative prognosticators of safe laparoscopic hepatocellular carcinoma resection in advanced cirrhosis: a propensity score matching population-based analysis of 1799 western patients. *J Gastrointest Surg.* (2019) 23:1157–65. doi: 10.1007/s11605-019-04139-7
3. Cillo U, Noaro G, Vitale A, Neri D, D'Amico F, Gringeri E, et al. Laparoscopic microwave ablation in patients with hepatocellular carcinoma: a prospective cohort study. *HPB.* (2014) 16:979–86. doi: 10.1111/hpb.12264
4. Cillo U, Bertacco A, Fasolo E, Carandina R, Vitale A, Zanus G, et al. Videolaparoscopic microwave ablation in patients with HCC at a European high-volume center: results of 815 procedures. *J Surg Oncol.* (2019) 120:956–65. doi: 10.1002/jso.25651
5. Golse N, Ducerf C, Rode A, Gouillat C, Baulieux J, Mabrut JY, et al. Transthoracic approach for liver tumors. *J Visc Surg.* (2012) 149:e11–22. doi: 10.1016/j.jviscsurg.2011.10.009
6. Izzo F, Granata V, Grassi R, Fusco R, Palaia R, Delrio P, et al.. Radiofrequency ablation and microwave ablation in liver tumors: an update. *Oncologist.* (2019) 24:e990–1005. doi: 10.1634/theoncologist.2018-0337
7. Clavien PA, Barkun J, de Oliveira ML, Vauthey JN, Dindo D, Schulick RD, et al. The Clavien-Dindo classification of surgical complications: five-year experience. *Ann Surg.* (2009) 250:187–96. doi: 10.1097/SLA.0b013e3181b13ca2
8. Eisenhauer EA, Therasse P, Bogaerts J, Schwartz LH, Sargent D, Ford R, et al. New response evaluation criteria in solid tumours: revised RECIST guideline (version 1.1). *Eur J Cancer.* (2009) 45:228–47. doi: 10.1016/j.ejca.2008.10.026
9. Zanus G, Boetto R, Gringeri E, Vitale A, D'Amico F, Carraro A, et al. Microwave thermal ablation for hepatocarcinoma. *Tranplantat Proc.* (2011). 43:1091–4. doi: 10.1016/j.transproceed.2011.02.044
10. Gigot JF, Glineur D, Santiago Azagra J, Goergen M, Ceuterick M, Morino M, et al. Laparoscopic liver resection for malignant liver tumors: preliminary results of a multicenter European study. *Ann Surg.* (2002) 236:90–7. doi: 10.1097/00000658-200207000-00014
11. Liu Y, Li S, Wan X, Li Y, Li B, Zhang Y, et al. Efficacy and safety of thermal ablation in patients with liver metastases. *Eur J Gastroenterol Hepatol.* (2013) 25:442–6. doi: 10.1097/MEG.0b013e32835cb566
12. Shibata T, Shibata T, Maetani Y, Kubo T, KyoItoh, Togashi K, et al. Transthoracic percutaneous radiofrequency ablation for liver tumors in the hepatic dome. *J Vasc Interv Radiol.* (2004) 15:1323–7. doi: 10.1097/01.RVI.0000132297.97113.C4
13. D'Amico F, Serafini S, Finotti M, Di Bello M, Di Renzo C, Cillo U. One-lung ventilation to treat hepatic dome lesion - a further step towards minimally invasive surgery: a case report. *J Med Case Rep.* (2019) 13:83. doi: 10.1186/s13256-019-1999-6
14. Fujiwara H, Arai Y, Ishii H, Kanazawa S. Computed tomography-guided radiofrequency ablation for sub-diaphragm hepatocellular carcinoma: safety and efficacy of inducing an artificial pneumothorax. *Acta Med Okayama.* (2016) 70:189–95. doi: 10.18926/AMO/54418
15. Kang CM, Ko HK, Song SY, Kim KS, Choi JS, Lee WJ, et al. Multimedia manuscript. Dual-scope guided (simultaneous thoraco-laparoscopic) transthoracic transdiaphragmatic intraoperative radiofrequency ablation for hepatocellular carcinoma located beneath the diaphragm. *Surg Endosc.* (2008) 22:541. doi: 10.1007/s00464-007-9410-x
16. Bassanello M, Vitale A, Ciarleglio FA, Brolese A, Zanus G, D'Amico F, et al. Adjuvant chemotherapy for transplanted hepatocellular carcinoma patients: impact on survival or HCV recurrence timing. *Transplant Proc.* (2003) 35:2991–4. doi: 10.1016/j.transproceed.2003.10.075
17. Lubner MG, Brace CL, Hinshaw JL, Lee FT. Microwave tumor ablation: mechanism of action, clinical results, and devices. *J Vasc Interv Radiol.* (2010) 21(Suppl. 8):S192–203. doi: 10.1016/j.jvir.2010.04.007
18. Martin RC, Scoggins CR, McMasters KM. Microwave hepatic ablation: initial experience of safety and efficacy. *J Surg Oncol.* (2007) 96:481–6. doi: 10.1002/jso.20750
19. Meloni MF, Chiang J, Laeseke PF, Dietrich CF, Sannino A, Solbiati M, et al. Microwave ablation in primary and secondary liver tumours: technical and clinical approaches. *Int J Hyperthermia.* (2017) 33:15–24. doi: 10.1080/02656736.2016.1209694
20. Ogata Y, Uchida S, Hisaka T, Horiuchi H, Mori S, Ishibashi N, et al. Intraoperative thermal ablation therapy for small colorectal metastases to the liver. *Hepatogastroenterology.* (2008) 55:550–6.
21. Qin S, Liu GJ, Huang M, Huang J, Luo Y, Wen Y, et al. The local efficacy and influencing factors of ultrasound-guided percutaneous microwave ablation in colorectal liver metastases: a review of a 4-year experience at a single center. *Int J Hyperthermia.* (2019) 36:36–43. doi: 10.1080/02656736.2018.1528511
22. Yamashita Y, Sakai T, Maekawa T, Watanabe K, Iwasaki A, Shirakusa T. Thoracoscopic transdiaphragmatic microwave coagulation therapy for a liver tumor. *Surg Endosc.* (1998) 12:1254–8. doi: 10.1007/s004649900831
23. Ishikawa T, Kohno T, Shibayama T, Fukushima Y, Obi S, Teratani T, et al. Thoracoscopic thermal ablation therapy for hepatocellular carcinoma located beneath the diaphragm. *Endoscopy.* (2001) 33:697–702. doi: 10.1055/s-2001-16216
24. Lee NN, O'Rourke RW, Cheng J, Hansen PD. Transthoracic hepatic radiofrequency ablation. *Surg Endosc.* (2004) 18:1672–4. doi: 10.1007/s00464-004-8110-z

25. Kurokohchi K, Hirai S, Ohgi T, Ono M, Yoshitake A, Ebara K, et al. Thoracoscopic ethanol injection and radiofrequency ablation for the treatment of hepatocellular carcinoma located immediately under the diaphragm. *Int J Oncol.* (2006) 29:375–80. doi: 10.3892/ijo.29.2.375
26. Park SW, Kim Y, Kang HY, You AH, Jeon JM, Woo H, et al. Transthoracic radiofrequency ablation for hepatic tumor located beneath the diaphragm under one-lung ventilation: a case report. *Medicine.* (2018) 97:e13863. doi: 10.1097/MD.0000000000013863
27. Qin L, Fei L, YongGang W, Bo L. Use of transthoracic transdiaphragmatic approach assisted with radiofrequency ablation for thoracoscopic hepatectomy of hepatic tumor located in segment VIII. *J Gastrointest Surg.* (2019) 23:1547–8. doi: 10.1007/s11605-019-04172-6
28. Teramoto K, Kawamura T, Takamatsu S, Noguchi N, Nakamura N, Arii S. Laparoscopic and thoracoscopic partial hepatectomy for hepatocellular carcinoma. *World J Surg.* (2003) 27:1131–6. doi: 10.1007/s00268-003-6936-5
29. Tanaka K, Kojima T, Hiraguchi E, Hashida H, Noji T, Hirano S. Laparoscopy-guided transthoracic transdiaphragmatic radiofrequency ablation for hepatic tumors located beneath the diaphragm. *J Laparoendosc Adv Surg Tech A.* (2016) 26:180–4. doi: 10.1089/lap.2015.0380

22

Efficacy of Liver Resection for Single Large Hepatocellular Carcinoma in Child-Pugh A Cirrhosis: Analysis of a Nationwide Cancer Registry Database

Suk Kyun Hong, Kwang-Woong Lee, Su young Hong, Sanggyun Suh, Kwangpyo Hong, Eui Soo Han, Jeong-Moo Lee, YoungRok Choi, Nam-Joon Yi and Kyung-Suk Suh*

Department of Surgery, Seoul National University College of Medicine, Seoul, South Korea

***Correspondence:**
Kwang-Woong Lee
kwleegs@gmail.com

Background: Therapeutic strategies and good prognostic factors are important for patients with single large hepatocellular carcinoma (HCC). This retrospective study aimed to identify the prognostic factors in patients with single large HCC with good performance status and Child-Pugh A cirrhosis using a large national cancer registry database and to recommend therapeutic strategies.

Methods: Among 12139 HCC patients registered at the Korean Primary Liver Cancer Registry between 2008 and 2015, single large (≥ 5 cm) HCC patients with Eastern Cooperative Oncology Group (ECOG) performance status 0 and Child-Pugh score A were selected.

Results: Overall, 466 patients were analyzed. The 1-,2-,3-, and 5-year survival rates after initial treatment were 84.9%, 71.0%, 60.1%, and 51.6%, respectively, and progression-free survival rates were 43.6%, 33.0%, 29.0%, and 26.8%, respectively. Platelet count $< 100 \times 10^9$/L ($P < 0.001$), sodium level < 135 mmol/L ($P = 0.002$), maximum tumor diameter ≥ 10 cm ($P = 0.001$), and treatment other than resection (transarterial therapy vs. resection: $P < 0.001$, others vs. resection: $P = 0.002$) were significantly associated with poorer overall survival; sodium < 135 mmol/L ($P = 0.015$), maximum tumor diameter ≥ 10 cm ($P < 0.001$), and treatment other than resection (transarterial therapy vs. resection: $P < 0.001$, others vs. resection: $P = 0.001$) were independently associated with poorer progression-free survival.

Conclusion: Resection as an initial treatment should be considered when possible, even in patients with single large HCC with good performance status and mild cirrhosis. Caution should be exercised in patients with low platelet level ($< 100 \times 10^9$/L), low serum sodium level (< 135 mmol/L), and maximum tumor diameter ≥ 10 cm.

Keywords: hepatocellular carcinoma, hepatectomy, prognosis, survival, recurrence

INTRODUCTION

Surveillance programs for detecting hepatocellular carcinoma (HCC) vary with each country depending on the prevalence of HCC. Since hepatitis B virus is endemic to Korea and Japan, the prevalence of HCC is high. The recommended surveillance programs for HCC detection include liver ultrasonography and monitoring serum alpha-fetoprotein (AFP) levels (1, 2). However, despite surveillance programs, the proportion of diagnosis of large HCC is still substantial (3). When treating HCC, tumor factors including number, size, and aggressiveness, together with underlying liver function and performance status should be considered. Liver resection can be considered as the first-line treatment in patients with single HCC confined to the liver without cirrhosis in cases where the residual liver function is expected to be sufficient even with cirrhosis (4–6). The most recent version of the combined American Joint Committee on Cancer (AJCC)/Union for International Cancer Control (UICC) TNM staging system from 2017 states that patients with multiple tumors, any of which are > 5 cm, are categorized as T3 (7). Previous studies have reported that although the 5-year survival was similar in patients with and without cirrhosis who had single HCC ≤ 5 cm, it was worse in patients with cirrhosis with HCC > 5 cm (8). However, recent studies demonstrated that microvascular invasion was not observed in about one-third of patients with tumor size > 10 cm and positive outcomes were reported after resection in these patients; thus, resection should not be considered based on solely the size of the tumor (3, 9). However, these studies had limitations, such as small sample sizes, lack of comparison groups, and/or selection bias. Moreover, treatment for single large (≥ 5 cm) HCCs is still debated, with limited data available.

This study aimed to identify prognostic factors for single large HCC using a large, nationwide cancer registry database. To focus on the effectiveness of resection and to minimize selection bias, we restricted the cohort to patients with Child-Pugh class A and an Eastern Cooperative Oncology Group (ECOG) PERFORMANCE STATUS OF 0.

MATERIALS AND METHODS

Patients and Methods

The present study was approved by the Institutional Review Board of the Seoul National University Hospital (IRB No. 2101-088-1189). Due to the retrospective nature of the study, the requirement for patient consent was waived. The study population was obtained from the Korean Primary Liver Cancer Registry (KPLCR), which represents a national, random sample of approximately 15% of patients registered in the Korean Central Cancer Registry (KCCR). Considering that KCCR accounts for more than 95% of all cancer cases in Korea, the KPLCR represents a group of patients with newly diagnosed HCC. The following data were obtained from the KPLCR database: age, sex, height, weight, smoking history, alcohol history, medical history of diabetes and hypertension, underlying liver disease, performance status, Child-Pugh score, Model for End-Stage Liver Disease (MELD) score, laboratory results, including AFP and proteins induced by vitamin K absence-II (PIVKA-II), diagnosis date, tumor number, maximum size, macrovascular invasion, distant metastasis, initial treatment modality and date, secondary treatment modality and date, and survival outcome.

Figure 1 shows the flowchart for the selection of study population. Between 2008 and 2015, 12139 liver tumor patients were registered in the KPLCR from 54 hospitals. The potential cohort included all the patients registered under KPLCR, except those without a follow-up or missing treatment dates. Of these, 1457 patients had single large (≥ 5 cm) HCCs. Patients with distant metastasis or macrovascular invasion were excluded from the study. Furthermore, patients with ECOG performance status other than 0 and Child-Pugh grade other than grade A were also excluded. Finally, 466 patients were included in the study. The duration of survival was measured from the date of initial treatment to the date of death or the last follow-up date. The duration of progression-free survival was measured from the initial treatment date to the second or last follow-up date. The cut-off values of continuous variables were selected considering previous publications.

Statistical Analysis

Results are expressed as mean ± standard deviation or median (range) for continuous data and as numbers with percentages for categorical data. Survival and progression-free survival were calculated using the Kaplan-Meier method and compared using the log-rank test. Multivariate Cox proportional hazards regression with backward selection was used to determine the effect of statistically significant variables in the univariate analysis. A *P*-value of < 0.05 was considered significant. Statistical analysis was performed using the SPSS software (version 25; SPSS Inc., Chicago, IL, USA).

RESULTS

Baseline Characteristics

There were 466 HCC patients with single and large (≥ 5 cm) tumors with Child A, performance status of 0, but without distant metastasis and macrovascular invasion. **Table 1** summarizes the demographic characteristics of these patients. The mean age was 61.3 years, and the mean body mass index (BMI) was 24.0 kg/m^2. More than half of the patients (56.0%) tested positive for hepatitis B surface antigen. The mean Child-Pugh score was 5.2, whereas all the patients were Child grade A according to the selection criteria of this study. The mean platelet count was 201.9 × 10^9/L, and the mean total bilirubin level was 0.8 mg/dL. The median serum AFP was 34.6 ng/mL (0.4-200000.0) and median PIVKA-II was 936.0 mAU/mL (5.0-95926.0). The most common initial treatment modality was resection (52.8%), followed by transarterial therapy, most of which was transarterial chemoembolization (TACE) (43.8%).

Overall Survival Rates and Progression-Free Survival Rates

Kaplan-Meier analysis showed that the 1-,2-,3-, and 5-year survival rates after initial treatment were 84.9%, 71.0%, 60.1%,

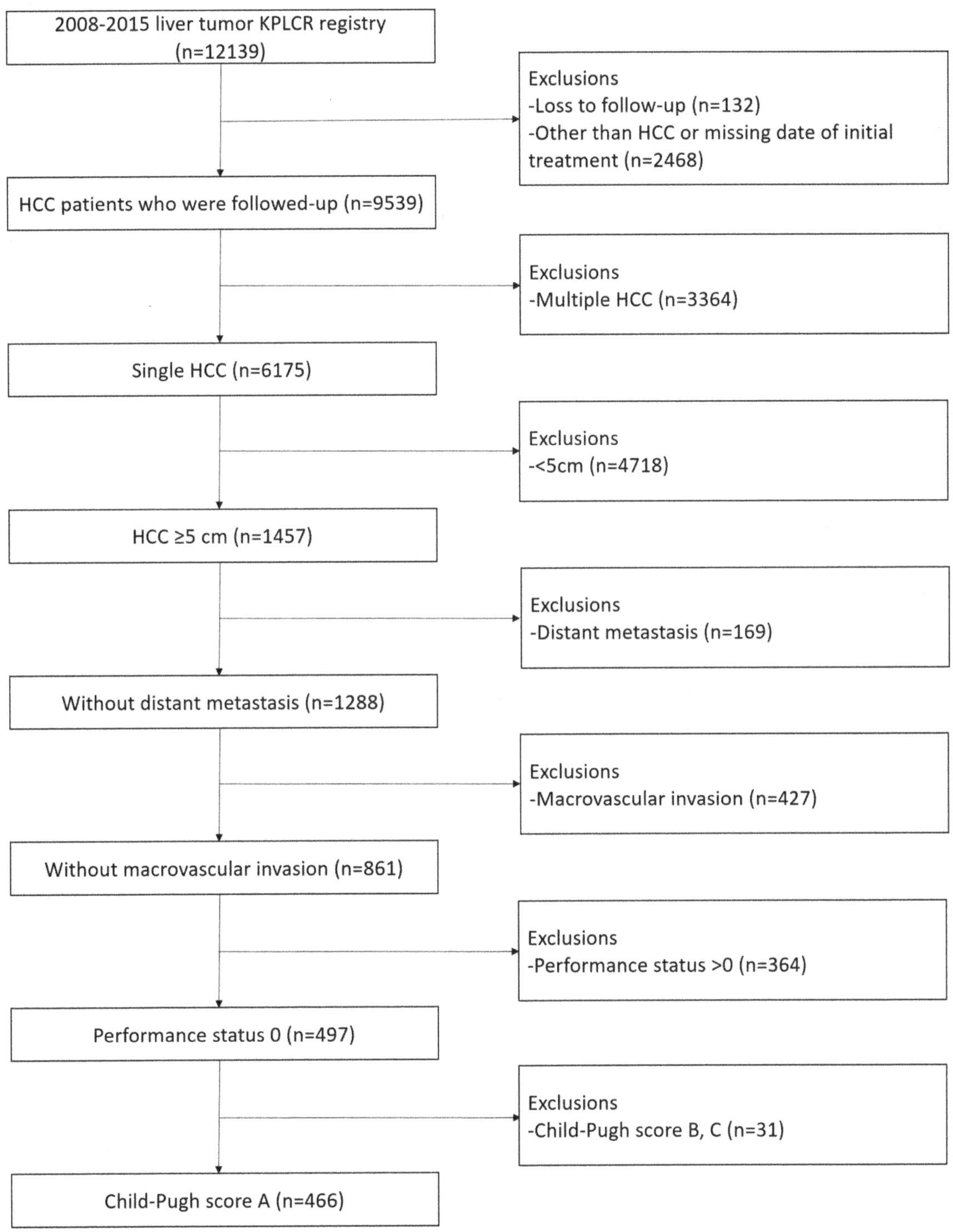

FIGURE 1 | Flowsheet of the enrolled patients.

and 51.6%, respectively (**Figure 2A**), and the 1-,2-,3-, and 5-year progression-free survival rates were 43.6%, 33.0%, 29.0%, and 26.8%, respectively (**Figure 2B**). The 1-,2-,3-, and 5-year survival rates after resection were 92.6%, 81.1%, 73.7%, and 65.6%, and the 1-,2-,3-, and 5-year progression-free survival rates were 62.8%, 50.0%, 45.0%, and 43.2%, respectively.

TABLE 1 | Demographic and clinical characteristics of the included patients.

Variables	N = 466
Demographic variables	
Age (year)	61.3 ± 11.9
Male: Female	388: 78
BMI (kg/m^2)	24.0 ± 3.5
Smoking	214 (45.9)
Alcohol	149 (32.0)
Diabetes	118 (25.3)
Hypertension	184 (39.5)
Etiology	
HBV*	261 (56.0)
HCV*	40 (8.6)
Non-B Non-C	156 (33.5)
Child-Pugh score	5.2 ± 0.4
MELD score	8.0 ± 2.0
Laboratory variable	
Platelet count (10^9/L)	201.9 ± 85.3
Total bilirubin (mg/dL)	0.8 ± 0.4
Serum albumin (g/dL)	4.1 ± 0.5
Alanine aminotransferase (IU/L)	48.1 ± 55.7
Prothrombin time (INR)	1.1 ± 0.1
Creatinine (mg/dL)	1.0 ± 0.8
Sodium (mmol/L)	139.6 ± 3.2
Alpha-fetoprotein (ng/mL)	34.6 (0.4-200000.0)
PIVKA-II (mAU/mL)	936.0 (5.0- 95926.0)
Tumor variable	
Maximum tumor diameter (cm)	8.0 ± 3.0
Treatment variable	
Initial treatment	
Resection	246 (52.8)
Transarterial therapy	204 (43.8)
Chemotherapy	8 (1.7)
Local ablative therapy	3 (0.6)
Radiation	3 (0.6)
Liver transplantation	2 (0.4)

**Four patients had underlying hepatitis B and C coinfections.*
BMI, body mass index; HBV, hepatitis B virus; HCV, hepatitis C virus; MELD, Model for End-Stage Liver Disease; PIVKA-II, protein induced by vitamin K absence-II.

Factors Affecting Overall Survival and Progression-Free Survival

Univariate analysis showed that the Child-Pugh score, MELD score, platelet count, total bilirubin, serum albumin, sodium, maximum tumor diameter, and initial treatment modality were associated with survival rate (**Table 2**). Among these factors, platelet count < 100 × 10^9/L (P < 0.001), sodium level < 135 mmol/L (P = 0.002), maximum tumor diameter ≥ 10 cm (P = 0.001), and treatment other than resection (transarterial therapy vs. resection, P < 0.001; others vs. resection, P = 0.002) (**Figure 3A**) were significantly associated with poorer overall survival.

Another univariate analysis identified that hepatitis C virus infection as an underlying liver disease (P = 0.037), Child-Pugh score 6 (P = 0.001), platelet count < 100 × 10^9/L (P < 0.001), serum albumin < 3.5 g/dL (P = 0.007), sodium level < 135 mmol/L (P < 0.001), PIVKA-II level ≥ 1000 mAU/mL (P = 0.008), maximum tumor diameter ≥ 10 cm (P < 0.001), and initial treatment other than resection (P < 0.001) were associated with poorer progression-free survival after initial treatment. Multivariate analysis revealed that sodium < 135 mmol/L (P = 0.015), maximum tumor diameter ≥ 10 cm (P < 0.001), and treatment other than resection (transarterial therapy vs. resection, P < 0.001; others vs. resection, P = 0.001) (**Figure 3B**) were independently associated with poorer progression-free survival.

DISCUSSION

Liver resection is widely recognized as the first-line treatment in patients with HCC when feasible, considering patient performance status, remnant liver function, and tumor factors (4–6). According to previous studies, liver resection in Child A patients showed good results, with an average 5-year survival of over 60% and long-term intrahepatic control rates of over 40% (10, 11). The patients in our study had large HCC with performance status 0 and Child A cirrhosis. Among them, 246 (52.8%) patients underwent resection, and showed similar 5-year survival (65.6%) and progression-free survival (43.2%) rates. This is in line with previous studies that demonstrated comparable outcomes in large HCC patients and proposed considering resection not based solely on tumor size (3, 9). Lin et al. reported that Barcelona Clinic Liver Cancer (BCLC) stage B, Child A showed better survival rates in patients who underwent resection than in those who underwent TACE (12).

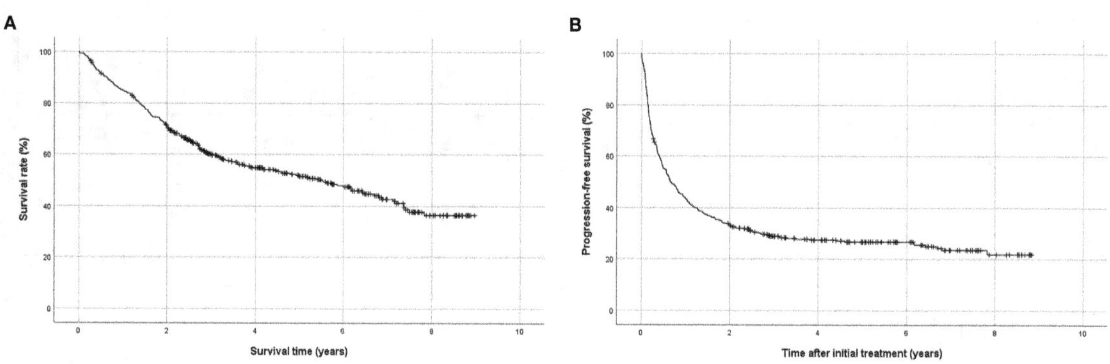

FIGURE 2 | Kaplan-Meier analysis of survival using the Korean Primary Liver Cancer Registry database. **(A)** Overall survival, **(B)** progression-free survival.

TABLE 2 | Univariate and multivariate analyses of factors affecting overall survival and progression-free survival.

Demographic variables			N = 466	Overall survival				Progression-free survival			
				Univariate	Multivariate			Univariate	Multivariate		
				P-value	HR	95% CI	P-value	*P*-value	HR	95% CI	*P*-value
Age (year)											
	<60		203								
	≥60		263	0.233				0.186			
Sex											
	Male		388								
	Female		78	0.091				0.500			
BMI (kg/m^2)											
	<25		296								
	≥25		159	0.216				0.059			
Smoking											
	No		251								
	Yes		214	0.760				0.058			
Alcohol											
	No		311								
	Yes		149	0.990				0.288			
Diabetes											
	No		348								
	Yes		118	0.859				0.275			
Hypertension											
	No		282								
	Yes		184	0.588				0.480			
Etiology											
	HBV										
		No	195								
		Yes	261	0.481				0.312			
	HCV										
		No	400						Reference		
		Yes	40	0.058				0.037	–	–	0.533
Child-Pugh score											
	5		368		Reference				Reference		
	6		98	<0.001	–	–	0.155	0.001	–	–	0.214
MELD score											
	<9		333		Reference						
	≥9		128	0.033	–	–	0.165	0.254			
Laboratory variables											
Platelet count (10^9/L)											
	<100		40		Reference				Reference		
	≥100		425	<0.001	0.452	0.306-0.668	<0.001	<0.001	–	–	0.484
Total bilirubin (mg/dL)											
	<1.2		386		Reference						
	≥1.2		50	0.010	–	–	0.248	0.242			
Serum albumin (g/dL)											
	<3.5		54		Reference				Reference		
	≥3.5		412	0.008	–	–	0.561	0.007	–	–	0.101
Alanine aminotransferase (IU/L)											
	<50		338								
	≥50		127	0.845				0.482			
Prothrombin time (INR)											
	<1.2		429		Reference						
	≥1.2		37	0.003	–	–	0.162	0.308			
Creatinine (mg/dL)											
	<1.0		300								
	≥1.0		164	0.607				0.721			
Sodium (mmol/L)											
	<135		24		Reference				Reference		
	≥135		438	<0.001	0.468	0.292-0.750	0.002	<0.001	0.477	0.263-0.864	0.015
Alpha-fetoprotein (ng/mL)											
	<1000		343								
	≥1000		102	0.075				0.604			
PIVKA-II (mAU/mL)											

(Continued)

TABLE 2 | Continued

Demographic variables		N = 466	Overall survival				Progression-free survival			
			Univariate	Multivariate			Univariate	Multivariate		
			P-value	HR	95% CI	P-value	*P*-value	HR	95% CI	*P*-value
	<1000	171						Reference		
	≥1000	166	0.450				0.008	–	–	0.118
Tumor variables										
Maximum tumor diameter (cm)										
	<10	367		Reference				Reference		
	≥10	99	0.005	1.693	1.243-2.306	0.001	<0.001	1.891	1.369-2.611	<0.001
Treatment variable										
Initial treatment			<0.001				<0.001			
	Resection	246		Reference				Reference		
	Transarterial therapy	204		2.167	1.623-2.893	<0.001		3.736	2.821-4.949	<0.001
	Others	16		2.660	1.413-5.006	0.002		3.113	1.591-6.091	0.001

BMI, body mass index; CI, confidence interval; HBV, hepatitis B virus; HCV, hepatitis C virus; HR, hazard ratio; MELD, Model for End-Stage Liver Disease; PIVKA-II, protein induced by vitamin K absence-II.

Several other recent studies showed survival benefit of resection for BCLC stage B HCC (13–19). Hwang et al. demonstrated that resection followed by active recurrence treatment improved survival even in patients with HCC ≥ 10 cm (3). Multivariate analysis in our study also showed that resection was associated with significantly better survival and progression-free survival than other treatments, most of which were transarterial therapy.

Although the outcomes of patients with single large (≥ 5 cm) HCC who underwent resection as the initial treatment were comparable with previous reports, multivariate analysis demonstrated that a maximum tumor diameter ≥ 10 cm showed poorer overall survival and progression-free survival than a maximum tumor diameter < 10 cm. A recent study also reported poorer 5-year overall survival and recurrence-free survival in patients with huge HCC (≥ 10 cm) than in patients with HCC < 10 cm and identified tumor size ≥ 10 cm as an independent risk factor of initial extrahepatic recurrence. Although this study does not contain any information on the location or pattern of recurrence, it can be roughly inferred from the second treatment. Out of the 466 patients, 266 (57.1%) underwent a second treatment due to disease progression. Of the 266 patients, more than half underwent transarterial treatment (64.7%) as the second treatment, followed by local ablation (10.5%), chemotherapy (10.2%), resection (9.8%), and radiation (4.9%). Considering the increased proportion of chemotherapy and radiation in the second treatment compared to the initial treatment, disease progression in our study may not be limited to the liver.

Of the 204 patients who underwent transarterial treatment as initial treatment, 22 underwent resection as a secondary treatment. Considering that 13 of the 22 patients underwent resection after transarterial treatment within 2 months, these patients may have been intentionally treated with TACE before surgery. Their overall survival was similar to that of patients who underwent resection as initial treatment ($P = 0.430$) (**Figure 4A**), suggesting that resection after transarterial therapy can be another possible therapeutic option for patients with single large HCC with tolerable liver function. This finding was similar to that of other studies that show that resection after TACE may be considered as an effective method in some intermediate-stage HCC patients (20, 21).

Two patients underwent liver transplantation (LT) as initial treatment. One patient with a maximum tumor diameter of 8 cm, AFP level of 5.3 ng/mL, and PIVKA-II 500 mAU/mL

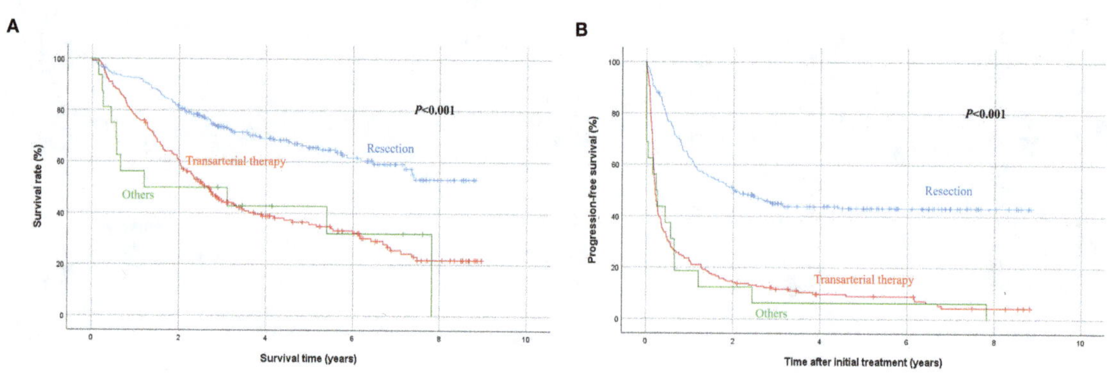

FIGURE 3 | Kaplan-Meier analysis of survival according to initial treatment modality. **(A)** Overall survival, **(B)** progression-free survival.

survived 7.8 years after LT without recurrence until death. Another patient with a maximum tumor diameter of 12 cm, AFP level of 18 ng/mL, and PIVKA-II 19 mAU/mL died 1.2 years after LT without recurrence until death. These patients must have undergone LT as per the Milan criteria based on biologic markers, such as AFP and PIVKA-II (22). However, due to the small number of patients, the efficacy of LT in single large HCC should be further studied using the national LT database.

Several studies have reported the association between preoperative low platelet count and poor prognosis in different kinds of cancer, including HCC (23, 24). Preoperative thrombocytopenia was reported to be associated with overall survival as well as recurrence-free survival in HCC patients (25–28). Although the exact reason for poor outcome in HCC with low platelet count needs to be studied further, one of the possible explanations could be the frequent occurrence of thrombocytopenia in cirrhotic patients with portal hypertension (29–32). Portal hypertension reflects the severity of cirrhosis, which is a well-known risk factor related to late recurrence in patients with HCC. The mechanism of late recurrence can be explained by multicentric recurrence in the remnant liver (31, 32). Regarding surgical resection, liver fibrosis and significant portal hypertension are risk factors for postoperative hepatic decompensation, which is a serious complication after resection (30). According to our study, multivariate analysis revealed that preoperative low platelet counts significantly affected poor overall survival. Although the cohort in the study included only patients with Child A, the low platelet count among these patients still affected poor survival. However, even though a low platelet count was associated with poor progression-free survival in the univariate analysis, it was not statistically significant in the multivariate analysis.

Hyponatremia due to splanchnic vasodilatation, which reduces the effective circulating blood volume, is frequently seen in cirrhotic patients (33–36). Serum sodium levels tend to decrease as liver cirrhosis progresses (34–36). Several studies have previously reported the prognostic role of serum sodium levels in patients with HCC (33, 37). Min et al. reported that sodium levels were an independent risk factor for post-TACE acute hepatic failure (38). Nishikawa et al. analyzed 1170 HCC patients with liver cirrhosis and revealed that serum sodium level was independently associated with overall survival (33). According to their study, 804 patients had Child A cirrhosis and 41 of them (5.1%) had serum sodium levels < 135 mmol/L. In the present study, which included only Child A patients, 24 (5.2%) patients had hyponatremia (< 135 mmol/L). Similar to previous reports, the present study also revealed that serum sodium levels < 135 mmol/L were independently associated with poor overall survival and progression-free survival.

When performing subgroup analysis limited to patients with platelet count < 100 × 10^9/L, there was no significant difference in survival between resection and transarterial therapy as initial treatment (P = 0.688) (**Figure 4B**). Another subgroup analysis limited to patients with serum sodium < 135 mmol/L also showed no significant survival difference between resection and transarterial therapy as initial treatment (P = 0.728) (**Figure 4C**). The survival benefit of resection disappeared when the patients had a low platelet count < 100 × 10^9/L or serum sodium level < 135 mmol/L.

This study has several limitations that should be considered. First, it was a retrospective study using a national registry database that relied on the completeness of medical records. There are risks of data loss and differences between centers with regard to data recording. However, the patients in the KPLCR were selected from the KCCR using the probability proportional to size method to minimize selection bias, and thus became representative of all Korean HCC patients. Second, in some instances, relevant data, including comorbidities other than smoking, alcohol history, and complications after treatment were missing. Third, the database contains the date of initial treatment and the date of the second treatment, which allowed the calculation of disease progression-free survival. However, recurrence-free survival could not be assessed because second treatment does not entail recurrence. Moreover, data for progression-free survival may be biased since the second treatment date or the date of death as reference for progression can be inappropriate and inaccurate considering the nationwide retrospective nature of this study. Despite these limitations, a notable strength of this study is that it is a large study using a national registry database focused on single large HCC patients with performance status 0 and Child A. There are only few studies with sufficient sample size that have been analyzed in this particular patient group.

The outcomes of single large HCC patients with Child A were satisfactory, which is consistent with the results of previous

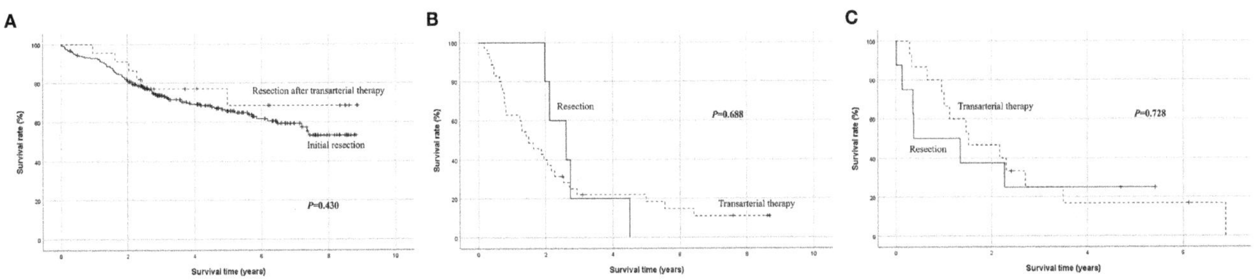

FIGURE 4 | Subgroup Kaplan-Meier analysis of overall survival. **(A)** Initial resection vs. resection after transarterial therapy, **(B)** resection vs. transarterial therapy in patients with low platelet count < 100 × 10^9/L, **(C)** resection vs. transarterial therapy in patients with low serum sodium < 135 mmol/L.

worldwide studies. Resection should be initially considered whenever possible, and not dismissed based only on tumor size. Patients with low serum sodium levels (< 135 mol/L) and HCCs ≥ 10 cm had a higher risk of poor overall survival and disease progression-free survival.

AUTHOR CONTRIBUTIONS

SKH and K-WL made the concept and design. SKH, K-WL, SYH, and SS acquired, analyzed, and interpreted the data. SKH drafted the manuscript. SKH, K-WL, SYH, SS, KH, EH, J-ML, YC, NY, and K-SS critically revised the manuscript for important intellectual content. All authors contributed to the article and approved the submitted version.

ACKNOWLEDGMENTS

The database used in this study was provided by the Korean Central Cancer Registry, Ministry of Health and Welfare, South Korea, and the Korean Liver Cancer Association.

REFERENCES

1. Korean Liver Cancer Study Group (KLCSG). National Cancer Center, Korea (Ncc). 2014 KLCSG-NCC Korea Practice Guideline for the Management of Hepatocellular Carcinoma. *Gut Liver* (2015) 9:267–317. doi: 10.5009/gnl14460
2. Kokudo N, Makuuchi M. Evidence-Based Clinical Practice Guidelines for Hepatocellular Carcinoma in Japan: The J-HCC Guidelines. *J Gastroenterol* (2009) 44:119–21. doi: 10.1007/s00535-008-2244-z
3. Hwang S, Lee YJ, Kim KH, Ahn CS, Moon DB, Ha TY, et al. Long-Term Outcome After Resection of Huge Hepatocellular Carcinoma ≥10 Cm: Single-Institution Experience With 471 Patients. *World J Surg* (2015) 39:2519–28. doi: 10.1007/s00268-015-3129-y
4. Poon RT, Fan ST, Lo CM, Ng IO, Liu CL, Lam CM, et al. Improving Survival Results After Resection of Hepatocellular Carcinoma: A Prospective Study of 377 Patients Over 10 Years. *Ann Surg* (2001) 234:63–70. doi: 10.1097/00000658-200107000-00010
5. Capussotti L, Muratore A, Massucco P, Ferrero A, Polastri R, Bouzari H. Major Liver Resections for Hepatocellular Carcinoma on Cirrhosis: Early and Long-Term Outcomes. *Liver Transpl* (2004) 10:64–8. doi: 10.1002/lt.20035
6. Lang H, Sotiropoulos GC, Dömland M, Frühauf NR, Paul A, Hüsing J, et al. Liver Resection for Hepatocellular Carcinoma in non-Cirrhotic Liver Without Underlying Viral Hepatitis. *Br J Surg* (2005) 92:198–202. doi: 10.1002/bjs.4763
7. AJCC. Ajcc Cancer Staging Manual. In: *Eighth Edition Updates and Corrections*. New York: Springer (2017). Available at: www.cancerstaging.org.
8. Poon RT, Fan ST, Lo CM, Liu CL, Ng IO, Wong J. Long-Term Prognosis After Resection of Hepatocellular Carcinoma Associated With Hepatitis B-related Cirrhosis. *J Clin Oncol* (2000) 18:1094–101. doi: 10.1200/JCO.2000.18.5.1094
9. Zhou YM, Li B, Xu DH, Yang JM. Safety and Efficacy of Partial Hepatectomy for Huge (≥10 Cm) Hepatocellular Carcinoma: A Systematic Review. *Med Sci Monit* (2011) 17:RA76–83. doi: 10.12659/msm.881443
10. Chen HY, Juan CC, Ker CG. Laparoscopic Liver Surgery for Patients With Hepatocellular Carcinoma. *Ann Surg Oncol* (2008) 15:800–6. doi: 10.1245/s10434-007-9749-1
11. Yin Z, Fan X, Ye H, Yin D, Wang J. Short- and Long-Term Outcomes After Laparoscopic and Open Hepatectomy for Hepatocellular Carcinoma: A Global Systematic Review and Meta-Analysis. *Ann Surg Oncol* (2013) 20:1203–15. doi: 10.1245/s10434-012-2705-8
12. Lin CT, Hsu KF, Chen TW, Yu JC, Chan DC, Yu CY, et al. Comparing Hepatic Resection and Transarterial Chemoembolization for Barcelona Clinic Liver Cancer (BCLC) Stage B Hepatocellular Carcinoma: Change for Treatment of Choice? *World J Surg* (2010) 34:2155–61. doi: 10.1007/s00268-010-0598-x
13. Zhong JH, Ke Y, Wang YY, Li LQ. Liver Resection for Patients With Hepatocellular Carcinoma and Macrovascular Invasion, Multiple Tumours, or Portal Hypertension. *Gut* (2015) 64:520–1. doi: 10.1136/gutjnl-2014-308139
14. Lei JY, Zhong JJ, Yan LN, Zhu JQ, Wang WT, Zeng Y, et al. Response to Transarterial Chemoembolization as a Selection Criterion for Resection of Hepatocellular Carcinomas. *Br J Surg* (2016) 103:881–90. doi: 10.1002/bjs.9864
15. Zhong JH, Ke Y, Gong WF, Xiang BD, Ma L, Ye XP, et al. Hepatic Resection Associated With Good Survival for Selected Patients With Intermediate and Advanced-Stage Hepatocellular Carcinoma. *Ann Surg* (2014) 260:329–40. doi: 10.1097/SLA.0000000000000236
16. Vitale A, Burra P, Frigo AC, Trevisani F, Farinati F, Spolverato G, et al. Survival Benefit of Liver Resection for Patients With Hepatocellular Carcinoma Across Different Barcelona Clinic Liver Cancer Stages: A Multicentre Study. *J Hepatol* (2015) 62:617–24. doi: 10.1016/j.jhep.2014.10.037
17. Yin L, Li H, Li AJ, Lau WY, Pan ZY, Lai EC, et al. Partial Hepatectomy vs. Transcatheter Arterial Chemoembolization for Resectable Multiple Hepatocellular Carcinoma Beyond Milan Criteria: A RCT. *J Hepatol* (2014) 61:82–8. doi: 10.1016/j.jhep.2014.03.012
18. Jianyong L, Lunan Y, Wentao W, Yong Z, Bo L, Tianfu W, et al. Barcelona Clinic Liver Cancer Stage B Hepatocellular Carcinoma: Transarterial Chemoembolization or Hepatic Resection? *Medicine* (2014) 93:e180. doi: 10.1097/MD.0000000000000180
19. Kim H, Ahn SW, Hong SK, Yoon KC, Kim HS, Choi YR, et al. Survival Benefit of Liver Resection for Barcelona Clinic Liver Cancer Stage B Hepatocellular Carcinoma. *Br J Surg* (2017) 104:1045–52. doi: 10.1002/bjs.10541
20. Lee HS, Kim KM, Yoon JH, Lee TR, Suh KS, Lee KU, et al. Therapeutic Efficacy of Transcatheter Arterial Chemoembolization as Compared With Hepatic Resection in Hepatocellular Carcinoma Patients With Compensated Liver Function in a Hepatitis B Virus-Endemic Area: A Prospective Cohort Study. *J Clin Oncol* (2002) 20:4459–65. doi: 10.1200/JCO.2002.02.013
21. Chen J, Lai L, Lin Q, Huang W, Cai M, Zhu K, et al. Hepatic Resection After Transarterial Chemoembolization Increases Overall Survival in Large/Multifocal Hepatocellular Carcinoma: A Retrospective Cohort Study. *Oncotarget* (2017) 8:408–17. doi: 10.18632/oncotarget.13427
22. Hong SK, Lee KW, Kim HS, Yoon KC, Yi NJ, Suh KS. Living Donor Liver Transplantation for Hepatocellular Carcinoma in Seoul National University. *HepatoBiliary Surg Nutr* (2016) 5:453–60. doi: 10.21037/hbsn.2016.08.07
23. Buergy D, Wenz F, Groden C, Brockmann MA. Tumor-Platelet Interaction in Solid Tumors. *Int J Cancer* (2012) 130:2747–60. doi: 10.1002/ijc.27441
24. Levin J, Conley CL. Thrombocytosis Associated With Malignant Disease. *Arch Intern Med* (1964) 114:497–500. doi: 10.1001/archinte.1964.03860100079008
25. Ozcelik F, Yiginer O, Özgün A. Relationship Between Thrombocytopenia and Extrahepatic Metastasis of Hepatocellular Carcinoma: A Different Perspective. *Liver Int* (2016) 36:614. doi: 10.1111/liv.13062
26. Amano H, Tashiro H, Oshita A, Kobayashi T, Tanimoto Y, Kuroda S, et al. Significance of Platelet Count in the Outcomes of Hepatectomized Patients With Hepatocellular Carcinoma Exceeding the Milan Criteria. *J Gastrointest Surg* (2011) 15:1173–81. doi: 10.1007/s11605-011-1538-2
27. Khorana AA, Francis CW, Culakova E, Lyman GH. Risk Factors for Chemotherapy-Associated Venous Thromboembolism in a Prospective Observational Study. *Cancer* (2005) 104:2822–9. doi: 10.1002/cncr.21496
28. Simanek R, Vormittag R, Ay C, Alguel G, Dunkler D, Schwarzinger I, et al. High Platelet Count Associated With Venous Thromboembolism in Cancer Patients: Results From the Vienna Cancer and Thrombosis Study (Cats). *J Thromb Haemost* (2010) 8:114–20. doi: 10.1111/j.1538-7836.2009.03680.x
29. Cheng Z, Yang P, Qu S, Zhou J, Yang J, Yang X, et al. Risk Factors and Management for Early and Late Intrahepatic Recurrence of Solitary Hepatocellular Carcinoma After Curative Resection. *HPB* (2015) 17:422–7. doi: 10.1111/hpb.12367

30. Rajakannu M, Cherqui D, Ciacio O, Golse N, Pittau G, Allard MA, et al. Liver Stiffness Measurement by Transient Elastography Predicts Late Posthepatectomy Outcomes in Patients Undergoing Resection for Hepatocellular Carcinoma. *Surgery* (2017) 162:766–74. doi: 10.1016/j.surg.2017.06.006
31. Du ZG, Wei YG, Chen KF, Li B. Risk Factors Associated With Early and Late Recurrence After Curative Resection of Hepatocellular Carcinoma: A Single Institution's Experience With 398 Consecutive Patients. *Hepatobiliary Pancreat Dis Int* (2014) 13:153–61. doi: 10.1016/s1499-3872(14)60025-4
32. Jung KS, Kim JH, Kim SU, Song K, Kim BK, Park JY, et al. Liver Stiffness Value-Based Risk Estimation of Late Recurrence After Curative Resection of Hepatocellular Carcinoma: Development and Validation of a Predictive Model. *PloS One* (2014) 9:e99167. doi: 10.1371/journal.pone.0099167
33. Nishikawa H, Kita R, Kimura T, Ohara Y, Sakamoto A, Saito S, et al. Hyponatremia in Hepatocellular Carcinoma Complicating With Cirrhosis. *J Cancer* (2015) 6:482–9. doi: 10.7150/jca.11665
34. Ginès P, Guevara M. Hyponatremia in Cirrhosis: Pathogenesis, Clinical Significance, and Management. *Hepatology* (2008) 48:1002–10. doi: 10.1002/hep.22418
35. Gianotti RJ, Cardenas A. Hyponatraemia and Cirrhosis. *Gastroenterol Rep* (2014) 2:21–6. doi: 10.1093/gastro/got037
36. Yu C, Sharma N, Saab S. Hyponatremia: Clinical Associations, Prognosis, and Treatment in Cirrhosis. *Exp Clin Transplant* (2013) 11:3–11. doi: 10.6002/ect.2012.0147
37. Biolato M, Miele L, Vero V, Racco S, Di Stasi C, Iezzi R, et al. Hepatocellular Carcinoma Treated by Conventional Transarterial Chemoembolization in Field-Practice: Serum Sodium Predicts Survival. *World J Gastroenterol* (2014) 20:8158–65. doi: 10.3748/wjg.v20.i25.8158
38. Min YW, Kim J, Kim S, Sung YK, Lee JH, Gwak GY, et al. Risk Factors and a Predictive Model for Acute Hepatic Failure After Transcatheter Arterial Chemoembolization in Patients With Hepatocellular Carcinoma. *Liver Int* (2013) 33:197–202. doi: 10.1111/liv.12023

23

Prognostic Factors of Survival of Advanced Liver Cancer Patients Treated with Palliative Radiotherapy

Qingling Hua[1†]*, Dejun Zhang*[1†]*, Yunqiao Li*[2†]*, Yue Hu*[1]*, Pian Liu*[1]*, Guangqin Xiao*[1]*,*
Tao Zhang[1*] *and Jun Xue*[1*]

[1] *Cancer Center, Union Hospital, Tongji Medical college, Huazhong University of Science and Technology, Wuhan, China,* [2] *Department of Geriatrics, Union Hospital, Tongji Medical College, Huazhong University of Science and Technology, Wuhan, China*

Correspondence:
Jun Xue
xjunion@126.com
Tao Zhang
taozhangxh@hust.edu.cn

[†]*These authors have contributed equally to this work*

Aims: Survival benefit of liver cancer patients who undergo palliative radiotherapy varies from person to person. The present study aims to identify indicators of survival of advanced liver cancer patients receiving palliative radiotherapy.

Patients and Methods: One hundred and fifty-nine patients treated with palliative radiotherapy for advanced liver cancer were retrospectively assessed. Of the 159 patients, 103 patients were included for prediction model construction in training phase, while other 56 patients were analyzed for external validation in validation phase. In model training phase, clinical characteristics of included patients were evaluated by Kaplan-Meier curves and log-rank test. Thereafter, multivariable Cox analysis was taken to further identify characteristics with potential for prediction. In validation phase, a separate dataset including 56 patients was used for external validation. Harrell's C-index and calibration curve were used for model evaluation. Nomograms were plotted based on the model of multivariable Cox analysis.

Results: Thirty-one characteristics of patients were investigated in model training phase. Based on the results of Kaplan-Meier plots and log-rank tests, 6 factors were considered statistically significant. On multivariable Cox regression analysis, bone metastasis (HR = 1.781, $P = 0.026$), portal vein tumor thrombus (HR = 2.078, $P = 0.015$), alpha-fetoprotein (HR = 2.098, $P = 0.007$), and radiation dose (HR = 0.535, $P = 0.023$) show significant potential to predict the survival of advanced liver cancer patients treated with palliative radiotherapy. Moreover, nomograms predicting median overall survival, 1- and 2-year survival probability were plotted. The Harrell's C-index of the predictive model is 0.709 (95%CI, 0.649-0.769) and 0.735 (95%CI, 0.666-0.804) for training model and validation model respectively. Calibration curves of the 1- and 2-year overall survival of the predictive model indicate that the predicted probabilities of OS are very close to the actual observed outcomes both in training and validation phase.

Conclusion: Bone metastasis, portal vein tumor thrombus, alpha-fetoprotein and radiation dose are independent prognostic factors for the survival of advanced liver cancer patients treated with palliative radiotherapy.

Keywords: liver cancer, palliative radiotherapy, prognostic factors, nomograms, multivariable Cox regression

INTRODUCTION

Liver cancer (LC) is one of the most common malignancies and the fourth leading cause of cancer-related death worldwide (1). When diagnosed with LC, about 70% patients are in advanced stage, resulting in a poor five year overall survival (OS) rate (approximately 5%) (2). Most advanced LC patients are incurable (3), thereafter it is important to provide beneficial non-curative therapies for those patients (4, 5).

Palliative radiotherapy is one of the non-curative treatments for LC, which mainly aims to alleviate symptoms and improve the quality of life (QoL) (3, 6). Interestingly, occasional success of survival prolongation can be seen in patients receiving palliative radiation. More intensive treatment regimens should be recommended if those patients who will benefit from palliative radiotherapy can be identified. Inversely, patients with poor prognosis should not receive too much radiation treatment (7, 8). Therefore, it is essential to identify predictive indicators for the survival of advanced LC patients treated with radiation, which will be convenient for clinicians to distinguish those patients who will benefit from palliative radiotherapy.

We performed a retrospective study to develop several predictive factors and construct a predictive model by analyzing the characteristics of LC patients receiving palliative radiation. Nomograms for the survival prediction of cancer patients have been widely used. It can help clinicians to predict the prognosis of cancer patients by using a convenient numerical estimation model instead of complex statistical models. In this study, nomograms were also plotted based on the identified predictive factors and model.

METHODS

Patient Selection

We retrospectively evaluated LC patients treated with palliative radiotherapy in our hospital between January 2017 and July 2020 following inclusion criteria: 1) age ≥ 18 years; 2) diagnosed by pathology or clinical evidences; 3) palliative radiotherapy for tumor in liver or distant metastatic sites; 4) stage IIIB-IV according to Chinese stage system of LC. The exclusion criteria consist of 1) curative radiotherapy; 2) metastatic tumor in liver from other cancers. The most recent follow-up date was July 26, 2020. Included patients were divided to be analyzed in model training phase and external validation phase. The training set comprised 103 advanced LC patients receiving palliative radiotherapy between November 2017 and July 2020. The external validation set comprised 56 similar patients treated between January 2017 and July 2020.

Clinical characteristics such as age, sex, stage, metastasis, radiation techniques, radiation dose, toxicity and other 25 variables were collected. Toxicities were recorded in accordance with the CTCAE (version 5.0). The primary end point was OS that was calculated from the time of palliative radiation to the time of death, or last follow-up (July 26, 2020). The requirement for informed consent from the patients was waived since this study is retrospective.

Statistical Analysis

Statistical analysis was performed by using R software packages (version 3.6). Median follow-up time was estimated by reverse Kaplan-Meier curves. Kaplan-Meier curves and log-rank test were used to identify the factors associated with OS, and statistically potential factors were confirmed by multivariable Cox regression analysis. Proportional hazards (PH) assumption of multivariable Cox regression analysis was checked by Kaplan-Meier plot for category variables, while schoenfeld residuals were calculated for continuous variables (9). To confirm the assumption of proportionality, time-dependent covariate analysis was used. Martingale residual was calculated to assess nonlinearity of continuous variables. The continuous variables will be converted to category variables if they have no linearity. Variables with high co-linearity were not included in the same regression model. Hazards ratio (HR) and 95% confidence interval (CI) were calculated for each of the variables. Then, predictive model for OS was developed by using multivariable Cox regression analysis. After that, nomograms were constructed based on the predictive model (10). Harrell's C-index and calibration curves were used to assess the feasibility of the predictive model (11). A two-tailed P value of <0.05 was considered statistically significant.

RESULTS

Clinical Characteristics of Included Patients

The detailed patients inclusion process was illustrated in **Figure 1**. Briefly, 159 patients who met the inclusion criteria were finally included, with a median age of 55 years (range, 24-84 years). Men accounted for 85.5% and women accounted for 14.5%. All patients were diagnosed by pathology. One hundred and three patients were included for predictive model training, while other 56 patients treated with palliative radiotherapy in the same time-period were used for external validation. The median follow-up time was 13.7 months (range: 0.7-64.2 months). The baseline demographic characteristics of the patients were shown in **Table 1**. Most patients have evident symptoms including pain,

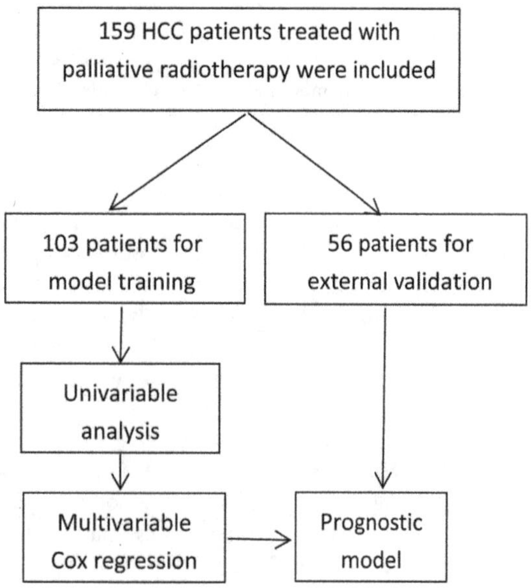

FIGURE 1 | Flowchart of patients inclusion.

shortness of breath, abdominal discomfort, nausea, or fatigue. After palliative radiation treatment, about half of patients have improvement in symptoms. Most patients have no or grade I-II toxicity. Grade III blood toxicity was recorded in 2 patients and no patients have grade IV toxicity.

Univariable Cox Regression Analyses

The median OS of LC patients receiving palliative radiotherapy is 14.8months (**Supplementary Figure 1**). In model training phase, thirty-one characteristics were investigated by Kaplan-Meier curves and log-rank tests. Six factors (bone metastasis, portal vein tumor thrombus, alpha-fetoprotein, radiation of tumor in liver, radiation dose and biologically effective dose) were considered potentially significant ($P < 0.05$) (**Table 2** and **Figure 2**). Patients with bone metastasis have a median OS of 9.5 months, which is shorter than patients without bone metastasis (17.1 months). Patients with portal vein tumor thrombus (PVTT) have a median OS of 6.8 months, while the median OS of patients without PVTT is 15.1 months. Patients with and without high alpha-fetoprotein (AFP) have a median OS of 9.0 and 16.4 months, respectively. Patients with low radiation dose (< 40 Gy) have a shorter median OS (6.6 months) than patients with high radiation dose (≥40 Gy) (16.8 months). Patients with radiation of tumor in liver have longer survival (30.2 months) compared to patients without radiation of tumor in liver (12.9 months). Patients with higher biologically effective dose (BED ≥ 60 Gy) have a better median OS (20.6 months) compared to patients with low BED (< 60 Gy) (10.1 months).

Multivariable Cox Regression Analyses

BED was excluded in multivariable Cox regression analysis because of the high co-linearity between BED and radiation dose ($P< 0.05$). Thereafter, the remaining five variables were included in the multivariable Cox regression model. Four factors including bone metastasis (HR = 1.781, $P = 0.026$), PVTT (HR = 2.078, $P = 0.015$), AFP (HR = 2.098, $P = 0.007$) and radiation dose (HR = 0.535, $P = 0.023$) have significant potential to predict survival (**Table 2**). Harrell's C-index of the predictive model is 0.709 (95%CI, 0.649-0.769), which indicates good discriminative ability. Additionally, calibration curves of the 1- and 2-year OS of the predictive model indicate that the predicted probabilities of OS are very close to the actual observed outcomes (**Supplementary Figure 2**). For external validation, the Harrell's C-index is 0.735 (95%CI, 0.666-0.804) and calibration curves also indicate good feasibility of the predictive model (**Supplementary Figure 3**).

Assessment of Robustness of Predictive Model by Stratified Analyses

Two radiation treatment techniques including conventional fraction and stereotactic body radiation therapy (SBRT) were used for included patients during the study period. The OS of these two groups of patients have no statistical difference (**Supplementary Figure 4**). Stratified analyses show that predictive model based on bone metastasis, PVTT, AFP, and radiation dose was robust both for patients treated with SBRT or conventional fraction radiation (**Supplementary Table 1**). Metastatic tumors in different organs including liver, lung, bone, and others were radiated. To further investigate the robustness of our predictive model for patients with metastatic tumors in different organs, stratified analyses were conducted and the results demonstrate that our predictive model perform good for all patients (**Supplementary Table 1**).

Nomograms for Survival of LC Patients

Coefficients obtained from the multivariable Cox regression model were taken to establish nomograms for median survival time and 1- and 2-year OS probability (**Figure 3**). Each variable included in the model was assigned a score by locating it to the point scale. The total score of all the variables determines the prediction of a patient's outcome by drawing a vertical line from the total score to the median survival time scale and survival probability scale, respectively. As shown in the **Figure 3**, more total score means better prognosis of patients.

DISCUSSION

To prevent LC patients receiving palliative radiation from over- or under-treatment, survival prediction of patients should be considered before decision making. In this study, 6 clinical characteristics were indicated to be associated with OS of patients according to univariable analysis, and 4 (bone metastasis, PVTT, AFP and radiation dose) of them were statistically significant in multivariable Cox regression analysis.

Bone metastasis often leads to skeletal-related events, such as severe bone pain, pathological fractures, spinal cord compression

TABLE 1 | Clinical characteristics of patients.

Clinical characteristics	Training set (n=103) N (%)	Validating set (n=56) N (%)
Sex (Male/Female)	88 (85.4%)/15 (14.6%)	48 (85.7%)/8 (14.3%)
Age at radiotherapy (< 55/≥ 55 years)	49 (47.6%)/54 (52.4%)	37 (66.1%)/19 (33.9%)
Tobacco (No/Yes)	78 (75.7%)/25 (24.3%)	37 (66.1%)/19 (33.9%)
Alcohol (No/Yes)	59 (57.3%)/44 (42.7%)	35 (62.5%)/21 (37.5%)
Viral hepatitis		
No	22 (21.4%)	15 (26.8%)
B type	76 (73.8%)	36 (64.3%)
Other types	5 (4.8%)	5 (8.9%)
Cirrhosis (No/Yes)	48 (46.6%)/55 (53.4%)	26 (46.4%)/30 (53.6%)
Chinese stage (IIIB/IV)	95 (92.2%)/8 (7.8%)	52 (92.9%)/4 (7.1%)
Tumor sites in liver		
Left lobe	17 (16.5%)	10 (17.9%)
Right lobe	52 (50.5%)	32 (57.1%)
Caudate lobe	11 (10.7%)	3 (5.4%)
≥ 2 lobes	23 (22.3%)	11 (19.6%)
Diagnostic type (Pathological/Clinical)	68 (66.0%)/35 (34.0%)	23 (41.1%)/33 (58.9%)
Metastatic sites		
Liver (No/Yes)	34 (33%)/69 (67%)	21 (37.5%)/35 (62.5%)
Bone (No/Yes)	55 (53.4%)/48 (46.6%)	34 (60.7%)/22 (39.3%)
Lung (No/Yes)	54 (52.4%)/49 (47.6%)	31 (55.4%)/25 (44.6%)
Others (No/Yes)	47 (45.6%)/56 (54.4%)	29 (51.8%)/27 (48.2%)
PVTT (No/Yes)	80 (77.7%)/23 (22.3%)	31 (55.4%)/25 (44.6%)
IVCT (No/Yes)	96 (93.2%)/7 (6.8%)	50 (89.3%)/6 (10.7%)
Tumor in liver (No/Yes)	23 (22.3%)/80 (77.7%)	10 (17.9%)/46 (82.1%)
AFP (Normal/High)	70 (68.0%)/33 (32.0%)	35 (62.5%)/21 (37.5%)
Early therapies		
Surgery (No/Yes)	47 (45.6%)/56 (54.4%)	36 (64.3%)/20 (35.7%)
Radiofrequency ablation (No/Yes)	79 (76.7%)/24 (23.3%)	46 (82.1%)/10 (17.9%)
Intervention therapy (No/Yes)	65 (63.1%)/38 (36.9%)	37 (66.1%)/19 (33.9%)
Target therapy (No/Yes)	87 (84.5%)/16 (15.5%)	51 (91.1%)/5 (8.9%)
Chemotherapy (No/Yes)	81 (78.6%)/22 (21.4%)	49 (87.5%)/7 (12.5%)
BED (< 60 Gy/≥ 60 Gy)	49 (47.6%)/54 (52.4%)	16 (28.6%)/40 (71.4%)
Radiation dose (< 40/≥ 40 Gy)	44 (42.7%)/59 (57.3%)	14 (25.0%)/42 (75.0%)
Fraction (Conventional/SBRT)	39 (37.9%)/64 (62.1%)	17 (30.4%)/39 (69.6%)
Radiation of tumor in		
Liver	28 (27.2%)	17 (30.4%)
Bone	28 (27.2%)	16 (28.6%)
Lung	26 (25.2%)	14 (25.0%)
Others	21 (20.4%)	9 (16.1%)
Target therapy combination (No/Yes)	97 (94.2%)/6 (5.8%)	53 (94.6%)/3 (5.4%)
Chemotherapy combination (No/Yes)	91 (88.3%)/12 (11.7%)	50 (89.3%)/6 (10.7%)
Toxicity		
Hepatic (No/Yes)	91 (88.3%)/12 (11.7%)	53 (94.6%)/3 (5.4%)
Gastroenterological (No/Yes)	89 (86.4%)/14 (13.6%)	53 (94.6%)/3 (5.4%)
Hematological (No/Yes)	82 (79.6%)/21 (20.4%)	52 (92.9%)/4 (7.1%)

PVTT, portal vein tumor thrombus; IVCT, inferior vena cava thrombosis; AFP, alpha-fetoprotein; BED, biologically effective dose; SBRT, stereotactic body radiation therapy.

and hypercalcemia. Habermehl et al.'s study showed that the median OS of LC patients with bone metastasis was 4.2 months after palliative radiation (range, 0.2-38.9 months) (6). In line with Habermehl et al.'s study, we found that bone metastasis can significantly reduce the OS of LC patients (HR = 1.781, P = 0.026). Moreover, about 10%-40% of LC patients have macrovascular invasion (MVI) including portal and/or hepatic veins when they were initially diagnosed (12–14). MVI is an independent predictive factor of poor OS in LC patients. The median OS of LC patients with MVI is significantly lower than those without MVI (2-4 months vs.10-24 months). Similarly, in our study, PVTT can significantly reduce survival of LC patients (HR = 2.078, P = 0.015). Patients with PVTT have a median OS of 6.8 months, which is shorter than patients without PVTT (15.1 months). Furthermore, Elevated AFP before palliative radiotherapy is associated with poor survival. Numerous studies use AFP as a biomarker to predict survival of LC patients. Czauderna et al.'s study shows that high pre-treatment AFP predicts reduced OS in LC (15). In our study, high AFP before palliative radiotherapy also can be an indicator of poor OS (HR = 1.098, P = 0.007). In addition, our study shows that high radiation dose can reduce death rate of advanced liver cancer patients (HR = 0.535, P = 0.023). Similarly, in Kong et al.'s study, the median OS of LC patients treated with high-dose radiation was better than that patients with low-dose radiotherapy (42 months vs. 19 months) (16).

TABLE 2 | Univariable and multivariable Cox regression analysis.

Characteristics	Univariable (*P* value)	Multivariable Cox regression analysis		
		HR	95%CI	*P* value
Bone metastasis (Yes)	0.000	1.781	1.070-2.966	0.026
PVTT (Yes)	0.025	2.078	1.150-3.755	0.015
AFP (High)	0.002	2.098	1.220-3.608	0.007
Radiation of tumor in liver (Yes)	0.036	1.168	0.605-2.257	0.644
Radiation dose ≥ 40 Gy	0.000	0.535	0.311 -0.919	0.023
BED ≥ 60 Gy	0.006	–	–	–

PVTT, portal vein tumor thrombus; AFP, alpha-fetoprotein; BED, biologically effective dose.

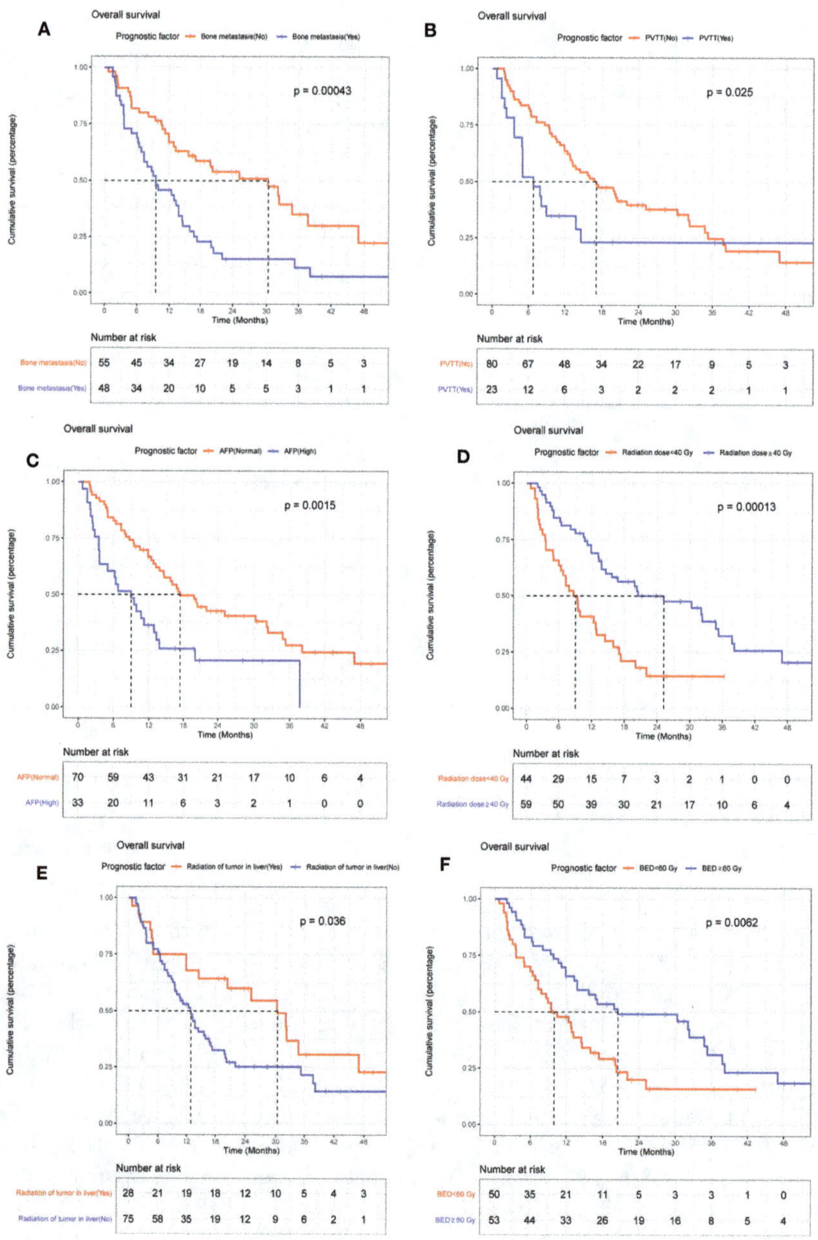

FIGURE 2 | Kaplan-Meier plots of overall survival stratified by bone metastasis **(A)**, portal vein tumor thrombus **(B)**, alpha-fetoprotein **(C)**, radiation dose **(D)**, radiation of tumor in liver **(E)**, and BED **(F)**.

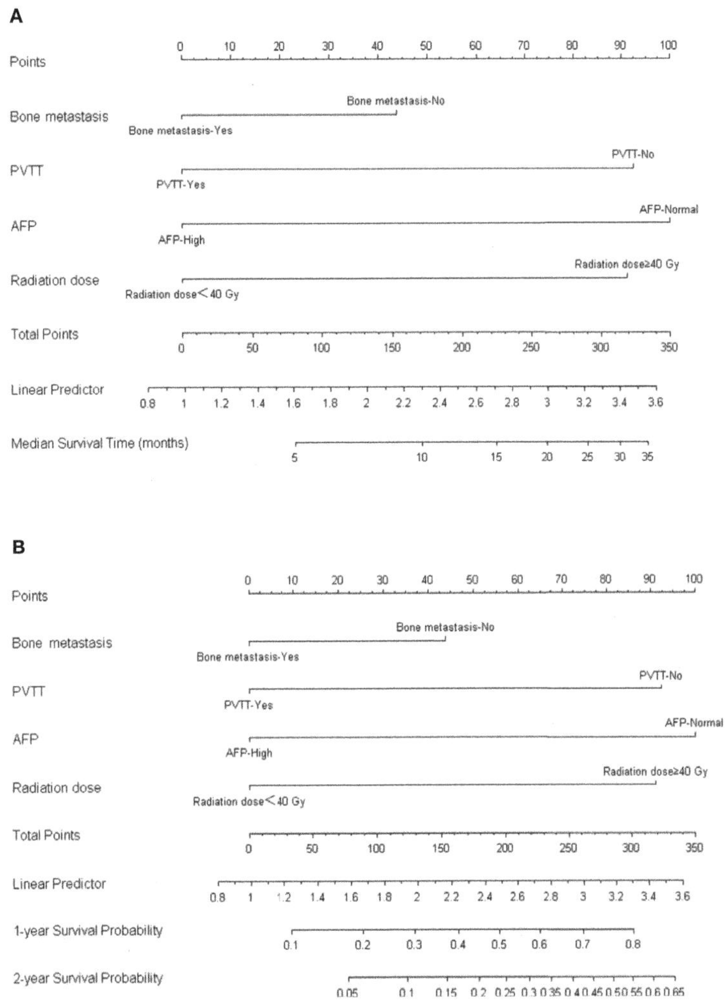

FIGURE 3 | Nomogram for predicting the median OS **(A)** and 1-year/2-year survival probability **(B)**.

There are several limitations should be stated in our article. Firstly, our findings should be interpreted with caution due to the retrospective design of our study. Moreover, all the patients included in our study were treated in a single hospital, which means that potential selection bias may diminish the accuracy of our conclusions. Secondly, different early therapies including surgery, chemotherapy, Intervention therapy and targeted therapy may increase the heterogeneity of included patients. Thirdly, different radiation techniques including SBRT and conventional radiation were taken to treat patients. Although our stratified analyses indicate that our predictive model perform good both for patients treated with conventional radiation and SBRT, our model may fail to predict the OS of patients treated with other radiation techniques. Fourthly, elaborative data of symptoms and QoL was absent, leading to absence of quantitative assessment of symptoms and QOL improvement by scale tools. Finally, several patients received both of palliative radiation and target therapy/chemotherapy during the study time period. According to our univariable analysis, target therapy or chemotherapy combined with palliative radiation have no significant effect on the OS of LC patients compared with patients received single palliative radiation. However, this conclusion should be further investigated in the future because of the small number of patients (6 patients with target therapy and 12 patients with chemotherapy).

Conclusively, four predictive factors of survival of advanced LC patients treated with palliative radiotherapy were identified. These factors were bone metastasis, PVTT, AFP and radiation dose. Recommendations for an individualized palliative radiotherapy for advanced LC patients could be made based on these four factors.

AUTHOR CONTRIBUTIONS

QH, DZ, and YL analyzed the data and draft the manuscript. YH, PL, and GX contributed to the collection of data. TZ and JX contributed to the design of the research. All authors contributed to the article and approved the submitted version.

SUPPLEMENTARY MATERIAL

Supplementary Figure 1 | Kaplan-Meier curve of overall survival of included patients.

Supplementary Figure 2 | Calibration curves of the 1- **(A)** and 2-year **(B)** OS of the predictive model in training phase.

Supplementary Figure 3 | Calibration curves of the 1- **(A)** and 2-year **(B)** OS of the predictive model in validation phase.

Supplementary Figure 4 | Kaplan-Meier curves of overall survival of patients treated with SBRT or conventional radiation.

REFERENCES

1. Siegel RL, Miller KD, Jemal A. Cancer Statistics, 2020. *CA Cancer J Clin* (2020) 70(1):7–30. doi: 10.3322/caac.21590
2. Wu B, Zhou J, Ling G, Zhu D, Long Q. CalliSpheres Drug-Eluting Beads *Versus* Lipiodol Transarterial Chemoembolization in the Treatment of Hepatocellular Carcinoma: A Short-Term Efficacy and Safety Study. *World J Surg Oncol* (2018) 16(1):69. doi: 10.1186/s12957-018-1368-8
3. Mutsaers A, Greenspoon J, Walker-Dilks C, Swaminath A. Systematic Review of Patient Reported Quality of Life Following Stereotactic Ablative Radiotherapy for Primary and Metastatic Liver Cancer. *Radiat Oncol* (2017) 12(1):110. doi: 10.1186/s13014-017-0818-8
4. Amini A, Gamblin TC. Palliation: Treating Patients With Inoperable Biliary Tract and Primary Liver Tumors. *Surg Oncol Clin N Am* (2014) 23(2):383–7. doi: 10.1016/j.soc.2013.10.008
5. Cunningham SC, Choti MA, Bellavance EC, Pawlik TM. Palliation of Hepatic Tumors. *Surg Oncol* (2007) 16(4):277–91. doi: 10.1016/j.suronc.2007.08.010
6. Habermehl D, Haase K, Rieken S, Debus J, Combs SE. Defining the Role of Palliative Radiotherapy in Bone Metastasis From Primary Liver Cancer: An Analysis of Survival and Treatment Efficacy. *Tumori* (2011) 97(5):609–13. doi: 10.1177/030089161109700512
7. Hayashi S, Tanaka H, Hoshi H. Palliative External-Beam Radiotherapy for Bone Metastases From Hepatocellular Carcinoma. *World J Hepatol* (2014) 6 (12):923–9. doi: 10.4254/wjh.v6.i12.923
8. Zeng ZC, Tang ZY, Fan J, Zhou J, Qin LX, Ye SL, et al. Radiation Therapy for Adrenal Gland Metastases From Hepatocellular Carcinoma. *Jpn J Clin Oncol* (2005) 35(2):61–7. doi: 10.1093/jjco/hyi020
9. Rulli E, Ghilotti F, Biagioli E, Porcu L, Marabese M, D'Incalci M, et al. Assessment of Proportional Hazard Assumption in Aggregate Data: A Systematic Review on Statistical Methodology in Clinical Trials Using Time-to-Event Endpoint. *Br J Cancer* (2018) 119(12):1456–63. doi: 10.1038/s41416-018-0302-8
10. Zhang Z, Kattan MW. Drawing Nomograms With R: Applications to Categorical Outcome and Survival Data. *Ann Transl Med* (2017) 5(10):211. doi: 10.21037/atm.2017.04.01
11. Hu JQ, Yu PC, Shi X, Liu WL, Zhang TT, Lei BW, et al. Prognostic Nomograms for Predicting Overall Survival and Cancer-Specific Survival of Patients With Major Salivary Gland Mucoepidermoid Carcinoma. *J Cancer* (2019) 10(18):4380–8. doi: 10.7150/jca.27992
12. Cheung TK, Lai CL, Wong BC, Fung J, Yuen MF. Clinical Features, Biochemical Parameters, and Virological Profiles of Patients With Hepatocellular Carcinoma in Hong Kong. *Aliment Pharmacol Ther* (2006) 24(4):573–83. doi: 10.1111/j.1365-2036.2006.03029.x
13. Minagawa M, Makuuchi M. Treatment of Hepatocellular Carcinoma Accompanied by Portal Vein Tumor Thrombus. *World J Gastroenterol* (2006) 12(47):7561–7. doi: 10.3748/wjg.v12.i47.7561
14. Llovet JM, Bustamante J, Castells A, Vilana R, Ayuso Mdel C, Sala M, et al. Natural History of Untreated Nonsurgical Hepatocellular Carcinoma: Rationale for the Design and Evaluation of Therapeutic Trials. *Hepatology* (1999) 29(1):62–7. doi: 10.1002/hep.510290145
15. Czauderna C, Schmidtmann I, Koch S, Pilz L, Heinrich S, Otto G, et al. High Pre-Treatment Static and Dynamic Alpha-Fetoprotein Values Predict Reduced Overall Survival in Hepatocellular Carcinoma. *United Eur Gastroenterol J* (2021) 9(3):388–97. doi: 10.1177/2050640620972611
16. Kong XQ, Dong YP, Wu JX, He JY, Le YY, Du KX, et al. High-Biologically Effective Dose Palliative Radiotherapy for a Tumor Thrombus Might Improve the Long-Term Prognosis of Hepatocellular Carcinoma: A Retrospective Study. *Radiat Oncol* (2017) 12(1):92. doi: 10.1186/s13014-017-0831-y

24

Diagnostic Performance of Theranostic Radionuclides Used in Transarterial Radioembolization for Liver Cancer

Rou Li[1,2], Danni Li[1], Guorong Jia[1], Xiao Li[1], Gaofeng Sun[1] and Changjing Zuo[1,2*]*

[1] Department of Nuclear Medicine, Shanghai Changhai Hospital, Shanghai, China, [2] School of Medical Imaging, Xuzhou Medical University, Xuzhou, China

***Correspondence:**
Gaofeng Sun
sgf1256@163.com
Changjing Zuo
changjing.zuo@qq.com*

Primary liver tumor with hepatocellular carcinoma accounting for 75–80% of all such tumors, is one of the global leading causes of cancer-related death, especially in cirrhotic patients. Liver tumors are highly hypervascularized *via* the hepatic artery, while normal liver tissues are mainly supplied by the portal vein; consequently, intra-arterially delivered treatment, which includes transarterial chemoembolization (TACE) and transarterial radioembolization (TARE), is deemed as a palliative treatment. With the development of nuclear technology and radiochemistry, TARE has become an alternative for patients with hepatic cancer, especially for patients who failed other therapies, or for patients who need tumor downstaging treatment. In practice, some radionuclides have suitable physicochemical characteristics to act as radioactive embolism agents. Among them, ^{90}Y emits β rays only and is suitable for bremsstrahlung single photon emission computed tomography (BS SPECT) and positron emission tomography (PET); meanwhile, some others, such as ^{131}I, ^{153}Sm, ^{166}Ho, ^{177}Lu, ^{186}Re, and ^{188}Re, emit both β and γ rays, enabling embolism beads to play a role in both therapy and single photon emission computed tomography (SPECT) imaging. During TARE, concomitant imaging provide additive diagnostic information and help to guide the course of liver cancer treatment. Therefore, we review the theranostic radionuclides that have been used or could potentially be used in TARE for liver cancer and focus on the clinical benefits of diagnostic applications, including real-time monitoring of embolism beads, evaluating irradiation dose, predicting therapy effects, and corresponding adjustments to TARE.

Keywords: liver cancer, diagnostic performance, theranostic radionuclides, transarterial radioembolization, nuclear imaging

INTRODUCTION

The primary liver tumor often occurs in patients with liver cirrhosis, with hepatitis virus being the most common risk factor for liver cirrhosis (1). As the most common type of liver cancer, hepatocellular carcinoma (HCC) is the fifth most common cancer worldwide and the second leading cause of cancer-related mortality (2).

Nowadays, there are many options for the treatment of liver cancer according to the guidelines in the Barcelona Clinic Liver Cancer (BCLC) algorithm (3). However, because of the underlying liver dysfunction and its often-late diagnosis, only approximately 30% of patients when initially diagnosed are eligible for curative treatments (resection, percutaneous ablation, etc). Additionally, due to locally advanced diseases, poor liver function, or additional comorbidities, recurrence or metastasis are common after major curative treatment. Hence, various palliative treatments are considered for intermediate-advanced stage liver cancer, especially in inoperable cases. Taking advantage of the fact that the tumor is supplied by the hepatic artery while the surrounding normal liver tissue is mainly supplied by the portal system, transarterial radioembolization (TARE) appears as one of the attractive treatment options.

TARE intra-arterially delivers therapeutic radioactive agents to the tumor, which can achieve embolization of the feeding artery and radiation killing effect on tumor cells simultaneously during the treatment of liver cancer. Different from external radiotherapy, TARE limits systemic irradiation and preserves the healthy liver to a maximum extent. Additionally, the incidence of postembolization syndrome in TARE is relatively rare and mild compared to TACE (transarterial chemoembolization). TARE has been demonstrated to be feasible in treating patients at different stages or with postoperative recurrence, and serves as a downstaging strategy prior or as a bridge to transplantation (4). Meanwhile, TARE is an alternative treatment for those may be contraindication to other treatments.

Prior to TARE, structural imaging, such as computed tomography (CT) or magnetic resonance (MR), shows the size and location of the tumor and its relationship with the surrounding tissue. Besides, x-ray angiography is also vital before TARE, which can provide the blood supply of the tumor and the travel, distribution and variation of blood vessels. Single photon emission computed tomography/computed tomography (SPECT/CT) is also common imaging method during TARE. All these imaging technologies are helpful to guide treatment planning (e.g., the method of delivery, suitable treatment dose) and even predict treatment efficacy. After injecting the theranostic radionuclide into the hepatic artery, therapeutic effect is achieved by internal exposure around the tumor. Meanwhile, real-time or post-therapeutic nuclear imaging, such as SPECT/CT, provides information on verification of treatment delivery, the biodistribution of radioconjugates, integral radiation dose at tumor site and organs of interest (lung, liver, thyroid gland, etc) and prediction of treatment outcome. Later post-therapeutic imaging mainly observes the therapeutic effect on the tumor and monitors other organs for complications. Furthermore, positron emission tomography/computed tomography (PET/CT) is also a potential imaging modality for TARE. It realizes functional imaging before and after treatment by showing the glucose metabolism of the tumor and sensitively finding metastasis. Hence, imaging plays a key role in drug development and clinical evaluation, and is conducive to developing adaptive TARE plans according to the metabolic mode.

Theranostic radionuclides integrating imaging and treatment during radioembolization are the most important component of TARE for liver cancer. Based on how TARE works, radionuclides that emit α rays are not suitable because of their pathlengths are relatively short and thus have a limited range in tissue. Radionuclides emiting β rays can provide substantial radiation therapy for liver tumors due to their pathlengths ranging from millimeters to centimeters. Meanwhile, emitted γ rays are helpful in monitoring embolization beads using nuclear imaging. Considering the therapeutic purpose, the half-life of nuclides ranging from one to several days is suitable, allowing the tumor to be exposed to sufficient radiation while avoiding radiation damage in the process of excretion. Thus far, only two ^{90}Y based microspheres (MSs) and ^{131}I-lipiodol are approved for clinical use, while many others are still in the pre-clinical or basic research stage. Recently, the use of additional theranostic nuclides in TARE has been explored. **Table 1** summarizes the critical characteristics (nuclear property and imaging type) of theranostic nuclides that have been used and those that have shown potential in TARE for hepatic cancer. At the same time, the theranostic effects, especially the diagnostic performance of those theranostic radionuclides will be summarized by nuclides and presented here. Among them, ^{90}Y is the most important.

YTTRIUM-90

Yttrium-90, which has favorable physicochemical characteristics, is presently the most widely used nuclide for TARE of liver cancer clinically. Yttrium-90 is a pure β emitter and has a half-life of 64.2 h. The average energy of β emission is 0.937 MeV with a mean tissue penetration of 2.5 mm. High energy, short tissue penetration distance and relatively short half-life make ^{90}Y a suitable nuclide in TARE. Compared with other radionuclide compounds, ^{90}Y-labeled MSs (^{90}Y-MSs) are already clinically available for liver cancer in some countries. The two currently commercially available ^{90}Y-MS products are glass MSs (TheraSphere) and resin MSs (SIR-Spheres). Because of the different physical and chemical properties, the treatment dose calculation for ^{90}Y-MS TARE differs significantly according to the MS type (5).

Blood supply and hepatic collateral circulation of tumor are essential for the efficacy and safety of treatment. Current clinical ^{90}Y-MS BS SPECT (bremsstrahlung single photon emission computed tomography) is hindered by image quality, while ^{90}Y-MS PET is extremely challenging due to low activity concentrations in the lungs and the low positron yield of ^{90}Y. Hence, ^{99m}Tc-MAA (Technetium-99m macroaggregated albumin) is a surrogate of ^{90}Y for pre-treatment imaging. Intra-arterially delivery of ^{99m}Tc-MAA is able to simulate the distribution of therapeutic drugs in the liver, by measuring the radiation intensity of cancerous and non-cancerous liver tissue respectively, the ratio of tumor/non-tumor (T/NT) can be calculated more accurately (6). That provides a quantitative index for evaluating the abundance of tumor blood supply and the ability of cancer tissue to absorb therapeutic drugs through hepatic artery. Patients should undergo ^{99m}Tc-MAA examination before ^{90}Y-MS TARE, which offers important preprocedural information. In ^{99m}Tc-MAA SPECT/CT, ^{99m}Tc-MAA (4–5 mCi) is injected into the hepatic artery to assess extra-hepatic depositions and lung shunting, and can provide the calculation of the lung shunt

TABLE 1 | Major radionuclides used for radioembolization of hepatocellular carcinoma.

Radionuclides	Emission and energy (MeV)	Half-life	Maximum tissue penetration (mm)	Imaging type
^{90}Y	β 2.28 (100%) γ/	2.7 d	12	BS SPECT/ PET
^{32}P	β 1.71 (100%) γ/	14.3 d	7.9	BS SPECT/ PET
^{131}I	β 0.607 (99%) γ 0.364 (1%)	8.04 d	2	SPECT
^{188}Re	β 2.12 (71.6%) 1.96 (25.1%) γ 0.155 (15%)	16.9 h	11	SPECT
^{166}Ho	β 1.84 (50.5%) 1.74 (48.7%) γ 0.081 (6.2%) 0.00138(0.93%)	1.1 d	8.7	SPECT/MR
^{177}Lu	β 0.176 (12.2%) 0.497 (78.6%) 0.384 (9.1%) γ 0.113 (6.4%) 0.208 (11%)	6.7 d	2.2	SPECT
^{153}Sm	β 0.81 (20%) 0.71 (30%) 0.64 (50%) γ 0.103 (28%)	46.3 h	3	SPECT
^{186}Re	β 2.13 (70%) 1.98 (26%) γ 0.155 (16.2%) 0.633 (1.6%)	3.8 d	4.5	SPECT

absorbed dose, which guides dosimetry to avoid radiation pneumonitis. Moreover, accurate superselective angiography should be performed to evaluate the targeted vascular territory and anatomic variants or extra-hepatic vessels should accept prophylactic embolization, which can avoid ectopic embolization of non-targeted organs. However, the concordance between ^{99m}Tc-MAA and ^{90}Y-MSs remains controversial. Many studies have reported both similarity (7) and differences (8) between ^{99m}Tc-MAA and ^{90}Y-MSs uptake. The inconsistent concordance may be due to several factors (the different size, shape, and number of MAA relative to microspheres, flow dynamics during delivery, etc), for which the post-therapy images of ^{90}Y-activity distribution is considered appropriate to determine the tumor dose-response. Apart from SPECT/CT, CT or MR imaging are also be used to assess the volume, location, and relationship with surrounding hepatic tissues of the tumor before TARE.

^{99m}Tc-MAA scanning and superselective angiography are often performed before ^{90}Y-MS TARE to guide dosimetry, although accumulating evidence has improved the safety and efficacy of using radioembolization with ^{90}Y-labeled resin or glass MSs for the management of hepatic tumors (9). A study of 1,652 patients (1,124 TACE, 528 ^{90}Y-TARE) showed that ^{90}Y-MS TARE increased the 2-year overall survival (OS) rates relative to the observational subgroup and resulted in better objective response (OR) rates than treatment with TACE. Furthermore, a lower risk of adverse events was observed in ^{90}Y-TARE than in TACE (10). Many studies have demonstrated that ^{90}Y-MS TARE is an effective choice and results in significantly fewer severe adverse events when treating HCC patients with portal vein thrombosis (PVT), which is a contraindication for most traditional therapies (11).

For post-treatment imaging, compared with the majority of the radionuclides used in TARE, ^{90}Y is a pure β emitter and lacks discrete-energy photon emissions, such as γ rays and/or characteristic fluorescence x-rays (12). The β particles emitted by ^{90}Y produce secondary bremsstrahlung radiation, which may be imaged to locate the ^{90}Y-MSs. Commonly, BS SPECT is used after radioembolization to exclude extra-hepatic activity deposition and to assess intra-hepatic MSs distribution. Ahmadzadehfar et al. performed BS SPECT/CT imaging on 188 patients who accepted ^{90}Y-MS TARE 24 h prior, to assess the capability of BS SPECT/CT in detecting and positioning of extrahepatic accumulation (gastrointestinal complications). Gastroduodenoscopy served as reference standards. The results showed that the positive predictive values, sensitivity, specificity and the accuracy of BS SPECT/CT were 100, 87, 100, and 99%, respectively (13). Furthermore, BS SPECT/CT after radioembolization is beneficial to evaluate tumor dose-response characteristics and predict treatment response for the management of patients (14). Potrebko et al. demonstrated that voxel-based dosimetry for ^{90}Y microsphere therapy allows for quantitative quality assurance of the delivered treatment using deformable image registration, calculated isodose distributions, and dose-volume histograms (DVHs). Since β-radiation emitted by ^{90}Y interacts with body tissues resulting in bremsstrahlung radiation, SPECT/CT has traditionally been regarded as the gold-standard modality to image the biodistribution of this radionuclide. However, the limitations of the BS SPECT image are poor spatial resolution (11–15 mm) and limited quantitative accuracy because of the low photon yield and continuous nature of the BS X-ray spectrum. The absence of some correction techniques leads to a further reduction in the image contrast. Many efforts have been made to improve BS SPECT/CT imaging qualitatively and quantitatively, in which Monte Carlo simulation is frequently accepted. However, it is not commercially available and cannot be easily implemented clinically (15).

Interestingly, the ^{90}Y decay process is of a very small branching to the excited state of stable ^{90}Zr. The internal pair production (positron) generated during the decay scheme of ^{90}Y allows quantitative monitoring on itself *via* PET (16, 17). Compared with BS SPECT, ^{90}Y PET imaging provides better image quality in contrast and resolution (4–5 mm). Elschot et al. quantitatively demonstrated that the image quality of PET was superior to that of BS SPECT for the assessment of ^{90}Y-MS distribution after radioembolization in a study of estimated liver dose distributions in 5 patients (18) (**Figure 1B**). The **Figure 1A** showed that the PET-based CDVH (cumulative dose-volume histograms) of the spherical region-of-interest followed the true CDVH more closely than the SPECT-based CDVH. Moreover, calculating the tumor dose on imaging may predict the response to the treatment. A study published in 2013 demonstrated that tumor and non-target tissue absorbed dose quantification using ^{90}Y PET was accurate and yielded radiobiologically meaningful dose-response information to guide adjuvant or mitigative action (23). The true definitions of the minimal effective tumor dose and maximum tolerated non-tumor dose remain challenges for each tumor and MS type, and ^{90}Y PET may be a potential solution.

Undoubtedly, ^{90}Y is the most suitable theranostic radionuclide for TARE of liver cancer so far. ^{90}Y, as a pure β emitter, has high energy and relatively small radiation range, which can effectively kill tumor cells while avoiding damage to surrounding healthy tissue, and no requiring subsequent isolation of patients is needed. Although BS SPECT and PET can match the imaging requirements, there are still many unsolved technological issues restricting the accuracy of images and widespread clinical use. For example, low true-coincidence count-rate for positron emission results in relatively longer acquisition times for ^{90}Y PET imaging. Besides, standardization and uniform implementation of reconstruction and correction techniques are urgently needed. The necessity of specialized nuclear reactors and relatively long transportation times to each hospital limit the use of ^{90}Y. Importantly, ^{90}Y is still not be approved and available in many countries, such as in China. Serious complications caused by ectopic embolization of ^{90}Y-MS may also occur, which needs high attention in clinical application.

IODINE-131

The nuclide ^{131}I ($T_{1/2} = 8.04d$) emits both β and γ rays. Its β particles have a maximum energy of 0.6 MeV and a maximum path length in tissue of 2.3 mm. Utilizing the characteristics of iodine lipiodol, which selectively deposits in nodules of hepatocellular carcinoma, radioactive lipiodol accumulates in cancer tissues and decreases irradiation damage to non-cancer tissues. Hence, ^{131}I-lipiodol was often studied for TARE of liver cancer before. In a representative clinical study of 50 patients, the median survival of patients treated with ^{131}I-lipiodol was 24 weeks longer than that of the untreated group and no radiotoxic effect was found, especially interstitial pneumonia (19) (**Figure 1C**).

In addition to lipiodol, ^{131}I can also be used to label embolism beads, normally in the form of MSs, which are often prepared in stepwise procedures for multiple theranostic applications. Liu et al. incorporated hollow CuS nanoparticles into PLGA (poly lactic-co-glycolic acid) MSs to produce HCuSNPs-loaded MSs, which were then labeled with ^{131}I to form ^{131}I-HCuSNPs-MSs (24). After the intra-arterial embolization with ^{131}I-HCuSNPs-MSs delivered into the hepatic artery of liver tumor-bearing rats, SPECT imaging confirmed that MSs were mainly located in liver tumor and only minimal accumulation was detected in other organs, particularly in the lungs. SPECT imaging findings qualitatively manifested the success of TARE operation and avoidance of damage potentially resulting from the leakage of embolism beads. The follow-up SPECT scan proved that effective embolization lasted for up to 48 h. The predictive results aided understanding of the entire treatment process and prognosis, which was more timely to figure out the primary outcome than traditional follow-up diagnosis, such as blood tests and CT.

Regarding diagnostic performance, ^{131}I-based imaging provides qualitative information on whole-body distribution, including tumor accumulation, and even permits semi-quantitative analysis (25). Becker et al. reported that 7 days after the injection, 61% of ^{131}I-lipiodol was distributed in the liver tumor, 23% was distributed in non-tumoral liver, and 16% was distributed in the lungs, which highlighted that the clinical toxicities of ^{131}I-lipiodol were more commonly affected the lungs (20). More importantly, tumor radioactivity dosimetry helps to define an absorbed dose threshold, especially when the accumulation of the radioactive embolism agent was recorded dynamically (**Figure 1D**). That would predict a therapeutic effect, thus providing guidance for the subsequent therapeutic approach and optimizing the activity to be injected.

There are still some deficiencies in the TARE transformation of ^{131}I. Compared to ^{90}Y, possible extra managements are needed for the patient's excreta (such as urine) due to the longer half-life of ^{131}I. Besides, non-therapeutic rays (γ rays) with high energy and long path length probably damage the surrounding normal tissue. In addition, too many scattered rays produced by ^{131}I lead to relatively low contrast and resolution of SPECT image that are not conducive to quantitative analysis and barely suitable for qualitative analysis. Moreover, defects in terms of *in vivo* stability still exist in ^{131}I compounds produced using iodized oil replacement or labeling methods.

OTHER POTENTIAL THERANOSTIC RADIONUCLIDES FOR TARE

Rhenium-188

^{188}Re is obtained from $^{188}W/^{188}Re$ generators in a convenient and comparatively cheap way, and its radioactivity yield can recover to 80% at 40 h postelution. The product of ^{188}Re is ^{188}Os by β decay, with a half-life of 16.9 h. ^{188}Re with a shorter half-life and similar energy of β rays compared ^{90}Y, is a promising radionuclide proposed for TARE of hepatic tumors. Similar to

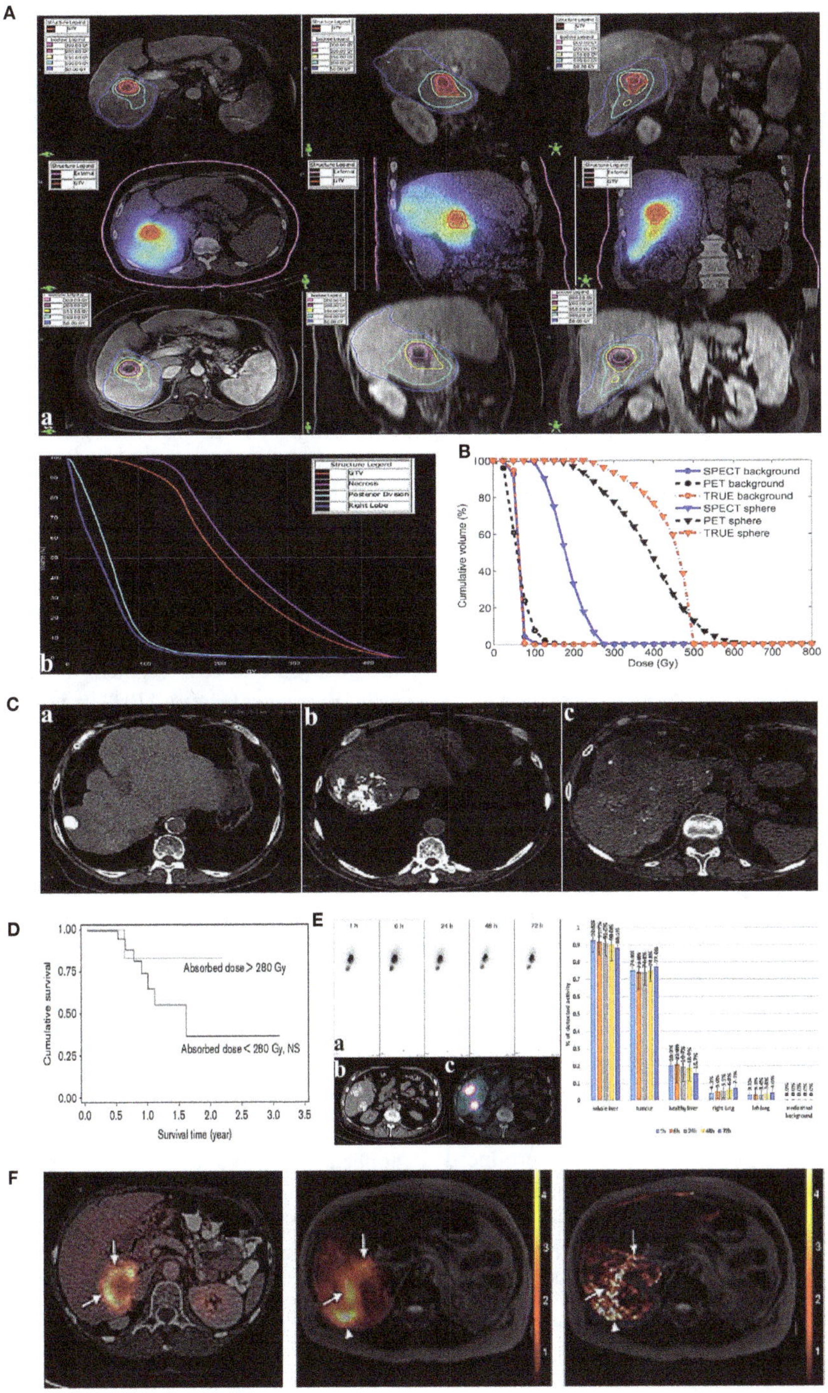

FIGURE 1 | Examples of post-therapeutic imaging of liver tumor. **(A)** The dose of each ROI (regions of interest) in pre-treatment diagnostic MR (top), post-treatment SPECT/CT (middle), and 5-week follow-up MR (bottom) for one patient with HCC (a). Dose-volume histograms of the GTV (gross target volume), necrotic region, posterior division, and right lobe (on the right) (b). Adapted from Potrebko et al. (14). **(B)** CDVH of the phantom (a method of image reconstruction) background ROI and the ROI of the 37-mm diameter sphere. Adapted from Elschot et al. (18). **(C)** Lipiodol tumor accretion at 1 month after intra-arterial injection: complete accretion (49 patients): (a) complete accumulation in 5 patients (10%), (b) partial defect in 15 (31%), (c) faint accumulation in 29 patients (59%). Adapted from Gaultier et al. (19). **(D)** Survival in terms of tumoural absorbed dose (threshold=280 Gy) calculated in tomographic mode. Adapted from Becker et al. (20). **(E)** Intra-arterial injection of ^{188}Re-SSS Lipiodol on hepatocellular carcinoma patients. Adapted from Delaunay et al. (21). The left shows whole-body scintigraphic studies (mean geometric) of patient by (a) SPECT, (b) CT, (c) fused SPECT/CT. The right is the average biodistribution profile of patients treated ^{188}Re-SSS lipiodol by SPECT/CT image. **(F)** The picture shows intrahepatic biodistribution of ^{166}Ho-microspheres on liver tumor patient by ^{18}F-FDG PET/CT, SPECT and MR imaging (from left to right). Adapted from Smits et al. (22).

^{131}I, the γ ray emission of ^{188}Re allows post-therapeutic SPECT imaging.

Early available ^{188}Re embolism agents were the lipiodol conjugates as well. ^{188}Re-chelator mixed with lipiodol, such as ^{188}Re-HDD/lipiodol, ^{188}Re-DEDC/lipiodol, and ^{188}Re-SSS/lipiodol, has been tested in humans to date. Some studies showed that TARE with ^{188}Re-HDD/lipiodol is a safe, effective, and promising method. Meanwhile, ^{188}Re was also used to label MSs as embolism beads. A study of 10 patients (3 patients with unresectable colorectal liver metastases and 7 patients with hepatocellular cancer), who received treatment with ^{188}Re-human serum albumin MSs, displayed considerable survival rates and tolerable toxicity (26). Other reported ^{188}Re-MSs include ^{188}Re-PLGA (27), ^{188}Re-poly(L-lactic acid) (PLLA) (28), ^{188}Re-glass-MSs, and ^{188}Re-resin-MSs.

Regarding diagnostic performance, embolization evaluation and related dosimetry in nuclear imaging are helpful for the treatment plan. In a study of 6 patients with unresectable HCC who accepted intra-arterial ^{188}Re-SSS/lipiodol, whole-body planar scintigraphy and SPECT were used during therapy (21) and revealed curative hepatic uptake; 90.7 ± 1.6% of radioactivity was detected in the liver with 74.9 ± 1.8% of detected radioactivity in the tumor and 9.3 ± 1.6% of radioactivity was detected in the lungs (**Figure 1E**). The average T/NT uptake ratio was 42.7 ± 7.8 on SPECT. These quantitative data provided a definite diagnosis to conclude that ^{188}Re-SSS/lipiodol had satisfactory embolization characteristics, guaranteeing *in vivo* therapeutic application.

Because of its short half-life, much more activities are needed for ^{188}Re than ^{90}Y to achieve a comparable therapeutic effect, which may produce acute radiation damage to normal tissue. Notably, ^{188}Re labeling relies on a relatively complicated reaction, which partially restricts the synthesis of the ^{188}Re embolism agents and clinical transformation.

Holmium-166

^{166}Ho emits high-energy β rays, with a comparatively short half-life (1.1 days) (29). Due to its short half-life, ^{166}Ho is suitable for patients in urgent need of downstaging treatment compared to the longer radiation therapy time of ^{90}Y. ^{166}Ho can be produced by two methods, in a nuclear reactor or by neutron activation of ^{164}Dy; hence its production is both fast and relatively cheap. Additionally, its outstanding advantage over ^{90}Y, ^{131}I, and ^{188}Re is that ^{166}Ho is paramagnetic and emits low-energy γ radiation, which enables the dual MR and SPECT imaging.

^{166}Ho-labeled lipiodol has rarely been reported. Das et al. prepared radiolabeled lipiodol by dispersing ^{166}Ho-oxine complex in lipiodol (30). For *in vivo* evaluation, the imaging studies of ^{166}Ho-lipiodol revealed satisfactory hepatic retention and insignificant uptake was detected in other major organs or tissues except skeleton. ^{166}Ho-MSs were extensively studied. Several ^{166}Ho-MSs have been prepared so far, including glass, resin, phosphate, and polymer MSs, and all of them have shown good prospects for TARE, especially polymer MSs, due to the advantage of near-plasma density, biodegradability, and biocompatibility (31). In a phase I trial including 15 patients with an unresectable and chemorefractory liver tumor, ^{166}Ho-PLLA-MS TARE was implemented in four cohorts of three to six patients, injecting 20 Gy, 40 Gy, 60 Gy, and 80 Gy, respectively. At 6 weeks, treatment response was one patient with partial response, seven with stable disease and seven with disease progression (32). Similarly, ^{166}Ho-chitosan MSs and ^{166}Ho-alginate MSs (33) that were prepared for radioembolization behaved feasibly and safely.

What is noteworthy is that, due to favorable nuclear imaging characteristics of ^{166}Ho, a scout dose (250 MBq) of ^{166}Ho is used as an alternative before ^{166}Ho-MS TARE, which is superior in calculating the lung shunt fraction compared to ^{99m}Tc MAA (34). Considering controversy over the concordance of ^{99m}Tc MAA and ^{90}Y-MSs, ^{166}Ho itself can be used in pre-treatment imaging, for which pre-treatment imaging planning dosimetry could potentially be more accurate. Regarding diagnostic performance, taking advantage of both SPECT and MR imaging, the estimated radiation absorbed dose could be evaluated more precisely in ^{166}Ho-complex liver radioembolization. In 2013, Smits et al. performed a phase I clinical trial to investigate the feasibility of quantitative imaging of ^{166}Ho radioembolization in 15 patients with unresectable liver cancer based on SPECT and MR imaging (22). The gross comparison yielded a strong correlation between MR and SPECT imaging and moderate agreement between the absorbed dose in each segment as evaluated based on MR and SPECT imaging (**Figure 1F**). The median overall T/NT ratio was 1.4 based on SPECT (range, 0.9–2.8) and 1.4 based on MR imaging (range, 1.1–3.1). In 40% patients (6/15), all T/NT ratios ≥1, indicating that dosimetry based on ^{166}Ho-MS SPECT and MR correlated well for the dose in liver segments and tumor tissue. There is no doubt that the use of two imaging modalities allows more informed decision making regarding treatment.

Due to the shorter half-life and lower energy of β rays of ^{166}Ho compared to ^{90}Y, similar to ^{188}Re, a larger administered doses are needed to achieve the dosimetry equivalent to that of ^{90}Y for treatment, which potentially cause acute damage to the surrounding normal tissue.

Lutecium-177

^{177}Lu, a popular theranostic nuclide in clinical studies and recently applied in many contexts, may also be the promising radionuclide in TARE for liver cancer treatment. ^{177}Lu has a similar half-life to ^{90}Y but emits relatively low energy β rays, which limits the radiation exposure to surrounding tissues. Regarding diagnostic performance, emitted γ rays are convenient for positioning observation and radiation dosimetry. As a potential theranostic radionuclide, ^{177}Lu has shown to be advantageous in peptide receptor radionuclide therapy (PRRT) of neuroendocrine tumors and peptide radioligand therapy (PRLT) of prostate cancers (35). As a source for TARE, ^{177}Lu still has many issues that need to be addressed in future studies. ^{177}Lu is produced using reactor irradiation, but few sources of supply and relatively high cost limit its broad application now.

Samarium-153

^{153}Sm emits both β and γ rays, meeting the requirements for theranostic radionuclides. Recent studies have shown that the absorbed doses of ^{153}Sm-labeled MSs in all organs can be controlled below 1 Gy and are safe for surrounding healthy tissues (36). Due to limited reports, its therapeutic potential in cancer treatment has not been widely studied, and its diagnostic performance is still not clear.

Rhenium-186

^{186}Re has an appropriate half-life and emits both β and γ rays. At present, ^{186}Re is clinically used to treat bone metastases caused by prostate cancer, rarely used in TARE for liver cancer. Due to its shared chemical properties and referential experience in embolism agent development with ^{188}Re, ^{186}Re is likely to be an ideal nuclide for TARE.

CONCLUSION

The incidence of liver cancer is increasing worldwide; nevertheless, effective therapeutic options are limited, and recurrence is common after preferred suitable treatment. Although TARE is not included in the BCLC staging system guidelines, current ongoing randomized clinical trials suggest that TARE is a safe, feasible, and palliative treatment for liver cancer, especially when other conventional treatments have failed. In some cases, where there may be contraindications for other treatments, TARE will be a safe and effective choice. It can achieve a similar or higher overall survival rate and slow down the progression of the disease compared to other routine treatments in the reported literature. Theranostic radionuclides in TARE allow for controlled high radiation doses to be supplied to hepatic tumors while the adjacent liver is relatively spared. In the meantime, diagnostic performance is attractive in the course of treatment. The qualitative or quantitative detection of effective embolization promotes the development of radioactive embolic agents, and assessment of the accumulated dose can guide the course of treatment using post-treatment partial or full body scan. In fact, due to the differences in the supply of nuclides around the world, the current status of clinical application of each radionuclide is not the same. In future, technical improvements and clinical studies are needed to promote the use of radionuclides in TARE. In terms of technology, the technique of radionuclide labeling, efficiency and technology of the acquisition of β and γ rays, and technology of image reconstruction all could be improved and developed for better diagnostic and therapeutic effect. In addition, besides ^{90}Y, other potential nuclides (^{166}Ho, ^{177}Lu, etc) still lack adequate clinical studies and applications for TARE.

Furthermore, except for theranostic radionuclides, embolism agents are also being widely developed and studied. Various new drug-eluting beads (such as, HepaSpheres, CalliSpheres, TANDEM, etc) have obtained certain verification in clinical trials. Natural biological materials, silk fibroin, is proposed to become a potential embolism agent for the treatment of liver cancer and still in basic research stage. In a word, future efforts should be aimed at personalizing TARE therapy depending on the characteristics of different theranostic radionuclides and embolism agents, which making TARE a more effective and safe treatment for liver cancer.

AUTHOR CONTRIBUTIONS

RL wrote the manuscript. RL, DL and GJ were responsible for searching related literature. XL, GS, and CZ were involved in revisions and proof-reading. All authors contributed to the article and approved the submitted version.

REFERENCES

1. Gomaa AI, Khan SA, Toledano MB, Waked I, Taylor-Robinson SD. Hepatocellular carcinoma: epidemiology, risk factors and pathogenesis. *World J Gastroenterol* (2008) 14(27):4300–8. doi: 10.3748/wjg.14.4300
2. Ferlay J, Soerjomataram I, Dikshit R, Eser S, Mathers C, Rebelo M, et al. Cancer incidence and mortality worldwide: sources, methods and major patterns in GLOBOCAN 2012. *Int J Cancer* (2015) 136(5):E359–86. doi: 10.1002/ijc.29210
3. Bruix J, Sherman M. Management of hepatocellular carcinoma: an update. *Hepatology* (2011) 53(3):1020–2. doi: 10.1002/hep.24199
4. Woodall CE, Scoggins CR, Ellis SF, Tatum CM, Hahl MJ, Ravindraet KV, et al. Is selective internal radioembolization safe and effective for patients with inoperable hepatocellular carcinoma and venous thrombosis? *J Am Coll Surg* (2009) 208(3):375–82. doi: 10.1016/j.jamcollsurg.2008.12.009
5. Saini A, Wallace A, Alzubaidi S, Knuttinen MG, Naidu S, Sheth R, et al. History and Evolution of Yttrium-90 Radioembolization for Hepatocellular Carcinoma. *J Clin Med* (2019) 8(1):55. doi: 10.3390/jcm8010055
6. Camacho JC, Kokabi N, Xing M, Schuster DM, Kim HS. PET Response Criteria for Solid Tumors Predict Survival at Three Months After Intra-Arterial Resin-Based ^{90}Yttrium Radioembolization Therapy for Unresectable Intrahepatic Cholangiocarcinoma. *Clin Nucl Med* (2014) 39:944–50. doi: 10.1097/RLU.0000000000000557
7. Chiesa C, Mira M, Maccauro M, Spreafico C, Romito R, Morosi C, et al. Radioembolization of hepatocarcinoma with ^{90}Y glass microspheres: development of an individualized treatment planning strategy based on dosimetry and radiobiology. *Eur J Nucl Med Mol Imaging* (2015) 42 (11):1718–38. doi: 10.1007/s00259-015-3068-8
8. Haste P, Tann M, Persohn S, LaRoche T, Aaron V, Mauxion T, et al. Correlation of Technetium-99m Macroaggregated Albumin and Yttrium-90 Glass Microsphere Biodistribution in Hepatocellular Carcinoma: A Retrospective Review of Pretreatment Single Photon Emission CT and Posttreatment Positron Emission Tomography/CT. *J Vasc Interv Radiol* (2017) 28(5):722–30. doi: 10.1016/j.jvir.2016.12.1221
9. Raoul JL, Boucher E, Rolland Y, Garin E. Treatment of hepatocellular carcinoma with intra-arterial injection of radionuclides. *Nat Rev Gastro Hepat* (2010) 7(1):41–9. doi: 10.1038/nrgastro.2009.202
10. Yang Y, Si T. Yttrium-90 transarterial radioembolization versus conventional transarterial chemoembolization for patients with hepatocellular carcinoma: a systematic review and meta-analysis. *Cancer Biol Med* (2018) 15(3):299–310. doi: 10.20892/j.issn.2095-3941.2017.0177
11. Cho YY, Lee M, Kim HC, Chung JW, Kim YH, Gwak GY, et al. Radioembolization Is a Safe and Effective Treatment for Hepatocellular Carcinoma with Portal Vein Thrombosis: A Propensity Score Analysis. *PloS One* (2016) 11(5):e0154986. doi: 10.1371/journal.pone.0154986
12. Siman W, Mikell JK, Kappadath SC. Practical reconstruction protocol for quantitative ^{90}Y bremsstrahlung SPECT/CT. *Med Phys* (2016) 43(9):5093–103. doi: 10.1118/1.4960629
13. Ahmadzadehfar H, Muckle M, Sabet A, Wilhelm K, Kuhl C, Biermann K, et al. The significance of bremsstrahlung SPECT/CT after yttrium-90 radioembolization treatment in the prediction of extrahepatic side effects. *Eur J Nucl Med Mol Imaging* (2012) 39:309–15. doi: 10.1007/s00259-011-1940-8
14. Potrebko PS, Shridhar R, Biagioli MC, Sensakovic WF, Andl G, Poleszczuk J, et al. SPECT/CT image-based dosimetry for Yttrium-90 radionuclide therapy: Application to treatment response. *J Appl Clin Med Phys* (2018) 19(5):435–43. doi: 10.1002/acm2.12400

15. Du XRY, Ljungberg M, Rault E, Vandenberghe S, Frey EC. Development and evaluation of an improved quantitative ^{90}Y bremsstrahlung SPECT method. *Med Phys* (2012) 39(5):2346–58. doi: 10.1118/1.3700174
16. Kallini JR, Gabr A, Salem R, Lewandowski RJ. Transarterial Radioembolization with Yttrium-90 for the Treatment of Hepatocellular Carcinoma. *Adv Ther* (2016) 33(5):699–714. doi: 10.1007/s12325-016-0324-7
17. Kao YH, Tan EH, Lim KY, Ng CE, Goh SW. Yttrium-90 internal pair production imaging using first generation PET/CT provides high-resolution images for qualitative diagnostic purposes. *Br J Radiol* (1015) 2012) 85:1018–9. doi: 10.1259/bjr/33524085
18. Elschot M, Vermolen BJ, Lam MG, de Keizer B, van den Bosch MAAJ, de Jong HWAM. Quantitative Comparison of PET and Bremsstrahlung SPECT for Imaging the In Vivo Yttrium-90 Microsphere Distribution after Liver Radioembolization. *PloS One* (2013) 8(2):e55742. doi: 10.1371/journal.pone.0055742
19. Gaultier AL, Perret C, Ansquer C, Euge`nec T, Bode´re FK, Frampas E. Intra-arterial injection of ^{131}I-labeled Lipiodol for advanced hepatocellular carcinoma: a 7 years' experience. *Nucl Med Commun* (2013) 34(7):674–81. doi: 10.1097/MNM.0b013e32836141a0
20. Becker S, Laffonta S, Vitry F, Rolland Y, Lecloirec J, Boucher E, et al. Dosimetric evaluation and therapeutic response to internal radiation therapy of hepatocarcinomas using iodine-131-labelled lipiodol. *Nucl Med Commun* (2008) 29(9):815–25. doi: 10.1097/MNM.0b013e32830439c6
21. Delaunay K, Edeline J, Rolland Y, Lepareur N, Laffont S, Palard X, et al. Preliminary results of the Phase 1 Lip-Re I clinical trial: biodistribution and dosimetry assessments in hepatocellular carcinoma patients treated with ^{188}Re-SSS Lipiodol radioembolization. *Eur J Nucl Med Mol I* (2019) 46 (7):1506–17. doi: 10.1007/s00259-019-04277-9
22. Smits ML, Elschot M, van den Bosch MA, van de Maat GH, van het Schip AD, Zonnenberg BA, et al. In Vivo Dosimetry Based on SPECT and MR Imaging of ^{166}Ho-Microspheres for Treatment of Liver Malignancies. *J Nucl Med* (2013) 54(12):2093–100. doi: 10.2967/j.113.119768
23. Kao YH, Steinberg JD, Tay YS, Lim GK, Yan J, Townsend DW, et al. Post-radioembolization yttrium-90 PET/CT-part 2: dose-response and tumor predictive dosimetry for resin microspheres. *EJNMMI Res* (2013) 3(1):57. doi: 10.1186/2191-219X-3-57
24. Liu QF, Qian YY, Li PL, Zhang SH, Liu JJ, Sun XG, et al. ^{131}I-labeled copper sulfide-loaded microspheres to treat hepatic tumors via hepatic artery embolization. *Theranostics* (2018) 8(3):785–99. doi: 10.7150/thno.21491
25. Lambert B, Van de Wiele C. Treatment of hepatocellular carcinoma by means of radiopharmaceuticals. *Eur J Nucl Med Mol Imaging* (2005) 32(8):980–9. doi: 10.1007/s00259-005-1859-z
26. Liepe, Brogsitter C, Leonhard J, Wunderlich G, Hliscs R, Pinkert J, et al. Feasibility of High Activity Rhenium-188-Microsphere in Hepatic Radioembolization. *JPN J Clin Oncol* (2007) 37(12):942–50. doi: 10.1093/jjco/hym137
27. Vega JCDL, Esquinas PL, Rodríguez-Rodríguez C, Bokharaei M, Moskalev I, Liu D, et al. Radioembolization of Hepatocellular Carcinoma with Built-In Dosimetry: First in vivo Results with Uniformly-Sized, Biodegradable Microspheres Labeled with ^{188}Re. *Theranostics* (2019) 9(3):868–83. doi: 10.7150/thno.29381
28. Jamre M, Shamsaei M, Erfani M, Sadjadi S, Ghannadi Maragheh M. Preparation and evaluation of ^{188}Re sulfide colloidal nanoparticles loaded biodegradable poly (L-lactic acid) microspheres for radio-embolization therapy. *J Labelled Compd Rad* (2018) 61(8):586–94. doi: 10.1002/jlcr.3627
29. Reinders MTM, Smits MLJ, Roekel CV, Braat AJAT. Holmium-166 Microsphere Radioembolization of Hepatic Malignancies. *Semin Nucl Med* (2019) 49(3):237–43. doi: 10.1053/j.semnuclmed.2019.01.008
30. Das T, Chakraborty S, Sarma HD, Venkatesh M, Banerjee S. Preparation of ^{166}Ho-oxine-lipiodol and its preliminary bioevaluation for the potential application in therapy of liver cancer. *Nucl Med Commun* (2009) 30 (5):362–7. doi: 10.1097/MNM.0b013e328329981a
31. Bouvry C, Palard X, Edeline J, Ardisson V, Loyer P, Garin E, et al. Transarterial Radioembolization (TARE) Agents beyond ^{90}Y-Microspheres. *BioMed Res Int* (2018) 2018:1–14. doi: 10.1155/2018/1435302
32. Smits ML, Nijsen JF, van den Bosch MA, Lam MG, Vente MD, Huijbregts JE, et al. Holmium-166 radioembolization for the treatment of patients with liver metastases: design of the phase I HEPAR trial. *J Exp Clin Canc Res* (2010) 29 (1):70. doi: 10.1186/1756-9966-29-70
33. Zielhuis SW, Seppenwoolde JH, Bakker CJ, Jahnz U, Zonnenberg BA, van het Schip AD, et al. Characterization of holmium loaded alginate microspheres for multimodality imaging and therapeutic applications. *J BioMed Mater Res* (2007) 82A(4):892–8. doi: 10.1002/jbm.a.31183
34. Prince JF, Rooij RV, Bol GH, de Jong HW, van den Bosch MAJ, Lam MEH. Safety of a Scout Dose Preceding Hepatic Radioembolization with ^{166}Ho Microspheres. *J Nucl Med* (2015) 56:817–23. doi: 10.2967/jnumed.115.155564
35. Ceci F, Castellucci P, Cerci JJ, Fanti S. New Aspects of Molecular Imaging in Prostate Cancer. *Methods* (2017) 130:36–41. doi: 10.1016/j.ymeth.2017.07.009
36. Aziz Hashikin1 NA, Yeong CH, Abdullah BJ, Ng KH, Chung LY, Dahalan R, et al. Neutron Activated Samarium-153 Microparticles for Transarterial Radioembolization of Liver Tumour with Post-Procedure Imaging Capabilities. *PloS One* (2015) 10(9):e0138106. doi: 10.1371/journal.pone.0138106

Permissions

All chapters in this book were first published Frontiers; hereby published with permission under the Creative Commons Attribution License or equivalent. Every chapter published in this book has been scrutinized by our experts. Their significance has been extensively debated. The topics covered herein carry significant findings which will fuel the growth of the discipline. They may even be implemented as practical applications or may be referred to as a beginning point for another development.

The contributors of this book come from diverse backgrounds, making this book a truly international effort. This book will bring forth new frontiers with its revolutionizing research information and detailed analysis of the nascent developments around the world.

We would like to thank all the contributing authors for lending their expertise to make the book truly unique. They have played a crucial role in the development of this book. Without their invaluable contributions this book wouldn't have been possible. They have made vital efforts to compile up to date information on the varied aspects of this subject to make this book a valuable addition to the collection of many professionals and students.

This book was conceptualized with the vision of imparting up-to-date information and advanced data in this field. To ensure the same, a matchless editorial board was set up. Every individual on the board went through rigorous rounds of assessment to prove their worth. After which they invested a large part of their time researching and compiling the most relevant data for our readers.

The editorial board has been involved in producing this book since its inception. They have spent rigorous hours researching and exploring the diverse topics which have resulted in the successful publishing of this book. They have passed on their knowledge of decades through this book. To expedite this challenging task, the publisher supported the team at every step. A small team of assistant editors was also appointed to further simplify the editing procedure and attain best results for the readers.

Apart from the editorial board, the designing team has also invested a significant amount of their time in understanding the subject and creating the most relevant covers. They scrutinized every image to scout for the most suitable representation of the subject and create an appropriate cover for the book.

The publishing team has been an ardent support to the editorial, designing and production team. Their endless efforts to recruit the best for this project, has resulted in the accomplishment of this book. They are a veteran in the field of academics and their pool of knowledge is as vast as their experience in printing. Their expertise and guidance has proved useful at every step. Their uncompromising quality standards have made this book an exceptional effort. Their encouragement from time to time has been an inspiration for everyone.

The publisher and the editorial board hope that this book will prove to be a valuable piece of knowledge for researchers, students, practitioners and scholars across the globe.

List of Contributors

Weiqi Zhang, Wen Zhu, Jian Yang, Nan Xiang, Ning Zeng, Haoyu Hu and Chihua Fang
Department of Hepatobiliary Surgery, Zhujiang Hospital, Southern Medical University, Guangzhou, China
Guangdong Provincial Clinical and Engineering Center of Digital Medicine, Guangzhou, China

Fucang Jia
Research Laboratory for Medical Imaging and Digital Surgery, Shenzhen Institutes of Advanced Technology, Chinese Academy of Sciences, Shenzhen, China

Tao Wang, Jinfu Zhang, Xianwei Yang, Shu Shen and Wentao Wang
Department of Liver Surgery and Liver Transplantation Center, West China Hospital of Sichuan University, Chengdu, China

Wanxiang Wang
Department of Hepatobiliary, Pancreatic, and Splenic Surgery, The Affiliated Hospital of Inner Mongolia Medical University, Hohhot, China

Ying Liu, Yuzhu Wang, Qianzhou Lv and Xiaoyu Li
Department of Pharmacy, Zhongshan Hospital, Fudan University, Shanghai, China

Xinkun Guo
Deparment of Hepatic Oncology, Zhongshan Hospital, Fudan University, Xiamen, China

Yifeng He, Jian Zhou and Xiaowu Huang
Department of Liver Surgery and Transplantation, Liver Cancer Institute, Zhongshan Hospital, Fudan University, Shanghai, China
Key Laboratory of Carcinogenesis and Cancer Invasion, Ministry of Education, Shanghai, China

Rong-Rui Huo, Hao-Tian Liu, Zhu-Jian Deng, Xiu-Mei Liang, Wen-Feng Gong, Lu-Nan Qi, Xue-Mei You, Bang-De Xiang, Le-Qun Li, Liang Ma and Jian-Hong Zhong
Hepatobiliary Surgery Department, Guangxi Liver Cancer Diagnosis and Treatment Engineering and Technology Research Center, Guangxi Medical University Cancer Hospital, Nanning, China

Jie Mei, Shao-Hua Li, Liang-He Lu, Jing-Wen Zou, Wen-Ping Lin, Yu-Hua Wen, Wei Wei and Rong-Ping Guo
Department of Hepatobiliary Oncology, Sun Yat-sen University Cancer Center, Guangzhou, China
State Key Laboratory of Oncology in South China, Guangzhou, China
Collaborative Innovation Center for Cancer Medicine, Guangzhou, China

Qiao-Xuan Wang
State Key Laboratory of Oncology in South China, Guangzhou, China
Collaborative Innovation Center for Cancer Medicine, Guangzhou, China
Department of Radiation Oncology, Sun Yat-sen University Cancer Center, Guangzhou, China

Yi-Hong Ling
State Key Laboratory of Oncology in South China, Guangzhou, China
Collaborative Innovation Center for Cancer Medicine, Guangzhou, China
Department of Pathology, Sun Yat-sen University Cancer Center, Guangzhou, China

Yiming Liu, Yanqiao Ren, Sangluobu Ge, Bin Xiong, Guofeng Zhou, Gansheng Feng, Songlin Song and Chuansheng Zhen
Department of Radiology, Union Hospital, Tongji Medical College, Huazhong University of Science and Technology, Wuhan, China
Hubei Provinve Key Laboratory of Molecular Imaging, Wuhan, China

Jiamin Zhou, Xigan He, Miao Wang, Yiming Zhao, Ning Zhang, Longrong Wang, Anrong Mao and Lu Wang
Department of Hepatic Surgery, Shanghai Cancer Center, Fudan University, Shanghai, China
Department of Oncology, Shanghai Medical College, Fudan University, Shanghai, China

Yeting Lin
Anesthesiology Department, Ningbo Yinzhou No. 2 Hospital, Ningbo, China

Yuexiu Si
School of Basic Medical Sciences, Zhejiang Chinese Medical University, Hangzhou, China

Jinhang Zhang
Surgery Department, Fenghua Hospital of Traditional Chinese Medicine, Ningbo, China

Qiu-Qiang Zhang, Pan-Yi-Sha Wu, Mugahed ALBahde, Lu-Fei Zhang and Yu-Feng Li
Department of Hepatobiliary and Pancreatic Surgery, The Second Affiliated Hospital, Zhejiang University School of Medicine, Hangzhou, China
Clinical Medicine Innovation Center of Precision Diagnosis and Treatment for Hepatobiliary and Pancreatic Disease of Zhejiang University, Hangzhou, China

Zhu-Ha Zhou
Department of General Surgery, School of Medicine, Sir Run Run Shaw Hospital, Zhejiang University, Hangzhou, China

Hua Liu
Department of Hepatobiliary and Pancreatic Surgery, The First Affiliated Hospital, Zhejiang University School of Medicine, Hangzhou, China

Wei-Lin Wang
Department of Hepatobiliary and Pancreatic Surgery, The Second Affiliated Hospital, Zhejiang University School of Medicine, Hangzhou, China
Clinical Medicine Innovation Center of Precision Diagnosis and Treatment for Hepatobiliary and Pancreatic Disease of Zhejiang University, Hangzhou, China
Key Laboratory of Precision Diagnosis and Treatment for Hepatobiliary and Pancreatic Tumor of Zhejiang Province, Hangzhou, China
Research Center of Diagnosis and Treatment Technology for Hepatocellular Carcinoma of Zhejiang Province, Hangzhou, China
Clinical Research Center of Hepatobiliary and Pancreatic Diseases of Zhejiang Province, Hangzhou, China

Kai-Xuan Liu, Jian-Guo Hong, Rui Wu, Zhao-Ru Dong, Ya-Fei Yang, Yu-Chuan Yan, Chun-Cheng Yang, Lun-Jie Yan, Sheng-Yu Yao, Hai-Chao Li , Xu-Ting Zhi and Tao Li
Department of General Surgery, Qilu Hospital, Shandong University, Jinan, China

Hui Dong, Hao Peng, Wenjing Xu and Zhe Fan
School of Medicine, Southeast University, Nanjing, China

Jitao Wang
School of Medicine, Southeast University, Nanjing, China
Xingtai Institute of Cancer Control, Xingtai People's Hospital, Xingtai, China

Yong Liao, Jinlong Li, Fengxiao Gao, Chengyu Liu and Dengxiang Liu
Xingtai Institute of Cancer Control, Xingtai People's Hospital, Xingtai, China

Zhi Li
Department of Infection Management, Xingtai General Hospital of North China Healthcare Group, Xingtai, China

Yewei Zhang
School of Medicine, Southeast University, Nanjing, China
Department of Hepatobiliary and Pancreatic Surgery, The Second Affiliated Hospital of Nanjing Medical University, Nanjing, China

Jiaxuan Xu, Jiaze Hong, Yiran Wang and Yujing He
The Second Clinical Medical College, Zhejiang Chinese Medical University, Hangzhou, China

Lingling Zhou
The First Clinical Medical College, Wenzhou Medical University, Wenzhou, China

Binbin Xu
Department of Nutrition, HwaMei Hospital, University of Chinese Academy of Sciences, Ningbo, China

Yizhou Chen
Emergency Medical Center, Ningbo Yinzhou No. 2 Hospital, Ningbo, China

Jiang Li
Hepatic Surgery Center, Tongji Hospital, Tongji Medical College, Huazhong University of Science and Technology, Wuhan, China
Hepatobiliary Surgery, The First Affiliated Hospital, College of Medicine, Shihezi University, Shihezi, China

Wei-wei Sheng
Department of General Surgery, People's Hospital of Wuning County, Jiujiang, China

Xiaozhun Huang, Lin Xu, Teng Ma, Xin Yin, Zhangkan Huang and Caibin Wang
Department of Hepatobiliary Surgery, National Cancer Center/National Clinical Research Center for Cancer/Cancer Hospital and Shenzhen Hospital, Chinese Academy of Medical Sciences and Peking Union Medical College, Shenzhen, China

Yibin Liu
Department of General Surgery, Longgang District Central Hospital of Shenzhen, Shenzhen, China

Zhen Huang and Xinyu Bi
Department of Hepatobiliary Surgery, National Cancer Center/National Clinical Research Center for Cancer/Cancer Hospital, Chinese Academy of Medical Sciences and Peking Union Medical College, Beijing, China

Xu Che
Department of Hepatobiliary Surgery, National Cancer Center/National Clinical Research Center for Cancer/Cancer Hospital and Shenzhen Hospital, Chinese Academy of Medical Sciences and Peking Union Medical College, Shenzhen, China
Department of Gastrointestinal and Pancreatic Surgery, National Cancer Center/National Clinical Research Center for Cancer/Cancer Hospital, Chinese Academy of Medical Sciences and Peking Union Medical College, Beijing, China

Yun Yang, Meng-chao Wang, Tao Tian, Jian Huang, Sheng-xian Yuan, Lei Liu, Peng Zhu, Fang-ming Gu, Si-yuan Fu, Bei-ge Jiang, Fu-chen Liu, Ze-ya Pan and Wei-ping Zhou
Eastern Hepatobiliary Surgery Hospital, Shanghai, China

Jin-Kai Feng, Zong-Tao Chai, Kang Wang, Jie Shi, Wei-Xing Guo, Meng-Chao Wu and Shu-Qun Cheng
Department of Hepatic Surgery VI, Eastern Hepatobiliary Surgery Hospital, Second Military Medical University, Shanghai, China

Xiu-Ping Zhang
Department of Hepatic Surgery VI, Eastern Hepatobiliary Surgery Hospital, Second Military Medical University, Shanghai, China
Faculty of Hepato-Biliary-Pancreatic Surgery, The First Medical Center of Chinese People's Liberation Army (PLA) General Hospital, Beijing, China

Teng-Fei Zhou
Department of Oncology, The No. 313 Hospital of PLA, Huludao, China

Zi-Yang Sun
Department of Hepatic Surgery VI, Eastern Hepatobiliary Surgery Hospital, Second Military Medical University, Shanghai, China
College of Basic Medical Sciences, Second Military Medical University, Shanghai, China

Zuo-Jun Zhen
Department of Hepatobiliary Surgery, Foshan First People's Hospital, Foshan, China

Dong Zhou
Department of Hepatobiliary Surgery, Fujian Cancer Hospital, Fuzhou, China

Fan Zhang
Department of Hepatobiliary Surgery, Affiliated Hospital of Binzhou Medical College, Binzhou, China

Yi-Ren Hu
Department of General Surgery, Wenzhou People's Hospital, Wenzhou, China

Cheng-Qian Zhong
Department of Hepatobiliary Surgery, LongYan First Hospital, Affiliated to Fujian Medical University, Longyan, China

Zhen-Hua Chen
Department of General Surgery, Zhejiang Provincial Armed Police Corps Hospital, Hangzhou, China

Wan Yee Lau
Department of Hepatic Surgery VI, Eastern Hepatobiliary Surgery Hospital, Second Military Medical University, Shanghai, China
Faculty of Medicine, The Chinese University of Hong Kong, Hong Kong, SAR China

Cheng-Maw Ho, Rey-Heng Hu and Po-Huang Lee
Department of Surgery, National Taiwan University Hospital and College of Medicine, Taipei, Taiwan

Chih-Hsin Lee
Division of Pulmonary Medicine and Pulmonary Research Center, Wanfang Hospital, Taipei Medical University, Taipei, Taiwan

Ming-Chia Lee
Department of Pharmacy, New Taipei City Hospital, New Taipei City, Taiwan
School of Pharmacy, College of Pharmacy, Taipei Medical University, Taipei, Taiwan

Jun-Fu Zhang
Biostatistics Center, College of Management, Taipei Medical University, Taipei, Taiwan
Big Data Center, Lo-Hsu Medical Foundation, Lotung Poh-Ai Hospital, Yilan, Taiwan

Chin-Hua Chen
Biostatistics Center, College of Management, Taipei Medical University, Taipei, Taiwan
Graduate Institute of Data Science, College of Management, Taipei Medical University, Taipei, Taiwan
Department of Medical Education and Research, Wanfang Hospital, Taipei Medical University, Taipei, Taiwan

Jann-Yuan Wang
Department of Internal Medicine, National Taiwan University Hospital, and College of Medicine, Taipei, Taiwan

Yue-Lin Zhang, Tan-Yang Zhou, Guan-Hui Zhou, Tong-Yin Zhu, Xin-Hua Chen, Bao-Quan Wang, Zi-Niu Yu and Li Jing
Hepatobiliary and Pancreatic Interventional Treatment Center, Division of Hepatobiliary and Pancreatic Surgery, The First Affiliated Hospital, Zhejiang University School of Medicine, Hangzhou, China
Zhejiang Clinical Research Center of Hepatobiliary and Pancreatic Diseases, Hangzhou, China

Chun-Hui Nie, Sheng-Qun Chen, Hong-Liang Wang and Zhi-Min He
Hepatobiliary and Pancreatic Interventional Treatment Center, Division of Hepatobiliary and Pancreatic Surgery, The First Affiliated Hospital, Zhejiang University School of Medicine, Hangzhou, China
Zhejiang Provincial Research Center for Diagnosis and Treatment of Hepatobiliary Diseases, Hangzhou, China

Jun-Hui Sun
Hepatobiliary and Pancreatic Interventional Treatment Center, Division of Hepatobiliary and Pancreatic Surgery, The First Affiliated Hospital, Zhejiang University School of Medicine, Hangzhou, China
Zhejiang Clinical Research Center of Hepatobiliary and Pancreatic Diseases, Hangzhou, China
Zhejiang Provincial Research Center for Diagnosis and Treatment of Hepatobiliary Diseases, Hangzhou, China

Feng Chen
Department of Radiology, The First Affiliated Hospital, Zhejiang University School of Medicine, Hangzhou, China

Ling Tan, Fei Liu, Zi-lin Liu and Jiang-wei Xiao
Department of Gastrointestinal Surgery, Clinical Medical College and the First Affiliated Hospital of Chengdu Medical College, Chengdu, China

Hai-su Tao, Er-lei Zhang, Jian Li, Wen-qiang Wang, Jin Gu and Zhi-yong Huang
Hepatic Surgery Center, Tongji Hospital, Tongji Medical College, Huazhong University of Science and Technology, Wuhan, China

Umberto Cillo, Michele Finotti, Chiara Di Renzo, Alessandro Vitale, Giacomo Zanus, Enrico Gringeri, Alessandra Bertacco and Marina Polacco
Department of Surgery, Oncology and Gastroenterology, Hepatobiliary Surgery and Liver Transplantation, Padova University, Padova, Italy

Francesco D'Amico
Department of Surgery, Oncology and Gastroenterology, Hepatobiliary Surgery and Liver Transplantation, Padova University, Padova, Italy
Department of Surgery, Immunology and Transplantation Unit, Yale University, New Haven, CT, United States

Suk Kyun Hong, Kwang-Woong Lee, Su young Hong, Sanggyun Suh, Kwangpyo Hong, Eui Soo Han, Jeong-Moo Lee, YoungRok Choi, Nam-Joon Yi and Kyung-Suk Suh
Department of Surgery, Seoul National University College of Medicine, Seoul, South Korea

Qingling Hua, Dejun Zhang, Yue Hu, Pian Liu, Guangqin Xiao, Tao Zhang and Jun Xue
Cancer Center, Union Hospital, Tongji Medical college, Huazhong University of Science and Technology, Wuhan, China

Yunqiao Li
Department of Geriatrics, Union Hospital, Tongji Medical College, Huazhong University of Science and Technology, Wuhan, China

Danni Li, Guorong Jia, Xiao Li and Gaofeng Sun
Department of Nuclear Medicine, Shanghai Changhai Hospital, Shanghai, China

Rou Li and Changjing Zuo
School of Medical Imaging, Xuzhou Medical University, Xuzhou, China

Index

www.ingramcontent.com/pod-product-compliance
Lightning Source LLC
LaVergne TN
LVHW081034210926
848485LV00004B/1021